AF294684

Bone Densitometry and Osteoporosis

Springer

Berlin
Heidelberg
New York
Barcelona
Hongkong
London
Mailand
Paris
Singapur
Tokio

H. K. Genant, G. Guglielmi, M. Jergas (Eds.)

Bone Densitometry and Osteoporosis

With Contributions by
S. Adami, J. Adams, L.V. Avioli, C. Berkovich, E. Bonucci, V. Braga,
M. Cammisa, E. Canalis, R. Civitelli, M.T. DiMuzio, K. Engelke,
L.K. Fattore, D. Felsenberg, J.L. Ferretti, T. Fuerst, H.K. Genant,
C. Gennari, V. Gilsanz, G. Guglielmi, D. Hans, S.T. Harris, K. Houki,
M. Jergas, O. Johnell, W. Kalender, M. Kleerekoper, C. van Kuijk,
T.F. Lang, Y. Lu, S. Majumdar, G. Martini, A. Mathur, P.D. Miller, S. Mora,
R. Nuti, S. Ortolani, R. Pacifici, C. Reiners, P.D. Ross, P. Schneider,
C. Trevisan, M. Uffmann, C.B. Westlund, A. Zallone Zambonin,
G. Zambonin, K. Ziambaras

With 132 Figures and 34 Tables

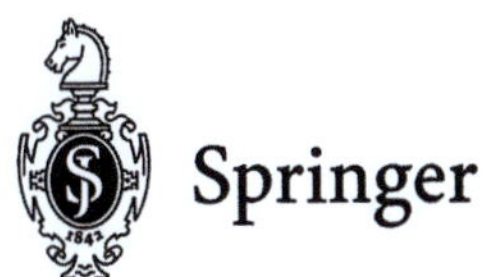 Springer

Editors:

Professor Dr. Harry K. Genant
Chief, Musculoskeletal Radiology
Professor of Radiology, Medicine, Epidemiology & Orthopadic Surgery
Executive Director, Osteoporosis & Arthritis Research Group
University of California, San Francisco, CA 94143-0628, USA

Giuseppe Guglielmi, M.D.
Scientific Institute Hospital „Casa Sollievo della Sofferenza",
Department of Radiology
Viale Cappuccini, 71013 San Giovanni Rotondo (FG), Italy

Michael Jergas, M.D.
St. Josef-Hospital, Department of Radiology
Gudrunstraße 56, 44791 Bochum, Germany

ISBN-13:978-3-642-80442-7

Library of Congress Cataloging-in-Publication Data
Bone densitometry and osteoporosis / H. K. Genant, G. Guglielmi, M. Jergas (eds.).
Includes bibliographical references and index.
ISBN-13:978-3-642-80442-7   e-ISBN-13:978-3-642-80440-3
DOI: 10.1007/978-3-642-80440-3

1. Osteoporosis. 2. Bone densitometry.
I. Genant, Harry K. II. Guglielmi, G. (Giuseppe). III. Jergas, M. (Michael)
[DNLM: 1. Osteoporosis–diagnosis. 2. Osteoporosis–therapy. 3. Densitometry-methods.
4. BoneDensity-physiology. WE 250 B7119 1998]
RC931.073B654 1998   616.7'16–dc21   DNLM/DLC.

Cover design: Springer-Verlag, E. Kirchner, Heidelberg
Typesetting: Dataconversion by MEDIO GmbH, Berlin
SPIN:10698732   21/3020 - 5 4 3 2 1 - Printed on acid-free paper

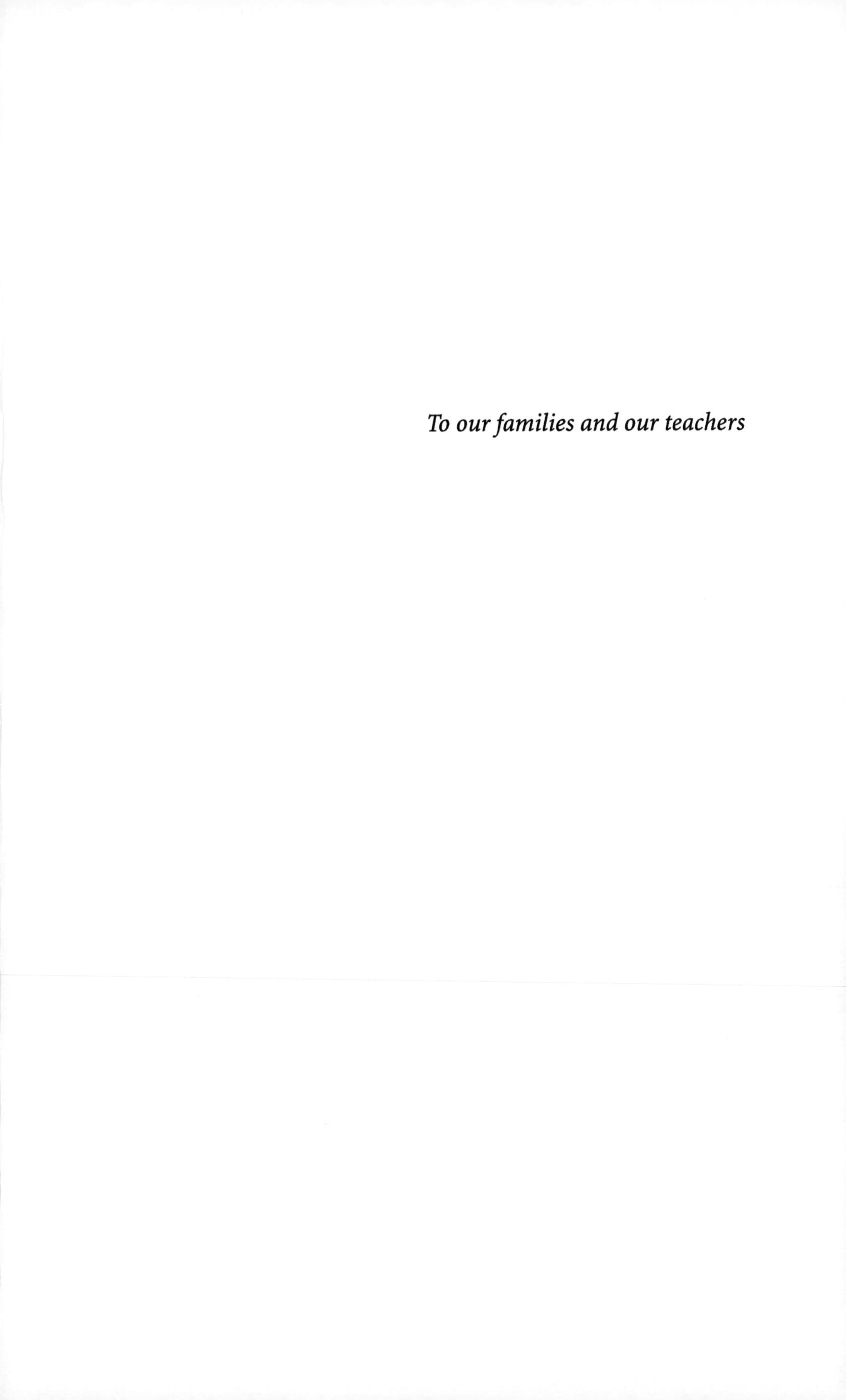

To our families and our teachers

Sponsorship from Nycomed, Italy, is gratefully acknowledged.

Preface

The diagnosis of osteoporosis and the determination of fracture risk has always been a challenge for radiologists, epidemiologists, and clinicians as well as other researchers and health care professionals working in the field. It is bone mineral density that is closely related to bone fragility, and the advent of techniques to quantitatively assess bone density has been welcomed. It has reduced the subjectivity inherent to conventional radiologic assessment of osteoporosis. The ongoing technical process has made various techniques to assess bone density widely available. However, these measurement techniques have also incurred some criticism because bone densitometry has sometimes been applied without specific indications and without appropriate clinical ramifications.

The purpose of this text is to provide a perspective on the current status of bone densitometry and ist relevance to osteoporosis diagnosis and management. Therefore, this book will give the reader an introduction to the nature of osteoporosis, its pathophysiology and epidemiology, and the clinical consequences of performing bone densitometry. Aside from standard bone densitometry, newer technologies such as quantitative ultrasound techniques, magnetic resonance imaging and bone structure analysis are discussed in the context of diagnosing osteoporosis.

The excellent cooperation with the publisher has made possible a short interval between the receipt of manuscripts and publication of this volume. Therefore, the chapters included are as close as possible to the current state of knowledge in this field. In this regard, we would like to thank Ms. Adelheid Duhm, Ms. Doris Engelhardt and Dr. Ute Heilmann from Springer-Verlag and Ms. Regine Schädlich from ProduServ Verlagsservice. We would also like to thank all of the authors for their excellent contributions that will make this volume a worthy read for clinicans, radiologists, physicists, and all researchers in the field of osteoporosis.

Harry K. Genant, San Francisco
Giuseppe Guglielmi, San Giovanni Rotondo
Michael Jergas, Bochum

Contents

7 Determinants of Bone Loss ... 127

S. ADAMI AND V. BRAGA

8 Biomechanical Properties of Bone ... 143

J. L. FERRETTI

Contributors

S. Adami
C.O.C. di Valeggio, University of Verona, 37067 Valeggio s/M, Verona, Italy

J. Adams
Department of Diagnostic Radiology, The University of Manchester, Stopford Building, Oxford Road, Manchester M13 9PT, UK

L. V. Avioli
Departments of Medicine and Orthopaedic Surgery, Washington University School of Medicine, 216 South Kingshighway Blvd., Ms, Mo 63110, St. Louis, Missouri, and Department of Internal Medicine, Wayne State University School of Medicine, Detroit Michigan, USA

C. Berkovich
Department of Periodontics, Northwestern University Dental School, 240 E. Hurons, Chicago, IL 60611, USA

E. Bonucci
Dipartimento di Medicina Sperimentale e Patologia, Sezione die Anatomia Patologica, Policlinico Umberto I, Viale Regina Elena 324, 00161 Roma, Italy

V. Braga
C.O.C. di Valeggio, University of Verona, 37067 Valeggio s/M, Verona, Italy

M. Cammisa
Department of Radiology, Scientific Institute Hostpital „CSS", 71013 San Giovanni Rotondo, Italy

E. Canalis
Saint Francis Hospital and Medical Center, 114 Woodland Street, Hartford, CT 06105-1299, USA

R. Civitelli
Division of Bone and Mineral Diseases, Washington University School of Medicine, and Barnes-Jewish Hospital, North Campus, 216 S. Kingshighway Blvd., St. Louis, MO 63110, USA

M. T. DiMuzio
Highland Park Hospital, 718 Glenview Avenue, Highland Park, IL 60035-2497,
USA

K. Engelke
University of Erlangen, Institute of Medical Physics (IMP), Krankenhausstraße
12, 91054 Erlangen, Germany

L. K. Fattore
Department of Geriatric Dentistry, Northwestern University Dental School, Chicago, IL 60611, USA

D. Felsenberg
Department of Radiology, Klinikum Benjamin Franklin of the Free University of
Berlin, Hindenburgdamm 30, 12200 Berlin, Germany

J. L. Ferretti
Center for P-Ca Metabolism Studies, National University of Rosario, Juan B. Justo 1427, 2000 Rosario, and Metabolic Research Institute, Libertad 836, 1er.piso,
1012 Buenos Aires, Argentina

T. Fuerst
Osteoporosis and Arthritis Research Group, Department of Radiology, University of California San Francisco, 505 Parnassus Avenue M-392, San Francisco, CA
94143-0628, USA

H. K. Genant
Osteoporosis and Arthritis Research Group, Department of Radiology, University of California San Francisco, 505 Parnassus Avenue M-392, San Francisco, CA
94143-0628, USA

C. Gennari
Istiuto di Patologia Speciale Medica, Universita di Siena, Policlinico Le Scotte,
Viale Bracci, 53100 Siena, Italy

V. Gilsanz
Department of Radiology, Childrens Hospital Los Angeles, Radiology Department MS# 81, 4650 Sunset Boulevard, Los Angeles, CA 90027, USA

G. Guglielmi
Department of Radiology, Scientific Institute Hospital „CSS", 71013 San Giovanni Rotondo, Italy

D. Hans
Osteoporosis and Arthritis Research Group, Department of Radiology, University of California San Francisco, 505 Parnassus Avenue M-392, San Francisco, CA 94143-0628, USA

S. T. Harris
University of California San Francisco, 350 Parnassus Ave., Suite # 706, USA, CA 94117-3608

K. Houki
Department of Geriastric Dentistry, Northwestern University Dental School, Chicago, IL 60611, USA

M. Jergas
Department of Radiology, St. Josef-Hospital, Ruhr-University Bochum, Gudrunstraße 56, 44791 Bochum, Germany

O. Johnell
Department of Orthopaedics, Malmö University Hospital, S-20502 Malmö, Sweden

W. Kalender
University of Erlangen, Institute of Medical Physics (IMP), Krankenhausstraße 12, 91054 Erlangen, Germany

M. Kleerekoper
Departments of Medicine and Orthopaedic Surgery, Washington University School of Medicine, St. Louis, Missouri, and Department of Internal Medicine, Wayne State University School of Medicine, Harper Hospital, 1 Webber South, 3990 John R, Detroit, Mi 48201 USA

C. van Kuijk
Osteoporosis and Arthritis Research Group, Department of Radiology, University of California San Francisco, 505 Parnassus Avenue M-392, San Francisco, CA 94143-0628, USA

T. F. Lang
Department of Radiology, University of California San Francisco, 505 Parnassus Avenue M-392, San Francisco, CA 94143-0628 USA

Y. Lu
Osteoporosis and Arthritis Research Group, Department of Radiology, University of California San Francisco, 505 Parnassus Avenue M-392, San Francisco, CA 94143-0628, USA

S. Majumdar
Osteoporosis and Arthritis Research Group, Department of Radiology, University of California San Francisco, 505 Parnassus Avenue M-392, San Francisco, CA 94143-0628, USA

G. Martini
Istituto di Patologia Speciale Medica, Universita di Siena, Policlinico Le Scotte, Viale Bracci, 53100 Siena, Italy

A. Mathur
Osteoporosis and Arthritis Research Group, Department of Radiology, University of California San Francisco, 505 Parnassus Avenue M-392, San Francisco, CA 94143-0628, USA

P. D. Miller
University of Colorado Health Sciences Center, Colorado Center for Bone Research, 3190 S Wadsworth # 250, Lakewood, CO 80227, USA

S. Mora
Division of Pediatrics, University of Milan Clinical Pediatrica 3, H. San Raffaele, Via Olgettina 60, Milan, 20132 Italy

R. Nuti
Istituto di Patologia Speciale Medica, Universita di Siena, Policlinico Le Scotte, Viale Bracci, 53100 Siena, Italy

S. Ortolani
Istituto Auxologico Italiano, Istituto di Ricovero e Cura a Carattere Scientifico, Via L. Ariosto, 13, 20145 Milano, Italy

R. Pacifici
Division of bone and Mineral Diseases, Barnes-Jewish Hospital St. Louis MO, 216 S. Kinghighway, St. Louis, MO 63110, USA

C. Reiners
Clinic for Nuclear Medicine, University of Würzburg, Josef-Schneider-Straße 2, 97080 Würzburg, Germany

P. D. Ross
Hawaii Osteoporosis Center, 401 Kamakee Street, Honolulu, HI 96814, USA

P. Schneider
Clinic for Nuclear Medicine, University of Würzburg, Josef-Schneider-Straße 2, 97080 Würzburg, Germany

C. Trevisan
Centro Auxologico Italiano, Istituto di Ricovero e Cura a Carattere Scientifico,
Via L. Ariosto, 13, 20145 Milano, Italy

M. Uffmann
Department of Radiology, St. Josef-Hospital, Ruhr-University Bochum, Gudrunstraße 56, 44791 Bochum, Germany

C. B. Westlund
Highland Park Hospital, 718 Glenview Avenue, Highland Park, IL 60035-2497,
USA

A. Zallone Zambonin
Istituto Anatomia Umana Normale, Policlinico, Piazza Giulio Cesare, 11, 70124
Bari, Italy

G. Zambonin
Istituto Anatomia Umana Normale, Policlinico, Piazza Giulio Cesare, 11, 70124
Bari, Italy

K. Ziambaras
Division of Bone and Mineral Diseases, Washington University School of Medi-
cine, and Barnes-Jewish Hospital, North Campus, 216 S. Kingshighway Blvd., St.
Louis, MO 63110, USA

1 Osteoporosis: The Clinical Problem

L. V. Avioli and M. Kleerekoper

Osteoporosis is a disease characterized by low bone mass and the development of nontraumatic or atraumatic fractures as a direct result of the low bone mass. A nontraumatic fracture has been arbitrarily defined as one occurring from trauma equal to or less than that of a fall from a standing height. In the preclinical state the disease is characterized simply by low bone mass without fractures. This totally asymptomatic state is often termed "osteopenia." Osteoporosis and osteopenia are the most common metabolic bone diseases in the developed countries of the world, whereas osteomalacia may be more prevalent in underdeveloped countries where nutrition is suboptimal and vitamin D deficiency common [1]. To be able to evaluate more fully the prevalence and incidence of osteoporosis worldwide, the World Health Organization (WHO) recently convened an expert panel to define osteoporosis on the basis of bone mass measurement [2]. The diagnostic categories for women that were established by that panel are as follows [1]:
- Normal: bone mineral density or bone mineral content less than 1 SD of the young adult reference mean
- Low bone mass: bone mineral density or bone mineral content between (osteopenia) –1.0 and –2.5 SD lower than the young adult reference mean
- Osteoporosis: bone mineral density or bone mineral content more than –2.5 SD below the young adult reference mean
- Severe (established): osteoporosis with one or more osteoporosis fragility fractures

Osteoporotic fractures may affect any part of the skeleton except the skull. Most commonly, fractures occur in the distal forearm (Colles' fracture), thoracic and lumbar vertebrae, and proximal femur (hip fracture).

Epidemiology

The incidence of osteoporotic fractures increases with age, is higher in whites than in blacks, and is higher in women than in men [3]. The female to male ratio is 1.5:1 for Colles' fracture, 7:1 for vertebral fractures, and 2:1 for hip fractures. Because most osteoporotic fractures do not require admission to the hospital, it is difficult to obtain precise figures on the true prevalence of this disease. Almost without exception, a hip fracture requires admission to a hospital, and current estimates indicate that there are 275 000 new osteoporotic hip fractures each year in the United States [4]. It has been estimated that after menopause a woman's lifetime risk of sustaining an osteoporotic fracture is one in three. Regrettably, despite improvements in surgical techniques and anesthesiology, most hip fractures require surgical intervention on a nonelective basis, and there is a 15%–20% excess mortality after an osteoporotic hip fracture. Perhaps more important, after such fractures less than one-third of the patients are restored to their prefracture functional state within 12 months of the fracture. Most patients require some form of ambulatory support, and many require institutional care. Attempts to define the multiple impairments that can result from vertebral compression fractures demonstrate reduced levels of functional performance in fracture subjects compared with controls with increased levels of assistance, pain and difficulty in activities [5]. Moreover, caution should be used in the assessment of benign appearing compression fractures in osteoporotic patients since neurological signs and symptoms are often delayed [6]. According to recent estimates at least 90% of all hip and vertebral fractures among elderly white women can be attributed to osteoporosis [7].

Health care expenditures attributable to osteoporotic fractures in 1995 were estimated at U.S. $13.8 billion, of which $10.3 billion (75%) was for the treatment of white women, $2.5 billion (18.4%) for white men, $0.7 billion (5.3%) for nonwhite women, and $0.2 billion (1.3%) for nonwhite men [8]. When costs for individual service sites are analyzed for 1995, $8.6 billion (62.4%) was spent for inpatient care, $3.9 billion (28.2%) for nursing home care, and $1.3 billion (9.4%) for outpatient services [8]. Moreover, these studies emphasize the fact that nonhip fracture contributes substantially to the morbidity and expenditures associated with osteoporosis, with 36.9% of the total expenditures used for this purpose alone. Although bone mineral density is considered an essential determinant for fracture, ethnic and life-style factors must also be considered. For example, although the bone mineral density when adjusted for height and weight are relatively comparable in Chinese and whites, the incidence of hip fractures is lower in Chinese than in whites [3]. In this case the difference has been ascribed at least in part to the fact that the hip axis length is lower in Chinese than in whites [3].

Pathogenesis

Once peak adult bone mass has been attained in the third, or possibly fourth, decade of life, bone mass at any point in time is the difference between peak adult bone mass and the loss of bone mass that has occurred since this was attained. Because age-related bone loss is a universal phenomenon in humans, any circumstance that limits an individual's ability to maximize peak adult bone mass increases the likelihood of developing osteoporosis later in life. Strategies for maximizing peak adult bone mass include maximizing calcium intake in growing children and young adults, minimizing the use of drugs which are potentially harmful to the skeleton and insuring normal gonadal function after menarche and puberty. The excessive bone loss that characterizes the pathogenesis of osteoporosis results primarily from abnormalities in the bone remodeling cycle. In brief, bone remodeling is a mechanism for keeping the skeleton "young" by a process of removal of old bone and replacement with new bone. The cycle is initiated by resorption of old bone, recruitment of osteoblasts, deposition of new matrix, and mineralization of that newly deposited matrix. It appears that with each cycle there is a slight, imperceptible deficit in bone formation. The total bone loss is therefore a function of the number of cycles in process at any one time.

Conditions that increase the rate of activation of the bone remodeling process thus increase the proportion of the skeleton undergoing remodeling at any one time and increase the rate of bone loss. In this circumstance, which is called "high-turnover" osteoporosis, the deficit per unit of remodeling is apparently constant. Most of the secondary causes of osteoporosis are associated with this increased rate of activation of the remodeling cycle:

- Genetic
- White or Asian ethnicity
- Positive family history
- Small body frame
- Life-style
- Smoking
- Inactivity
- Nulliparity
- Excessive exercise (producing amenorrhea)
- Early natural menopause
- Late menarche
- Nutritional factors
- Milk intolerance
- Lifelong low dietary calcium intake
- Vegetarian dieting
- Excessive alcohol intake
- Consistently high protein intake
- Medical disorders
- Anorexia nervosa
- Thyrotoxicosis
- Hyperparathyroidism
- Cushing's syndrome
- Type I diabetes
- Alterations in gastrointestinal and hepatobiliary function
- Occult osteogenesis imperfecta
- Mastocytosis
- Rheumatoid arthritis
- "Transient" osteoporosis
- Prolonged parenteral nutrition

- Prolactinoma
- Hemolytic anemia
- After organ transplantation
- Drugs
- Excessive dose of thyroid hormone
- Glucocorticoid drugs
- Anticoagulants
- Chronic lithium therapy
- Chemotherapy (breast cancer or lymphoma)
- Gonadotropin-releasing hormone agonist or antagonist therapy
- Anticonvulsants
- Chronic phosphate-binding antacid use
- Extended tetracycline use
- Diuretics producing calciuria
- Phenothiazine derivatives
- Cyclosporin A (not yet associated with decreased bone mass in humans, although identified as either toxic to bone in animals or as inducing calciuria or calcium malabsorption in humans)

In the normal aging process there appears to be a progressive impairment of the signaling between bone resorption and bone formation such that with every cycle of remodeling there is an increase in the deficit between resorption and formation because osteoblast recruitment is inefficient. Thus excessive bone loss can occur even when activation of the skeleton is not increased, and in fact even when activation of the skeleton is decreased. This gives rise to the concept of low- or normal-turnover osteoporosis.

Classifications of Osteoporosis

In addition to describing osteoporosis as being of the high- or low-turnover type, there are several other classification systems. The first is the classification into "primary" and "secondary," the latter being osteoporosis for which a clearly identifiable etiological mechanism is recognized. Primary osteoporosis is further characterized into "postmenopausal" and "senile." In "postmenopausal" osteoporosis there is an apparent excess loss of cancellous bone, with relative sparing of cortical bone, and the clinical syndromes involve Colles' fracture and vertebral fracture. In "senile" osteoporosis there is a more concordant loss of both cortical and cancellous bone. The pathogenesis of senile osteoporosis is uncertain, but it is postulated to result from an age-related decline in renal production of 1,25-dihydroxyvitamin D and calcium malabsorption, with subsequent secondary hyperparathyroidism. It is the hyperparathyroidism that is largely responsible for the excess cortical bone loss. Fracture syndrome often seen in the patient with senile osteoporosis characteristically involves the hip and pelvis.

Clinical Manifestations of Osteoporosis

As mentioned above, osteoporosis without fracture is often totally asymptomatic. This does not lessen its importance because the aim of all therapies should be to prevent even the first fracture, let alone subsequent fractures. When osteoporosis is complicated by the development of an osteoporotic fracture, the symptoms and signs are those related to the fracture itself. Osteoporotic vertebral fractures may represent a unique situation, and this is discussed separately here. Primary orthopedic management of peripheral fractures should not be influenced by the fact that the fracture results from osteoporosis. Management consists of immobilization and analgesia. There does not appear to be anything about an osteoporotic fracture that results in delayed fracture union. If delayed fracture union or fracture nonunion complicates an osteoporotic fracture, one needs to look for conditions other than osteoporosis, such as osteomalacia, hyperparathyroidism, diabetes, or occult forms of osteogenesis imperfecta. Immobilization should be for only a limited period of time, sufficient to ensure primary fracture healing. Longer immobilization leads to accelerated bone loss and must be avoided.

The brittleness of the osteoporotic skeleton may complicate open surgical repair of osteoporotic fractures, with limited purchase for pins, plates, screws, or nails. Restoration of the prefracture anatomic and functional state is the goal in the management of osteoporotic fractures of the appendicular skeleton. Regrettably, with respect to osteoporotic hip fractures, this is often not the outcome that is attained, given the excess morbidity and mortality discussed above. In general this is because surgical repair of an osteoporotic hip fracture is usually a non-elective procedure. Circumstances that appear to increase mortality after a hip fracture are related to the overall medical health and nutritional status of the subject sustaining the fracture. Frail, elderly subjects – particularly men – taking large numbers of medications and with mental impairment have the greatest mortality. Less than one-third of patients who survive the early operative intervention for an osteoporotic hip fracture are restored to their prefracture functional state, and the others require either institutionalized care or some form of ambulatory support. Recent analyses of hospital courses of hip fracture patients show that surgical repair within the first 2 days of hospitalization and more than five sessions per week of physical therapy are associated with better health outcomes.

Osteoporotic vertebral fractures are quite different from other osteoporotic fractures. Surveys of spine radiographs in older subjects suggest that many vertebral fractures occur in the absence of acute symptoms. If acute symptoms do occur at the time of fracture, these manifest as intense pain and limitation of motion. Operative intervention is seldom required for stabilization of these fractures. However, the principle of immobilization for a short time should still hold. The concept of placing the patient with an osteoporotic fracture in a back brace for years is to be decried. Similarly, the acute skeletal pain after an osteoporotic vertebral fracture should dissipate within 4–6 weeks. If skeletal tenderness persists much beyond this, other causes for the fracture (e.g., metastatic disease, multiple myeloma) should be considered. Osteoporotic fractures of the vertebral bodies rarely result in "referred nerve pain syndrome" or long tract symptoms or signs. Again, if a fracture is complicated by these symptoms or signs, causes other than osteoporosis should be considered.

Once a vertebral body has been fractured, restoration of normal anatomy is not possible. In fact, refracture of the same vertebra with further abnormalities of shape and size is often the outcome. As noted above, even those vertebral fractures that are not associated with any acute symptoms at the time of fracture give rise to chronic pain, disability, and often obvious deformity. All vertebral fractures are associated with loss of stature; in the thoracic spine this is associated with a progressive increase in the degree of kyphosis, and in the lumbar spine this is associated with a progressive flattening of the lordotic curve and scoliosis in some individuals. As the number of vertebrae involved increases and the severity of individual vertebral deformities progresses, these anatomic changes become more pronounced. There is gradual loss of the waistline contour and protuberance of the abdomen, and in severe cases the lower ribs approximate the pelvic rim and ultimately lie within the pelvis. Each of these progressive anatomic deformities is associated with symptoms.

The progressive loss of stature results in progressive "shortening" of the paraspinal musculature, that is, the paraspinal muscles are actively contracting, resulting in the pain of muscle fatigue. This is the major cause of the chronic back pain in spinal osteoporosis. Careful clinical examination reveals that the skeleton (spine) itself is not tender, and most patients indicate that the pain is paraspinal. The pain is worse with prolonged standing and is often relieved by walking. After an acute fracture, there may be associated paraspinal muscle spasm, but this dissipates with time. The loss of height and the protuberant abdomen are usually not associated with direct symptoms per se, but do give the patient the emotional discomfort of the altered body image. Many patients attempt to wear abdominal flattening girdles or go on weight-reduction diets, both of which are of limited benefit and potential harm. It is important that the patient be advised of the irreversible nature of these anatomic changes. One common complaint of patients with advanced disease is vague gastrointestinal distress aggravated by eating. This can be alleviated somewhat by having the patient consume frequent, smaller meals. This is a particularly vexing problem for patients with chronic airway disease who have osteoporosis as a result of therapy with corticosteroids. In these patients the flattened diaphragm coupled with the shortened spinal column results in marked diminution in the size of their abdominal cavity.

There are several important approaches to the long-term management of patients with these chronic deformities from spinal osteoporosis. Of particular importance is educating the patient to understand the nature of the deformity so that he or she can have realistic expectations concerning body image and the anticipated goals of therapy (relief of pain, restoration of function, maintenance of a reasonable quality of life, and prevention of further fractures). The major focus of therapy should be rehabilitation and analgesia aimed at lessening the chronic back pain. However, caution must be used with analgesics and non-steroidal anti-inflammatory agents, many of which cause significant constipation. Straining of the stool to relieve constipation from narcotic analgesics tends to aggravate back pain substantially. In this regard it is worth noting that many generic calcium preparations also tend to cause vague gastrointestinal symptoms, including constipation in some patients. It is equally important to instruct the patient adequately in activities of daily living so that he or she bends, lifts, and stoops in a manner that does not increase strain on the brittle skeleton. Nurses, physical therapists, and occupational therapists become important partners in the management of the patient with spinal osteoporosis. In many respects this nonpharmacological approach to these patients is far more important than the pharmacological therapy.

Diagnostic Studies in Osteoporosis

The same diagnostic approach should be taken with patients suspected of having osteoporosis regardless of whether they have already sustained an osteoporotic fracture. These studies should be undertaken only after an appropriate history and physical examination have been completed. The history, physical examination, and studies should all be conducted with the aim of determining the extent and severity of disease, pathogenesis of the bone loss, and physiology of the skeleton at the time of presentation. Although postmenopausal and senile osteoporosis are the most prevalent forms of the disease, it must be remembered that as many as 20% of women who otherwise appear to have postmenopausal osteoporosis have other etiological factors in addition to their age, gender, and ethnic background. Many of these secondary causes of osteoporosis (see above) can be suggested from the history and physical examination so that appropriate testing parameters can be ordered.

If an osteoporotic fracture is suspected, it is imperative that radiographs be taken of the appropriate part of the skeleton. However, there is no clear indication for radiographs of the skeleton if fracture is not suspected. All patients suspected of having osteoporosis, with or without fracture, should have bone mineral density measurements. The one possible exception is the patient with very advanced disease clinically and radiographically. Because osteoporosis may be the only manifestation of many of the secondary causes listed above, it is appropriate to perform simple screening studies looking for these causes in each patient. A biochemical profile provides information about renal and hepatic function, primary hyperparathyroidism, and possible malnutrition. A hematological profile might also provide clues to the presence of myeloma and malnutrition. The precise role of hyperthyroidism, particularly exogenous, in the pathogenesis of accelerated bone loss and osteoporosis remains unresolved. Nonetheless, for the time being at least it seems prudent to obtain a sensitive thyroid-stimulating hormone assay in all patients with documented bone loss. A 24-h urine collection for measurement of calcium (which should always be accompanied by measurement of creatinine and sodium) detects patients with hypercalciuria, which may be the end result of excess skeletal loss or may contribute to excess skeletal loss. In contrast, a very low urine calcium level (50 mg or less for 24 h) may provide a clue to the presence of vitamin D malnutrition or malabsorption [1]. In general, the intensity with which one looks for occult secondary causes of accelerated bone loss should be related to any unusual features of the clinical presentation, such as rapid bone loss in premenopausal women, in women very early in menopause, in others who are losing bone during estrogen therapy, and in men without obvious hypogonadism. One should also pay particular attention to patients whose fractures occur at sites other than the vertebrae or hips.

Calcitropic Hormones and Biochemical Markers of Bone Remodeling

In most cases of osteoporosis there is no need to measure the calcitropic hormones (parathyroid hormone, calcitriol, or calcitonin) unless there is a specific indication for these measurements based on the history, physical examination, and biochemical screening. Although there are reports of abnormalities in some of these measurements when compared with published reference ranges, this is often not the case when the reference values are appropriately adjusted for age, gender, and ethnic background.

In contrast, it is becoming increasingly important to monitor the biochemical markers of bone remodeling that are discussed in detail in Chap. 6. The control of normal bone turnover is detailed in Chap. 3, and the role of abnormalities in the remodeling cycle in the pathogenesis of osteoporosis presented in Chap. 5. There is an analogy between turnover abnormalities leading to osteoporosis and abnormalities in the red cell life cycle leading to anemia. High-turnover bone loss with increased resorption and increased, but insufficient, formation is analogous to hemolytic anemia with increased red cell destruction and increased (but insufficient) red cell formation, characterized by the increased reticulocyte count in this type of anemia. Low-turnover bone loss with normal resorption and subnormal formation is analogous to anemia of chronic disease. It should be recognized in this regard that bone remodeling does not decline after menopause in osteoporotic fracture-prone individuals [10].

There is increasing evidence that biochemical markers of bone formation and resorption are a useful adjunct in predicting the rate of bone loss and the response to therapy. Table 1-1 lists biochemical markers of bone resorption and formation which are currently available through commercial diagnostic laboratories. Table 1-1 also provides details of the reference intervals for these tests in healthy premenopausal white women. Theoretically, patients with high-turnover osteoporosis with increased levels of resorption and formation markers should be experiencing bone loss at an accelerated rate [11] and should respond best to therapy with drugs that inhibit bone resorption [12]. In contrast, those with low- or nor-

Table 1-1 Biochemical markers of bone remodeling[a]

Marker	Reference interval[b]
Bone resorption	
Lysylpyridinoline	24–52 nM Pyd/mM Cr
Deoxylysylpyridinoline	2.5–6.2 nM Dpd/mM Cr
N-Telopeptide of the cross-links	5–65 nM/mM Cr of collagen based upon 95% CI
C-Telopeptide of the cross-links	13–96 nM/mM Cr of collagen
Bone formation	
Osteocalcin	Bone Gla 1.6–9.2 ng/ml protein
Bone-specific alkaline	11.6–30.6 BAP, U/l phosphatase
Carboxyterminal extension	45–190 µg/l peptide of type I procollagen

[a] All resorption markers are based on urine collected after an overnight fast. Usually a spot sample of the first or second voided urine is analyzed. Data are normalized for creatinine excretion. All formation markers are based on random serum samples. CI, confidence interval.

[b] Reference intervals are for premenopausal women.

mal-turnover osteoporosis should have normal or low levels of the markers, should not be losing bone at an accelerated rate, should respond less well to antiresorptive therapy, and should be treated preferentially with drugs that primarily enhance bone formation. The greatest difficulty has been demonstrating that the markers can be used to select therapy for individual patients [13,14], principally because the only therapies available are all antiresorptive. As therapeutic options broaden over the next several years, the usefulness of biochemical markers in this fashion will become more apparent.

At present the most practical use of these markers is to monitor the response to therapy. It has been demonstrated that changes in markers after only 3 months of therapy are significantly related to changes in bone mass after 24 months of therapy [15]. This is of considerable practical importance, particularly with respect to patient compliance with treatment, as changes in bone mass in response to therapy may not become apparent within 12 months of treatment. The markers may also provide confidence for dose adjustment, allowing the clinician to use a smaller than recommended dose of therapy if this proves sufficient to restore biochemical markers of remodeling to the normal premenopausal range.

In summary, the current approach to evaluation of the osteoporotic patient involves documentation of bone mass, documentation of fractures if present, a diligent search for secondary causes, and then a pragmatic evaluation of the biochemistry of skeletal remodeling.

Medical Therapy

At the time of this writing the only drugs approved by the United States Food and Drug Administration (FDA) for treatment of postmenopausal osteoporosis are estrogen, calcitonin, and the bisphosphonate alendronate. The FDA is evaluating a request for approval of a sustained-release sodium fluoride preparation.

Although calcitriol and etidronate are both approved by the FDA for use in the United States, osteoporosis is currently not an approved indication. Oral calcium supplements are not subject to FDA regulation, and sodium fluoride as a supplement is also not subject to FDA regulation. Although vertebral bone mineral loss occurs in estrogen-replete, calcium-replete premenopausal women [16], the primary role for estrogen in the prevention of early postmenopausal bone loss and the subsequent development of osteoporotic fractures has been well established. Despite the observation that estrogens improve bone density in osteoporotic women aged over 65 years [18], a definitive role for the use of estrogens in established osteoporosis with fractures needs further justification.

Estrogen is an "antiresorptive" agent in that it inhibits bone resorption by decreasing the frequency of activation of the bone remodeling cycle. Estrogen would be expected to be most efficient if bone remodeling or bone turnover were increased. This is why it is so effective in the early stages of menopause. In an individual patient with established osteoporosis who can be shown to have increased bone remodeling estrogen is effective in inhibiting remodeling, regardless of how long it has been since the patient had her menopause. Thus estrogen therapy slows the rate of bone loss in any estrogen-deficient woman so treated. However, the ability of estrogen to result in any net gain in bone mass is limited, a 2%–4% annual increase for 2 years, the average response in young postmenopausal women. Recent studies have suggested that older women may also receive benefit from estrogen of similar magnitude [18,19]. The usual starting dose is 0.625 mg of conjugated equine estrogen (Premarin) for 25 days per month or its equivalent (Table 1-2). Short-term complications of estrogen therapy in women include breast tenderness and vaginal bleeding [20]. If estrogens are given without progesterone, there is an increased likelihood of endometrial hyperplasia. Although the relationship between estrogen therapy and breast cancer is still debatable [21], most studies suggest that there is little if any increased risk of breast cancer during the first 5–10 years of therapy. As long as therapy is tolerated, estrogen therapy, once indicated, should be continued indefinitely with appropriate patient monitoring especially for maximal protection against fracture syndromes [22].

Table 1-2 Hormone replacement therapies approved for the prevention and treatment of osteoporosis in the United States

Drug	Dosage
Premarin[a]	0.625 mg per day
PremPro	0.625/2.5 mg per day
Premphase	0.625/5 mg per day
Ogen[a]	0.625 mg per day
Estrace[a]	0.5 mg per day
Estraderm[a]	0.05 mg twice a week

[a] Estrogen-only preparations, usually prescribed with progesterone in women with intact uterus.

Since compliance to estrogen therapy is often a problem, synthetic salmon calcitonin (Calcimar and Miacalcin) is available either as a subcutaneous injection or nasal spray formulation. As with estrogen, calcitonin inhibits bone resorption and slows the rate of bone loss. The ability of calcitonin to increase bone mass is a function of the rate of bone remodeling at the time that calcitonin therapy is initiated. The response is better in patients with increased bone turnover than in patients with low turnover [24]. Again, a beneficial effect is observed as long as the medication is used [24–30]. There is increasing evidence that calcitonin has inherent analgesic properties, and many physicians recommend its use for osteoporotic patients in the early postfracture period because of this effect [29]. The major side effects of calcitonin, which are transient flushing of the face and nausea, are all dose dependent and virtually disappear with nasal spray formulations. The recommended nasal spray dose is 200 IU daily [30] in postmenopausal women with decreased bone mass. Smaller doses have been used unsuccessfully in attempts to prevent bone loss in perimenopausal women [31]. Increased bone mass and decreased fracture incidence have been documented in patients using injectable calcitonin for 10 days each month over a 2-year period [32]. Therapy should be continued for as long as the drug is tolerated and is considered effective by monitoring either urinary biomarkers or vertebral bone mass measurements.

As discussed above, use of the biochemical markers may assist in finding a suitable dose of estrogen or calcitonin for individual patients, particularly if side effects or other concerns limit the recommended starting dose. For example, breast tenderness on estrogen is less likely in older women if initiated in a dose of Premarin 0.3 mg/day. If this dose can be demonstrated to have reduced the rate of resorption, dose adjustment might not be indicated. Similarly, if the markers of resorption have not changed appropriately (arbitrarily a 40%–50% reduction from baseline after 8–12 weeks of therapy), the patient might be more willing to consider a higher dose of therapy. This is equally appropriate when trying to maximize the dose of calcitonin in the therapy of the osteoporotic female.

Alendronate (Fosamax), an amino-bisphosphonate for which extensive clinical trials have been completed worldwide, was recently approved by the FDA for the treatment of osteoporosis. In the clinical trials there was a progressive increase in spine and hip bone mineral density during 3 years of daily therapy at a dose of 10 mg once a day [33, 34]. Fewer and less severe spinal and hip fractures were observed in patients receiving therapy than in those on placebo. The major potential problem with this therapy is poor gastrointestinal absorption (less than 1%) of an orally administered dose. This poor absorption is further impaired if the medication is taken with food, any liquid except water, and calcium supplements. These problems can be avoided if patients are advised to take the medication first thing in the morning with water and to delay breakfast for at least 30 min. The major side effect is esophagitis, which occurs in approximately 20% of patients [36].

Etidronate (Didronel), the first bisphosphonate to become clinically available in the United States, has been used in several clinical trials to stabilize or increase bone mass and also to possibly reduce the vertebral fracture rate [37, 38]. However, the effect on the vertebral fracture rate is currently still controversial and by no means well established. The treatment regimen for etidronate is 400 mg orally daily for 2 weeks followed by a 10- to 12-week etidronate-free period, with a repeat of this 3-month cycle for 2 years. As cited earlier for alendronate, this bisphosphonate is poorly absorbed orally, and because its absorption is obliterated when given concurrently with calcium, it is important to advise the patient not to ingest any calcium, either as a supplement or in food, for 4 h before or after ingestion of etidronate. Calcium (1000–1500 mg) as a daily supplement is administered during the etidronate-free periods. It is imperative that etidronate be used in this rigorous treatment cycle, and that the dose not be exceeded in amount or duration. Reports of defective mineralization during etidronate treatment of both Paget's disease of bone [39–41] and postmenopausal osteoporosis [42] should be acknowledged in this regard. Currently, although etidronate is often used as "off-label" therapy, this drug is not an FDA-approved therapy for osteoporosis in the United States. As noted earlier for calcitonin and estrogen, etidronate is an antiresorptive drug. Although there is very little formal evidence that its effectiveness is a function of remodeling activity at the time therapy is initiated, one can anticipate a gain of 2%–4% annually in vertebral bone mass.

Although calcitriol (Rocaltrol) in a dose of 0.25 mg/day has been shown in one study to reduce the vertebral fracture rate compared with a group of patients taking calcium alone [42], other clinical trials have not found calcitriol to be effective in this regard. However, because calcitriol is the most potent metabolite [43] of vitamin D, it does increase intestinal calcium absorption, often resulting in hypercalciuria or hypercalcemia. Patients should be cautioned to monitor their calcium intake to avoid excessive amounts and should also be monitored every 6–8 weeks for development of hypercalciuria or hypercalcemia, because clinical symptoms and signs of these conditions may be very subtle and not evident until irreversible renal damage has occurred. It is unclear what specific effect calcitriol has on bone mass, although in some instances, increments in bone mass of 1%–2% per annum have been recorded [44].

The effects of calcium supplementation on bone mass and vertebral fracture rate in established osteoporotic syndromes are variable. A few retrospective reviews and prospective studies reveal that calcium supplementation in postmenopausal women does decrease the rate of bone loss when administered in doses of 1000–1500 mg/day, especially in individuals with histories of marginally low calcium intake [45–48]. A combination of calcium supplements and exercise has also proven effective in stabilizing skeletal bone loss rates in postmenopausal women. Obviously it is important to maintain a calcium intake of 1000–1500 mg/ day in addition to the active drug during estrogen, calcitonin, or alendronate therapeutic interventions because it is difficult to mineralize newly formed matrix fully in the absence of adequate calcium.

In doses of 50–75 mg/day the increase in vertebral bone mass achieved with sodium fluoride approximates 8% per year, twice that seen with either estrogen, calcitonin, or bisphosphonates. However, there is little evidence from properly conducted prospective clinical trials that this increase in bone mass translates into a reduction in vertebral fractures. Moreover, sodium fluoride is associated with a significant degree of gastrointestinal distress and also a painful lower-extremity syndrome believed to represent stress fractures induced by fluoride [49]. Recent studies with a lower dose of a slow-release sodium fluoride preparation administered cyclically have indicated a beneficial effect on vertebral fracture rates [50]. The best results were reported in those osteoporotic patients with the highest bone mass (>65% of peak adult bone mass). Therapy was most effective in preventing fractures in previously nonfractured vertebrae; there was no significant effect on the progression of fractures in vertebra that were already fractured before initiation of treatment. It should be emphasized that these patients were also subjected to estrogen therapy. Currently sodium fluoride is still not approved by the United States FDA for either the treatment or prevention of osteoporosis.

There are isolated reports that the prevalence of osteoporotic hip fractures decreases in hypertensive patients receiving long-term therapy with hydrochlorothiazide [51–54]. To our knowledge, there are no formal prospective studies of thiazide diuretic therapy in osteoporotic or postmenopausal normotensive populations. Until such studies are recorded and show them to be effective, thiazide diuretics should not be used as therapy for osteoporosis. However, a case could be made for selecting thiazides as the diuretic of choice in patients with osteoporosis, should diuretic therapy be otherwise indicated, for example, in early hypertensive syndromes. Because thiazides decrease renal excretion of calcium and, uncommonly, lead to mild hypercalcemia, extreme caution should be used when considering calcitriol therapy in a patient taking thiazides, or thiazide therapy in a patient taking calcitriol. Side effects such as hypomagnesemia, hyperglycemia, hypercholesterolemia, and hypokalemia preclude advocating thiazide drugs as potentially therapeutic for osteoporotic patients who are not hypertensive [55].

Newer generations of bisphosphonates, synthetic parathyroid hormone, selective estrogen receptor modulators (SERMs), and various combinations and treatment regimens of these experimental drugs, are currently undergoing extensive clinical trials. At present the safety and efficacy of these various drugs and their potential combinations are not well established. Consequently their use cannot be recommended. One exception is the antiestrogen tamoxifen. This drug is widely prescribed for women with breast cancer to minimize the likelihood of recurrence. Tamoxifen as a SERM drug inhibits bone resorption in the same manner as estrogen and is effective in preserving bone mass. However, because of reported side effects, not the least of which is endometrial carcinoma, its use should be restricted to women for whom it is prescribed as adjunctive therapy for breast cancer.

Selecting a Therapy and Monitoring the Response to Therapy

At a minimum every patient with established osteoporosis, with or without fractures, should be given supplemental calcium at 1000–1500 mg/day. Specific therapy for osteoporosis in the United States should be restricted to estrogen, calcitonin, and alendronate, given that these drugs are approved by the FDA for an osteoporosis indication. Bone mass, which should always be measured at baseline, should be monitored at the end of 12 months of therapy. A decrease in bone mass of 2% or greater should prompt a change in therapy, either a change in dose or a change in medication. After a patient has experienced 1 full year of successful therapy, that is, 1 year of therapy with either an increase in bone mass or less than a 2% decrease, monitoring can be restricted to biannual measurement of bone mass. At present there is no indication that therapy should be discontinued as long as the patient is tolerating the medication, and there is no progressive decrement in bone mass. It should be noted that the antifracture efficacy of each of these drugs during the early therapeutic phase is not well established, and the occurrence of an osteoporotic fracture within the first 6–12 months of therapy should not be taken as an indication of failed therapy. The patient should be made completely aware of this before initiation of therapy.

It is deemed appropriate that each patient have a baseline measurement of biochemical markers of bone remodeling before initiating therapy. The patient should be seen and clinically evaluated 6–8 weeks later to ascertain compliance and possible side effects from therapy. It is also appropriate to repeat the biomarker test at this time to confirm that there is indeed a decrease in the rate of bone remodeling. If there is no satisfactory change in the biochemistry, one should consider increasing the dose. If the dose of medication is changed for whatever reason, clinical and biochemical evaluation should be repeated in 6–8 weeks until a satisfactory response is achieved. If there is no response to 3 months of therapy, one should consider a change in medication. Studies confirming the scientific rationale for monitoring biochemical markers of bone remodeling have not been fully completed. However, available data suggest that the anticipated early (3 months or less) change in several of the markers, in response to successful therapy, is greater than the precision error of the biochemical measurement. This is in contrast to serial measurement of bone mineral density, for which even a good response to therapy cannot be detected within 1 year in most patients because the anticipated change is close to the precision limits of the methods. Furthermore, there is evidence that early (3 months) changes in biochemical markers reliably predict later (24 months) changes in bone mass.

Most patients and their treating physicians are reluctant to take therapy for 12 months before measurable feedback is available, and this practical consideration may dictate the frequency with which biochemical markers are monitored. As far as is known, there are no ill effects of long-term use of calcitonin or alendronate in the treatment schedules described above. Cost and convenience become important factors in long-term patient acceptance of these drugs. Because of the potential association between long-term estrogen therapy and development of endometrial and breast cancer, appropriate monitoring for these complications must be continued. Patients must be instructed in the technique of monthly breast self-examination and must undergo an annual examination by a clinician and an annual mammogram. All episodes of unexplained vaginal bleeding must be fully evaluated by a gynecologist. In women with an intact uterus, progesterone should be given along with estrogen; most patients soon develop either amenorrhea or a stable, recognizable bleeding pattern, which should not give rise to concern or investigation.

It is important to reemphasize that drug therapy should never be substituted for the commonsense approaches to daily living discussed in some detail in the above sections. This includes emphasizing safety and fall prevention, avoiding drugs such as sedatives, hypnotics, and antihypertensives, which might predispose to sedation, ataxia, or postural hypotension and recognizing the need to use supplements of vitamin D of 800 IU/day in the elderly [1, 56, 57]. Patients should all be encouraged to become involved in a regular active exercise/rehabilitation program. With appropriate medical, nursing, and rehabilitation care, most patients, except for those with the most advanced disease with multiple vertebral compression fractures, can be expected to be restored to reasonable functional health with a good quality of life. Likewise, an anticipated goal of therapy should be to prevent even the first osteoporotic fracture in patients whose therapy is initiated early.

References

1. Villareal DT, Civitelli R, Chines A, Avioli LV (1991) Subclinical vitamin D deficiency in postmenopausal women with low vertebral bone mass. J Clin Endocrinol Metab 72:628–634
2. World Health Organization (1994) Assessment of fracture risk and its application to screening for postmenopausal osteoporosis. Report of a WHO Study Group. World Health Organ Tech Rep Ser 843:1–129
3. Lau EMC, Cooper C (1996) The epidemiology of osteoporosis. The Oriental perspective in a world context. Clin Orthop Related Res 323:65–74
4. Avioli LV (1991) Significance of osteoporosis: a growing international health care problem. Calcif Tissue Int 49:S5–S7
5. Lyles KW, Gold DT, Shipp KM, Pieper CF, Martinez S, Mulhausen PL (1993) Association of osteoporotic vertebral compression fractures with impaired functional status. Am J Med 94:595–601
6. Heggeness MH (1993) Spine fracture with neurological deficit in osteoporosis. Osteoporosis Int 3:215–221
7. Melton LJ III, Thamer M, Ray NF, Chan JK, Chesnut CH III, Einhorn TA, Johnston CC, Raisz LG, Silverman SL, Siris ES (1997) Fractures attributable to osteoporosis: report from the National Osteoporosis Foundation. J Bone Miner Res 12:16–23

8. Fay NF, Chan JK, Thamer M, Melton LJ III (1997) Medical expenditures for the treatment of osteoporotic fractures in the United States in 1995: report from the National Osteoporosis Foundation. J Bone Miner Res 12:24–35

9. Hoenig H, Rubenstein LV, Sloane R, Horner R, Kahn K (1997) What is the role of timing in the surgical and rehabilitative care of community-dwelling older persons with acute hip fracture? Arch Intern Med 157:513

10. Wand JS, Green JR, Hesp R, Bradbeer JN, Sambrook PN, Smith T, Hampton L, Zanelli JM, Reeve J (1992) Bone remodeling does not decline after menopause in vertebral fracture osteoporosis. Bone Miner 17:361–375

11. Hanson DA, Weis MAE, Bollen AM, Maslan SL, Singer FR, Eyre DR (1992) A specific immunoassay for monitoring human bone resorption: quantitation of Type I collagen cross-linked N-telopeptides in urine. J Bone Miner Res 7:1251–1258

12. Lyritis GP, Magiasis B, Tsakalakos N (1995) Prevention of bone loss in early nonsurgical and nonosteoporotic high turnover patients with salmon calcitonin: the role of biochemical bone markers in monitoring high turnover patients under calcitonin treatment. Calcif Tissue Int 56:38–41

13. Cosman F, Nieves J, Wilkinson C, Schnering D, Shen V, Lindsay R (1996) Bone density change and biochemical indices of skeletal turnover. Calcif Tissue Int 58:236–243

14. Lotz J, Steeger D, Hafner G, Ehrenthal W, Heine J, Prellwitz W (1995) Biochemical bone markers compared with bone density measurement by dual energy X-ray absorptiometry. Calcif Tissue Int 57:253–257

15. Garnero P, Shih WJ, Gineyts E, Karpf DB, Delmas PD (1994) Comparison of new biochemical markers of bone turnover in late postmenopausal women in response to alendronate treatment. J Clin Endocrinol Metab 79:1693–1700

16. Citron JT, Ettinger B, Genant HK (1995) Spinal bone mineral loss in estrogen-replete, calcium-replete premenopausal women. Osteoporosis Int 5:228–233

17. The Writing Group for the PEPI Trial (1996) Effects of hormone therapy on bone mineral density. JAMA 276:1389–1396

18. Marx CW, Dailey GE III, Cheney C, Vint VC II, Muchmore DB (1992) Do estrogens improve bone mineral density in osteoporotic women over age 65? J Bone Miner Res 7:1275–1279

19. Lufkin EG, Wahner HW, O'Fallon WM et al (1992) Treatment of postmenopausal osteoporosis with transdermal estrogen. Ann Intern Med 117:1–9

20. Prince RL, Smith M, Dick IM et al (1991) Prevention of postmenopausal osteoporosis. Comparative study of exercise, calcium supplementation, and hormone replacement therapy. N Engl J Med 325:1189–1195

21. Belchetz P (1989) Hormone replacement treatment: deserves wider use. BMJ 298:1467

22. Cauley JA, Seeley DG, Ensrud K, Ettinger B, Black D, Cummings SR (1995) Estrogen replacement therapy and fractures in older women. Ann Intern Med 122:9–16

23. Cano A (1995) Compliance to hormone replacement therapy in menopausal women controlled in a third level academic centre. Maturitas 20:91–99
24. Civitelli R, Gonnelli S, Zacchei F et al (1988) Bone turnover in postmenopausal osteoporosis. J Clin Invest 82:1268–1274
25. Avioli LV (1991) Heterogeneity of osteoporotic syndromes and the response to calcitonin therapy. Calcif Tissue Int 49 [Suppl 2]:S16–S19
26. Rico H, Hernandez ER, Diaz-Mediaville J et al (1990) Treatment of multiple myeloma with nasal spray calcitonin: a histomorphometric and biochemical study. Bone Miner 8:231–237
27. Mazzuoli GF, Passeri M, Gennari C et al (1986) Effects of salmon calcitonin in postmenopausal osteoporosis: a controlled double-blind clinical study. Calcif Tissue Int 38:3–8
28. Overgaard K, Riis BJ, Christiansen C et al (1989) Effect of calcitonin given intranasally on early postmenopausal bone loss. BMJ 299:477–479
29. Lyritis GP, Tsakalakos S, Magiasis B et al (1991) Analgesic effect of salmon calcitonin on osteoporotic vertebral fractures. Double-blind, placebo-controlled study. Calcif Tissue Int 49:369–372
30. Ellerington MC, Hillard TC, Whitcroft SIJ, Marsh MS, Lees B, Banks LM, Whitehead MI, Stevenson JC (1996) Intranasal salmon calcitonin for the prevention and treatment of postmenopausal osteoporosis. Calcif Tissue Int 59:6–11
31. Arnala I, Saastamoinen J, Alhava EM (1996) Salmon calcitonin in the prevention of bone loss at perimenopause. Bone 4:629–632
32. Rico H, Hernandez ER, Revilla M, Gomez-Castresana F (1992) Salmon calcitonin reduces vertebral fracture rate in the postmenopausal crush fracture syndrome. Bone Miner 16:131–138
33. Devogelaer JP, Broll H, Correa-Rotter R, Cumming DC, Nagant De Deuxchaisnes C, Geusens P, Hosking D, Jaeger P, Kaufman JM, Leite M, Leon J, Liberman U, Menkes CJ, Meunier PJ, Reid I, Rodriguez J, Romanowicz A, Seeman E, Vermeulen A, Hirsch LJ, Lombardi A, Plezia K, Santora AC, Yates AJ, Yuan W (1996) Oral alendronate induces progressive increases in bone mass of the spine, hip, and total body over 3 years in postmenopausal women with osteoporosis. Bone 18:141–150
34. Liberman UA, Weiss SR, Brull J, Minne HW, Quan H, Bell NH, Rodriguez-Portales J, Downs RW Jr, Dequeker J, Favus M, Seeman E, Recker RR, Shah RV, Hirsch LJ, Karpf DB (1995) Effect of oral alendronate on bone mineral density and the incidence of fractures in postmenopausal osteoporosis. N Eng J Med 333:1437–1443
35. Black DN, Cummings SR, Karpf DB, Cualey JA, Thompson DE, Nevitt MC, Bauer DC, Genant HK, Haskell WL, Marcus R, Ott SM, Torner JC, Quandt SA, Reiss TF, Ensrud KE (1996) Randomised trial of effect of alendronate on risk of fracture in women with existing vertebral fractures. Lancet 348:1535–1541
36. DeGroen PC, Lubbe DF, Hirsch LJ, Daifotis A, Stephenson W, Freedholm D, Pryor-Tillotson S, Seleznick MJ, Pinkas H, Wang KK (1996) Esophagitis associated with the use of alendronate. N Engl J Med 335:1016–1021

37. Storm T, Thamsborg G, Steiniche T, Genant HK, Sorensen OH (1990) Effect of intermittent cyclical etidronate therapy on bone mass and fracture rate in women with postmenopausal osteoporosis. N Engl J Med 322:1265–1271

38. Watts NB, Harris ST, Genant HK et al (1990) Intermittent cyclical etidronate treatment of postmenopausal osteoporosis. N Engl J Med 323:73–79

39. Krane SM (1982) Etidronate disodium in the treatment of Paget's disease of bone. Ann Intern Med 96:619–625

40. Nagant de Deuxchaisnes C, Rombouts-Lindemans C, Huaux JP, Dovogelaer JP (1982) Diphosphonates and inhibition of bone mineralization. Lancet 2:607–608

41. Alexandre C, Meunier PJ, Edouard C et al (1981) Effect of ethane-1 hydroxy-1,1-diphosphonate (5 mg/kg/day dose) on quantitative bone histology in Paget's disease of bone. Metab Bone Dis 3:309–315

42. Simalawansa SJ (1995) Combined therapy with estrogen and etidronate has an additive effect on bone mineral density in the hip and vertebrae: Four-year randomized study. Am J Med 99:36–42

43. Ott SM, Chesnut CH III (1989) Calcitriol treatment is not effective in post-menopausal osteoporosis. Ann Intern Med 110:267–274

44. Gallagher JC (1993) Prevention of bone loss in postmenopausal and senile osteoporosis with vitamin D analogues. Osteoporosis Int 1:S172–175

45. Dawson-Hughes B (1991) Calcium supplementation and bone loss: a review of controlled clinical trials. Am J Clin Nutr 54:274S–280S

46. Dawson-Hughes B, Dallal GE, Krall EA, Sadowski L, Sahyoun N, Tannenbau S (1990) Controlled trial of the effect of calcium supplementation on bone density in postmenopausal women. N Engl J Med 323:878–883

47. Elders PJM, Netelenbos JC, Lips P et al (1991) Calcium supplementation reduces vertebral bone loss in perimenopausal women: a controlled trial in 248 women between 46 and 55 years of age. J Clin Endocrinol Metab 73:533–540

48. Licata AA, Jones-Gall DJ (1992) Effect of supplemental calcium on serum and urinary calcium in osteoporotic patients. J Am Coll Nutr 11:164–167

49. Hedlund LR, Gallagher JC (1989) Increased incidences of fractures in osteo-porosis patients treated with sodium fluoride. J Bone Miner Res 4:223–225

50. Pak YC, Sakhaee K, Adams-Huet B, Piziak V, Peterson RD, Poindexter JR (1995) Treatment of postmenopausal osteoporosis with slow-release sodium fluoride. Final report of a randomized controlled trial. Ann Intern Med 123:401–408

51. Jones G, Nguyen T, Sambrook PN, Eisman JA (1995) Thiazide diuretics and fractures: can meta-analysis help? J Bone Miner Res 10:106–111

52. LaCroix AZ, Wienpahl J, White LR et al (1990) Thiazide diuretic agents and the incidence of hip fracture. N Engl J Med 322:286–290

53. Peh CA, Horowitz M, Wishart JM, Need AG, Morris HA, Nordin BEC (1993) The effect of chlorothiazide on bone-related biochemical variables in nor-mal post-menopausal women. J Am Geriatr Soc 41:513–516

54. Sowers MR, Clark MK, Jannausch ML, Wallace RB (1993) Body size, estogen use and thiazide diuretic use affect 5-year radial bone loss in postmenopausal women. Osteoporosis Int 3:314–321
55. Martin BJ, Milligan K (1987) Diuretic associated hypomagnesemia in the elderly. Arch Intern Med 147:1768–1771
56. Van der Wielen RPJ, Lowik MRH, van den Berg H, de Groot L, Haller J, Moreiras O, van Staveren WA (1995) Serum vitamin D concentrations among elderly people in Europe. Lancet 346:207–210
57. Chapuy MC, Schott AM, Garnero P, Hans D, Delmas PD, Meunier PJ, Epidos Study Group (1996) Healthy elderly French women living at home have secondary hyperparathyroidism and high bone turnover in winter. J Clin Endocrinol Metab 81:1129–1133

2 Epidemiology of Osteoporosis

P. D. Ross

Introduction

Fractures related to osteoporosis affect more than half of women and about one-third of men in the United States during their lifetimes, making it one of the most prevalent chronic health conditions among the elderly. Many persons currently have low bone density and are at risk but have not yet experienced fractures. This chapter reviews how common osteoporosis is, based on two criteria (low bone density and frequency of fractures), and also reviews the extent of health and economic impacts.

Osteoporosis has been defined by the 1990 Consensus Development Panel as a "disease characterized by low bone mass and microarchitectural deterioration of bone tissue, leading to enhanced bone fragility and a consequent increase in fracture risk" [1]. This is a useful concept, but an operational definition is required for clinical use. Some have argued that a history of nonviolent fracture should be required for diagnosis. However, this would be comparable to requiring a history of stroke for diagnosing hypertension. Other proposed definitions have been based on bone mineral density (BMD) measurements alone. The rationale for this is that a woman with low BMD has a high risk of fractures – while she may have no fractures one day, she could easily have a nonviolent fracture the next day. Relatively few hypertensive patients have had strokes at any given point in time. Similarly, only a small proportion of patients at risk have already had nonviolent fractures. Measurements of BMD can identify patients at risk before fractures have occurred and can also monitor disease progression and treatment efficacy.

The World Health Organization has defined three categories, recognizing that low bone density and a history of previous fractures both contribute to increased risk of future fractures [2–6]:

- Low bone mass, or osteopenia, defined as BMD values between 1.0 and 2.5 SD below the mean for young healthy adults (aged 30–40 years). Persons with osteopenia currently have a moderate risk of fractures but deserve watchful monitoring and possibly treatment to ensure that subsequent bone loss does not increase their risk dramatically.
- Osteoporosis, defined as BMD values more than 2.5 SD below the mean for young adults. These people have not yet had fractures, but are already at high risk, warranting immediate attention.

- Severe (or established) osteoporosis, with low BMD (more than 2.5 SD below the mean for young adults) plus history of nonviolent fracture. These patients require treatments designed to increase bone density and prevent subsequent loss, to reduce their already high risk of fractures.

These categories are somewhat misleading in that fracture risk is a continuum. Fracture probability increases approximately exponentially with declining levels of bone density. Thus persons whose bone density is 4.1 SD below the mean for young adults have a much higher risk than those who are 2.6 SD below the mean, even though both are considered to have severe osteoporosis on the basis of the above definition. Likewise, patients with three preexisting vertebral fractures have a much higher risk than others with single fractures, who are in turn at greater risk than persons without any fractures [3–6]. Furthermore, osteoporosis is multifactorial; there are a multitude of other risk factors which contribute to fracture risk independently of bone density. Nevertheless, the WHO criteria provide a simple, useful tool for characterizing the presence and severity of this disease. Therefore the frequency of low bone density and fractures are discussed below because both are components of the WHO definition, and both contribute independently to fracture risk.

Skeletal Development and Aging

Skeletal Development

Skeletal development, which begins in utero and continues past the age of 20 years, plays an important role in the later risk of osteoporosis [7–9]. Skeletal size and mass both increase during development but at differing rates depending on gen-

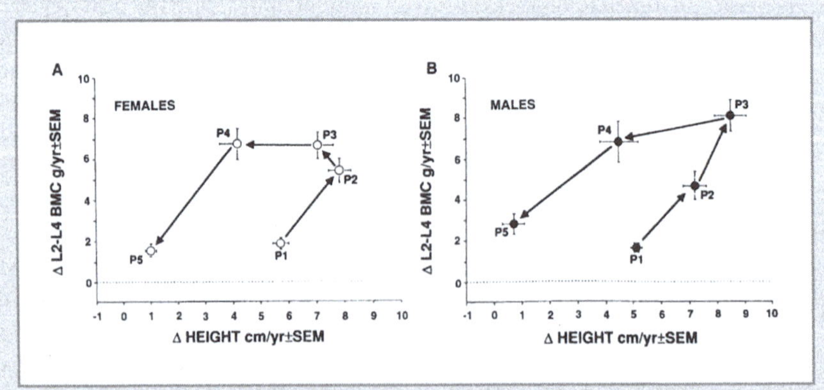

Fig. 2-1 Annual changes in bone mass (L2–4 bone mineral content, *BMC*) plotted against concomitant changes in stature (height), according to pubertal stages. *Each symbol*, mean ± SEM of the differences. Note that relatively large increases in height occur during Tanner stage P1 with little coincident increase in BMD, causing bone mass to be dispersed over a larger skeletal area. (From [150] with permission)

der, age, skeletal site, and pubertal stage [9, 10]. Girls experience greater annual increases in spine bone mass and density than boys between the ages of 10 and 13 years, but annual increases at the spine and femur are greater among boys after the age of 14 [11]. During Tanner pubertal stage P1 there is a rapid increase in stature, but little concomitant increase in bone mass (Fig. 2-1). This dispersion and redistribution of bone mineral over a larger skeleton may partly explain the transient increase in fracture incidence during childhood [12]. Consequently stature and bone mass both increase during Tanner stages P2–P4. In stage P5 there is little increase in stature, but bone mass continues to increase.

After the skeleton has ceased growing in size externally (approximately age 18 years), bone density continues to increase during a period of "consolidation," reaching a plateau during midlife [13–15]. Attainment of maximal skeletal mass helps to protect against fractures later in life by providing additional skeletal reserves to limit the effects of subsequent bone loss. Heredity, diet, and physical activity are recognized as important determinants of peak skeletal mass [10, 15–22].

Prevalence of Low Bone Density

Some studies have reported that bone density is stable at some skeletal sites prior to menopause, whereas others have reported declines among healthy premenopausal women that are accentuated by ovulatory disturbances [14, 23–28]. However, the rate of decline is most rapid (approximately 2%–3% per year) soon after menopause in women [14, 24, 27, 29, 30]. The rate of bone loss gradually slows to approximately 1%–2% per year within about 5 years after the menopause, but bone loss continues throughout the remainder of life [23, 24, 31–33]. Among men bone loss begins by at least age 60, and continues through the remainder of life at a rate approximately half that of women. Some evidence suggests that the rate of loss may increase after age 70 for both men and women, possibly due to declining physical activity, worsening health, or other factors [31, 34–37].

There is a wide variation in bone density between individuals, corresponding to differences in fracture risk of at least 10–15 times at a given age [38]. Wide variations in bone loss rates also exist between individuals [31, 32, 39]. Some people may have stable bone density over a 10-year period, whereas others can lose 25% or more of their bone mass during the same period of time. During an average lifetime bone density declines by more than 50% in women, and more than 30% in men [40]. Thus bone loss rate and baseline bone density both contribute to fracture risk, resulting in very large differences in risk between individuals when the entire age range is considered [38, 41, 42].

Using the WHO criterion, only 0.6% would be classified as having osteoporosis. However, approximately 15% of young women would be classified with osteopenia (between 1.0 and 2.5 SD below the mean for ages 30–40). The typical menopause-related bone loss causes many of these women to sink into the high risk osteoporotic category if untreated. Bone density declines at all skeletal sites after menopause (Fig. 2-2) [31, 43]. However, the apparent rate of loss is less at the spine than other sites after age 65 because of spine bone density measurement errors related to arthritic changes and soft-tissue calcification [43, 44]. The progressive loss of bone density with age results in large proportions of elderly women with osteoporosis and associated fractures (Fig. 2-3). Surveys indicate that almost a third of all women ages 60–70 in the United States currently have osteoporosis (more than 2.5 SD below the young adult mean with or without fractures), and that most of the remaining women have osteopenia; only one out of nine have "normal" bone density. After age 80 about 70% of women have osteoporosis [2, 45–47]. Hopefully these numbers will decrease if a sufficient number of women receive treatment. In the meantime there are approximately 16.8 million women in the United States with osteopenia (54% of all postmenopausal white women), and another 9.4 million have osteoporosis. More than half of those with osteoporosis have already had fractures.

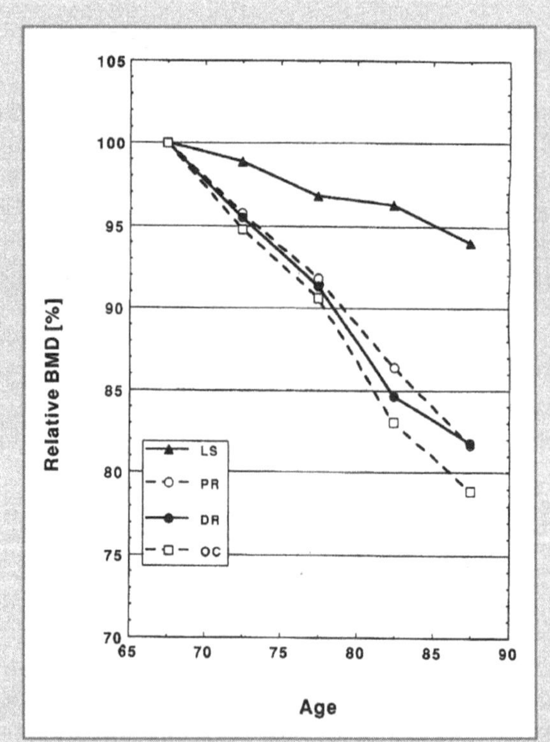

Fig. 2-2 Declines in bone density at the lumbar spine (LS), proximal radius (PR), distal radius (DR), and calcaneus (os calcis, OC) among women older than 65 years. Note that the spine exhibits less decrease with age than peripheral sites because arthritis and soft-tissue calcification cause an artifactual increase in apparent bone density among many women in this age range. (From [43] with permission)

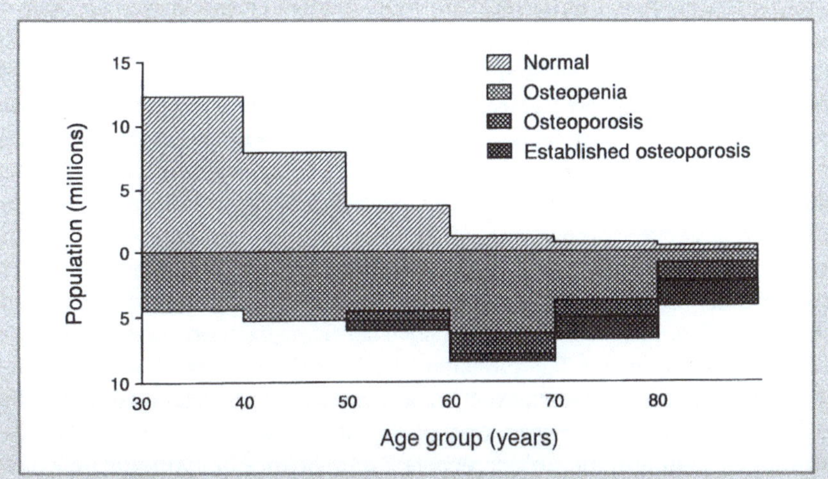

Fig. 2-3 Estimated skeletal status of United States white women in 1990, by age group. Osteopenia is bone density of the hip, spine, or distal forearm more than 1.0 but less than 2.5 SD below the young normal mean (ages 30–40). Osteoporosis is bone density at one or more of these sites more than 2.5 SD below the young adult mean (ages 30–40) and, when linked with a history of fracture, is deemed established osteoporosis. Above 0, the number of women with normal BMD for each age group; below 0, the number of women in the three categories of osteopenia and osteoporosis in proportion to the corresponding shaded regions. (From [46], with permission)

Fracture Incidence and Prevalence

Most fractures among the elderly are caused by mild to moderate trauma, such as a fall from standing height or less. Such nonviolent forces account for approximately 90% of hip and Colles' fractures among the elderly [48, 49].

Vertebral Fractures

The incidence of vertebral fractures is greater than any other skeletal site [50]. Some studies have examined the incidence of diagnosed vertebral fractures, usually based on medical record surveillance [51–53]. Most vertebral fractures (85%) identified in these surveys were symptomatic; the remaining 15% were identified serendipitously during workup for other reasons. Other studies have used radiographic surveillance of population-based samples to ensure that all cases are identified. Whereas hip and other nonspine fractures are associated with severe pain and are usually diagnosed immediately, only about one-third of persons with radiographically evident vertebral fractures have been diagnosed and are aware of them [52–54]. Many vertebral fractures are not diagnosed because symptoms are often mild (or absent), or because the absence of a specific injury leads the patient (or the physician) to suspect back strain instead.

There have been few radiographic surveys of fracture incidence because they require serial radiographs of large numbers of persons over a period of years.

Typical radiographic criteria for identifying incident fractures are decreases in measured vertebral height of more than 15%–20% on serial radiographs; the 20% criterion identifies approximately 80% of the fractures identified using the 15% criterion [3, 5, 55, 56]. Vertebral fracture incidence is essentially zero prior to age 50 and increases approximately exponentially with age thereafter [50, 57, 58]. Extrapolating from the observed prevalence of vertebral fractures in a cross-sectional study of women in Minnesota, calculated incidence rates ranged from about 0.5% per year at ages 55–59 to more than 3% per year above age 85 [51]. The incidence of clinically diagnosed vertebral fractures in the same population was approximately one-third that of radiographically detected fratures [53]. Two longitudinal radiographic surveys [5, 56] have confirmed the rates estimated from the prevalence survey [51]. The annual incidence of new vertebral fractures among 503 women, diagnosed as vertebral height decreases of more than 20% on serial radiographs, was 0.4% between ages 65–69, and 1.9% after age 75 [5]. Another longitudinal radiographic survey reported an incidence of approximately 0.2% per year at age 60, increasing more than 15 times to approximately 3.3% per year by age 85 [56], based on a diagnostic criterion of vertebral height decreases more than 15% on serial radiographs.

Vertebral size and shape vary by location within the spine as well as by gender, geographic locality, and race [52, 59, 60]. Furthermore, the proposed definitions for diagnosing prevalent fractures overlap with the normal range, making it difficult to reliably diagnose prevalent fractures from a single radiograph. Incident fractures are easier to standardize because they do not rely on population distributions but are instead based on changes within the individual. Moreover, incident fractures are known to be of recent origin, whereas prevalent vertebral deformities might have been caused by trauma in the remote past, other disease conditions, or simply genetic variants, rather than osteoporotic fractures. Numerous proposed definitions as well as differences in population sampling have led to considerable differences in the reported prevalence [52]. Recognizing these limitations, prevalence surveys may still provide a useful picture of the burden of disease. The prevalence of vertebral fractures has been as high as 50% among women over age 80 in some reports. Furthermore, half of all women with vertebral fractures have multiple deformities, presumably because the incidence rate after age 65 is relatively high, and because existing vertebral deformities dramatically increase the risk of additional fractures [3–5, 52, 58, 61]. Surveys may underestimate the true prevalence because institutionalized persons and those with poor health are less likely to participate.

Hip Fractures

As with spine fractures, there is an approximately exponential increase in hip fracture incidence with age (Fig. 2-4) [62–65]. Among women in the United States the incidence increases from about 0.2% per year (2 cases for every 1000 patients followed for a single year) at age 65 to about 3% per year (30 cases per 1000 patient

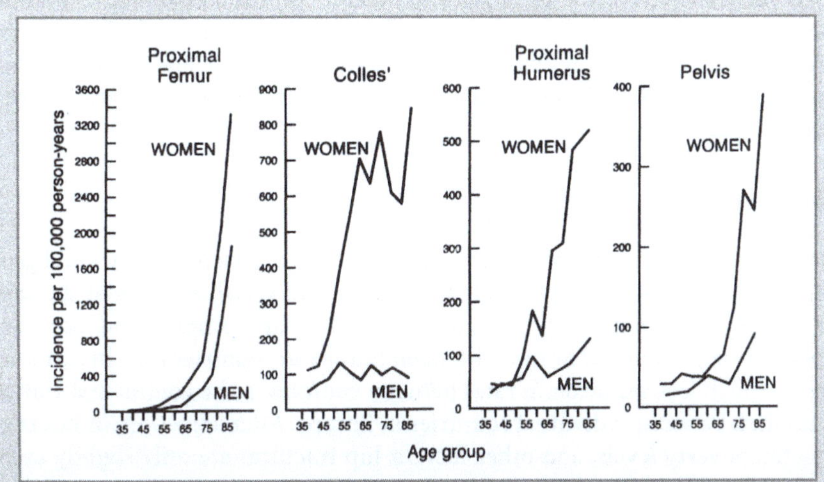

Fig. 2-4 Age- and sex-specific incidence rates among residents of Rochester, Minn., for four age-related fracture sites. Note that the vertical scale varies for each fracture site. (Reprinted by permission of Wiley-Liss, from [66]

years) above age 85 [65, 66]. The ratio of trochanteric to femoral neck fractures is approximately 1.0 but varies somewhat with age, gender, and other factors [67]. In 1986 the total number of hip fractures attributed to osteoporosis in the United States was approximately 238 000. This number is projected to double, or possibly triple, during the next 50 years as a result of increasing life expectancy and shifting of the age distribution in the United States and Europe, whereas it is projected to increase 6 to 12 times in other parts of the world [68–70].

A small increase in life expectancy results in a significant increase in hip fracture incidence, because the risk increases exponentially with age. It is a sobering fact that more than half of postmenopausal women live beyond age 80 and many age 90. As a result more than half (approximately 55%) of all hip fractures in the United States occur after age 80 and one-third after age 85 [71]. Although the incidence in women is only twice that in men of the same age, 80% of hip fractures in the United States occur among women because of their longer life expectancy [72].

Other Fractures

Almost all types of fractures among the elderly are associated with low bone density [73,74]. The incidence of most fractures increases progressively with age after menopause in women, but the rate of increase is greater for some skeletal sites than for others (Fig. 2-4) [75]. Although the incidence of wrist fractures increases rapidly among women after menopause, the rate levels off at approximately 0.7% per year after age 60 (Fig. 2-4) [50, 62, 66, 76, 77]. One hypothesis for this is that persons tend to fall down or backward as they become older, rather than forward on an outstretched hand [78]. Riggs and Melton [79] estimated that 1.2 million osteoporotic fractures occur each year in the United States, but this figure probably underestimates the actual total because only hip, wrist, and vertebral fractures were counted, and the incidence of vertebral fractures was based on the first occurrence only.

Secular Trends

There is a large range of hip fracture incidence rates between countries and geographic regions, suggesting that environmental and racial factors may account for a large proportion of hip fractures [72, 80, 81]. For example, incidence rates appear to vary sevenfold or more between European countries [81]. In contrast, there is much less variation in rates between counties in the continental United States than between individual countries in Europe. After adjusting for hours of sunlight, poverty levels, and other factors, hip fractures are only slightly more common (about 10%–20% higher) in the southern than in the northern United States [82]. Numerous studies have reported that age-specific hip fracture incidence rates among both men and women have increased by two to three times or more over time during the previous 10–50 years, again suggesting that environmental (nongenetic) factors play an important role. Similar trends have been reported for fractures at other skeletal sites, including the spine, distal radius, humerus, and ankle [83, 84]. These findings have been summarized elsewhere [72, 85]. In some studies the age-adjusted incidence appears to be stable, or decreasing [85–87].

Lifetime Risk

Cummings et al. [88] calculated that on average a 50-year-old woman has a 16% risk of experiencing a hip fracture, a 15% risk of Colles' fracture, and a 32% risk of vertebral fracture during her remaining lifetime. Similar results were reported by Lauritzen et al. [86], who also estimated that the lifetime risk of humeral fractures was 8% for a postmenopausal woman. Thus the risk of fractures is much greater than the lifetime risk of approximately 9% for breast cancer and 3% for endometrial cancer for a 50-year-old white woman in the United States [88]. Among those who live to age 90 the risk of hip fracture is about twice as high: 32% for women, and 17% for men [89].

Fractures can occur at a variety of sites, increasing the probability beyond those given above for individual sites. For example, approximately 40% of women experience one or more hip, wrist, or clinically diagnosed vertebral fractures during their lifetimes. The corresponding proportion of men who experience one or more of these fracture types is about 13% [47, 90]. The proportion of persons affected by osteoporotic fractures is probably higher than 50% for women and perhaps 30% for men because only about one-third of all vertebral fractures are diagnosed clinically, and because these hip, wrist, and spine fractures account for little more than one-third of all fractures associated with osteoporosis [73]. Furthermore, these figures do not reflect the total burden of fractures because many persons experience multiple fractures.

Mortality and Morbidity

Mortality

Increased mortality has been reported for patients with hip or vertebral fractures and for those with low bone density. Compared to persons of similar age without hip fractures, both men and women are two to five times more likely to die during the first 6–12 months after a hip fracture (Table 2-1) [63, 64, 71, 91, 92]. It is not certain to what extent the increased mortality is related to the fracture and complications, as opposed to preexisting poor health. One study reported that the most important predictors of mortality are serious concomitant illness and marked delirium at admission [92]. The lifetime risk of dying from a hip fracture is 2.8% for white women in the United States [88]. For comparison, the lifetime risk of dying from other causes are 31% for coronary heart disease, 2.8% for breast cancer, and 0.7% for endometrial cancer. However, these are average figures, and some individuals may have a greater risk of death from hip fracture than from heart disease if they have many risk factors for hip fracture, and few for heart disease.

Increased mortality rates have been reported for persons with vertebral fractures but not wrist fractures [91, 93]. Whereas the increased mortality associated with hip fractures is limited to the initial 12 months postfracture, excess mortality after vertebral fractures increased progressively over the 5 years for which data were available [91]. As with hip fractures, it is uncertain whether decreased survival among vertebral fracture cases is due to the fracture, to comorbid conditions, or somehow related to low bone density. Both men and women with low bone density have higher mortality than those with greater bone density. The increased risk of death appears to be related to an increased rate of stroke rather

Tabelle 2-1 Mortality rates (%/year) among hip fracture cases and people without hip fractures (data from United States Congress Office of Technology Assessment [71])

Age group	All patients		Male		Female	
	Nonfracture	Hip fracture	Nonfracture	Hip fracture	Nonfracture	Hip fracture
50–64	1%	NA	2%	NA	1%	7%
65–74	3%	14%	4%	22%	2%	10%
75–84	6%	21%	8%	34%	5%	17%
85+	16%	31%	18%	48%	14%	28%

NA= Not available.

than a consequence of fractures [94–96]. In one study mortality rate increased 20%, and risk of death from stroke increased 70% with each standard deviation decrease in bone density. These associations remained after adjusting for known risk factors for stroke (age, smoking, hypertension, prior stroke, diabetes, and hormone replacement therapy). One possibility is that both low BMD and risk of stroke are related to declines in health.

Economic Costs and Morbidity

It has been said that osteoporosis is a disease that does not usually kill, but rather a disease that one must live with – often for many years. Although mortality is increased, as noted above, osteoporosis is primarily a chronic condition. Physical impairment and declines in quality of life have been documented extensively for hip and spine fractures. Morbidity is usually greatest for hip fractures but can also be substantial for spine and other fractures as well. The cumulative morbidity due to fractures other than the hip may exceed that due to hip fractures alone because hip fractures represent less than 10% of all fractures, and many nonhip fractures occur earlier in life.

Hospitalization, Nursing Home Stays, and Health Care Costs.
Hip fracture cases incur large medical costs because almost all cases are hospitalized [71, 97, 98]. In Europe, the average length of hospitalization is approximately 20–30 days, whereas it has decreased to about 13 days in the United States during the past 15 years [92, 97, 99–101]. In the United States about half of hip fracture patients are discharged to a nursing home or other institution [92]. In one study [92] more than one-third of all hip fracture patients were hospitalized again after discharge, and the reason for the second hospitalization appeared to be related to the hip fracture in about half of these cases.

Hip fractures account for more than 250 000 hospitalizations, 3.4 million hospital bed-days, 60 000 admissions to nursing homes, and more than 7 million days of restricted activity each year in the United States [98, 102, 103]. Approximately 25% of hip fracture cases admitted to nursing homes stay longer than 6 months, and another 41% stay between 1 and 6 months [71]. However, hip fractures accounted for only 10% of the 2.3 million outpatient services and only about half of the hospitalizations related to osteoporosis in 1986 [102]. Approximately one-third of all vertebral fractures lead to physician visits, 8% to hospitalization, and 2% to nursing care; the number of hospitalizations for vertebral fractures is about half that for hip fractures [80, 149]. Thus both hip and other osteoporotic fractures represent a substantial public health burden.

The economic costs associated with osteoporotic fractures are enormous. Approximately half of the health care costs for hip fracture patients are attributable to nursing homes [71, 102]. Analysis of computerized national health data has yielded estimated annual costs of $2.8 billion for inpatient care, $2.1 billion for nursing home care, and $0.2 billion for outpatient care for all types of fractures (including hip) and complications related to osteoporosis in the United States for 1986 [102]. Other studies of United States data have estimated annual costs of $6–20 billion for all fractures combined, and $4.5 billion for spine, hip, and vertebral fractures alone [90, 103–105].

Pain, Physical Function, and Psychosocial Declines.
Hip fracture patients experience major declines in physical function [106–110]. One prospective study reported that among those able to function at baseline, 50% of cases were unable to walk independently 1 year after the fracture, and 87% were unable to climb stairs without assistance. Studies based on recall have found that 20%–60% are unable to perform certain activities after 6–12 months that they had been able to do prior to the fracture [106–110]. Most of the functional recovery occurs during the first 6 months after the fracture [108]. Predictors of poor recovery were older age, dementia, depression, postsurgical delirium, length of hospital stay, and rehospitalization [108, 109]. A long-term study of hip fracture patients found that 31% were bedridden and only 9% could walk outdoors by themselves 6 years after the fracture, whereas only 1.5% of the control group was bedridden and 55% of the controls could walk outdoors [111]. Pressure sores, urinary tract infections, and pneumonia also occur frequently among hip fracture cases [98, 112]. However, as many as 90% of hip fracture patients have preexisting comorbid conditions, and it is difficult to determine the extent to which health problems are directly attributable to the hip fracture itself [111, 112].

Numerous studies have also demonstrated physical and psychosocial declines as a result of vertebral fractures, the most frequent site of osteoporotic fractures. Vertebral fracture symptoms range widely in severity from mild to unbearable [51, 54, 113–130]. The crushing deformation typical of vertebral fractures would cause severe symptoms if it occurred at other skeletal sites. Indeed, acute pain is intolerable for up to one-third of clinically diagnosed patients, but approximately half of all radiologically evident fracture cases paradoxically do not report having had any pain [51, 54, 119, 122]. Reasons for the diversity in symptoms are not known, but may be related to the number, spinal location, and physical features of fractures. In one study, 40% of acute cases were initially misdiagnosed as sciatica or muscle strain, signalling a need for greater awareness among physicians and patients [119].

Chronic pain from vertebral fractures may persist for years [113, 126, 130]. Vertebral fractures also lead to decreased physical performance and permanent changes in appearance (kyphosis and stature loss) [115, 122, 123, 126, 127, 129, 131–145]. Some 60%–70% of symptomatic vertebral fracture cases with chronic pain reported problems with lifting, carrying, walking, housework, and shopping [145]. The risk of pain and physical impairment increase progressively with the number and severity of vertebral fractures (Table 2-2) [113, 125, 128, 132]. The odds of physical impairment are increased two to three times per vertebral fracture for fractures identified in radiographic population surveys, and three to four times per fracture for clinically diagnosed fractures (Table 2-3) [125, 132, 135]. Objective

Table 2-2 Proportion (%) of symptomatic women (n=2992) by number of vertebral fractures (data from Ettinger et al. [129]

	Number of severe fractures (vertebral height more than 4 SD below mean)			
Outcome	0	1	2	>2
Disability score greater than 6	4	7	14	27
Height loss more than 4 cm	23	43	67	81
Moderate/severe back pain	42	56	55	77

Table 2-3 Self-reported physical impairment associated with clinically diagnosed vertebral fractures (data from Greendale et al. [135])

Reported difficulty with	Odds ratio	95% Confidence Interval
Descending stairs	4.2	1.5–11.6
Lifting 10 lbs	3.4	1.2–9.5
Bending to floor	3.1	1.2–7.8
Walking a few blocks	2.7	1.0–7.4
Climbing stairs	2.2	0.7–6.7
Getting into/out of a car	2.1	0.8–5.6

measures of physical performance are also impaired. Objectively measured physical characteristics of vertebral fracture cases, relative to controls were [127]: 45% lower maximal trunk extension torque, 40% lower spinal range of motion, 33% longer time to walk 6 m, 22% shorter functional reach, 9 cm shorter stature, 2.2 times greater difficulty with activities. The mean age was 82 years; cases had an average of more than four vertebral fractures per patient.

Fractures other than the hip and spine also contribute to declines in physical function and quality of life. One study examined the impact of all fracture sites on physical function [135]. Women with fractures (which had occurred 7 years earlier on average) were two to six times more likely to report difficulty with activities such as climbing or descending stairs, reaching above the head, bending and lifting, walking, getting in or out of a car, cooking, shopping, putting on socks, and heavy housework. Moreover, these findings may underestimate associations because this sample represents community dwelling survivors; fracture cases with the worst outcomes may have been institutionalized or may have been unable or unwilling to participate. For wrist fracture cases physical function is poor or fair after 6 months for approximately half, and as many as 30% experience algodystrophy and increased risk of arthritis and neuropathy [146–148].

Declines in physical function lead to increased risk of falls and fear of falling, causing a downward spiral of further restrictions in activities and independence, and increased risk of institutionalization. In fact, Chrischilles et al. [149] calculated that fractures due to osteoporosis cause 6.7% of all women in the United States to become dependent in basic activities of daily living, and 7.8% to require long-term nursing home care for an average of 7.6 years; these outcomes were in addition to nursing care and lost independence expected for women of similar age without fractures.

Quality of life may be the most important outcome. Whereas some persons are able to adapt to physical challenges and maintain a positive attitude, the physical changes and chronic pain associated with osteoporotic fractures often lead to fears, anxiety, depression, loss of self-esteem, and declines in quality of life which may be just as important, or more important than measurable physical declines. People with osteoporosis appear to have serious declines in quality of life [128, 133, 144, 145]. Unfortunately, few studies to date have included controls for comparison, and the extent of decline relative to others of similar age is therefore uncertain.

Summary

Osteoporotic fractures affect a large segment of the population, and are projected to increase significantly as a result of increasing lifespan. The majority of elderly persons are already at high risk of fractures. Fractures cause serious acute and chronic declines in physical performance and physcial appearance, which all too often lead to physical dependence and impaired quality of life. Efforts to reduce fracture risk now will pay off in reduced health burdens from osteoporotic fractures in the future.

References

1. Consensus Development Conference (1991) Prophylaxis and treatment of osteoporosis. Am J Med 90:107–110
2. Kanis JA, Melton LJ III, Christiansen C, Johnston CC, Khaltev N (1994) The diagnosis of osteoporosis. J Bone Miner Res 9:1137–1141
3. Ross PD, Davis JW, Epstein RS, Wasnich RD (1991) Pre-existing fractures and bone mass predict vertebral fracture in women. Ann Intern Med 114:919–923
4. Ross PD, Genant HK, Davis JW, Miller P, Wasnich RD (1993) Predicting vertebral fracture incidence from prevalent fractures and bone density among non-black, osteoporotic women. Osteo Int 3:120–127
5. Black DM, Nevitt MC, Palermo L et al (1994) Prediction of new vertebral deformities (abstract). J Bone Miner Res 9:S135
6. Cummings SR, Nevitt MC, Browner WS et al (1995) Risk factors for hip fracture in white women. N Engl J Med 332:767–773
7. Hillman L (1996) Bone mineral acquisition in utero and during infancy and childhood. In: Marcus R, Feldman D, Kelsey J (eds) Osteoporosis. Academic, New York, pp 449–464
8. Recker RR, Davies KM, Hinders SM, Heaney RP, Stegman MR, Kimmel DB (1992) Bone gain in young adult women. JAMA 268:2403–2408

9.   Bonjour J-P, Rizzoli R (1996) Bone acquisition in adolescence. In: Marcus R, Feldman D, Kelsey J (eds) Osteoporosis. Academic, New York, pp 465–476

10. Lloyd T, Martel JK, Rollings N, Andon MB, Kulin H, Demers LM, Eggli DF, Kieselhorst K, Chinchilli VM (1996) The effect of calcium supplementation and Tanner stage on bone density and area in teenage women. Osteoporosis Int 6:276–283

11. Kröger H, Kotaniemi A, Kröger L, Alhava E (1993) Development of bone mass and bone density of the spine and femoral neck – a prospective study of 65 children and adolescents. Bone Miner 23:171–182

12. Hagino H, Yamamoto K, Teshima R, Kishimoto H, Nakamura T (1990) Fracture incidence and bone mineral density of the distal radius in Japanese children. Acta Orthop Trauma Surg 109:262–264

13. Teegarden D, Proux WR, Martin BR et al (1995) Peak bone mass in young women. J Bone Miner Res 10:711–716

14. Hagino H, Yamamoto K, Teshima R, Kishimoto H, Kagawa T (1992) Radial bone mineral changes in pre- and postmenopausal healthy Japanese women: cross-sectional and longitudinal studies. J Bone Miner Res 7:147–152

15. Parsons TJ, Prentice A, Smith EA, Cole TJ, Compston JE (1996) Bone mineral mass consolidation in young British adults. J Bone Miner Res 11(2):264–74

16. Turner JG, Gilchrist NL, Ayling EM et al (1992) Factors affecting bone mineral density in high school girls. N Z Med J 105:95–96

17. Cooper C, Cawley M, Bhalla A et al (1995) Childhood growth, physical activity, and peak bone mass in women. J Bone Miner Res 10(6):940–947

18. Ruiz JC, Mandel C, Garabedian M (1995) Influence of spontaneous calcium intake and physical exercise on the vertebral and femoral bone mineral density of children and adolescents. J Bone Miner Res 10:675–682

19. Slemenda CW, Miller JZ, Hui SL, Reister TK, Johnston CC Jr (1991) Role of physical activity in the development of skeletal mass in children. J Bone Miner Res 6:1227–1233

20. Kröger H, Heikkinen J, Laitinen K, Kotaniemi A (1992) Dual-energy X-ray absorptiometry in normal women: a cross-sectional study of 717 Finnish volunteers. Osteo Int 2:135–140

21. Kröger H, Kotaniemi A, Vainia P, Alhava E (1992) Bone density of the spine and femur in children by dual-energy X-ray absorptiometry. Bone Miner 17:75–85

22. Snow CM, Shaw JM, Matkin CC (1996) Physical activity and risk for osteoporosis. In: Marcus R, Feldman D, Kelsey J (eds) Osteoporosis. Academic, New York, pp 511–528

23. Prior JC, Vigna YM, Schechter MT, Burgess AE (1990) Spinal bone loss and ovulatory disturbances. N Engl J Med 323:1221–1227

24. Sowers MR, Clark MK, Hollis B, Wallace RB, Jannausch M (1992) Radial bone mineral density in pre- and postmenopausal women: a prospective study of rates and risk factors for loss. J Bone Miner Res 7:647–657

25. Prior JC, Vigna YM, Barr SI, Kennedy S, Schulzer M, Li DKB (1996) Ovula-

tory premenopausal women lose cancellous spinal bone: a five year prospective study. Bone 18(3):261–267

26. Riggs BL, Wahner HW, Melton LJ III, Richelson LS, Judd HL, Offord KP (1986) Rates of bone loss in the appendicular and axial skeletons of women: evidence of substantial vertebral loss before menopause. J Clin Invest 77:1487– 1491

27. Hui SL, Evans R, Johnston CC, Slemenda CW, Peacock M (1996) Patterns of growth and loss of BMD at the spine and hip in white females (abstract). J Bone Miner Res 11 [Suppl 1]:S104

28. Citron JT, Ettinger B, Genant HK (1995) Spinal bone mineral loss in estrogen-replete, calcium-replete premenopausal women. Osteoporosis Int 5:228–233

29. Elders PJM, Netelenbos JC, Lips P, van Ginkel FC, van der Stelt PF (1988) Accelerated vertebral bone loss in relation to the menopause: a cross-sectional study on lumbar bone density in 286 women of 46 to 55 years of age. Bone Miner 5:11–19

30. Nilas L, Christiansen C (1988) Rates of bone loss in normal women: evidence of accelerated trabecular bone loss after the menopause. Eur J Clin Invest 18:529–534

31. Davis JW, Ross PD, Wasnich RD, MacLean CJ, Vogel JM (1989) Comparison of cross-sectional and longitudinal measurements of age-related changes in bone mass. J Bone Min Res 4:351–357

32. Harris S, Dawson-Hughes B (1992) Rates of change in bone mineral density of the spine, heel, femoral neck and radius in healthy postmenopausal women. Bone Miner 17:87–95

33. Hansen MA, Overgaard K, Christiansen C (1995) Spontaneous post-menopausal bone loss in different skeletal areas – followed up for 15 years. J Bone Miner Res 10:205–210

34. Davis JW, Ross PD, Vogel JM, Wasnich RD (1991) Age-related changes in bone mass among Japanese-American men. Bone Miner 15:227–236

35. Ensrud KE, Palermo L, Black D et al (1994) Hip bone loss increases with advancing age: longitudinal results from the Study of Osteoporotic Fractures (abstract). J Bone Miner Res 9 [Suppl 1]:S153

36. Greenspan SL, Maitland LA, Myers ER, Krasnow MB, Kido TH (1994) Femoral bone loss progresses with age: a longitudinal study in women over age 65. J Bone Miner Res 9:1959–1965

37. Hannan MT, Kiel DP, Mercier CE, Anderson JJ, Felson DT (1994) Longitudinal bone mineral density (BMD) change in elderly men and women: the Framingham Osteoporosis Study (abstract). J Bone Miner Res 9 [Suppl 1]:S153

38. Ross PD (1994) Risk factors for fracture. In: Cooper C, Reeve J (eds) Spine. State of the art reviews: vertebral osteoporosis, vol 8. Hanley and Belfus, Philadelphia, pp 91–110

39. Ross PD, He Y-F, Davis JW, Epstein RS, Wasnich RD (1994) Normal ranges for bone loss rates. Bone Miner 26:169–180

40. Riggs BL, Wahner HW, Seeman E, Offord KP, Dunn WL, Mazess RB, Johnson KA, Melton LJ III (1982) Changes in bone mineral density of the proximal femur and spine with aging: differences between the postmenopausal and senile osteoporosis syndromes. J Clin Invest 70:716–723

41. Riis BJ, Hansen MA, Jensen AM, Overgaard K, Christiansen C (1996) Low bone mass and fast rate of bone loss at menopause: equal risk factors for future fracture: a 15-year follow-up study. Bone 19(1):9–12

42. Sklarin PM, Cummings SR, Nevitt MC, Ensrud K, Black DM (1996) Bone loss is an independent predictor of hip fracture in elderly women with low bone mass. Presented at the International Congress of Endocrinology, June 1996

43. Steiger P, Cummings SR, Black DM, Spencer NE, Genant HK (1992) Age-related decrements in bone mineral density in women over 65. J Bone Miner Res 7:625–632

44. Ross PD, Wasnich RD, Vogel JM (1988) Detection of pre-fracture spinal osteoporosis using bone mineral absorptiometry. J Bone Miner Res 3(1):1–11

45. Looker AC, Johnston CC Jr, Wahner HW et al (1995) Prevalence of low femoral bone density in older women from NHANES III. J Bone Miner Res 10:796–802

46. Melton LJ III (1995) How many women have osteoporosis now? J Bone Miner Res 10:175–177

47. Melton LJ, Chrischilles EA, Cooper C, Lane AW, Riggs BL (1992) How many women have osteoporosis? J Bone Miner Res 7:1005–1010

48. Owen RA, Melton LJ III, Johnson KA, Ilstrup DM, Riggs BL (1982) Incidence of Colles' fracture in a North American community. Am J Public Health 72:605–607

49. Melton LJ III, Ilstrup DM, Riggs BL, Beckenbaugh RD (1982) Fifty-year trend in hip fracture incidence. Clin Orthop 162:144–149

50. Melton LJ III, Cummings SR (1987) Heterogeneity of age-related fractures: implications for epidemiology. Bone Miner 2:321–331

51. Melton LJ III, Kan SH, Frye MA, Wahner HW, O'Fallon WM, Riggs BL (1989) Epidemiology of vertebral fractures in women. Am J Epidemiol 129:1000–1011

52. Cooper C (1994) Epidemiology of vertebral fractures in western populations. In: Cooper C, Reeve J (eds) Spine. State of the art reviews: vertebral osteoporosis, vol 8. Hanley and Belfus, Philadelphia, pp 1–21

53. Cooper C, Atkinson EJ, O'Fallon WM, Melton LJ III (1992) Incidence of clinically diagnosed vertebral fractures: a population-based study in Rochester, Minnesota, 1985–1989. J Bone Miner Res 7:221–227

54. Ross PD, Davis JW, Epstein RS, Wasnich RD (1994) Pain and disability associated with new vertebral fractures and other spinal conditions. J Clin Epidemiol 47:231–239

55. Cummings SR, Melton LJ III, Felsenberg D et al (1995) Report: assessing vertebral fractures. J Bone Miner Res 10:518–523

56. Ross PD, Huang C, Davis JW et al (1995) Predicting vertebral deformity

using bone densitometry at various skeletal sites and calcaneus ultrasound. Bone 16:325–332

57. Ross PD, Wasnich RD, Vogel JM (1988) Detection of pre-fracture spinal osteoporosis using bone mineral absorptiometry. J Bone Miner Res 3:1–11

58. Ross PD, Fujiwara S, Huang C et al (1995) Japanese women in Hiroshima have greater vertebral fracture prevalence than Caucasians or Japanese-Americans in the US. Int J Epidemiol 24(6):1171–1177

59. Ross PD, Wasnich RD, Davis JW, Vogel JM (1991) Vertebral dimension differences between Caucasian populations, and between Caucasians and Japanese. Bone 12:107–112

60. O'Neill TW, Varlow J, Felsenberg D et al (1994) Variation in vertebral height ratios in population studies. J Bone Miner Res 9:1895–1907

61. Kiel DP, Hannan MT, Genant HK, Felson DT (1994) Prevalence and incidence of vertebral fractures in the elderly: initial results from the Framingham Study (abstract). J Bone Miner Res 9 [Suppl 1]:S129

62. Melton LJ III, Riggs BL (1985) Risk factors for injury after a fall. Clin Geriatr Med 1(3):525–539

63. Fisher ES, Baron JA, Malenka DJ et al (1991) Hip fracture incidence and mortality in New England. Epidemiology 2:116–122

64. Gallagher JC, Melton LJ III, Riggs BL, Bergstrath E (1980) Epidemiology of fractures of the proximal femur in Rochester, Minnesota. Clin Orthopaed Relat Res 150:163–171

65. Farmer ME, White LR, Brody JA, Bailey KR (1984) Race and sex differences in hip fracture incidence. Am J Publ Health 74:1374–1380

66. Melton LJ III (1993) Epidemiology of age-related fractures. In: Avioli LV (ed) The osteoporotic syndrome. Detection, prevention, and treatment, 3rd edn. Wiley-Liss, New York, pp 17–38

67. Karagas MR, Lu-Yao GL, Barrett JA, Beach ML, Baron JA (1996) Heterogeneity of hip fracture: age, race, sex, and geographic patterns of femoral neck and trochanter fractures among the US elderly. Am J Epidemiol 143:677–682

68. Schneider EL, Guralnik JM (1990) The ageing of America: impact on health care costs. JAMA 263:2335–2340

69. Cummings SR, Rubin SM, Black D (1990) The future of hip fractures in the United States: numbers, costs, and potential effects of postmenopausal estrogen. Clin Orthop 252:163–166

70. Cooper C, Campion G, Melton LJ III (1992) Hip fractures in the elderly: a world-wide projection. Osteoporosis Int 2:285–289

71. US Congress, Office of Technology Assessment (1994) Hip fracture outcomes in people age fifty and over – background paper, OTA-BP-H-120. US Government Printing Office, Washington DC

72. Cooper C, Melton LJ III (1996) Magnitude and impact of osteoporotic fractures. In: Marcus R, Feldman D, Kelsey J (eds) Osteoporosis. Academic, San Diego, pp 419–434

73. Seeley DG, Browner WS, Nevitt MC, Genant HK, Scott JC, Cummings SR

(1991) Which fractures are associated with low appendicular bone mass in elderly women? Ann Intern Med 115:837–842

74. Seeley DG, Browner WS, Nevitt MC, Genant HK, Cummings SR (1995) Almost all fractures are osteoporotic (abstract). J Bone Miner Res 10 [Suppl 1]:S468

75. Kanis JA, Pitt FA (1992) Epidemiology of osteoporosis. Bone 13:S7–S15

76. Hayes WC, Myers ER, Morris JN, Gerhart TN, Yett HS, Lipsitz LA (1993) Impact near the hip dominates fracture risk in elderly nursing home residents who fall. Calcif Tissue Int 52:192–198

77. Sølgaard S, Petersen VS (1985) Epidemiology of distal radius fractures. Acta Orthop Scand 56:391–393

78. Nevitt MC, Cummings SR (1993) Type of fall and risk of hip and wrist fractures: the study of osteoporotic fractures. The Study of Osteoporotic Fractures Research Group. J Am Geriatr Soc 41:1226–1234

79. Riggs BL, Melton LJ (1986) Involutional osteoporosis. N Engl J Med 314:1676– 1686

80. Jacobsen SJ, Cooper C, Gottlieb MS, Goldberg J, Yahnke DP, Melton LJ III (1992) Hospitalization with vertebral fracture among the aged: a national population-based study, 1986–1989. Epidemiology 3:515–518

81. Johnell O, Gullberg B, Allander E, Kanis JA, the MEDOS Study Group (1992) The apparent incidence of hip fracture in Europe: a study of national register sources. Osteoporosis Int 2:298–302

82. Jacobsen SJ, Goldberg J, Miles TP, Brody JA, Stiers W, Rimm AA (1990) Regional variation in the incidence of hip fracture: US white women aged 65 years and older. JAMA 264:500–502

83. Obrant KJ, Bengner U, Johnell O, Nilsson BE, Sernbo I (1989) Increasing age-adjusted risk of fragility fractures. Calcif Tissue Int 44:157–167

84. Cooper C, Atkinson EJ, Kotowicz M, O'Fallon WM, Melton LJ III (1992) Secular trends in the incidence of postmenopausal osteoporosis. Calcif Tissue Int 51:100–104

85. Melton LJ III, O'Fallon WM, Riggs BL (1987) Secular trends in the incidence of hip fractures. Calcif Tissue Int 41:57–64

86. Lauritzen JB, Schwarz P, Lund B, McNair P, Transbol I (1993) Changing incidence and residual lifetime risk of common osteoporosis-related fractures. Osteoporosis Int 3:127–132

87. Spector TD, Cooper C, Lewis AF (1990) Trends in admissions for hip fracture in England and Wales, 1968–85. BMJ 300:1173–1174

88. Cummings SR, Black DM, Rubin SM (1989) Lifetime risks of hip, Colles', or vertebral fracture and coronary heart disease among white postmenopausal women. Arch Intern Med 149:2445–2448

89. Grisso JA, Chiu GY, Maislin G, Steinmann WC, Portale J (1991) Risk factors for hip fractures in men: a preliminary study. J Bone Miner Res 6:865–868

90. Chrischilles EA, Shireman T, Wallace R (1994) Costs and health effects of osteoporotic fractures. Bone 15:377–386

91. Cooper C, Atkinson EJ, Jacobsen SJ, O'Fallon WM, Melton LJ III (1993) Population-based study of survival after osteoporotic fractures. Am J Epidemiol 137:1001–1005

92. Magaziner J, Simonsick EM, Kashner TM, Hebel JR, Kenzora JE (1989) Survival experience of aged hip fracture patients. Am J Public Health 79:274–278

93. Weiss NS, Liff JM, Ure CL, Ballard JH, Abbott GH, Daling JR (1983) Mortality in women following hip fracture. J Chron Dis 36:879–882

94. Browner WS, Seeley DG, Vogt TM, Cummings SR (1991) Non-trauma mortality in elderly women with low bone mineral density. Lancet 338:355–358

95. Browner WS, Pressman AR, Nevitt MC, Cauley JA, Cummings SR (1993) Association between low bone density and stroke in elderly women. The Study of Osteoporotic Fractures. Stroke 24:940–946

96. Gärdsell P, Johnell O (1993) Bone mass–a marker of biologic age? Clin Orthop 287:90–93

97. Kanis JA (1993) The incidence of hip fracture in Europe. Osteoporosis Int [Suppl] 1:S10–S15

98. Melton LJ III (1993) Hip fractures: a worldwide problem today and tomorrow. Bone 14 [Suppl]:S1–S8

99. Jensen JS, Tøndevold E, Sørensen PH (1980) Costs of treatment of hip fractures. Acta Orthop Scand 51:289–296

100. Fitzgerald JF, Fagan LF, Tierney WM, Dittus RS (1987) Changing patterns of hip fracture care before and after implementation of the Prospective Payment System. JAMA 258:218–221

101. Fitzgerald JF, Moore PS, Dittus RS (1988) The care of elderly patients with hip fracture. Changes since implementation of the Prospective Payment System. N Engl J Med 319:1392–1397

102. Phillips S, Fox N, Jacobs J, Wright WE (1988) The direct medical costs of osteoporosis for American women aged 45 and older, 1986. Bone 9:271–279

103. Holbrook TL, Grazier K, Kelsey JL, Stauffer RN (1984) The frequency of occurrence, impact, and cost of selected musculoskeletal conditions in the United States. American Academy of Orthopaedic Surgeons, Chicago

104. Peck WA, Riggs BL, Bell NH et al (1988) Research directions in osteoporosis. Am J Med 84:275–282

105. Praemer A, Furner S, Rice DP (1992) Musculoskeletal conditions in the United States. American Academy of Orthopaedic Surgeons, Park Ridge

106. Marotolli RA, Berkman LF, Cooney LM (1992) Decline in physical function following hip fracture. J Am Geriatr Soc 40:861–866

107. Cummings SR, Phillips SL, Wheat ME et al (1988) Recovery of function after hip fracture. J Am Geriatr Soc 36:801–806

108. Magaziner J, Simonsick EM, Kashner TM, Hebel JR, Kenzora JE (1990) Predictors of functional recovery one year following hospital discharge for hip fracture: a prospective study. J Gerontol Med Sci 45:M101–M107

109. Mossey JM, Mutran E, Knott K, Craik R (1989) Determinants of recovery 12

months after hip fracture: the importance of psychosocial factors. Am J Public Health 79:279–285

110. Ceder L, Thorngren K-G, Walden B (1980) Prognostic indicators and early home rehabilitation in elderly patients with hip fractures. Clin Orthop Rel Res 287:173–184

111. Jalovaara P, Virkkunen H (1991) Quality of life after hemiarthroplasty for femoral neck fracture. Acta Orthop Scand 62:208–217

112. Versluysen M (1986) How elderly patients with femoral fracture develop pressure sores in hospital. BMJ 292:1311–1313

113. Huang C, Ross PD, Wasnich RD (1996) Vertebral fractures and other predictors of back pain among older women. J Bone Miner Res 11(7):1025–1031

114. Lyritis GP, Mayasis B, Tsakalakos N, Lambropoulos A, Gazi S, Karachalios TH, Tsekoura M, Yiatzides A (1989) The natural history of the osteoporotic vertebral fracture. Clin Rheumatol 8 [Suppl 2]:66–69

115. Gold DT (1996) The clinical impact of vertebral fractures: quality of life in women with osteoporosis. Bone 18 [Suppl]:185S–189S

116. Hallal J (1991) Back pain with postmenopausal osteoporosis and vertebral fractures. Geriatr Nurs 7:285–287

117. Sato K (1984) Spinal deformity and back pain in spinal osteoporosis. Jpn J Geriatr 21:303–306

118. Silverman SL (1992) The clinical consequences of vertebral compression fracture. Bone 13 [Suppl]:S27–S31

119. Patel U, Skingle S, Campbell GA, Crisp AJ, Boyle IT (1991) Clinical profile of acute vertebral compression fractures in osteoporosis. Br J Rheumatol 30:418–421

120. Ryan PJ, Evans P, Gibson T, Fogelman I (1992) Osteoporosis and chronic back pain: a study with single-photon emission computed tomography bone scintigraphy. J Bone Miner Res 7(12):1455–1460

121. Ryan PJ, Blake G, Herd R, Fogelman I (1994) A clinical profile of back pain and disability in patients with spinal osteoporosis. Bone 15:27–30

122. Leidig G, Minne HW, Sauer P, Wuster C, Wuster J, Lojen M, Raue F, Ziegler R (1990) A study of complaints and their relation to vertebral destruction in patients with osteoporosis. Bone Miner 8:217–229

123. Scane AC, Sutcliffe AM, Francis RM (1994) The sequelae of vertebral crush fractures in men. Osteoporosis Int 4:89–92

124. Raspe H-H (1993) Back pain. In: Silman AJ, Hochberg MC (eds) Epidemiology of the rheumatic diseases. Oxford University Press, New York, pp 330–374

125. Nevitt M, Ettinger B, Black D, Stone K, Genant H, Cummings S (1996) Functional impact of first and recurrent vertebral fracture: a prospective study. Osteoporosis Int 6 [Suppl 1]:86

126. Ross PD, Davis JW, Epstein RS, Wasnich RD (1994) Pain and disability associated with new vertebral fractures and other spinal conditions. J Clin Epidemiol 47:231–239

127. Lyles KW, Gold DT, Shipp KM, Pieper CF, Martinez S, Mulhausen PL (1993) Association of osteoporotic vertebral compression fractures with impaired functional status. Am J Med 94:595–601

128. Ettinger B, Block JE, Smith R, Cummings SR, Harris ST, Genant HK (1988) An examination of the association between vertebral deformities, physical disabilities, and psychosocial problems. Maturitas 10:283–296

129. Ettinger B, Black DM, Palermo L, Nevitt MC et al (1992) Contribution of vertebral deformities to chronic back pain and disability. J Bone Miner Res 7(4):449–456

130. Itoi E, Sakurai M, Mizunashi K, Sato K, Kasama F (1990) Long-term observations of vertebral fractures in spinal osteoporosis. Calcif Tissue Int 47:202–208

131. Gold DT, Drezner MK (1995) Quality of life. In: Riggs BL, Melton LJ III (eds) Osteoporosis: etiology, diagnosis, and management, 2nd edn. Lippincott-Raven, Philadelphia

132. Huang C, Ross PD, Wasnich RD (1996) Vertebral fracture and other predictors of physical impairment and health care utilization. Arch Intern Med 156:2469–2475

133. Ross PD, Ettinger B, Davis JW, Melton LJ III, Wasnich RD (1991) Evaluation of adverse health outcomes associated with vertebral deformities. Osteoporosis Int 1(3):134–140

134. Huang C, Ross PD, Davis JW, Wasnich RD (1996) Contributions of vertebral fractures to stature loss among elderly Japanese-American women in Hawaii. J Bone Miner Res 11(3):408–411

135. Greendale GA, Barrett-Connor E, Ingles S, Haile R (1995) Late physical and functional effects of osteoporotic fracture in women: the Rancho Bernardo Study. J Am Geriatr Soc 43:955–961

136. Spector TD, McCloskey EV, Doyle DV, Kanis JA (1993) Prevalence of vertebral fracture in women and the relationship with bone density and symptoms: the Chingford Study. J Bone Miner Res 8(7):817–822

137. Davies KM, Recker RR, Stegman MR, Heaney RP (1991) Tallness versus shrinkage: do women shrink with age or grow taller with recent birth date? J Bone Miner Res 6:1115–1120

138. Davies KM, Heaney RP, Ryan RR (1996) Height loss in older women (abstract). J Bone Miner Res 10 [Suppl 1]:S357

139. Liberman UA, Weiss SR, Broll J et al (1995) Effect of oral alendronate on bone mineral density and the incidence of fractures in postmenopausal osteoporosis. N Engl J Med 333:1437–1443

140. Kleerekoper M, Nelson DA, Peterson EL, Tilley BC (1992) Outcome variables in clinical trials. Bone 13 [Suppl 1]:S29–S34

141. Leech JA, Dulberg C, Kellie S, Pattee L, Gay J (1990) Relationship of lung function to severity of osteoporosis in women. Am Rev Respir Dis 141(1):68–71

142. Xu L, Cummings SR, Qin MW, Stone K, Zhao XH, Chen XS, Jergas M, Richmond H, Nevitt MC, the Beijing Osteoporosis Project (1995) Vertebral osteo-

porosis in China: the first population-based study (abstract). J Bone Miner Res 10 [Suppl 1]:S467

143. Ensrud KE, Nevitt MC, Yunis C, Cauley JA, Seeley DG, Fox KM, Cummings SR (1994) Correlates of impaired function in older women. J Am Geriatr Soc 42:481–489

144. Greendale GA, Barrett-Connor E (1996) Outcomes of osteoporotic fractures. In: Marcus R, Feldman D, Kelsey J (eds) Osteoporosis. Academic, San Diego, pp 635–643

145. Cook DJ, Guyatt GH, Adachi JD et al (1993) Quality of life issues in women with vertebral fractures due to osteoporosis. Arthritis Rheum 36:750–756

146. Atkins RM, Duckworth T, Kanis JA (1990) Algodystrophy following Colles' fracture. J Bone Joint Surg 72 B:105–110

147. de Bruijn HP (1987) The Colles' fracture, review of literature, chap 3. Acta Octhop Scand 58 [Suppl 223]:7–25

148. Kaukonen J-P, Karaharju EO, Porras M, Luthje P, Jakobsson A (1988) Functional recovery after fractures of the distal forearm. Ann Chir Gynacol 77:27–31

149. Chrischilles EA, Butler CD, Davis CS, Wallace RB (1991) A model of lifetime osteoporosis impact. Arch Intern Med 151:2026–2032

150. Theintz G, Buchs B, Rizzoli R et al (1992) Longitudinal monitoring of bone mass accumulation in healthy adolescents: Evidence for a marked reduction after 16 years of age at the levels of lumbar spine and femoral neck in female subjects. J Clin Endocrinol Metab 75:1060–1065

3 The Pysiology of Bone Turnover

R. Pacifici

Introduction

Bone is remodeled by a sequence of cellular events which occur in discrete locations known as bone remodeling units. This process begins with the activation of mature osteoclasts adhering to the bone surfaces usually covered by lining osteoblasts and with an expansion of the osteoclastic pool. Through the interaction of preexisting and newly formed osteoclasts with osteoblasts, resorption is initiated in discrete areas. This phase, which lasts 2–4 weeks, leads to the formation of focal areas of bone resorption which reach a depth of about 30 µm [1]. Toward the end of the resorption phase mononuclear cells, an important source of cytokines, are typically found at the bottom of the resorption cavity [1]. The transition from resorption to formation is called reversal. This phase is characterized by the accumulation of osteoblast precursors and of a thin layer of inorganic matrix, known as cement line, at the bottom of the resorption pit. The cement line is rich in osteopontin, a RGD-rich protein which may be involved in signaling the cessation of osteoclastic activity. This is followed by the replacement of the removed bone by osteoblasts which accumulate at the base of the resorption lacunae and subsequently fill in the resorption cavity with newly formed bone.

Since receptors for systemic and locally produced factors capable of stimulating bone resorption are expressed in larger abundance by osteoblasts and osteoblast precursors of the stromal lineage than by osteoclasts, it is commonly accepted that bone resorption is initiated and regulated by osteoblasts [2]. More recent studies have also demonstrated that bone resorption is regulated primarily by the rate of osteoclast formation [3]. Since this process requires the integrated interaction of stromal cells and/or osteoblasts with hematopoietic osteoclast precursors [3, 4], the key regulatory role of osteoblasts and their precursors appears to be further substantiated. The proliferation, differentiation, and secretory activity of these cells is under the control of cytokines and growth factors. These molecules are produced by bone marrow and bone cells and are capable of regulating both the formation and functional activities of osteoclasts and the differentiation of osteoblasts.

Cytokines and Bone Remodeling

At present the production of a large number of cytokines in the bone microenvironment has been documented, and the complex and overlapping effects of these factors on both bone formation and resorption identified. Among these factors are (Table 3-1) interleukin (IL) 1α and 1β [5–9], IL-6 [10–12], tumor necrosis factor (TNF) α and β [13, 14], macrophage (M-) [15, 16], and granulocyte-macrophage (GM-) colony-stimulating factor (CSF) [17, 18].

IL-1 and TNF are among the most powerful stimulators of bone resorption known and well-recognized inhibitors of bone formation [9, 13, 19]. These cytokines promote bone resorption in vitro [6] and cause bone loss and hypercalcemia when infused in vivo [20–22]. IL-1 and TNF activate mature osteoclasts indirectly via a primary effect on osteoblasts [14] and inhibit osteoclast apoptosis [23]. In addition, they markedly enhance osteoclast formation by stimulating osteoclast precursor proliferation both directly [24] and by stimulating the pro-osteoclastogenic activity of stromal cells [25, 26].

A specific competitive inhibitor of IL-1, known as IL-1 receptor antagonist (IL-1ra), has also been identified [27, 28]. IL-1ra, which has a 26% amino acid sequence homology with IL-1β, binds to cells expressing primarily the 87-kDa type I IL-1 receptor with nearly the same affinity as IL-1 and competes with either IL-1α or IL-1β on these cells without detectable IL-1 agonist effects [29]. The type I IL-1 receptor is expressed in T cells, tissue macrophages, endothelial cells, and bone cells [30, 31]. IL-1ra also binds, although with a lower affinity, to the type II IL-1 receptor which is expressed mainly in blood neutrophils and B cells [30]. Since the binding of 5 molecules IL-1 per cell is sufficient to induce a full biological response, a 50% IL-1 inhibition in bone cells requires amounts of IL-1ra up to 100 times in excess of the amounts of IL-1α or IL-1β present.

The interpretation of the biological effects of IL-1 is further complicated by the fact that the binding of IL-1 to the type I receptor is antagonized not only by IL-1ra [30, 32] but also by soluble type I (sIL-1 RI) and type II IL-1 receptor (sIL-1 RII) [33, 34], anti-IL-1α autoantibodies [35] and IL-1β binding proteins [36].

Table 3-1 Effects of cytokines on bone resorption

Cytokine	Effects on osteoclast formation	Effects on activity resorption of mature osteoclasts	Effects on in vivo bone resorption in conditions of estrogen deficiency
IL-1	↑	↑	↑
IL-6	↑	–	–
IL-11	↑	–	–
TNF	↑	↑	↑
M-CSF	↑	–	↑
GM-CSF	↑	–	–
TGFβ	↑/↓	↓	–
IL-1ra	↑	↓	↓

Moreover, while sIL-1 RI antagonizes the effects of IL-1ra [34], sIL-1 RII binds IL-1β, but does not bind IL-1ra [33, 34]. Thus sIL-1 RII can compete with cell-associated receptors for IL-1β and potentiate the inhibitory action of IL-1ra. Recognition that the biological effects of IL-1 are not only a function of net concentration of IL-1 molecules but rather of the fine balance between agonist and antagonist molecules may facilitate the interpretation of contrasting data obtained measuring IL-1 activity by bioassay and IL-1 concentrations by enzyme-linked immunosorbent assays or immunoradiometric assays. For example, an association between estrogen deficiency and increased IL-1 activity was demonstrated in studies conducted by measuring IL-1 activity by bioassay [37–43]. Conversely, this association was not observed when IL-1 was measured by enzyme-linked immunosorbent assay or immunoradiometric assay [44, 45].

Another cytokine which has received considerable attention for its pro-osteoclastogenic effects is IL-6. This factor exerts its effects via a cell surface receptor that consists of a ligand binding chain (IL-6R) and a signal transducing chain known as gp130. Although IL-6 alone does not stimulate osteoclast formation [46], when bound to soluble IL-6R, IL-6 stimulates the early stages of osteoclastogenesis in human and murine cultures [47, 48], presumably by forming a complex with gp130 expressed on either stromal cell or osteoblasts [46, 49]. Interestingly, corticosteroids have been found to increase the stromal cell expression of IL-6R, suggesting the possibility that steroid-induced bone loss may be due at least in part to increased stromal cell responsiveness to IL-6 [46]. IL-6 increases in vitro bone resorption in systems rich in osteoclast precursors, such as the mouse fetal metacarpal assay [50], whereas it has no effect in organ cultures in which more mature cells predominate, such as murine fetal radii [48]. This suggests that IL-6 is more potent in increasing the formation of osteoclasts from hemopoietic precursors than in activating mature osteoclasts. Nevertheless, the effects of IL-6 on bone resorption in vivo remain controversial because blocking of IL-6 does not decrease in vivo bone resorption [51], IL-6 levels are not correlated with indices of bone turnover in postmenopausal women [52], and osteoporosis is not a feature of transgenic mice overexpressing IL-6 or IL-6R [46, 53, 54]. However, this cytokine does cause hypercalcemia in nude mice [35].

The essential role of CSFs in the proliferation and differentiation of osteoclast precursors is best demonstrated by the presence of osteopetrosis in a natural M-CSF knock out, the op/op mouse [25]. These mice, which are cured by the administration of M-CSF [55], have an additional thymidine inserted within the coding region of the M-CSF gene, a mutation that generates a stop codon within the coding sequence [56], thereby resulting in the production of a defective M-CSF [25]. The formation of osteoclasts in bone marrow cultures is also increased by GM-CSF [57, 58]. This factor stimulates the early stages of osteoclastogenesis in cooperation with IL-3 [18, 59]. Utilizing a novel culture system which induces the differentiation of peripheral blood stem cells into mature osteoclasts in the absence of stromal cells, we have recently found that GM-CSF is the most potent pro-osteoclastogenic factor among the known growth factors and cytokines

[60]. Thus, although in the mouse osteoclast formation is completely blocked by anti-M-CSF but not anti-GM-CSF antibodies [16], GM-CSF is critical for the proliferation and differentiation of human osteoclast precursors [60].

Although most bone cell-targeting cytokines are produced by either bone and bone marrow cells, mononuclear cells of the monocyte/macrophage lineage are recognized as the major source of IL-1 and TNF [30]. In contrast, pro-osteoclastogenic "downstream" cytokines are mainly produced by stromal cells and osteoblasts [61, 62]. Thus osteoclastogenesis requires the hierarchical interaction of mononuclear cells, stromal cells, and/or osteoblasts and hematopoietic osteoclast precursors as well as the conditioning effect of numerous cytokines.

Role of the Bone Matrix in the Regulation of Bone Turnover

Several lines of evidence suggest that bone matrix contributes to the regulation of bone turnover. Moreover, studies have also revealed that monocytes accumulate at the bottom of resorption pits just before the reversal phase. Thus a monocyte/bone matrix interaction is likely to play a critical role in the regulation of bone turnover. The adherence of monocytes to bone is in fact recognized as a potent stimulator of cytokine secretion [63]. This means of regulation was explored in studies aimed to investigate the effect of the bone matrix on the monocytic production of IL-1. These studies revealed that collagen and its fragments stimulate IL-1 production. This effect is mediated by the $\alpha_2\beta_1$ integrin, a collagen receptor expressed in monocytes [64]. Another important constituent of bone matrix, fibronectin, although not directly capable of inducing IL-1 release, potentiates the effects of collagen on IL-1 production by binding to the fibronectin receptor $\alpha_5\beta_1$ [65]. This, in turn, generates a signal transduced by the intracellular region of $\alpha_5\beta_1$ and protein kinase C and activates the $\alpha_2\beta_1$ receptor [66]. Interestingly, the bone matrix constituents capable of stimulating IL-1 activity are all released in the local microenvironment during bone resorption. Moreover, adherence proteins containing the Arg-Gly-Asp (RGD) sequence [67, 68], and osteocalcin, the most abundant noncollagen bone protein, have been hypothesized to participate in cell attachment to mineralized matrix because they bind tightly to collagen [67], and because vitamin K depletion prevents cell adherence to bone [69]. Thus, important functional differences exist among the bone fragments produced with bone resorption. Some adherence proteins and osteocalcin may in fact play a role in regulating the homing and attachment of mononuclear cells, while collagen and its fragments may be particularly important for regulating the secretion of cytokines active in bone resorption, such as IL-1.

These observations suggest that bone turnover could also be regulated both by the amounts of matrix fragments released locally and by the degree of mononuclear cells responsiveness to these fragments. The latter type of regulation is suggested by the ability of ovarian steroids and $1,25(OH)_2D_3$ to regulate mononuclear cell IL-1 activity [70–73] and the expression of collagen receptors on monocytic cells [74], respectively. Therefore the increase in bone resorption occurring

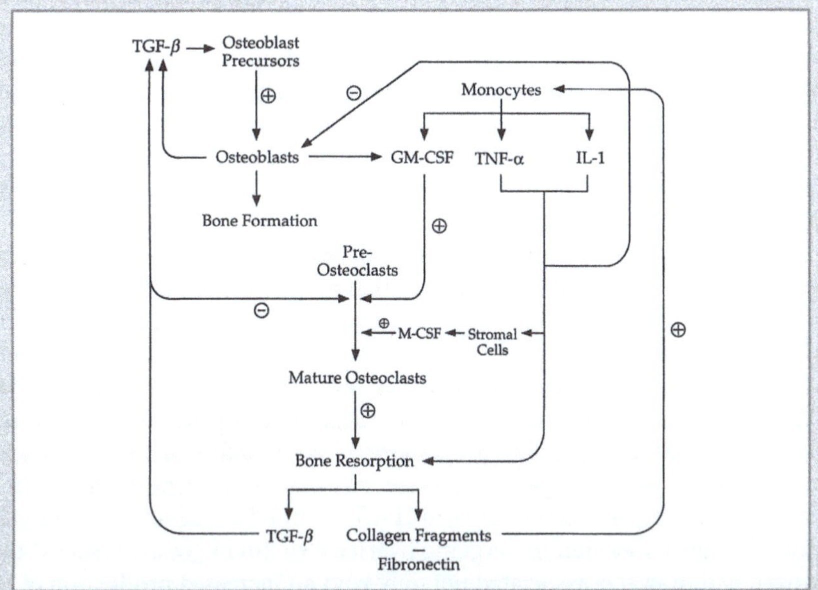

Fig. 3-1 Hypothetical view of the effects of the monocyte/bone matrix interactions on bone resorption. In conditions of estrogen deficiency the adherence of monocytes to the bone matrix triggers an increased production of IL-1, TNF, and GM-CSF. These cytokines stimulate bone resorption by promoting osteoclastogenesis and stimulating the resorbing activity of mature osteoclasts. This in turns leads to the release of constituents of the bone matrix such as collagen fragments, fibronectin, and TGFβ which are chemotactic for monocyte and stimulate further cytokine release, thereby potentiating bone resorption. The release of TGFβ may be relevant for both inhibiting osteoclastogenesis and stimulating bone formation

after the menopause could be visualized (Fig. 3-1) as the result of an enhanced responsiveness of marrow mononuclear cells to the release of bone matrix fragments and the resulting increase in cytokine secretion. More specifically, with estrogen deficiency cytokines active on bone resorption are released at specific sites, upon activation of new remodeling units, as a result of a local interaction between mononuclear cells and bone matrix fragments. Because of the autocrine effect [75] and the powerful bone-resorbing activity of IL-1 [5, 6], a cascade of events leading to an amplification of bone resorption and further cytokine production could be initiated. Estrogen replacement would then decrease the monocytic secretory response to bone matrix fragments, resulting in a lower number of mature osteoclasts available for activation of new remodeling units.

Effect of Menopause and Estrogen Replacement on the Production of Bone Resorbing Cytokines

Since menopause is associated with a significant increase in the rate of bone remodeling, a great deal of attention has been devoted to investigating the mechanism by which estrogen regulates bone turnover and the role of cytokines in this process. Evidence has now accumulated which suggests that IL-1, IL-6, TNF, M-CSF, and GM-CSF are produced in greater abundance in conditions of estrogen deficiency. Moreover, estrogen also increases the steady-state level of TGFβ mRNA and release of TGFβ protein from osteoblasts [76]. Since TGFβ is a potent inhibitor of osteoclastic function and an osteoblast mitogen [77], these data provides an example of "positive" effects of estrogen in bone which may result in decreased bone resorption. All of these cytokines are therefore potential mediators of the effects of estrogen in bone.

The cytokines first recognized as estrogen regulated were IL-1 and TNF. This observation was prompted by the finding that monocytes of patients with "high turnover" osteoporosis, the histological hallmark of postmenopausal osteoporosis, secrete increased amounts of IL-1 [70]. Cross-sectional and prospective comparisons of pre and postmenopausal women revealed that monocytic production of IL-1 and TNF increases after natural and surgical menopause and is decreased by treatment with estrogen and progesterone [38, 71]. Subsequent observations showed that the postmenopausal increase in IL-1 activity results from an effect of estrogen on the production of both IL-1β and the IL-1 inhibitor IL-1ra [78]. Studies in normal women undergoing ovariectomy (ovx) [37, 41] revealed that estrogen withdrawal is associated not only with an increased production of IL-1 and TNF, but also of GM-CSF. The changes in these cytokine levels occur in a temporal sequence consistent with a causal role of IL-1, TNF, and GM-CSF in the pathogenesis of ovx induced bone loss [37]. Moreover, since the increase in GM-CSF production precedes the increase in IL-1 and TNF [37], the data suggest that the increased production of GM-CSF is not a result of enhanced secretion of IL-1 and TNF, but rather a direct effect of estrogen withdrawal [37].

Conditions characterized by increased production of IL-1 and/or TNF such as rheumatoid arthritis [79], endometriosis [80], fasting (resorptive) hypercalciuria [81] are all associated with rapid bone loss [81–84]. More direct evidence in support of a link between cytokines and pathogenesis of osteoporosis has been provided by data from Rolston et al. [85] which demonstrate that IL-1, TNF and IL-6 mRNAs are expressed more frequently in bone cells from untreated postmenopausal women than in those from women on estrogen replacement. That the increased monocytic production of cytokines plays a direct role in inducing bone resorption was later demonstrated by Choen-Solal et al. [86] by examining the bone resorption activity of cultured supernatants from monocytes obtained from pre and postmenopausal women. Using this approach they found that the culture media of monocytes obtained from postmenopausal women have an increased in vitro bone resorption activity that is blocked by the addition of IL-1ra and anti-TNF antibody.

Subsequent studies conducted to determine whether estrogen regulates the production of IL-6 revealed that in murine stromal and osteoblastic cells IL-1- and TNF- induced IL-6 production is inhibited by the addition of estrogen [10] and stimulated by estrogen withdrawal [12]. In vivo studies also revealed that the production of IL-6 is increased in cultures of bone marrow cells from ovx mice [11].

This effect is mediated, at least in the mouse, by an indirect effect of estrogen on the transcription activity of the proximal 225-bp sequence of the IL-6 promoter [87, 88].

Interestingly, although studies with human cell lines demonstrated an inhibitory effect of estrogen on the human IL-6 promoter [89], three independent groups have failed to demonstrate an inhibitory effect of estrogen on IL-6 production from human bone cells and stromal cells expressing functional estrogen receptors [62, 90, 91]. These data raise the possibility that the production of human IL-6 protein does not increase in conditions of estrogen deficiency. This is further supported by a report that in humans surgical menopause is not followed by an increase in IL-6, although it causes an increase in soluble IL-6 receptor [92].

A regulatory effect of estrogen on the production of soluble IL-6R and on the expression of gp130 on bone cells could modulate the responsiveness of osteoclast and osteoblast precursors to IL-6 and to other cytokines which utilize gp130 as a signal transducer. Among them are IL-11 and the pro-osteoblastogenic cytokine, leukemia inhibitory factor. Thus, additional mechanisms by which estrogen controls bone turnover may include regulation of bone cell responsiveness to cytokines which utilizes gp130, and modulation of cytokine binding to activating soluble receptors.

Attempts to demonstrate that menopause increases circulating levels of IL-1, TNF, and IL-6 have for the most part been unsuccessful [93, 94], presumably because only a small fraction of the cytokines produced in the bone marrow "leak" into the peripheral circulation. The lack of increased serum cytokine levels in estrogen deficient women is also consistent with the notion that since cytokine release requires the adherence of cells to a solid substrate [63, 65], estrogen deficiency is unlikely to stimulate cytokine production from circulating cells.

Recent studies have further clarified the role of IL-1 and TNF and IL-6 in bone remodeling by inducing a functional block of these cytokines via infusion of the IL-1 antagonist, IL-1ra, the TNF antagonist, TNF binding protein (TNFbp) or anti-IL-6 antibodies in intact and ovariectomized animals.

This experimental strategy has revealed that in mature rats simultaneous treatment with IL-1ra and the TNFbp is required to completely prevent the bone loss and the increase in bone resorption induced early after ovariectomy [95]. In contrast, treatment of mature rats with IL-1ra, started late after ovx is sufficient to block bone loss and bone resorption and to fully reproduce the effects of estrogen replacement [96, 97]. These data demonstrate that IL-1 and TNF play a critical causal role in the pathogenesis of ovx-induced bone loss, and that the contribution of individual factors varies as time elapses after ovx. The specific contribution of IL-1 and TNF to ovx-induced bone loss is also species dependent as illustrated in the mouse, by treatment with TNFbp alone in the early postovx period, which duplicates the bone-sparing effect of estrogen [98]. In contrast, administration of TNFbp alone in the rat decreases, but does not completely block, ovx-induced bone loss [95]. The critical role of TNF in the mouse model is further documented by the failure of ovx to induce bone loss in transgenic mice which overexpress soluble TNF receptor [99]. Conversely, infusion of anti-IL-6 antibody does not prevent bone loss and the increase in in vivo bone resorption induced by ovx [98], although it decreases the formation of osteoclasts and their precursors [colony-forming units (CFU)-GM] in vivo and in vitro [11, 51]. These data clearly demonstrate that the block of IL-6 decreases osteoclastogenesis but does not prevent ovariectomy-induced bone loss. This is because IL-6 is not required for inducing the production of other "upstream" estrogen regulated factors, such as IL-1 and TNF. Consequently in conditions of estrogen deficiency IL-1 and TNF stimulate bone resorption and induce bone loss even in the absence of IL-6.

Studies have also revealed that treatment with either IL-1ra or TNFbp alone blocks the increase in ex vivo osteoclast formation induced by ovx [51]. Thus, IL-1 and TNF must possess either synergistic or sequential effects on osteoclastogenesis, the primary mechanism underlying long-term elevations of bone resorption [100, 101]. In contrast, since inhibition of both IL-1 and TNF is required to prevent the increase in bone resorption observed in the early postovx period, IL-1 and TNF are likely to have independent and redundant stimulatory effects on osteoclast activation, the primary mechanism by which bone resorption increases acutely after ovx.

Another approach to prove the existence of a causal relationship between cytokines, bone loss, and estrogen deficiency is to demonstrate that the deficiency or the functional block of a cytokine prevents the bone loss induced by menopause or ovx.

The development of transgenic mice has made it possible to link genes to specific phenotypes and determine the function of numerous proteins. Although this approach has been used in an attempt to determine which cytokines are causative factors in ovx-induced bone loss, it should be emphasized that postmenopausal osteoporosis results from the impact of estrogen deficiency on a normally developed skeleton. The lack of deactivatable promoters does not allow a "switch off" of gene when an animal reaches maturity. Thus knockout mice are characterized by bone modeling and remodeling defects that ensue during fetal development and lead to the formation of an abnormal mature skeleton. This is because the absence of a single gene is known to alter expression of other genes and developmental programs [102]. Moreover, the phenomenon of "gene compensation" may induce unstable phenotypes and make the recognition of the function of a factor problematic [102]. In spite of these limitations it was found that ovariectomy does not induce bone loss in IL-6 deficient mice. However, more recent observations from the same investigators indicate that IL-6 deficient mice of the third generation, which express a more stable phenotype, are not protected from the effects of ovariectomy on bone loss (G. Balena, personal communication). Thus, additional studies on well-characterized phenotypes of IL-6 deficient mice are necessary to determine the contribution of IL-6 to ovariectomy-induced bone loss.

Effect of Menopause on the Stromal Cell Responsiveness to Cytokines

The ability of estrogen to block the monocytic production of bone resorbing cytokines [37,38,103] is consistent with the reported expression of estrogen receptors in these cells. However, the presence of estrogen receptors in stromal cells [104] and osteoclasts [105, 106] indicate that estrogen is likely to regulate bone resorption not only by stimulating the production of cytokines in mononuclear cells but also by directly targeting the cells involved in osteoclastogenesis.

Osteoclastogenesis is a complex phenomenon which is facilitated by the interaction of bone marrow stromal cells with hematopoietic osteoclast precursors [25]. Such precursors are, or are related to, either CFU-GM or CFU-M [25]. Stromal cells contribute to osteoclastogenesis by providing a physical support for nascent osteoclasts and by producing soluble and membrane-associated factors which stimulate the proliferation and/or the differentiation of hematopoietic osteoclast precursors [16, 25]. The role of IL-1 and TNF in this process is that of increasing the pro-osteoclastogenic activity of stromal cells. This is in turn the result of the ability of these cytokines to stimulate the stromal cell production of factors which induce the proliferation and the differentiation of hematopoietic osteoclast precursors such as IL-6, IL-11, and M-CSF [25, 107].

Evidence has now accumulated which suggests that estrogen regulates the sensitivity or responsiveness of stromal cells to pro-osteoclastogenic cytokines, thereby resulting in decreased osteoclast production. This evidence includes the fact than when stromal cells from either ovariectomized or sham-operated mice are cocultured with hematopoietic osteoclast precursors from the opposite group, the number of mature osteoclasts generated by these cocultures is a function solely of the estrogen status of the stromal cell donor. The cocultures which produce the largest number of osteoclasts are in fact those containing stromal cells from ovariectomized mice [108]. Cocultures containing stromal cells from sham-operated mice produce a low number of osteoclasts regardless of the origin of the osteoclast precursors.

Among the factors produced by stromal cells which participate in inducing osteoclastogenesis, M-CSF plays the most critical role in inducing the proliferation and differentiation of the hemopoietic osteoclast precursor [16]. Moreover, the secretion of M-CSF from stromal cells is greatly stimulated by IL-1 and TNF. Because of these characteristics M-CSF appears an ideal target of estrogen regulation. Indeed, studies have shown that stromal cells from ovariectomized mice produce higher M-CSF levels and express more M-CSF mRNA in response to IL-1 and TNF than those from either sham-operated mice or estrogen-treated ovariectomized mice [108]. This does not exclude the possibility that estrogen may have other effects on stromal cells relevant to the osteoclast formation process. For example, it has been suggested that estrogen may regulate the expression of gp 130, the signal-transducing subunit of the receptor for IL-6 and IL-11 [109], a phenomenon which could decrease the pro-osteoclastogenic activity of stromal cells.

The existence of two sequential estrogen regulated steps (monocytic production of cytokines and stromal cell response to these cytokines) explains the marked sensitivity of the osteoclast formation process to estrogenic regulation.

Conclusions

Modulation of bone turnover appears to be particularly complex as it involves the regulated production of cytokines from mononuclear cells and bone cells [77, 107] and the responsiveness of stromal cells to these cytokines. Although many details of this process remain to be defined, it is now clearly established that IL-1 and TNF produced by bone marrow monocytes play a critical role in regulating bone turnover, especially in conditions of estrogen deficiency.

Numerous other local and systemic factors are likely to participate in the regulation of bone turnover. Probable candidates are IL-6 and TGFβ. The exact contribution of IL-6 remains unclear because of insufficient data demonstrating that the block of IL-6 decreases bone resorption in vivo and bone loss in a bona fide experimental model of postmenopausal osteoporosis. However, the exact role of IL-6 as well as that of TGFβ is likely to be defined in the near future.

References

1. Rodan GA (1996) Coupling of bone resorption and formation during bone remodeling. In: Marcus R, Feldman D, Kelsey J (eds) Osteoporosis. Academic, San Diego, pp 289–299
2. Chambers TJ (1980) The cellular basis for bone resorption. Clin Orthop Relat Res 151:283–293
3. Roodman GD (1996) Advances in bone biology: the osteoclast. Endocr Rev 17:308–332
4. Suda T, Udagawa N, Nakamura I, Miyaura C, Takahashi N (1995) Modulation of osteoclast differentiation by local factors. Bone 17:S87–S91
5. Gowen M, Wood DD, Ihrie EJ, McGuire MKB, Russell RGG (1983) An interleukin-1-like factor stimulates bone resorption in vitro. Nature 306:378–380
6. Lorenzo JA, Sousa SL, Alander C, Raisz LG, Dinarello CA (1987) Comparison of the bone-resorbing activity in the supernatants from phytohemaglutinin-stimulated human peripheral blood mononuclear cells with that of cytokines through the use of an antiserum to interleukin 1. Endocrinology 121:1164–1170
7. Gowen M, Wood DD, Russell RGG (1985) Stimulation of the proliferation of human bone cells in vitro by human monocyte products with interleukin-1 activity. J Clin Invest 75:1223–1229
8. Canalis E (1986) Interleukin-1 has independent effects on deoxyribonucleic acid and collagen synthesis in cultures of rat calvariae. Endocrinology 118:74–81
9. Stashenko P, Dewhirst FE, Rooney ML, Desjardins LA, Heeley JD (1987) Inter-

leukin-1β is a potent inhibitor of bone formation in vitro. J Bone Miner Res 2:559–565

10. Girasole G, Jilka RL, Passeri G, Boswell S, Boder G, Williams DC, Manolagas SC (1992) 17β-estradiol inhibits interleukin-6 production by bone marrow-derived stromal cells and osteoblasts in vitro: a potential mechanism for the antiosteoporotic effect of estrogens. J Clin Invest 89:883–891

11. Jilka RL, Hangoc G, Girasole G, Passeri G, Williams DC, Abrams JS, Boyce B, Broxmeyer H, Manolagas SC (1992) Increased osteoclast development after estrogen loss: mediation by interleukin-6. Science 257:88–91

12. Passeri G, Girasole G, Jilka RL, Manolagas SC (1993) Increased interleukin-6 production by murine bone marrow and bone cells after estrogen withdrawal. Endocrinology 133:822–828

13. Bertolini DR, Nedwin GE, Bringman TS, Smith DD, Mundy GR (1986) Stimulation of bone resorption and inhibition of bone formation in vitro by human tumor necrosis factor. Nature 319:516–518

14. Thomson BM, Mundy GR, Chambers TJ (1987) Tumor necrosis factor α and β induce osteoblastic cells to stimulate osteoclastic bone resorption. J Immunol 138:775–779

15. Takahashi N, Udagawa N, Akatsu T, Tanaka H, Shionome M, Suda T (1991) Role of colony-stimulating factors in osteoclast development. J Bone Miner Res 6:977–985

16. Tanaka S, Takahashi N, Udagawa N, Tamura T, Akatsu T, Stanley ER, Kurokawa T, Suda T (1993) Macrophage colony-stimulating factor is indispensable for both proliferation and differentiation of osteoclast progenitors. J Clin Invest 91:257–263

17. Schneider GB, Relfson M (1989) Pluripotent hemopoietic stem cells give rise to osteoclasts in vitro: effect of rGM-CSF. Bone Miner 5:129–138

18. Kurihara N, Suda T, Miura Y, Nakauchi H, Kodama H, Hiura K, Hakeda Y, Kumegawa M (1989) Generation of osteoclasts from isolated hematopoietic progenitor cells. Blood 74:1295–1302

19. Nguyen L, Dewhirst FE, Hauschka PV, Stashenko P (1991) Interleukin-1β stimulates bone resorption and inhibits bone formation in vivo. Lymphokine Cytokine Res 10:15–21

20. Boyce BF, Aufdemorte TB, Garrett IR, Yates AJP, Mundy GR (1989) Effects of interleukin-1 on bone turnover in normal mice. Endocrinology 125:1142–1150

21. Sabatini, M, Boyce B, Aufdemorte T, Bonewald L, Mundy GR (1988) Infusions of recombinant human interleukin 1 alpha and beta cause hypercalcemia in normal mice. Proc Natl Acad Sci USA 85:5235–5239

22. Johnson RA, Boyce BF, Mundy GR, Roodman GD (1989) Tumors producing human tumor necrosis factor induce hypercalcemia and osteoclastic bone resorption in nude mice. Endocrinology 124:1424–1427

23. Hughes DE, Jilka RL, Manolagas S, Dallas SL, Bonewald LF, Mundy GR, Boyce BF (1995) Sex steroids promote osteoclast apoptosis in vitro and in vivo. J Bone Miner Res 10:48 (abstract)

24. Pfeilschifter J, Chenu C, Bird A, Mundy GR, Roodman GD (1989) Interleukin-1 and tumor necrosis factor stimulate the formation of human osteoclast-like cells in vitro. J Bone Miner Res 4:113–118

25. Suda T, Takahashi N, Martin TJ (1992) Modulation of osteoclast differentiation. Endocr Rev 13:66–80

26. Srivastava S, McHugh K, Kimble R, Ross FP, Pacifici R (1995) Estrogen down regulates the expression of M-CSF mRNA in bone marrow stromal cells by stimulating the production of the transcription factor EGR-1. J Bone Miner Res 10 [Suppl 1]:S18

27. Carter DB, Deibel MR Jr, Dunn C J, Tomich C-S C, Laborde AL, Slightom JL, Berger AE, Bienkowski MJ, Sun FF, McEwan RN, Harris PKW, Yem AW, Waszak GA, Chosay JG, Sieu LC, Hardee MM, Zurcher-Neely HA, Reardon IM, Heinrikson RL, Truesdell SE, Shelly JA, Eessalu TE, Taylor BM, Tracey DE (1990) Purification, cloning, expression and biological characterization of an interleukin-1 receptor antagonist protein. Nature 344:633–638

28. Hannum CH, Wilcox CJ, Arend WP, Joslin FG, Dripps DJ, Heimdal PL, Armes LG, Sommer A, Eisenberg SP, Thompson RC (1990) Interleukin-1 receptor antagonist activity of a human interleukin-1 inhibitor. Nature 343:336–340

29. Arend WP (1991) Interleukin 1 receptor antagonist: a new member of the interleukin 1 family. J Clin Invest 88:1445–1451

30. Dinarello CA (1991) Interleukin-1 and interleukin-1 antagonism. Blood 77:1627–1652

31. Seckinger P, Klein-Nulend J, Alander C, Thompson RC, Dayer J-M, Raisz LG (1990) Natural and recombinant human IL-1 receptor antagonists block the effects of IL-1 on bone resorption and prostaglandin production. J Immunol 145:4181–4184

32. Thompson RC, Dripps DJ, Eisenberg SP (1991) IL-1ra: properties and uses of an interleukin-1 receptor antagonist. Agents Actions [Suppl] 35:41–49

33. Symons JA, Young PR, Duff GW (1995) Soluble type iI interleukin 1 (il-1) receptor binds and blocks processing of il-1-beta precursor and loses affinity for il-1 receptor antagonist. Proc Natl Acad Sci USA 92:1714–1718

34. Burger D, Chicheportiche R, Giri JG, Dayer JM (1995) The inhibitory activity of human interleukin-1 receptor anatgonist is enhanced by type II interleukin-I soluble receptor and hindered by type I interleukin-1 soluble receptor. J Clin Invest 96:38–41

35. Hansen MB, Svenson M, Bendtzen K (1990) Human anti-interleukin 1α antibodies. Immunol Lett 30:133–140

36. Simon JA, Eastgate JA, Duff GW (1990) A soluble binding protein specific for interleukin 1β is produced by activated mononuclear cells. Cytokine 2:190–198

37. Pacifici R, Brown C, Puscheck E, Friedrich E, Slatopolsky E, Maggio D, McCracken R, Avioli LV (1991) Effect of surgical menopause and estrogen replacement on cytokine release from human blood mononuclear cells. Proc Natl Acad Sci 88:5134–5138

38. Pacifici R, Rifas L, McCracken R, Vered I, McMurtry C, Avioli LV, Peck WA (1989) Ovarian steroid treatment blocks a postmenopausal increase in blood monocyte interleukin 1 release. Proc Natl Acad Sci USA 86:2398–2402

39. Pioli G, Basini G, Pedrazzoni M, Musetti G, Ulietti V, Bresciani D, Villa P, Bacci A, Hughes D, Russell G, Passeri M (1992) Spontaneous release of interleukin-1 and interleukin-6 by peripheral blood monocytes after ovariectomy. Clin Sci 83:503–507

40. Ralston SH, Russell RGG, Gowen M (1990) Estrogen inhibits release of tumor necrosis factor from peripheral blood mononuclear cells in postmenopausal women. J Bone Miner Res 5:983–988

41. Fiore CE, Falcidia E, Foti R, Motta M, Tamburino C (1993) Differences in the time course of the effects of oophorectomy in women on parameters of bone metabolism and interleukin-1 levels in the circulation. Bone Miner 20:79–85

42. Matsuda T, Matsui K, Shimakoshi Y, Aida Y, Hukuda S (1991) 1-Hydroxyethilidene-1, 1-bisphosphonate decreases the postovariectomy-enhanced interleukin-1 production by peritoneal macrophages in adult rats. Calcif Tissue Int 49:403–406

43. Kaneki M, Nakamura T, Masuyama A, Chen JT, Seimiya Y, Shiraki M, Ouchi Y, Orimo H (1991) The effect of menopause on IL-1 and IL-6 release from peripheral blood monocytes. J Bone Miner Res 6:76 (abstract)

44. Zarrabeitia MT, Riancho JA, Amado JA, Napal J, Gonzales-Macias J (1991) Cytokine production by blood cells in postmenopausal osteoporosis. Bone Miner 14:161–167

45. Hustmyer FG, Walker E, Yu XP, Girasole G, Sakagami Y, Peacock M, Manolagas SC (1993) Cytokine production and surface antigen expression by peripheral blood mononuclear cells in postmenopausal osteoporosis. J Bone Miner Res 8:51–59

46. Udagawa N, Takahashi N, Katagiri T, Tamura T, Wada S, Findlay DM, Martin TJ, Hirota H, Tada T, Kishimoto T, Suda T (1995) Interleukin (IL)-6 induction of osteoclast differentiation depends on IL-6 receptors expressed on osteoblastic cells but not on osteoclast progenitors. J Exp Med 182:1461–1468

47. Kurihara N, Civin C, Roodman GD (1991) Osteotropic factor responsiveness of highly purified populations of early and late precursors for human multinucleated cells expressing the osteoclast phenotype. J Bone Miner Res 6:257–261

48. Roodman GD (1992) Interleukin-6: an osteotropic factor? J Bone Miner Res 7:475–478

49. Tamura T, Udagawa N, Takahashi N, Miyaura C, Tanaka S, Yamada Y, Koishihara Y, Ohsugi Y, Kumaki K, Taga T, Kishimoto T, Suda T (1993) Soluble interleukin-6 receptor triggers osteoclast formation by interleukin-6. Proc Natl Acad Sci USA 90:11924–11928

50. Lowik CWGM, van der Pluijm G, Bloys H, Hoekman K, Bijvoet OL, Aarden LA, Papapoulos SE (1989) Parathyroid hormone (PTH) and PTH-like protein (PLP) stimulate IL-6 production by osteogenic cells: a possible role of

interleukin-6 in osteoclastogenesis. Biochem Biophys Res Commun 162:1546–1552

51. Kitazawa R, Kimble RB, Vannice JL, Kung VT, Pacifici R (1994) Interleukin-1 receptor antagonist and tumor necrosis factor binding protein decrease osteoclast formation and bone resorption in ovariectomized mice. J Clin Invest 94:2397–2406

52. Kania DM, Binkley N, Checovich M, Havighurst T, Schilling M, Ershler WB (1995) Elevated plasma levels of interleukin-6 in postmenopausal women do not correlate with bone density. J Am Geriatr Soc 43:236–239

53. Woodroofe C, Muller W, Ruther U (1992) Long-term consequences of interleukin-6 overexpression in transgenic mice. DNA Cell Biol 11:587–592

54. Suematsu S, Matsuda T, Aozasa K, Akira S, Nakano T, Kishimoto T (1989) IgG1 plasmacytosis in interleukin-6 transgenic mice. Proc Natl Acad Sci USA 86:7547–7551

55. Felix R, Cecchini MG, Fleish H (1990) Macrophage colony-stimulating factor restores in vivo bone resorption in the op/op osteopetrotic mouse. Endocrinology 127:2592–2597

56. Yoshida HS, Hayashi S, Kunisada T, Ogawa M, Nishikawa S, Okamura H, Sudo T, Schultz LD (1990) The murine mutation osteopetrosis is in the coding region of macrophage colony stimulating factor gene. Nature 345:442–444

57. Macdonald BR, Mundy GR, Clark S, Wang EA, Kuehl TJ, Stanley ER, Roodman GD (1986) Effects of human recombinant CSF-GM and highly purified CSF-1 on the formation of multi-nucleated cells with osteoclast characteristics in long-term bone marrow cultures. J Bone Miner Res 1:227–232

58. Lorenzo JA, Souss SL, Fonseca JM, Hock JM, Medlock ES (1987) Colony-stimulating factors regulate the development of multinucleated osteoclasts from recently replicated cells in vitro. J Clin Invest 160:164–160

59. Kurihara N, Chenu C, Miller M, Civin C, Roodman GD (1990) Identification of committed mononuclear precursors for osteoclast-like cells formed in long term human marrow cultures. Endocrinology 126:2733–2741

60. Matayoshi A, Brown C, DiPersio J, Haugh J, Abu-Amer Y, Liapis H, Kuestner R, Pacifici R (1996) Human blood-mobilized hematopoietic precursors differentiate into osteoclasts in the absence of stromal cells. Proc Natl Acad Sci USA 93:10785–10790

61. Fibbe WE, Van Damme J, Billiau A, Goselink HM, Vogt PJ, Van Eeden PR, Altroch BW, Falkenburg JHF (1988) Intereleukin-1 induces human marrow stromal cells in long term cultures to produce G-CSF and M-CSF. Blood 71:431–435

62. Rifas L, Kenney JS, Marcelli M, Pacifici R, Dawson LL, Cheng S, Avioli LV (1995) Production of interleukin-6 in human osteoblasts and human bone marrow stromal cells: evidence that induction by interleukin-1 and tumor necrosis factor-α is not regulated by ovarian steroids. Endocrinology 136:4056–4067 (abstract)

63. Pacifici R, Carano A, Santoro SA, Rifas L, Jeffrey JJ, Malone JD, McCracken R, Avioli LV (1991) Bone matrix constituents stimulate interleukin-1 release from human blood mononuclear cells. J Clin Invest 87:221–228

64. Hemler ME (1988) Adhesive protein receptors on hematopoietic cells. Immunol Today 9:109–113

65. Pacifici R, Basilico C, Roman J, Zutter MM, Santoro SA, McCracken R (1992) Collagen-induced release of interleukin 1 from human blood mononuclear cells Potentiation by fibronectin binding to the alpha 5 beta 1 integrin. J Clin Invest 89:61–67

66. Pacifici R, Roman J, Kimble R, Civitelli R, Brownfield CM, Bizzarri C (1994) Ligand binding to monocyte $\alpha_5\beta_1$ integrin activates the $\alpha_2\beta_1$ receptor via the α_5 subunit cytoplasmatic domain and protein kinase C. J.Immunol 153:2222–2233

67. Hynes RO (1986) Fibronectins. Sci Am 254:42–51

68. Oldberg A, Franzen A, Heinegard D (1986) Cloning and sequence analysis of rat bone sialoprotein (osteopontin) cDNA reveals an Arg-Gly-Asp cell binding sequence. Proc Natl Acad Sci USA 83:8819–8823

69. Lian JB, Dunn K, Key LL Jr (1986) In vitro degradation of bone particles by human monocytes is decreased with the depletion of the vitamin K-dependent bone protein from the matrix. Endocrinology 118:1636–1642

70. Pacifici R, Rifas L, Teitelbaum S, Slatopolsky E, McCracken R, Bergfeld M, Lee W, Avioli LV, Peck WA (1987) Spontaneous release of interleukin 1 from human blood monocytes reflects bone formation in idiopathic osteoporosis. Proc Natl Acad Sci USA 84:4616–4620

71. Pacifici R, Brown C, Rifas L, Avioli LV (1990) TNFα and GM-CSF secretion from human blood monocytes: effect of menopause and estrogen replacement. J Bone Miner Res 5:145 (abstract)

72. Schulof RS, Nayor PH, Sztein MB, Goldstein AL (1987) Thymic physiology and biochemistry. Adv Clin Chem 26:203–292

73. Paavonen T, Andersson LC, Adlercreutz H (1981) Sex hormone regulation of in vitro immune response. Estradiol enhances human B cell maturation via inhibition of suppressor T cells in pokeweed mitogen-stimulated cultures. J Exp Med 154:1935–1945

74. Polla BS, Healy AM, Byrne M, Krane SM (1987) 1,25-Dihydroxyvitamin D_3 induces collagen binding to the human monocyte line U937. J Clin Invest 80:962–969

75. Dinarello CL, Ikejima T, Warner SJC, Orencole SF, Lonneman G, Cannon JG, Libby P (1987) Interleukin-1 induces interleukin-1. I. Induction of circulating interleukin-1 in rabbits in vivo and in human mononuclear cells in vitro. J Immunol 139:1902–1908

76. Oursler MJ, Cortese C, Keeting P, Anderson MA, Bonde SK, Riggs BL, Spelsberg TC (1991) Modulation of transforming growth factor-beta production in normal human osteoblast-like cells by 17 beta-estradiol and parathyroid hormone. Endocrinology 129:3313–3320

77. Turner RT, Riggs BL, Spelsberg TC (1994) Skeletal effects of estrogen. Endocr Rev 15:275–300

78. Pacifici R, Vannice JL, Rifas L, Kimble RB (1993) Monocytic secretion of interleukin-1 receptor antagonist in normal and osteoporotic women: effect of menopause and estrogen/progesterone therapy. J Clin Endocrinol Metab 77:1135–1141

79. Tan P, Shore A, Leary P, Keystone EC (1984) Interleukin abnormalities in recently active rheumatoid arthritis. J Rheumatol 11:593–596

80. Fakih H, Baggett B, Holtz G, Tsang K-Y, Lee JC, Williamson HO (1987) Interleukin 1: a possible role in the infertility associated with endometriosis. Fertil Steril 47:213–217

81. Pacifici R, Rothstein M, Rifas L, Lau KH, Baylink DJ, Avioli LV, Hruska K (1990) Increased monocyte interleukin-1 activity and decreased vertebral bone density in patients with fasting idiopathic hypercalciuria. J Clin Endocrinol Metab 71:138–145

82. Sambrook PN, Reeve J (1988) Bone disease in rheumatoid arthritis. Clin Sci 74:225–230

83. Comite F, Delman M, Hutchinson-Williams K, DeCherney AH, Jensen P (1989) Reduced bone mass in reproductive-aged women with endometriosis. J Clin Endocrinol Metab 69:837–842

84. Pacifici R (1997) Idiopathic hypercalciuria and osteoporosis. Distinct clinical manifestations of increased cytokine-induced bone resorption? J Clin Endocrinol Metab 82:29–31

85. Ralston SH (1994) Analysis of gene expression in human bone biopsies by polymerase chain reaction: evidence for enhanced cytokine expression in postmenopausal osteoporosis. J Bone Miner Res 9:883–890

86. Cohen-Solal ME, Graulet AM, Denne MA, Gueris J, Baylink D, de Vernejoul MC (1993) Peripheral monocyte culture supernatants of menopausal women can induce bone resorption: Involvement of cytokines. J Clin Endocrinol Metab 77:1648–1653

87. Pottratz ST, Bellido T, Mocharia H, Crabb D, Manolagas S (1994) 17β-Estradiol inhibits expression of human interleukin-6 promoter-reporter constructs by a receptor-dependent mechanism. J Clin Invest 93:944–950

88. Ray A, Prefontaine KE, Ray P (1994) Down-modulation of interleukin-6 gene expression by 17 beta-estradiol in the absence of high affinity DNA binding by the estrogen receptor. J Biol Chem 269:12940–12946

89. Stein B, Yang MX (1995) Repression of the interleukin-6 promoter by estrogen receptor is mediated by NF-kappa-B and C/EBP beta. Mol Cell Biol 15:4971–4979

90. Rickard D, Russell G, Gowen M (1992) Oestradiol inhibits the release of tumour necrosis factor but not interleukin 6 from adult human osteoblasts in vitro. Osteoporosis Int 2:94–102

91. Chaudhary LR, Spelsberg TC, Riggs BL (1992) Production of various cytokines by normal human osteoblast-like cells in response to interleukin-1β and

tumor necrosis factor-α: lack of regulation by 17β-estradiol. Endocrinology 130:2528–2534

92. Girasole G, Pedrazzoni M, Giuliani N, Passeri G, Passeri M (1995) Increased serum soluble interleukin-6 receptor levels are induced by ovariectomy, prevented by estrogen replacement and reversed by alendronate administration. J Bone Miner Res 10:A86

93. McKane R, Khosla S, Peterson J, Egan K, Riggs BL (1993) Effect of age and menopause on serum interleukin-1β and intereleukin-6- levels in women. J Bone Miner Res 8:162A

94. Khosla S, Peterson JM, Egan K, Jones JD, Riggs LB (1994) Circulating cytokine levels in osteoporotic and normal women. J Clin Endocrinol Metab 79:707–711

95. Kimble RB, Matayoshi AB, Vannice JL, Kung VT, Williams C, Pacifici R (1995) Simultaneous block of interleukin-1 and tumor necrosis factor is required to completely prevent bone loss in the early post-ovariectomy period. Endocrinology 136:3054–3061

96. Kimble RB, Vannice JL, Bloedow DC, Thompson RC, Hopfer W, Kung V, Brownfield C, Pacifici R (1994) Interleukin-1 receptor antagonist decreases bone loss and bone resorption in ovariectomized rats. J Clin Invest 93:1959–1967

97. Kimble RB, Matayoshi AB, Vannice JL, Pacifici R (1994) Long-term treatment with IL-1 receptor antagonist (IL-1ra) blocks bone loss in ovariectomized rats. J Bone Miner Res 9: (in press) (abstract)

98. Kimble RB, Bain SD, Pacifici R (1997) The functional block of TNF but not of IL-6 prevents bone loss in ovariectomized mice. J Bone Miner Res 12:935–941

99. Ammann P, Garcia I, Rizzoli R, Meyer JM, Vassali P, Bonjour JP (1995) Transgenic mice expressing high levels of soluble tumor necrosis factor receptor-1 fusion protein are protected from bone loss caused by estrogen deficiency. J Bone Miner Res 10 [Suppl 1]:1 (abstract)

100. Wronski TJ, Dann LM, Qi H, Yen CF (1993) Skeletal effects of withdrawal of estrogen and diphosphonate treatment in ovariectomized rats. Calcif Tissue Int 53:210–216

101. Kimble RB, Vannice JL, Brownfield C, Pacifici R (1994) Persistent bone-sparing effect of interleukin-1 receptor antagonist: a hypothesis on the role of IL-1 in ovariectomy induced bone loss. Calcif Tissue Int 55:260–265

102. Routtenberg A (1995) Knockout mouse fault lines (letter). Nature 374:314–315

103. Pacifici R (1992) Is there a causal role of IL-1 in postmenopausal bone loss? Calcif Tissue Int 50:295–299

104. Bellido T, Girasole G, Passeri G, Yu X P, Mocharla A, Jilka RL, Notides A, Manolagas SC (1993) Demonstration of estrogen and vitamin D receptors in bone marrow-derived stromal cells: up-regulation of the estrogen receptor by 1,25-dihydroxyvitamin-D3. Endocrinology 133:553–562

105. Oursler MJ, Osdoby P, Pyfferoen J, Riggs BL, Spelsberg TC (1991) Avian osteoclasts as estrogen target cells. Proc Natl Acad Sci USA 88:6613–6617

106. Oursler MJ, Pederson L, Pyfferoen J, Osdoby P, Fitzpatrick L, Spelsberg TC (1993) Estrogen modulation of avian osteoclast lysosomal gene expression. Endocrinology 132:1373–1380
107. Horowitz M (1993) Cytokines and estrogen in bone: anti-osteoporotic effects. Science 260:626–627
108. Kimble RB, Srivastava S, Ross FP, Matayoshi A, Pacifici R (1996) Estrogen deficiency increases the ability of stromal cells to support osteoclastogenesis via an IL-1 and TNF mediated stimulation of M-CSF production. J Biol Chem 271:28890–28897
109. Bellido T, Girasole G, Passeri G, Jilka RL, Manolagas SC (1994) gp130 mRNA is increased by PTH and cytokines and decreased by sex steroids in stromal/osteoblastic cells. J Bone Miner Res 9:12 (abstract)

4 Growth Factors and the Skeleton

E. Canalis

Introduction

Bone remodeling is a process regulated by systemic hormones and locally synthesized factors. Bone remodeling consists of bone resorption and bone formation. These two functions are coupled, and local factors are probably important in the coupling of the resorptive and forming phases of bone remodeling. Agents that regulate bone formation may act either by increasing or decreasing the number of cells available to form new bone or by modifying the differentiated function of the bone forming cell, the osteoblast. Similarly, bone resorption can be regulated by agents that alter the number of osteoclasts or modify the function of these cells. The number of mature osteoblasts or osteoclasts can be regulated by increasing or decreasing the replication of precursor cells or by altering their differentiation into mature cells.

Hormones regulate bone formation and bone resorption, acting directly on skeletal cells, or modifying the synthesis or activity of locally produced factors (Canalis 1983). Skeletal cells synthesize insulin-like growth factors (IGF) I and II, transforming growth factors (TGF) β_1, β_2, and β_3, acidic and basic fibroblast growth factors (FGFs), platelet-derived growth factors (PDGFs) AA and BB, selected bone morphogenetic proteins (BMPs), or osteogenic proteins and a variety of cytokines (Canalis et al. 1993b). Selected cytokines have an important function in immune responses and are relevant to changes in bone resorption but play a limited role in the regulation of bone formation (Goldring and Goldring 1991). Frequently, growth factors synthesized by skeletal cells are also present in the systemic circulation. IGF I and IGF II circulate in serum bound to IGF binding proteins (IGFBPs), primarily IGFBP-3, and an acid labile subunit (Daughaday and Rotwein 1989). The source of the circulating IGF is the liver and the serum levels of IGF I and IGFBP-3 are growth hormone-dependent. The synthesis of IGF I in extrahepatic tissues is dependent on other hormones and growth factors. For example, in endometrial cells IGF I synthesis is increased by estrogens and in bone by estrogens and parathyroid hormone (PTH) (Ernst and Rodan 1991; McCarthy et al. 1989a). Selected growth factors such as PDGF and TGF-β are present in platelet granules and are released following platelet aggregation (Hart et al. 1990). This may suggest that they play a role in wound and fracture healing (Canalis 1996). Locally synthesized growth factors act either in an autocrine or in a paracrine fashion. Autocrine factors act on the cell of origin whereas paracrine factors act on adjacent cells. Growth factors regulate bone formation by modifying cell number or the differentiated function of the osteoblast. Some factors, such as IGFs, have limited mitogenic properties and act mostly by enhancing the differentiated function of the osteoblast. Other factors, such as PDGF, are primarily mitogens with limited activity on the differentiated function of the osteoblast (Canalis et al. 1993b).

A number of models have been developed to study the actions of growth factors in the skeletal system. Primary cultures of skeletal cells or of cell lines and organ cultures can be used to define their effects in vitro. Topical and systemic administration of growth factors can be used to determine their effects in vivo. Transgenic animals in which growth factors are overexpressed are also useful to define the actions of a growth factor in vivo. In this model a factor can be expressed in a specific cell by driving its gene with a cell-specific promoter. For instance, genes driven by the osteocalcin promoter are selectively expressed in osteoblasts. Gene disruption or knockout models define the phenotype of animals not expressing a gene and allow its function to be determined. The combination of in vitro and in vivo models has allowed investigators to define the function of growth factors in the skeletal system.

Platelet-Derived Growth Factors

PDGF is a polypeptide growth factor with a molecular mass of 30 000 (Heldin and Westermark 1993). There are two PDGF genes: PDGF A and B, and the mature PDGF polypeptide consists of two chains, which can be derived from either gene so that there are three possible PDGF isoforms: PDGF AA, BB, and AB (Betsholtz et al. 1986; Collins et al. 1985). The three isoforms have similar biological activity although PDGF BB is more potent than PDGF AA, and PDGF AB has intermediate potency (Canalis 1996; Centrella et al. 1991c). PDGF has a variety of actions in bone cells. PDGF stimulates bone cell replication, and as a result of its mitogenic actions PDGF increases the number of cells that synthesize bone collagen and noncollagen protein (Canalis et al. 1989b). However, on a cellular basis PDGF does not increase bone collagen and noncollagen protein synthesis. Histomorphometric analysis of calvariae labeled with [^{3}H]thymidine revealed that PDGF increases cell number although the effect is not specific to cells of the osteoblastic lineage (Hock and Canalis 1994). In fact close analysis of histological sections of calvariae treated with PDGF suggests a decrease in the number of differentiated osteoblasts. These effects are correlated with a decrease in the differentiated function of the osteoblast by PDGF, and histomorphometric analysis of calvariae radiolabeled with [^{3}H]proline revealed a dose-dependent decrease in matrix apposition rates. Although the immediate effects of PDGF are to inhibit the differentiated osteoblast, it is probable that its mitogenic effect results in an increased number of cells, which have the potential to differentiate into mature osteoblasts. Consequently the acute or immediate effects of a growth factor, such as PDGF, may not reflect its chronic and more permanent actions. These may become more apparent following transient instead of continuous exposure of the bone tissue to a given factor since transient treatment may allow the recently replicated cells to differentiate into mature functioning cells.

PDGF does not modify type I collagen gene expression, but it induces the expression of matrix metalloproteinases (MMP) (Varghese et al. 1996). These are a family of proteases which include collagenases. There are three known collagenases: collagenase 1 secreted by stimulated human osteoblasts, collagenase 2 secreted by neutrophils, and collagenase 3 secreted by rat osteoblasts and carcinoma of the breast cells (Matrisian and Hogan 1990). PDGF induces the expression of collagenase 1 or MMP 1 in fibroblasts and of collagenase 3 or MMP 13 in rat osteoblasts (Chua et al. 1985; Varghese et al. 1996). The stimulatory effect of PDGF on collagenase 3 transcripts in osteoblasts is dose and time dependent and is observed with PDGF BB but not with PDGF AA. PDGF BB also increases protease levels in the culture medium. The effect of PDGF on collagenase 3 expression occurs by transcriptional and posttranscriptional mechanisms (Varghese et al. 1996). PDGF increases collagenase 3 heterogeneous nuclear RNA (hnRNA) or unspliced RNA and the rates of gene transcription. PDGF also prolongs the half-life and stabilizes collagenase 3 mRNA in transcriptionally arrested osteoblasts. As a consequence of the increase in collagenase PDGF stimulates bone collagen degradation (Canalis et al. 1989b).

In addition to its effects on the collagen matrix, PDGF BB increases bone resorption (Cochran et al. 1993; Tashjian et al. 1982). The mechanism of the PDGF effect on bone resorption has not been explored and may involve the induction of prostaglandin E_2 in bone. PDGF also increases the expression of interleukin (IL) 6 mRNA and protein levels in osteoblast cultures (Franchimont and Canalis 1995). IL-6 increases bone resorption by increasing the recruitment of osteoclasts, and the stimulation of IL-6 synthesis by PDGF may be mechanistically relevant to its stimulatory effect on bone resorption (Tamura et al. 1993). The effect of PDGF on IL-6 expression is dose dependent, occurs immediately after exposure to the growth factor, and involves transcriptional mechanisms. PDGF increases IL-6 hnRNA levels, the rates of transcription and the activity of IL-6 promoter constructs transiently transfected into osteoblasts. IL-6 synthesis is autoregulated, and following its initial secretion the positive feedback may result in the production of significant concentrations of IL-6 in the bone microenvironment.

The effects of PDGF on bone metabolism in vivo have been examined in ovariectomized rats, and the results obtained are compatible with the actions observed in vitro (Mitlak et al. 1996). Systemically administered PDGF prevents bone loss in ovariectomized rats and increases bone mineral density. PDGF causes an increase in the number of osteoblasts but does not change the number of osteoclasts. This may be because osteoclastogenesis is already activated in conditions of estrogen deficiency where increased IL-6 secretion is present (Jilka et al. 1992). The systemic administration of PDGF to rodents causes fibrosis in extraskeletal tissues, a result consistent with the in vitro effects of PDGF in fibroblasts. There are no studies on the overexpression of PDGF A or B genes in osteoblasts. Disruption of the PDGF B or the PDGF-β receptor gene in mice results in hematological abnormalities, dilated heart, and impaired glomerular tuft formation in the kidney (Leveen et al. 1994; Soriano 1994). The knockout mice suffer premature death, but no skeletal abnormalities were found, suggesting that PDGF does not play a role in skeletal development in rodents. Examination of the actions of PDGF in vitro and in vivo suggests that PDGF plays a role in the remodeling of mature bone, particularly in the early phases of fracture healing. Following a fracture there is release of PDGF by the aggregating platelet with a consequent increase in cell replication. This serves to restore cells necessary for healing. The effects of PDGF on collagen degradation and resorption are also important in the early phases of fracture healing since bone fragments at the fracture site need to be resorbed before the process of fracture repair is underway. The lack of a stimulatory effect on the differentiated function of the osteoblast by PDGF suggests that this factor is not important in the maintenance of skeletal tissue and bone mass under physiological conditions. Furthermore, while PDGF is synthesized by normal osteoblasts, it is present at fracture sites, and its primary source is the circulating platelet, from where PDGF is released following injury and platelet aggregation (Andrew et al. 1995; Hart et al. 1990).

Normal osteoblasts as well as osteosarcoma cell lines express the PDGF A and B genes (Betsholtz et al. 1986; Graves et al. 1984, 1989; Rydziel et al. 1994; Rydziel and Canalis 1996). Peptide hormones, steroid and thyroid hormones do not regulate the synthesis of PDGF. The synthesis of PDGF is regulated by other growth factors (Rydziel et al. 1994; Rydziel and Canalis 1996). PDGF A mRNA and PDGF AA protein levels are increased by PDGF AA and BB and TGF-β. The autoregulation of PDGF AA may be important to produce significant levels of PDGF AA in the bone microenvironment once that its initial synthesis is induced, possibly by PDGF and TGF-β released from platelet granules after platelet aggregation. It is important to note that the levels of PDGF AA in the bone microenvironment are in the picomolar range (Rydziel et al. 1994). Consequently other factors may be necessary to obtain biologically active PDGF AA at the bone site. PDGF B transcripts are increased by TGF-β acting by transcriptional mechanisms (Rydziel and Canalis 1996). TGF-β increases the rates of gene transcription without modifying the half life of PDGF B mRNA in osteoblasts. In contrast to TGF-β, other growth factors such as PDGF BB, basic FGF, and IGF do not modify the expression of PDGF B transcripts in osteoblasts.

Osteoblasts express PDGF-α and -β receptors (Centrella et al. 1992). PDGF BB binds to both receptors whereas PDGF AA binds primarily to the PDGF-α receptor. Cytokines, such as IL-1 and tumor necrosis factor-α modify the binding and activity of PDGF AA to its receptor in rat osteoblasts (Centrella et al. 1992; Gilardetti et al. 1991; Kose et al. 1996; Tsukamoto et al. 1991). Since IL-1 and tumor necrosis factor-α are secreted during inflammation, it is possible that they modify the activity of PDGF AA in the bone microenvironment in conditions of inflammation. TGF-β decreases the binding of PDGF AA to osteoblasts. There are no specific binding proteins for PDGF. However, PDGF B chains bind to osteonectin or secreted protein acidic rich in cysteine (SPARC), and SPARC selectively blocks their activity (Lane and Sage 1994; Raines et al. 1992). The bone matrix is an abundant source of osteonectin or SPARC and glucocorticoids increase its expression in osteoblastic cells, whereas basic FGF is inhibitory (Ng et al. 1989). Changes in the abundance of osteonectin could modify the activity of PDGF B chains in bone.

At the present time there are no known skeletal diseases caused by mutations or activation of the PDGF A or B gene or the PDGF-α or PDGF-β receptor gene. PDGF has not been administered to humans and its value as a therapeutic agent is uncertain.

Fibroblast Growth Factors

FGFs are a family of at least nine genes encoding polypeptides with heparin binding properties (Baird and Klagsbrun 1991; Burgess and Maciag 1989). Acidic and basic FGF have a molecular mass of approximately 17 000 and are expressed by bone cells (Abraham et al. 1986; Globus et al. 1989). Basic and acidic FGF have similar biological activities in osteoblast cultures although basic FGF tends to be more potent than acidic FGF. In skeletal and nonskeletal cells the activity of FGF is enhanced by heparin, which induces dimerization of FGF receptors (McCarthy et al. 1989c; Faham et al. 1996). Basic and acidic FGF have mitogenic properties for cells of the osteoblastic lineage. As a consequence of an increased cell number FGFs increase protein synthesis. However, similarly to the actions of PDGF, neither acidic nor basic FGF causes an acute stimulatory effect on the differentiated function of the osteoblast (Hurley et al. 1993). Basic FGF inhibits type I collagen synthesis and alkaline phosphatase activity in osteoblast cultures, suggesting an inhibition of the differentiated function of this cell (Hurley et al. 1993; McCarthy et al. 1989a,b,c). It is important to note that cells that replicate under the influence of FGF can eventually differentiate into mature osteoblasts (Canalis et al. 1988). When intact calvariae are exposed to FGF for limited periods of time, collagen synthesis is increased following the removal of the growth factor, suggesting that cells dividing under the influence of FGF can differentiate into collagen producing osteoblasts. Similar to PDGF BB, basic FGF causes a time and dose-dependent increase in the expression of collagenase 3 in osteoblast cultures (Varghese et al. 1995). Basic FGF increases collagenase expression by transcriptional mechanisms and its actions involve protein kinase C dependent pathways. Acidic FGF has not been examined for its effects on collagenase expression.

The actions of FGF in vivo have been examined in an experimental fracture model in the rat (Kawaguchi et al. 1994). The administration of basic FGF resulted in accelerated fracture repair, and increased bone mineral content and bone strength at the fracture site. These effects were observed both in normal rats and in animals with experimental diabetes. These in vivo studies indicate a potential role for FGF in fracture healing, and a possible therapeutic value in this condition. It is probable that if growth factors, such as FGFs, are used to accelerate fracture repair, they will be applied topically since their systemic administration could result in nonspecific effects at extraskeletal sites and in serious side effects. An alternative would be the targeting of a growth factor to the skeletal tissue.

Transgenic animals overexpressing the basic FGF gene driven by the phosphoglycerase kinase promoter express a number of skeletal abnormalities (Coffin et al. 1995). These include chondrodysplasia, which is characterized by enlargement of the growth plate due to chondrocyte hyperplasia and increased extracellular matrix, as well as absence of chondrocytes in the differentiating zone. Mice overexpressing FGF have short and flat bones and macrocephaly. The counterpart of this phenotype is observed in mice with disruption of the FGF receptor 3 gene (Deng et al. 1996). These mice have abnormal endochondral ossification due to enhanced and prolonged endochondral bone growth secondary to an increase in proliferating and hypertrophic chondrocytes. Consequently bones of mice with FGF receptor 3 disruption are longer than those of wild-type animals indicating that the FGF receptor 3 is a negative regulator of bone growth that limits endochondral ossification.

Basic and acidic FGF, like PDGF, are regulated at the level of synthesis, receptor binding and possibly binding proteins. However, there is limited information about the regulation of acidic and basic FGF in skeletal cells. The synthesis of basic FGF in osteoblasts is increased by TGF-β and FGF itself (Hurley et al. 1994). Since PDGF increases the synthesis of FGF in nonskeletal cells, it is possible that it has similar effects in osteoblasts, although these have not been explored. There are four FGF receptors, but studies on their expression and regulation in skeletal cells have not been reported. A number of binding proteins or low-affinity FGF receptors can regulate the effective levels of FGF in various cellular systems, but there is no information about their synthesis and actions in bone.

There are various clinical disorders secondary to mutations of FGF receptor genes. Mutations of the extracellular domain of the FGF receptor 1 gene results in Pfeiffer's syndrome, which is characterized by craniosynostosis, resulting in a characteristic short tower head, widespread eyes and small nose, broad thumbs and toes, and syndactyly (Muenke et al. 1994). Mutations of the extracellular domain of the FGF receptor 2 gene result in Crouzon's syndrome, which is characterized by craniosynostosis with abnormal skull shape and proptosis (Reardon et al. 1994). Mutations of the extracellular domain of the FGF receptor 2 gene may also result in Jackson-Weiss syndrome, which is characterized by abnormal skull shape and hand and foot abnormalities. Mutations of the transmembrane domain of the FGF 3 receptor gene cause achondroplasia, the most common form of dwarfism, and macrocephaly (Shiang et al. 1994). In achondroplasia the FGF receptor 3 is activated in the absence of FGF, resulting in a negative regulation of skeletal growth.

Transforming Growth Factors-β

The TGF-β superfamily of polypeptides, consists of a group of proteins, which include TGF-β and the BMPs or osteogenic proteins (Barnard et al. 1990; Celeste et al. 1990; Kingsley 1994; Wang et al. 1990; Wozney et al. 1988). TGF-βs are polypeptides with an approximate molecular mass of 25 000, and are homodimers or heterodimers of the products of the TGF-β_1, -β_2, and -β_3 genes. TGF-β is secreted in an inactive form as a propetide bound to a binding protein (Miyazono et al. 1988). There are five TGF-β genes, and the genes for TGF-β_1, -β_2, and -β_3 are expressed by mammalian cells, including those of the skeletal tissue (Ogawa et al. 1992). The various isoforms of TGF-β have similar biological activity in osteoblasts and nonskeletal cells (Centrella et al. 1991b; Ten Dijke et al. 1990). In addition to TGF-β, multiple BMP genes have been reported. BMPs play a role in embryonic development and selected BMPs are expressed by skeletal cells. TGF-β has a dose-dependent biphasic mitogenic effect in osteoblasts (Centrella et al. 1987). The stimulation of cell replication is selective to cells of the osteoblastic lineage and in most cell cultures TGF-β inhibits cell division. In fact, TGF-β inhibits bone resorption probably by inducing osteoclast apoptosis (Chenu et al. 1988). TGF-β also increases type I collagen synthesis, acting by transcriptional mechanisms, but it does not increase all aspects of the differentiated function of the osteoblast since it does not stimulate alkaline phosphatase activity in cultured normal osteoblasts. Bone histomorphometric analysis of cultured calvariae revealed that TGF-β increases the replication of cells of the osteoblastic lineage and stimulates bone matrix apposition rates (Hock et al. 1990). These studies confirm that TGF-β enhances bone formation. BMPs have similar actions to those of TGF-β, although they likely act through different receptors (Penton et al. 1994). A difference between the effects of BMPs and TGF-β is the fact that BMPs induce the differentiation of cells of the osteoblastic lineage and enhance all parameters of the differentiated function of the osteoblast, including alkaline phosphatase activity (Chen et al. 1991).

TGF-β inhibits the expression of collagenase 1 or MMP 1 in fibroblast cultures acting by transcriptional mechanisms (Edwards et al. 1987). Similarly, TGF-β inhibits collagenase 3 or MMP 13 mRNA and protease levels in rat osteoblasts (Rydziel et al. 1997). The effect of TGF-β is time and dose dependent, and it is observed at picomolar concentrations of the growth factor. TGF-β inhibits collagenase 3 expression both by transcriptional and posttranscriptional mechanisms, since it inhibits the rates of transcription and destabilizes collagenase transcripts. The half-life of collagenase 3 is approximately 6 h in control transcriptionally arrested osteoblasts and less than 2 h in osteoblasts exposed to TGF-β. The gene elements responsible for the transcriptional effect of TGF-β on collagenase 3 lay in the region of −180 to +56, whereas the elements responsible for the destabilization of collagenase 3 transcripts have not been defined. BMP-2 also inhibits collagenase 3 mRNA and protease levels in rat osteoblasts (Varghese et al., unpublished observations). The effect is similar to that of TGF-β although BMP-2 does not destabilize collagenase 3 transcripts and acts solely by transcriptional mechanisms.

In vivo TGF-β has been administered topically and systemically to young and adult rats (Kalu et al. 1993; Rosen et al. 1994). In both circumstances TGF-β increased bone formation. In vivo TGF-β does not modify osteoclast number. Animals with disruption of the TGF-β1 gene develop a multifocal inflammatory disease affecting multiple tissues including the heart, the gastrointestinal system, and muscle (Shull et al. 1992). This inflammatory disease is characterized by tissue invasion of neutrophils and lymphocytes. In addition, TGF-β1 knockout mice have developmental retardation, defective vasculogenesis with inadequate capillary formation and defective hematopoiesis. However, they do not have skeletal abnormalities. Transgenic mice overexpressing the TGF-$β_2$ gene in osteoblasts have increased bone matrix, but decreased mineralization with consequent bone loss (Erlebacher and Derynck 1996). This phenotype, indicative of osteoporosis and in discrepancy with other known effects of TGF-β, has no obvious explanation. However, in the transgenic model the effects of TGF-β are examined in embryonic life and may represent developmental changes. In vivo, BMPs induce endochondral bone formation when implanted in soft tissues in the presence of demineralized bone pellets or of matrix carriers, indicating a role in endochondral ossification (Wang et al. 1990). Mice with disruption of the BMP-7 gene develop abnormalities in eye and kidney development but no obvious skeletal defects (Dudley et al. 1995; Luo et al. 1995).

In skeletal cells TGF-β is regulated at the level of synthesis, activation, and receptor binding. TGF-β is secreted as a large molecular weight complex consisting of TGF-β, a precursor peptide, and a binding protein (Miyazono et al. 1988). TGF-β is secreted in an inactive form and a way to regulate this growth factor is by activation. Bone resorbing hormones, such as PTH, and glucocorticoids activate TGF-β (Oursler et al. 1993; Pfeilschifter and Mundy 1987). Skeletal cells synthesize TGF-$β_1$, $β_2$, and $β_3$ although most studies carried out to examine the regulation of TGF-β synthesis and activity have examined the regulation of TGF-$β_1$. Basic FGF, TGF-β, and estrogens increase TGF-β1 synthesis (Kim et al. 1989; Liu et al. 1996; Noda and Vogel 1989; Oursler et al. 1991; van Obberghen- Schilling et al. 1988). TGF-β also can be regulated by changes in receptor binding. Osteoblasts express TGF-β I and II receptors, and both receptors are necessary for TGF-β signal transduction (Centrella et al. 1991a; Chen et al. 1993; Ebner et al. 1993; Laiho et al. 1990; Massague 1996). In addition, osteoblasts express betaglycan, which binds TGF-β, but has no signal transducing properties. Glucocorticoids increase the synthesis of betaglycan and shift the binding of TGF-β from signal transducing receptors I and II to betaglycan (Centrella et al. 1991a; Nakayama et al. 1994). As a consequence of this shift glucocorticoids oppose the biological actions of TGF-β on DNA and protein synthesis, possibly explaining some of the inhibitory actions of glucocorticoids on bone cell function. Other hormones, such as PTH, also regulate the binding of TGF-β to osteoblasts (Centrella et al. 1988).

No skeletal disorders have been associated to mutations in the genes of the members of the TGF-β family of peptides or of their receptors. A cross-sectional study demonstrated decreased concentrations of TGF-β in cortical bone of aging individuals (Nicolas et al. 1994). This finding as well as the demonstration of decreased TGF-β levels in bone from estrogen deficient animals suggests a possible role for TGF-β in the pathogenesis of osteoporosis (Finkelman et al. 1992). Overexpression of BMP-4 has been detected in lymphocytes from patients with fibrodysplasia ossificans progressiva (Shafritz et al. 1996).

Insulin-Like Growth Factors I and II

IGF I and IGF II are single-chain related polypeptides with a molecular mass of approximately 7500 (Daughaday and Rotwein 1989). IGFs are present in the systemic circulation bound to IGF binding proteins and an acid labile subunit. IGF I and IGF II are expressed by osteoblasts and osteoclasts and act as autocrine and paracrine regulators of bone cell function (Delany et al. 1994; Middleton et al. 1995). IGF I and IGF II are among the most abundant growth factors secreted by skeletal cells, and their levels in osteoblast cultures are in the nanomolar range. IGFs have important effects on bone cell function. IGF I is somewhat more potent than IGF II although both growth factors have similar actions (McCarthy et al. 1989b). IGFs increase the replication of cells of the osteoblastic lineage and these cells are capable of expressing the phenotype of the differentiated osteoblast. IGFs also enhance the function of the mature osteoblast, increasing the transcription of type I collagen and the synthesis of osteocalcin. Histomorphometric analysis of cultured calvariae confirms the modest mitogenic effect of IGF I and demonstrates that IGF I has an independent stimulatory effect on bone matrix apposition rates indicating that it enhances bone formation (Hock et al. 1988).

IGF I and IGF II inhibit collagenase 3 synthesis by the osteoblast, acting by transcriptional mechanisms (Canalis et al. 1995). As a consequence of this effect IGF I and IGF II inhibit bone collagen degradation. Therefore IGFs not only enhance bone matrix synthesis, but they also prevent its degradation and have a dual role in the maintenance of bone matrix. Recent studies from our laboratory revealed that IGFs are autologous suppressors of collagenase 3 expression (Delany et al. 1996). In experiments in which endogenous IGFs were blocked by the use of IGF neutralizing antibodies or of IGFBPs in excess, there was an overexpression of collagenase by the osteoblast. In addition, cells that do not express IGF I or IGF II, such as osteosarcoma cells, overexpress collagenase when compared to normal osteoblasts (Okazaki et al. 1995). This indicates an inverse correlation between collagenase and IGF I expression and confirms an autocrine role for IGFs in the down regulation of collagenase by osteoblastic cells.

The systemic administration of IGF I to normal rats causes a modest increase in bone formation. In unloaded rats IGF I has a more pronounced effect and increases bone formation, bone mineral apposition, and bone mineral density (Machwate et al. 1994). Administration of IGF I coupled to IGFBP-3 seems to be more effective, possibly because IGFBP-3 prevents the degradation of IGF I and prolongs its half life (Bagi et al. 1994). In humans the administration of IGF I causes an increase in serum levels of procollagen peptides, indicating an increase in bone formation, and in the urinary excretion of collagen cross-links, indicating enhanced collagen degradation and bone turnover. Transgenic animals overexpressing IGF I develop overgrowth, whereas IGF I or IGF II gene disruption results in dwarfism (Liu et al. 1993; DeChiara et al. 1990).

Skeletal IGF I and IGF II are regulated by changes in synthesis, receptor binding, and binding proteins. In osteoblasts IGF I synthesis is regulated by systemic hormones and local growth factors, whereas the synthesis of IGF II is modified by growth factors and not by hormones (Delany et al. 1994). PTH as well as other cyclic AMP inducers are major stimulators of IGF I expression in osteoblasts, and IGF I mediates the stimulatory effect of intermittent PTH on collagen synthesis in calvarial cultures (Canalis et al. 1989a). Estrogens also increase IGF I synthesis by osteoblasts whereas glucocorticoids are inhibitory (Delany and Canalis 1995; Ernst and Rodan 1991). This inhibition of IGF I synthesis by glucocorticoids occurs at the transcriptional level and may be important in the mechanism of the inhibitory action of these steroids on bone formation. Skeletal growth factors with mitogenic properties for cells of the osteoblastic lineage, such as TGF-β, PDGF BB, and basic FGF, inhibit IGF I and IGF II mRNA and protein levels in osteoblasts (Canalis et al. 1993a; Gabbitas et al. 1994). This inhibitory effect is not due to their mitogenic properties and is observed when the growth factors are tested in the presence or absence of the DNA synthesis inhibitor hydroxyurea. Growth factors that inhibit the differentiated function of the osteoblast, such as PDGF BB and basic FGF, inhibit the expression of IGF I and IGF II. In contrast, agents that enhance the differentiated function of the osteoblast, such as BMP-2, increase IGF I and IGF II expression (Canalis and Gabbitas 1994). These observations suggest that IGF I and IGF II not only are important in the maintenance of bone formation but are also relevant to the expression of the osteoblastic phenotype.

Osteoblasts express IGF I and IGF II receptors (Centrella et al. 1990). The IGF I receptor binds and mediates the anabolic actions of IGF I and IGF II in nonskeletal cells, and this is probably also the case in osteoblasts (Ewton et al. 1987; Furlanetto et al. 1987). The function of the IGF II receptor is less certain (Nissley et al. 1993). It binds IGF II but not IGF I, and the phenotype of IGF II receptor knockout mice suggests that the IGF II receptor acts as an IGF II binding protein (Lau et al. 1994). Disruption of the IGF II receptor gene results in high serum levels of IGF II, animal overgrowth, and death. These abnormalities are not manifested in mice with a disruption of the IGF II receptor and of the IGF II gene. This suggests that excessive IGF II is responsible for the manifestations observed in IGF II receptor knockout mice and that the IGF II receptor acts as a binding protein for IGF II. Glucocorticoids inhibit IGF II receptor transcription in osteoblasts, whereas vitamin D increases the binding of IGF I (Kurose et al. 1990; Rydziel and Canalis 1995).

Skeletal cells synthesize the six known IGFBPs (Delany et al. 1994; Hassager et al. 1992; Rechler 1993). IGFBP-1 is important in glucose homeostasis and in skeletal cells its synthesis is induced by glucocorticoids and decreased by insulin (Conover et al. 1996). IGFBP-2 is one of the most abundant binding proteins secreted by skeletal cells and at high doses it inhibits aspects of bone cell function. There is limited information on the regulation of IGFBP-2 synthesis in bone (McCarthy et al. 1994). IGFBP-3 is the most abundant circulating IGFBP, and at high doses it inhibits aspects of bone cell function (Raisz et al. 1993). However, under selected experimental conditions IGFBP-3 has stimulatory effects (Conover 1992). The synthesis of IGFBP-3 in osteoblasts is enhanced by growth hormone, vitamin D_3, and prostaglandin E_2 (McCarthy et al. 1994; Moriwake et al. 1992). IGFBP-4 is the most important inhibitory binding protein secreted by osteoblasts, and its levels are increased by PTH (LaTour et al. 1990; Mohan et al. 1995). IGFBP-5 is the only binding protein that increases bone cell growth and enhances the stimulatory effects of IGF I in bone (Andress and Birnbaum 1992). IGFBP-5 expression is maximal during active phases of bone cell replication and declines during cell differentiation (Thrailkill et al. 1995). The synthesis of IGFBP-5 is regulated by systemic hormones and by local growth factors. Glucocorticoids inhibit IGFBP-5 expression by transcriptional mechanisms and the elements responsible are located in the −70 to +120 region of the IGFBP-5 gene (Gabbitas et al. 1996). Mutations of the E-box contained in this region obliterate the inhibitory effects of glucocorticoids on IGFBP-5 transcription indicating that E-box consensus sequences are responsible for the inhibitory effect of glucocorticoids. Agents that induce osteoblastic differentiation, such as retinoic acid, or agents that enhance the differentiated function of the osteoblast, such as IGF I, increase IGFBP-5 expression by transcriptional mechanisms (Dong and Canalis 1995). IGF I also stabilizes the protein. Since IGFBP-5 stimulates bone cell growth and enhances the effects of IGF I this may be a positive feedback mechanism to increase the stimulatory actions of IGF I on bone formation. In contrast, skeletal growth factors with mitogenic properties, such as TGF-β, basic FGF, and PDGF BB decrease IGFBP-5 transcription (Canalis and Gabbitas 1995). This effect is correlated with an inhibition in IGF I and IGF II expression, suggesting a degree of coordination in the regulation of IGFBP-5 and IGF I and IGF II synthesis in osteoblasts (Canalis et al. 1993a; Gabbitas et al. 1994). This is confirmed by studies demonstrating that prostaglandin E_2 induces both IGF I and IGFBP-5 synthesis in osteoblasts (Pash et al. 1995; Pash and Canalis 1996). IGFBP-6 is secreted by osteoblasts, binds IGF II with 20–100 times more affinity than IGF I, and blocks the effects of IGF II on bone cell function (Kiefer et al. 1992). This selective trapping of IGF II by IGFBP-6 is a mode of regulating the amount of IGF II available to bone cells. The synthesis of IGFBP-6 is increased by retinoic acid and by glucocorticoids (Gabbitas and Canalis 1996a,b). Current information indicates that IGFBPs play a role in the transport of IGFs, increase their half-life, and modulate their activity and availability to target cells.

No metabolic bone disorders have been reported with mutations in the genes of IGF I, IGF II, their receptors, or binding proteins. Normally aging individuals have decreased levels of IGF I in serum and in cortical bone extracts, but no abnormalities in the synthesis or activity of IGF I or IGF II have been reported in osteoporosis (Hammerman 1987; Nicolas et al. 1994). IGF I but not IGF II has been administered to humans and causes an increase in bone remodeling (Ebeling et al. 1993).

Growth Factors and Clinical Medicine

It is apparent that selected growth factors, such as PDGF and FGF, have important mitogenic properties for bone cells and are likely important in wound and fracture healing. Other growth factors, such as IGFs appear to be more important in the maintenance of bone mass. It is conceivable that growth factors are relevant to the etiology of osteoporosis. There could be a decrease in the synthesis of selected growth factors, such as IGF I or IGF II, or abnormalities in receptor binding due to gene mutations in the receptors for selected growth factors. Changes in binding proteins are possible. There could be an increase in the levels of the inhibitory IGFBP-4 or a decrease in the levels of the stimulatory IGFBP-5. Since the distribution of IGFBPs is central to their actions in bone, changes in the distribution of selective binding proteins could result in changes in bone formation (Jones et al. 1993).

Growth factors can be used in the therapy of selected bone disorders. Their topical administration could enhance the process of fracture healing and bone repair. However, the value of the systemic administration of growth factors is somewhat uncertain, and it may be difficult to target them to bone cells. So far there is experience with the systemic administration of IGF I to humans. IGF I increases parameters of bone remodeling and may be of potential benefit in bone disorders (Ebeling et al. 1993; Grinspoon et al. 1995). However, it may need to be administered for limited periods of time. Prolonged exposure of nonskeletal tissues to IGF I may result in undesirable side effects. IGF I has the potential to cause hypoglycemia and causes salt and water retention with postural hypotension. IGF I has been administered for 2 years to children with growth hormone insensitivity syndrome. The adverse effects included lipohypertrophy at the injection site, thickening of soft tissues, increased intracranial pressure, thrombocytopenia, and hypokalemia (Backeljauw et al. 1996). Growth hormone is beneficial in the osteoporosis of patients with growth hormone deficiency, but less certain is its value in patients with idiopathic osteoporosis (Canalis 1995). Growth hormone counteracts the hypoglycemic effects of IGF I, and when administered simultaneously they have an additive generalized anabolic effect (Kupfer et al. 1993). This could suggest a possible benefit of combining IGF I and growth hormone therapy. An alternative to the administration of growth factors could be the use of agents that enhance the synthesis or activity of growth factors in bone. For instance, one could propose the use of parathyroid hormone or other cyclic AMP inducers selective to bone cells. PTH increases IGF I levels in the bone microenvironment and intermittent exposure of bones to PTH causes an increase in collagen synthesis, which is prevented by IGF antibodies (Canalis et al. 1989a). Administration of PTH to rats also causes increased bone formation, and in humans PTH increases serum levels of biochemical markers of bone formation and increases bone mineral density of the spine (Finkelstein et al. 1994; Reeve et al. 1991). Other therapeutic modalities could include agents that increase the receptor binding of local factors or that modify the synthesis or distribution of their binding proteins.

Acknowledgements. The work performed in the author's laboratory was supported by grants AR 21707 and DK 42424 from the National Institutes of Health. The author thanks Mrs. Margaret Nagle for valuable secretarial help.

References

Abraham JA, Whang JL, Tumolo A, Mergia A, Friedman J, Gospodarowicz J, Fiddes JC (1986) Human basic fibroblast growth factor: nucleotide sequence and genomic organization. EMBO J 5:2523–2528

Andress DL, Birnbaum RS (1992) Human osteoblast-derived insulin-like growth factor (IGF) binding protein-5 stimulates osteoblast mitogenesis and potentiates IGF action. J Biol Chem 267:22467–22472

Andrew JG, Hoyland JA, Freemont AJ, Marsh DR (1995) Platelet-derived growth factor expression in normally healing human fractures. Bone 16:455–460

Backeljauw PF, Underwood LE, the GHIS Collaborative Group (1996) Prolonged treatment with recombinant insulin-like growth factor-I in children with growth hormone insensitivity syndrome – a clinical research center study. J Clin Endocrinol Metab 81:3312–3317

Bagi CM, Brommage R, DeLeon L, Adams S, Rosen D, Sommer A (1994) Benefit of systemically administered rhIGF-I and rhIGF-IGFBP-3 on cancellous bone in ovariectomized rats. J Bone Miner Res 9:1301–1311

Baird A, Klagsbrun M (1991) The fibroblast growth factor family. Cancer Cells 3:239–243

Barnard JA, Lyons RM, Moses HL (1990) The cell biology of transforming growth factor β. Biochim Biophys Acta 1032:79–87

Betsholtz C, Johnsson A, C-H, Westermark B, Lind P, Urdea MS, Eddy R, Shows TB, Philpott K, Mellor AL, Knott TJ, Scott J (1986) cDNA sequence and chromosomal localization of human platelet-derived factor A-chain and its expression in tumor cell lines. Nature 320:695–699

Burgess WH, Maciag T (1989) The heparin-binding (fibroblast) growth factor family of proteins. Annu Rev Biochem 58:575–606

Canalis E (1983) The hormonal and local regulation of bone formation. Endocr Rev 4:62–77

Canalis E (1995) Growth hormone, skeletal growth factors and osteoporosis. Endocr Pract 1:39–43

Canalis E (1996) Platelet-derived growth factor and the skeleton. In: Bilezikian J, Raisz LG, Rodan GA (eds) Principles of bone biology. Academic, San Diego

Canalis E, Gabbitas B (1994) Bone morphogenetic protein-2 increases insulin-like growth factor I and II synthesis in bone cell cultures. J Bone Miner Res 9:1999–2005

Canalis E, Gabbitas B (1995) Skeletal growth factors regulate the synthesis of insulin-like growth factor binding protein-5 in bone cell cultures. J Biol Chem 270:10771–10776

Canalis E, Centrella M, McCarthy T (1988) Effects of basic fibroblast growth factor on bone formation vitro. J Clin Invest 81:1572–1577

Canalis E, Centrella M, Burch M, McCarthy TL (1989a) Insulin-like growth factor I mediates selected anabolic effects of parathyroid hormone in bone cultures. J Clin Invest 83:60–65

Canalis E, McCarthy TL, Centrella M (1989b) Effects of platelet-derived growth factor on bone formation in vitro. J Cell Physiol 140:530–537

Canalis E, Pash J, Gabbitas B, Rydziel S, Varghese S (1993a) Growth factors regulate the synthesis of insulin like growth factor I in bone cell cultures. Endocrinology 133:33–38

Canalis E, Pash J, Varghese S (1993b) Skeletal growth factors. Crit Rev Eukaryot Gene Expr 3:155–166

Canalis E, Rydziel S, Delany A, Varghese S, Jeffrey J (1995) Insulin-like growth factors inhibit interstitial collagenase synthesis in bone cell cultures. Endocrinology 136:1348–1354

Celeste AJ, Iannazzi JA, Taylor RC, Hewick RM, Rosen V, Wang EA, Wozney JM (1990) Identification of transforming growth factor β family members present in bone-inductive protein purified from bovine bone. Proc Natl Acad Sci USA 87:9843–9847

Centrella M, McCarthy TL, Canalis E (1987) Transforming growth factor beta is a bifunctional regulator of replication and collagen synthesis in osteoblast-enriched cell cultures from fetal rat bone. J Biol Chem 262:2869–2874

Centrella M, McCarthy TL, Canalis E (1988) Parathyroid hormone modulates transforming growth factor β activity and binding in osteoblast-enriched cell cultures from fetal rat parietal bone. Proc Natl Acad Sci USA 85:5889–5893

Centrella M, McCarthy TL, Canalis E (1990) Receptors for insulin-like growth factors I and II in osteoblast-enriched cultures from fetal rat bone. Endocrinology 126:39–44

Centrella M, McCarthy TL, Canalis E (1991a) Glucocorticoid regulation of transforming growth factor β_1 (TGF β_1) activity and binding in osteoblast-enriched cultures from fetal rat bone. Mol Cell Biol 11:4490–4496

Centrella M, McCarthy TL, Canalis E (1991b) Current concepts review. Transforming growth factor-beta and remodeling of bone. J Bone Joint Surg Am 73:1418–1428

Centrella M, McCarthy TL, Kusmik WF, Canalis E (1991c) Relative binding and biochemical effects of heterodimeric and homodimeric isoforms of platelet-derived growth factor in osteoblast-enriched cultures from fetal rat bone. J Cell Physiol 147:420–426

Centrella M, McCarthy TL, Kusmik WF, Canalis E (1992) Isoform-specific regulation of platelet-derived growth factor activity and binding in osteoblast-enriched cultures from fetal rat bone. J Clin Invest 89:1076–1084

Chen TL, Bates RL, Dudley A, Hammonds RG, Amento EP (1991) Bone morphogenetic protein-2b stimulation of growth and osteogenic phenotypes in rat osteoblast-like cells: comparison with TGF-β_1. J Bone Miner Res 6:1387–1393

Chen RH, Ebner R, Derynck R (1993) Inactivation of the type II receptor reveals two receptor pathways for the diverse TGF-β activities. Science 260:1335–1338

Chenu C, Pfeilschifter J, Mundy GR, Roodman GD (1988) Transforming growth factor β inhibits formation of osteoclast-like cells in long-term human marrow cultures. Proc Natl Acad Sci USA 85:5683–5687

Chua CC, Geiman DE, Keller GF, Ladda RL (1985) Induction of collagenase secretion in human fibroblast cultures by growth promoting factors. J Biol Chem 260:5213–5216

Cochran DL, Rouse CA, Lynch SE, Graves DT (1993) Effects of platelet-derived growth factor isoforms on calcium release from neonatal mouse calvariae. Bone 14:53–58

Coffin JD, Florkiewicz RZ, Neumann J, Mort-Hopkins T, Dorn II GW, Lightfoot P, German R, Howles PN, Kier A, O'Toole BA, Sasse J, Gonzalez AM, Baird A, Doetschman T (1995) Abnormal bone growth and selective translational regulation in basic fibroblast growth factor (FGF-2) transgenic mice. Mol Biol Cell 6:1861–1873

Collins T, Ginsburg D, Boss JM, Orkin SH, Pober JS (1985) Cultured human endothelial cells express platelet-derived growth factor β chain: cDNA cloning and structural analysis. Nature 316:748–750

Conover CA (1992) Potentiation of insulin-like growth factor (IGF) action by IGF-binding protein-3: studies of underlying mechanism. Endocrinology 130:3191–3199

Conover CA, Lee PDK, Riggs BL, Powell DR (1996) Insulin-like growth factor-binding protein 1 expression in cultured human bone cells: regulation by insulin and glucocorticoid. Endocrinology 137:3295–3301

Daughaday WH, Rotwein P (1989) Insulin-like growth factor I and II. Peptide, messenger ribonucleic acid and gene structures, serum, and tissue concentrations. Endocr Rev 10:68–91

DeChiara TM, Efstratiadis A, Robertson EJ (1990) A growth-deficiency phenotype in heterozygous mice carrying an insulin-like growth factor II gene disrupted by targeting. Nature 345:78–80

Delany AM, Canalis E (1995) Transcriptional repression of insulin-like growth factor I by glucocorticoids in rat bone cells. Endocrinology 136:4776–4781

Delany AM, Pash JM, Canalis E (1994) Cellular and clinical perspectives on skeletal insulin-like growth factor I. J Cell Biochem 55:1–6

Delany AM, Rydziel S, Canalis E (1996) Autocrine down regulation of collagenase-3 in rat bone cell cultures by insulin-like growth factors. Endocrinology 137:4665–4670

Deng C, Wynshaw-Boris A, Zhou F, Kuo A, Leder P (1996) Fibroblast growth factor receptor 3 is a negative regulator of bone growth. Cell 84:911–921

Dong Y, Canalis E (1995) Insulin-like growth factor I and retinoic acid induce the synthesis of insulin-like growth factor binding protein-5 in rat osteoblastic cells. Endocrinology 136:2000–2006

Dudley AT, Lyons KM, Robertson EJ (1995) A requirement for bone morphogenetic protein-7 during development of the mammalian kidney and eye. Genes Dev 9:2795–2807

Ebeling PR, Jones JD, O'Fallon WM, Janes CH, Riggs BL (1993) Short-term effects of recombinant human insulin-like growth factor-I on bone turnover in normal women. J Clin Endocrinol Metab 77:1384–1387

Ebner R, Chen RH, Shum L, Lawler S, Zioncheck TF, Lee A, Lopez AR, Derynck R (1993) Cloning of a type I TGF β-receptor and its effect on TGF-β binding to the type II receptor. Science 260:1344–1348

Edwards DR, Murphy G, Reynolds JJ, Whitham SE, Docherty AJP, Angel P, Heath JK (1987) Transforming growth factor beta modulates the expression of collagenase and metalloproteinase inhibitor. EMBO J 6:1899–1904

Erlebacher A, Derynck R (1996) Increased expression of TGF-β2 in osteoblasts results in an osteoporosis-like phenotype. J Cell Biol 132:195–210

Ernst M, Rodan GA (1991) Estradiol regulation of insulin-like growth factor-I expression in osteoblastic cells: evidence for transcriptional control. Mol Endocrinol 5:1081–1089

Ewton DZ, Falen SL, Florini JR (1987) The type II insulin-like growth factor (IGF) receptor has low affinity for IGF I analogs: pleiotypic actions of IGFs on myoblasts are apparently mediated by the type I receptor. Endocrinology 120:115–123

Faham S, Hileman RE, Fromm, JR, Linhardt RJ, Rees DC (1996) Heparin structure and interactions with basic fibroblast growth factor. Science 271:1116–1122

Finkelman RD, Bell NH, Strong DD, Demers LM, Baylink DJ (1992) Ovariectomy selectively reduces the concentration of transforming growth factor β in rat bone: implications for estrogen deficiency-associated bone loss. Proc Natl Acad Sci USA 89:12190–12193

Finkelstein JS, Klibanski A, Schaefer EH, Hornstein MD, Schiff I, Neer RM (1994) Parathyroid hormone for the prevention of bone loss induced by estrogen deficiency. N Engl J Med 331:1618–1623

Franchimont N, Canalis E (1995) Platelet-derived growth factor stimulates the synthesis of interleukin-6 in cells of the osteoblast lineage. Endocrinology 136:5469–5475

Furlanetto RW, DiCarlo JN, Wisehart C (1987) The type II insulin-like growth factor receptor does not mediate deoxyribonucleic acid synthesis in human fibroblasts. J Clin Endocrinol Metab 64:1142–1149

Gabbitas B, Canalis E (1996a) Cortisol enhances the transcription of insulin-like growth factor binding protein-6 in cultured osteoblasts. Endocrinology 137:1687–1692

Gabbitas B, Canalis E (1996b) Retinoic acid stimulates the transcription of insulin-like growth factor binding protein-6 in skeletal cells. J Cell Physiol 169:15–22

Gabbitas B, Pash J, Canalis E (1994) Regulation of insulin-like growth factor II synthesis in bone cell cultures by skeletal growth factors. Endocrinology 135:284–289

Gabbitas B, Pash JM, Delany AM, Canalis E (1996) Cortisol inhibits the synthesis of insulin-like growth factor binding protein-5 in bone cell cultures by transcriptional mechanisms. J Biol Chem 271:9033–9038

Gilardetti RS, Chaibi MS, Stroumza J, Williams SR, Antoniades HN, Carnes DC, Graves DT (1991) High-affinity binding of PDGF-AA and PDGF-BB to normal human osteoblastic cells and modulation by interleukin-1. Am J Physiol 261:C980–985

Globus RK, Plouet J, Gospodarowicz D (1989) Cultured bovine bone cells synthesize basic fibroblast growth factor and store it in their extracellular matrix. Endocrinology 124:1539–1547

Goldring MB, Goldring SR (1991) Cytokines and cell growth control. Crit Rev Eukaryot Gene Expr 1:301–326

Graves DT, Owen AJ, Barth RK, Tempst P, Winoto A, Fors L, Hood LE, Antoniades HN (1984) Detection of c-sis transcripts and synthesis of PDGF-like proteins by human osteosarcoma cells. Science 226:972–974

Graves DT, Valentin-Opran A, Delgado R, Valente AJ, Mundy G, Piche J (1989) The potential role of platelet-derived growth factor as an autocrine or paracrine factor for human bone cells. Connect Tissue Res 23:209–218

Grinspoon SK, Baum HBA, Peterson S, Klibanski A (1995) Effects of rhIGF-I administration on bone turnover during short-term fasting. J Clin Invest 96:900–906

Hammerman MR (1987) Insulin-like growth factors and aging. Endocrinol Metab Clin North Am 16:995–1008

Hart CE, Mason B, Curtis DA, Osborn S, Raines E, Ross R, Forstrom JW (1990) Purification of PDGF-AB and PDGF-BB from human platelet extracts and identification of all three PDGF dimers in human platelets. Biochemistry 29:166–172

Hassager C, Fitzpatrick LA, Spencer EM, Riggs BL, Conover CA (1992) Basal and regulated secretion of insulin-like growth factor binding proteins in osteoblast-like cells is cell line specific. J Clin Endocrinol Metab 75:228–233

Heldin C-H, Westermark B (1993) Platelet-derived growth factor. Acta Oncol 32:101–105

Hock J, Centrella M, Canalis E (1988) Insulin-like growth factor I (IGF-I) has independent effects on bone matrix formation and cell replication. Endocrinology 122:254–260

Hock JM, Canalis E (1994) Platelet-derived growth factor enhances bone cell replication but not differentiated function of osteoblasts. Endocrinology 134:1423–1428

Hock JM, Canalis E, Centrella M (1990) Transforming growth factor beta (TGF-beta-1) stimulates bone matrix apposition and bone cell replication in cultured fetal rat calvariae. Endocrinology 166:421–426

Hurley MM, Abreu C, Harrison JR, Lichtler AC, Raisz LG, Kream BE (1993) Basic fibroblast growth factor inhibits type I collagen gene expression in osteoblastic MC3T3-E1 cells. J Biol Chem 268:5588–5593

Hurley MM, Abreu C, Gronowicz G, Kawaguchi H, Lorenzo J (1994) Expression and regulation of basic fibroblast growth factor mRNA levels in mouse osteoblastic MC3T3-E1 cells. J Biol Chem 269:9392–9396

Jilka RL, Hangoc G, Girasole G, Passeri G, Williams DC, Abrams JS, Boyce B, Broxmeyer H, Manolagas SC (1992) Increased osteoclast development after estrogen loss: mediation by interleukin-6. Science 257:88–91

Jones JI, Gockerman A, Busby Jr WH, Camacho-Hubner C, Clemmons DR (1993) Extracellular matrix contains insulin-like growth factor binding protein-5: potentiation of the effects of IGF-I. J Cell Biol 121:679–687

Kalu DN, Salerno E, Higami Y, Liu CC, Ferraro F, Salih MA, Arjmand BH (1993) In vivo effects of transforming growth factor-beta 2 in ovariectomized rats. Bone Miner 22:209–220

Kawaguchi H. Kurokawa T, Hanada K, Hiyama Y, Tamura M, Ogata E, Matsumoto T (1994) Stimulation of fracture repair by recombinant human basic fibroblast growth factor in normal and streptozotocin-diabetic rats. Endocrinology 135:774–781

Kiefer MC, Schmid C, Waldvogel M, Schlapfer I, Futo E, Masiar FR, Green K, Barr PJ, Zapf J (1992) Characterization of recombinant human insulin-like growth factor binding proteins 4, 5, and 6 produced in yeast. J Biol Chem 267:12692–12699

Kim S-J, Jeang KT, Glick AB, Sporn MB, Roberts AB (1989) Promoter sequences of the human transforming growth factor-β1 gene responsive to transforming growth factor-β1 autoinduction. J Biol Chem 264:7041–7045

Kingsley DM (1994) The TGF-β superfamily: new members, new receptors, and new genetic tests of function in different organisms. Genes Dev 8:133–146

Kose KN, Xie JF, Carnes DL, Graves DT (1996) Pro-inflammatory cytokines downregulate platelet derived growth factor-α receptor gene expression in human osteoblastic cells. J Cell Physiol 166:188–197

Kupfer SR, Underwood LE, Baxter RC, Clemmons DR (1993) Enhancement of the anabolic effects of growth hormone and insulin-like growth factor I by use of both agents simultaneously. J Clin Invest 91:391–396

Kurose H, Yamaoka K, Okada S, Nakajima S, Seino Y (1990) 1,25-Dihydroxyvitamin D_3 [1,25-(OH)$_2$D$_3$] increases insulin-like growth factor I (IGF-I) receptors in clonal osteoblastic cells. Study on interaction of IGF-I and 1,25-(OH)$_2$D$_3$. Endocrinology 126:2088–2094

Laiho M, Weis FMB, Massague J (1990) Concomitant loss of transforming growth factor (TGF)-β receptor types I and II in TGFβ-resistant cell mutants implicates both receptor types in signal transduction. J Biol Chem 265:18518–18524

Lane TL, Sage EH (1994) The biology of SPARC, a protein that modulates cell-matrix interactions. FASEB J 8:163–173

LaTour D, Mohan S, Linkhart TA, Baylink DJ, Strong DD (1990) Inhibitory insulin-like growth factor-binding protein: cloning, complete sequence, and physiological regulation. Mol Endocrinol 4:1806–1814

Lau MMH, Stewart CEH, Liu Z, Bhatt H, Rotwein P, Stewart CL (1994) Loss of the imprinted IGF2/cation-independent mannose 6-phosphate receptor results in fetal overgrowth and perinatal lethality. Genes Dev 8:2953–2963

Leveen P, Pekny M, Gebre-Medhin S, Swolin B, Larsson E, Betsholtz C (1994) Mice deficient for PDGF B show renal, cardiovascular, and hematological abnormalities. Genes Dev 8:1875–1887

Liu C, Wallace K, Shi C, Heyner S, Komm B, Haddad JG (1996) Post-transcriptional stimulation of transforming growth factor β1 mRNA by TGF β1 treatment of transformed human osteoblasts. J Bone Miner Res 11:211–217

Liu J-P, Baker J, Perkins AS, Robertson EJ, Efstratiadis A (1993) Mice carrying null mutations of the genes encoding insulin-like growth factor I (IGF-1) and type 1 IGF receptor (IGF1R). Cell 75:59–72

Luo G, Hofmann C, Bronckers ALJJ, Sohocki M, Bradley A, Karsenty G (1995) BMP-7 is an inducer of nephrogenesis, and is also required for eye development and skeletal patterning. Genes Dev 9:2808–2820

Machwate M, Zerath E, Holy X, Pastoureau P, Marie PJ (1994) Insulin-like growth factor-I increases trabecular bone formation and osteoblastic cell proliferation in unloaded rats. Endocrinology 134:1031–1038

Massague J (1996) TGFβ signaling: receptors, transducers, and mad proteins. Cell 85:947–950

Matrisian LM, Hogan BLM (1990) Growth factor regulated proteases and extracellular matrix remodeling during mammalian development. Curr Top Dev Biol 24:219–259

McCarthy TL, Centrella M, Canalis E (1989a) Parathyroid hormone enhances the transcript and polypeptide levels of insulin-like growth factor I in osteoblast-enriched cultures from fetal rat bone. Endocrinology 124:1247–1253

McCarthy TL, Centrella M, Canalis E (1989b) Regulatory effects of insulin-like growth factor I and II on bone collagen synthesis in rat calvarial cultures. Endocrinology 124:301–309

McCarthy TL, Centrella M, Canalis E (1989c) Effects of fibroblast growth factors on deoxyribonucleic acid and collagen synthesis in rat parietal bone cells. Endocrinology 125:2118–2126

McCarthy T, Casinghino S, Centrella M, Canalis E (1994) Complex pattern of insulin-like growth factor binding protein expression in primary rat osteoblast enriched cultures: regulation by prostaglandin E_2, growth hormone, and the insulin-like growth factors. J Cell Physiol 160:163–175

Middleton J, Arnott N, Walsh S, Beresford J (1995) Osteoblasts and osteoclasts in adult human osteophyte tissue express the mRNAs for the insulin-like growth factors I and II and type 1 IGF receptor. Bone 16:287–293

Mitlak BH, Finkelman RD, Hill EL, Li J, Martin B, Smith T, D'Andrea M, Antoniades HN, Lynch SE (1996) The effect of systemically administered PDGF-BB on the rodent skeleton. J Bone Miner Res 11:238–247

Miyazono K, Hellman U, Wernstedt C, Heldin CH (1988) Latent high molecular weight complex of transforming growth factor-β1: purification from human platelets and structural characterization. J Biol Chem 263:6407–6415

Mohan S, Nakao Y, Honda Y, Landale E, Leser U, Dony C, Lang K, Baylink DJ (1995) Studies on the mechanisms by which insulin-like growth factor (IGF) binding protein-4 (IGFBP-4) and IGFBP-5 modulate IGF actions in bone cells. J Biol Chem 270:20424–20431

Moriwake T, Tanaka H, Kanzaki S, Higuchi J, Seino Y (1992) 1,25-dihydroxyvitamin D_3 stimulates the secretion of insulin-like growth factor binding protein 3 (IGFBP-3) by cultured human osteosarcoma cells. Endocrinology 130:1071–1073

Muenke M, Schell U, Hehr A, Robin NH, Losken HW, Schinzel A, Pulleryn LJ, Rutland P, Reardon W, Malcolm S, Winter RM (1994) A common mutation in the fibroblast growth factor receptor I gene in Pfeiffer syndrome. Nat Genet 8:269–274

Nakayama H, Ichikawa F, Andres JL, Massague J, Noda M (1994) Dexamethasone enhancement of betaglycan (TGF-β type III receptor) gene expression in osteoblast-like cells. Exp Cell Res 211:301–306

Ng KW, Manji SS, Young MF, Findlay DM (1989) Opposing influences of glucocorticoid and retinoic acid on transcriptional control in preosteoblasts. Mol Endocrinol 3:2079–2085

Nicolas V, Prewett A, Bettica P, Mohan S, Finkelman RD, Baylink DJ, Farley JR (1994) Age-related decreases of insulin-like growth factor-I and transforming growth factor-β in femoral cortical bone from both men and women: implications for bone loss with aging. J Clin Endocrinol Metab 78:1011–1016

Nissley P, Kiess W, Sklar M (1993) Developmental expression of the IGF-II/mannose-6-phosphate receptor. Mol Reprod Dev 35:408–413

Noda M, Vogel R (1989) Fibroblast growth factor enhances type beta 1 transforming growth factor gene expression in osteoblast-like cells. J Cell Biol 109:2529–2535

Ogawa Y, Schmidt DK, Dasch JR, Chang RJ, Glaser CB (1992) Purification and characterization of transforming growth factor-β2.3 and -β1.2 heterodimers from bovine bone. J Biol Chem 267:2325–2328

Okazaki R, Conover CA, Harris SA, Spelsberg TC, Riggs BL (1995) Normal human osteoblast-like cells consistently express genes for insulin-like growth factors I and II but transformed human osteoblast cells lines do not. J Bone Miner Res 10:788–795

Oursler MJ, Cortese C, Keeting P, Anderson MA, Bonde SK, Riggs BL, Spelsberg TC (1991) Modulation of transforming growth factor-β production in normal human osteoblast-like cells by 17β-estradiol and parathyroid hormone. Endocrinology 129:3313–3320

Oursler MJ, Riggs BL, Spelsberg TC (1993) Glucocorticoid-induced activation of latent transforming growth factor-β by normal human osteoblast-like cells. Endocrinology 133:2187–2196

Pash J, Delany AM, Adamo ML, Roberts Jr CT, LeRoith D, Canalis E (1995) Regulation of insulin-like growth factor I transcription by prostaglandin E_2 in osteoblast cells. Endocrinology 136:33–38

Pash JM, Canalis E (1996) Transcriptional regulation of insulin-like growth factor binding protein-5 by prostaglandin E$_2$ in osteoblast cells. Endocrinology 137:2375–2382

Penton A, Chen Y, Staehling-Hampton K, Wrana JL, Attisano L, Szidonya J, Cassill JA, Massague J, Hoffman FM (1994) Identification of two bone morphogenetic protein type I receptors in drosophila and evidence that Brk25D is a decapentaplegic receptor. Cell 78:239–250

Pfeilschifter J, Mundy GR (1987) Modulation of type B transforming growth factor activity in bone cultures by osteotropic hormones. Proc Natl Acad Sci USA 84:2024–2028

Raines EW, Lane TF, Iruela-Arispe ML, Ross R, Sage EH (1992) The extracellular glycoprotein SPARC interacts with platelet-derived growth factor (PDGF)-AB and -BB and inhibits the binding of PDGF to its receptors. Proc Natl Acad Sci USA 89:1281–1285

Raisz G, Fall M, Gabbitas BY, McCarthy TL, Kream BE, Canalis E (1993) Effects of prostaglandin E$_2$ on bone formation in cultured fetal rat calvariae; role of insulin-like growth factor I. Endocrinology 133:1504–1510

Reardon W, Winter RM, Rutland P, Pulleryn LJ, Jones BM, Malcolm S (1994) Mutations in the fibroblast growth factor receptor 2 gene cause Crouzon syndrome. Nat Genet 8:98–103

Rechler MM (1993) Insulin-like growth factor binding proteins. Vitam Horm 47:1–114

Reeve J, Bradbeer JN, Arlot M, Davies UM, Green JR, Hampton L, Eduoard C, Hesp R, Hulme P, Ashby JP (1991) hPTH 1-34 treatment of osteoporosis with added hormone replacement therapy: biochemical, kinetic and histological responses. Osteoporos Int 1:162–170

Rosen D, Miller SC, DeLeon E, Thompson AY, Bentz H, Mathews M, Adams S (1994) Systemic administration of recombinant transforming growth factor beta 2 (rTGF-β2) stimulates parameters of cancellous bone formation in juvenile and adult rats. Bone 15:355–359

Rydziel S, Canalis E (1995) Cortisol represses insulin-like growth factor II receptor transcription in skeletal cell cultures. Endocrinology 136:4254–4260

Rydziel S, Canalis E (1996) Expression and growth factor regulation of platelet-derived growth factor B transcripts in primary osteoblast cell cultures. Endocrinology (in press)

Rydziel S, Shaikh S, Canalis E (1994) Platelet-derived growth factors AA and BB enhance the synthesis of platelet-derived growth factor AA in bone cell cultures. Endocrinology 134:2541–2546

Rydziel S, Varghese S, Canalis E (1997) Transforming growth factor β1 inhibits collagenase 3 expression by transcriptional and post-transcriptional mechanisms in osteoblast cultures. J Cell Physiol (in press)

Shafritz AB, Shore EM, Gannon FH, Zasloff MA, Taub R, Muenke M, Kaplan FS (1996) Overexpression of an osteogenic morphogen in fibrodysplasia ossificans progressiva. N Engl J Med 335:555–561

Shiang R, Thompson LM, Zhu Y-Z, Church DM, Fielder TJ, Bocian M, Winokur SR, Wasmuth JJ (1994) Mutations in the transmembrane domain of FGFR3 cause the most common genetic form of dwarfism, achondroplasia. Cell 78:335–342

Shull MM, Ormsby I, Kier AB, Pawlowski S, Diebold RJ, Yin M, Allen R, Sidman C, Proetzel G, Calvin D, Annunziata N, Doetschman T (1992) Targeted disruption of the mouse transforming growth factor-β1 gene results in multifocal inflammatory disease. Nature 359:693–699

Soriano P (1994) Abnormal kidney development and hematological disorders in PDGF β-receptor mutant mice. Genes Dev 8:1888–1896

Tamura R, Udagawa N, Takahashi N, Miyaura C, Tanaka S, Yamada Y, Koishihara Y, Ohsugi Y, Kumaki K, Taga T, Kishimoto T, Suda T (1993) Soluble interleukin-6 receptor triggers osteoclast formation by interleukin 6. Proc Natl Acad Sci USA 90:11924–11928

Tashjian AH, Hohmann EL, Antoniades HN, Levine L (1982) Platelet-derived growth factor stimulates bone resorption via a prostaglandin-mediated mechanism. Endocrinology 111:118–124

Ten Dijke P, Iwata KK, Goddard C, Pieler C, Canalis E, McCarthy TL, Centrella M (1990) Recombinant transforming growth factor type β_3: biological activities and receptor binding activities in isolated bone cells. Mol Cell Biol 10:4473–4479

Thrailkill KM, Siddhanti SR, Fowlkes JL, Quarles LD (1995) Differentiation of MC3T3-E1 osteoblasts is associated with temporal changes in the expression of IGF-I and IGFBPs. Bone 17:307–313

Tsukamoto T, Matsui T, Nakata H, Ito M, Natazuka T, Fukase M, Fujita T (1991) Interleukin-1 enhances the response of osteoblasts to platelet-derived growth factor through the α receptor-specific up-regulation. J Biol Chem 266:10143–10147

van Obberghen-Schilling E, Roche NS, Flanders KC, Sporn MB, Roberts AB (1988) Transforming growth factor β1 positively regulates its own expression in normal and transformed cells. J Biol Chem 263:7741–7746

Varghese S, Ramsby ML, Jeffrey JJ, Canalis E (1995) Basic fibroblast growth factor stimulates expression of interstitial collagenase and inhibitors of metalloproteinases in rat bone cells. Endocrinology 136:2156–2162

Varghese S, Delany AM, Liang L, Gabbitas B, Jeffrey JJ, Canalis E (1996) Transcriptional and post-transcriptional regulation of interstitial collagenase by platelet-derived growth factor BB in bone cultures. Endocrinology 137:431–437

Wang EA, Rosen V, D'Alessandro JS, Bauduy M, Cordes P, Harada T, Israel DI, Hewick RM, Kerns KM, LaPan P, Luxenberg DP, McQuaid D, Moutsatsos IK, Nove J, Wozney JM (1990) Recombinant human bone morphogenetic protein induces bone formation. Proc Natl Acad Sci USA 87:2220–2224

Wozney JM, Rosen V, Celeste AJ, Mitsock LM, Whitters MJ, Kriz RW, Hewick RM, Wang EA (1988) Novel regulators of bone formation: molecular clones and activities. Science 242:1528–1534

5 Cellular Basis of Bone Resorption

A. Zambonin Zallone and G. Zambonin

Introduction

Bone remodeling is a finely tuned process that lasts throughout one's life. Old bone is removed, and new bone is formed according to the mechanical and metabolic needs of the body. Osteoblasts and osteoclasts are the cell types that take part in this complex task. The osteoblasts are very possibly, together with the osteocytes, responsible for selecting the area that is to be removed, while the osteoclasts are the cells that actually carry out the resorption. Newly formed osteoblasts are immediately thereafter recruited to repair and/or reorganize the tissue. This chapter describes principally the origin of the osteoclasts, the molecular mechanisms of bone resorption, and the current hypothesis about the coupling mechanism that joins osteoclast and osteoblast activity.

Osteoclast origin and differentiation. The osteoclasts are multinucleated cells arising from the hemopoietic stem cells of the granulocyte-monocyte lineage [1, 2]. The precursor cells migrate via the vascular pathway to the skeleton where osteoblasts, osteocytes, endothelial cells, and stromal cells are believed to provide the necessary microenvironment for "homing" of the precursors at the site of their final destination. Postmitotic cells differentiate into preosteoclasts and then fuse asynchronously to form mature multinucleated osteoclasts. Bone resorption thus also appears to be regulated by the mechanisms that control osteoclast precursor proliferation and differentiation. Research on osteopetrotic mutation has clarified some of the steps that produce the formation first of committed preosteoclasts and subsequently of fully differentiated active cells (for a complete review see [3]).

Colony-stimulating factor 1 (CSF-1) the growth factor for cells of the mononuclear phagocyte system, is essential for the development of osteoclasts [4, 5]. No biologically active CSF-1 is synthesized in the osteopetrotic (op) mouse due to a point mutation in the coding region of its gene. This leads to an almost complete lack of osteoclast development and to impaired bone resorption. Osteopetrosis also resulted from experimental gene disruption in mice. Targeted disruption of c-*src* proto-oncogene encoding a nonreceptor tyrosine kinase leads to a form of osteopetrosis in which osteoclasts are present but inactive [6]. Disruption of the c-*fos* proto-oncogene, a major component of the AP-1 transcription factor complex, leads to an osteopetrotic phenotype characterized by a complete absence of osteoclasts [7].

A number of agents are also known to modulate differentiation of osteoclast precursors. These belong to the cytokine family and include a variety of interleukins (ILs) and tumor necrosis factor (TNF) [8]. IL-1, IL-6, IL-11, and TNF stimulate bone resorption indirectly by increasing proliferation and differentiation of osteoclast precursors [9,10]. These molecules cross-regulate their production, as demonstrated by the fact that TNF amplifies IL-1 and parathyroid hormone-induced secretion of IL-6 [11]. IL-6 and IL-11 belong to a subfamily of cytokines in which signaling is mediated by receptors sharing a common subunit, gp130. Specificity is achieved by binding of each protein to separate subunits, which associate with gp130 to form the active signaling complex [12]. In the case of IL-6, an 80-kDa, soluble form of IL-6 binding subunit stimulates formation of osteoclasts in vitro [13]. Thus, increased osteoclastogenesis by IL-6 and IL-11 may arise from a common intracellular signal. Girasole et al. [14] showed that IL-11 dose-dependently stimulates osteoclast-like multinucleated cell formation in coculture of mouse osteoblasts and bone marrow cells. They reported that monoclonal anti-IL-11 antibody inhibits osteoclast formation induced by several osteotropic factors.

Steroid hormones, particularly 1,25 dihydroxyvitamin D_3 [1,25$(OH)_2D_3$] [15,16] and retinoic acid [17,18] are also critical for maturation of precursor cells. Thus it is not surprising that vitamin D receptors are present in osteoclast precursors and are lost upon formation of the terminally differentiated polykarions [19]. Additionally 1,25$(OH)_2D_3$ upregulates the estrogen receptor in human bone marrow stromal cells [20]. The ability of specific inhibitors of IL-1 and TNF to reverse the consequences of estrogen withdrawal [21] indicates that at least part of the effects of this steroid on osteoclast function are mediated via these cytokines. Osteoclast precursors very early express tartrate-resistant acid phosphatase and a high number of calcitonin receptors [22]. They also first express the $\alpha_v\beta_5$ integrin, that only at a later stage is substituted with $\alpha_v\beta_3$ [23,].

Osteoclast Morphology and Functions

The osteoclasts, being multinucleated motile cells, have a very distinct morphology. Moreover, they organize their membrane and cytoplasm in a different way depending on whether they are sitting on the bone, resorbing the bone matrix, or migrating toward or resting on bone surfaces. Nonresorbing cells have an almost homogeneous organization of their membrane, which can present wide infoldings in nonmigrating cells but fillopodia or undulating membrane during migration. Nuclei and organelles, mostly represented by numerous mitochondria, a few cisternae of rough endoplasmic reticulum, multiple Golgi apparati, and an elevated number of lysosomes, are usually equally distributed in the cell center [24].

Recruitment. In order to start resorption a sequence of well-controlled events occurs [25]. Osteoclasts recognize and adhere to the bone matrix proteins osteopontin and BSP. Osteocalcin, a small bone-specific protein, is believed to play a specific role in the first phases of the migration-adhesion process. It is the most abundant of the noncollagenous proteins of bone produced by osteoblasts and has several interesting features. It consist of a single chain of 46–50 amino acids and contains three vitamin K dependent gamma-carboxyglutamic residues (Gla) involved in its binding to calcium and hydroxylapatite. A potential role of this protein in the induction of bone resorption has been suggested by in vitro experiments showing that it has chemotactic activity for a number of cells including monocytes [26, 27]. Osteocalcin induces chemotaxis, in a dose-dependent manner, calcium-mediated intracellular signals, and the secretion of matrix proteins such as osteopontin, Bone sialsprotein (BSP), and fibronectin by osteoclast-like cells obtained from giant cell tumors of bone and characterized their osteoclast features [28–30]. Secretion of osteocalcin by osteoblasts is also regulated by vitamin D_3. Due to its small size this protein can diffuse and be a chemoactractive signal with a concentration gradient directed toward bone surfaces for preosteoclasts and osteoclasts.

Homing. Once arriving on the bone surfaces, osteoclasts recognize osteopontin and BSP through their integrin receptors. This recognition also triggers an intracellular calcium increase, but while the signals induced by osteocalcin are less pronounced and last longer before returning to baseline, the calcium increase triggered via integrin receptors is a prompt and transient response [31]. Osteoclasts, before starting their demolitive activity become polarized. How this polarization is accomplished, and why in certain circumstances osteoclasts sit on bone surfaces without being polarized, in a nonresorptive condition, while in other cases they polarize, i.e., dramatically change their organization and start to resorb bone actively, has not yet been understood.

Polarization and Resorption. It has recently been demonstrated that the osteoclast integrin $\alpha_v\beta_3$ can exist in two different conformations, both capable of ligand recognition, but possibly involved in different functions such as migration or tight adhesion [32]. It is possible that polarization-resorption is associated with one but not with both conformations of the $\alpha_v\beta_3$ integrin receptor. After polarization two well-defined areas of the plasma membrane have been identified: the apical, facing the bone and the basolateral in contact with the extracellular spaces [33]. The apical, bone-facing surface can be distinguished in two parts, namely, the sealing membrane that forms an outer ring and encircles an inner area, the ruffled border. A massive cytoskeletal rearrangement creates over the sealing membrane an actin-rich structure that outlines the entire bone-facing cell perimeter and encloses the specialized secretory membrane, which contains highly convoluted folds and has been called the ruffled border. The cytoplasm above the sealing membrane, also called the clear zone, is homogeneous and lacks cellular organelles, except free polyribosomes. Highly organized cytoskeletal and adhesive proteins have been demonstrated at this level, but their molecular anatomy is still controversial.

Lakkakorpi et al. [34] and Lakkakorpi and Vaananen [35] have described two circumferential rings of actin-containing microfilaments, separated by an intermediate ring of vinculin, and other authors [36-39] have demonstrated the presence of an anchorage ring formed by a number of highly dynamic, modified focal adhesions, the podosomes, which contain a number of cytoskeletal and regulatory proteins as well as integrin receptors, namely $\alpha_v\beta_3$ and $\alpha_2\beta_1$, engaged in bone matrix recognition and adhesion. The number of podosomes simultaneously observed in the clear zone may be extremely elevated; thus they may concurrently account for a tight but dynamic cell-matrix adhesion area.

The sealing membrane delimites an extracellular space, the resorbing lacuna, in which bone degradation takes place. The initial event in the resorption process, once the osteoclast is attached to the bone matrix, is the acidification of the extracellular resorptive microenvironment and is mediated by a vacuolar H^+-ATPase inserted in the ruffled membrane of the polarized cell. The structure and functional activity of this multienzyme complex is very similar to that of the analogous proton pump in the intercalated cell of the kidney [40]. The acidification step is critical, permitting not only mineral mobilization but also subsequent degradation of the organic phase of bone by acidic proteases such as cathepsins [33, 41, 42]. The intracellular pH is maintained by an energy-independent Cl^-/HCO_3^- exchanger similar to band 3 of the erythrocyte [43]. Electroneutrality is preserved by a plasma membrane Cl^- channel charge coupled to the H^+-ATPase, resulting in secretion of HCl into the resorptive microenvironment [45]. A major unsolved issue regarding osteoclast function concerns the detailed mechanism by which H^+-ATPase bearing vesicles are inserted into the ruffled border membrane. The fact that polarization follows attachment suggests that cell-matrix interactions produce a signal resulting in vesicular movement. The involvement of the c-*src* product in this process has been recently demonstrated [46].

It remaines unclear how osteoclasts handle the large amounts of inorganic and organic material released during the resorption event. Viral glycoproteins that in epithelial cells are targeted to the apical membrane are targeted in resorbing osteoclasts to a specific membrane area in the middle of the basolateral membrane [47]. Evidence has recently been provided that this unusual membrane domain is a target for membrane vesicles that are endocytosed from the ruffled border and contain bone degradation products [48, 49]. Both organic and inorganic degradation products are taken up and transcytosed along the same route. After transcytosis these vesicles reach the functional secretory domain and empty their contents through this membrane area. Intracellular trafficking of products resulting from tissue degradation may provide cells with a mechanism that can enable them to monitor and hence control proteolytic activity. It has been clearly demonstrated that a powerful osteoclast-inhibiting agent is the elevation of $[Ca^{2+}]_0$ [50–52]. This mechanism regulates calcium homeostasis by multiple targets. It is well established that increments in $[Ca^{2+}]_0$ simultaneously activate calcitonin release by thyroid C cells [53], inhibit parathyroid secretion by parathyroid glands [54], and block osteoclast activity. Elevated calcium is detected by osteoclasts via a unique, cell-surface expressed ryanodine receptor that is modulated by extracellular pH [55, 56]. The release of inorganic components of bone matrix via transcytotic vesicles may provide the osteoclasts with a local feedback mechanism that can directly control the resorbing activity.

Coupling Between Osteoclast and Osteoblast Activity

Bone formation and bone resorption do not occur at random; they are part of the turnover mechanism replacing old bone by new bone. In the normal adult skeleton bone formation occurs only where bone resorption has previously occurred. The sequence of events at the remodeling site is therefore activation-resorption-formation (ARF sequence). The cells responsible for bone resorption and formation at a given site are referred to as a bone-forming unit (BFU). This sequence of events caused several investigators to hypothesize the existence of a so-called "coupling factor" that links the osteoclast resorptive avtivity to the osteoblast new bone formation [57]. Some candidates have been suggested for such a factor(s). Transforming growth factor (TGF) β and other members of the TGFβ superfamily, such as bone morphogenetic proteins, are important regulators of bone morphogenesis and remodeling. TGFβ in particular may play a role as local regulator of the coupling process. It is secreted by osteoblasts and is present in the bone matrix in the latent state. It must be dissociated to release the active moiety and render it available to stimulate bone formation locally. It is released during bone resorption and can be activated by low pH produced by the osteoclasts in the resorbing compartment.

The transcytotic mechanism may explain the appearance of the active form in the site where resorption takes place, and its availability to osteoblasts and osteoblast precursors to stimulate new bone formation [58–60]. Hepatocyte growth factor (HGF) has also recently been suggested as a possible coupling factor. This is secreted by cells of mesodermal origin and has a mitogenic, morphogenetic, and morphogenic activity on several types of cells [61]. The HGF receptor is the tyrosine kinase encoded by the *met* proto-oncogene [62]. Both osteoclasts and osteoblasts express functional HGF receptors, and osteoclasts secrete active HGF. HGF induces biological responses both in osteoclasts and in osteoblasts. In osteoclasts it stimulates chemotactic-oriented migration. Cell migration is important in early steps of bone resorption. In osteoblasts HGF induces DNA synthesis.

The fact that HGF triggers proliferation of both bone-resorbing and bone-producing cells is only apparently a paradox. In fact it balances in this way the number of osteogenic cells required for bone remodeling [63]. The demonstrated newly angiogenic activity of HGF [64] completes this scenario, considering the critical role played by the newly formed capillary network in the organization of the haversian systems. The finding that osteoclasts themselves secrete HGF provides a simple mechanism to coordinate bone resorption and deposition by an autocrine-paracrine loop.

Systemic and Local Factors in Bone Remodeling

Systemic hormones and local factors regulate bone remodeling, and the aim of this continuous activity is to replace old bone, that is often not sufficiently vascularized or not in line with new mechanical situations of the body with new mineralized matrix. Systemic hormones include polypeptides, steroids, and thyroid hormones, while local factors include growth factors, cytokines, prostaglandins, and leukotrienes. Circulating hormones affect the whole skeleton, while local factors have effects mainly in the skeletal area where they are released, and their effects can be modulated by systemic hormones through the expression of cellular receptors (for a review see [65]).

Hormones involved in bone remodeling can be divided into (a) polypeptide hormones (parathyroid hormone, calcitonin, insulin, and growth hormone), (b) steroid hormones (vitamin D, corticosteroids, and sex steroids), and (c) thyroid hormones. Parathyroid hormone (PTH) stimulates bone resorption. This effect is mediated by osteoblasts since osteoclasts lack a parathyroid hormone receptor.

In vitro a continuous treatment inhibits bone formation while intermittent treatment stimulates bone synthesis. Calcitonin inhibits bone resorption and has no effects on bone formation. Insulin stimulates bone matrix synthesis and is necessary for its calcification. Growth hormone is necessary for maintenance of a normal bone mass, although its mechanism of action on bone cells is poorly understood. Vitamin D has multiple and complex actions on bone remodeling. It stimulates bone resorption and is necessary for calcification of osteoid matrix. Corticosteroids stimulate collagen synthesis after a short-term treatment, while after a long-term treatment they induce osteoporosis, which can be partially due to an increased stromal cell expression of the receptor for IL-6. Estrogens and androgens are important hormones for the prevention of bone loss decreasing the synthesis of cytokines that induces bone resorption. Thyroid hormones act primarily on cartilage formation and secondarily stimulate bone resorption. Local factors are produced in the bone microenvironment by bone marrow and bone cells and have only local effects [66].

Cytokines which are known to have effects on bone remodeling are IL-1α, IL-1β, IL-6, IL-11, TNFα, and TNFβ. IL-1 and TNF are very powerful stimulators of bone resorption and inhibitors of bone formation. These factors stimulate proliferation and differentiation of osteoclast precursors and enhance bone resorption by already differentiated osteoclasts either directly or by an osteoblast-mediated mechanism. IL-1 is antagonized by several factors such as a competitive inhibitor known as IL-1ra, the soluble type I IL-1 receptor (sIL-1RI), and type II IL-1 receptor (sIL-1RII), anti-IL-1α autoantibodies and IL-1β binding proteins, and thus the biological effects of IL-1 are the result of a complex balance between agonist and antagonist molecules.

Another cytokine with strong effect on osteoclast formation is IL-6. This molecule increases in vitro bone resorption in systems rich in osteoclast precursors but has no effect in culture composed predominantly of mature osteoclasts. The in vivo effects of IL-6 on bone resorption are still controversial since transgenic mice overexpressing IL-6 are not osteoporotic, but it causes hypercalcemia in nude mice. As with IL-6, IL-11 induces predominantly osteoclast formation and probably has no effect on bone resorption. Growth factors that have effects on bone remodeling are: insulin-like growth factor (IGF) I and II, TGFβ_1, -β_2, and -β_3, fibroblast growth factors (FGFs), platelet-derived growth factor (PDGF), and HGF. TGFβ, IGF I, and IGF II stimulate bone matrix synthesis and proliferation of cells of the osteoblast lineage, with IGF I four to seven times more potent than IGF II. FGF1 and FGF2 are angiogenic factors and stimulate osteoblast proliferation, while PDGF stimulates bone resorption and bone cell proliferation. These effects suggest that they could be important in the fracture healing process. In bone tissue HGF is synthetized by osteoclasts and has effects on osteoblasts and osteoclasts. On osteoblasts it induces cell proliferation, while on osteoclasts it increases intracellular Ca concentration, and induces chemotactic migration and cell proliferation. These effects suggest the possibility of an autocrine regulation of osteoclasts and a paracrine regulation of osteoblasts, both mediated by HGF. Prostaglandins and leukotrienes stimulate osteoclastic bone resorption.

References

1. Scheven BAA, Visser JWM, Nijweide PJ (1986) In vitro osteoclast generation from different bone marrow fractions, including a highly enriched haematopoietic stem cell population. Nature 321:79–81
2. Hagenaars CE, van der Kraan AAM, Kawilarang-de Haas EWM, Visser JWM, Nijweide PJ (1989) Osteoclast formation from cloned pluripotent haematopoietic stem cells. Bone Miner 6:179–189
3. Felix R, Hofstetter W, Cecchini MG (1996) Recent developments in the understanding of the pathophysiology of osteopetrosis. Eur J Endocrinol 134:143–156
4. Felix R, Cecchini MG, Fleisch H (1990) Macrophage colony stimulating factor restores in vivo bone resorption in the op/op osteopetrotic mouse. Endocrinology 127:2592–2594
5. Hofstetter W, Wetterwald A, Cecchini MC, Felix R, Fleich H, Muller C (1992) Detection of transcripts for the receptor for macrophage colony stimulating factor, c-fms in murine osteoclasts. Proc Natl Acad Sci USA 89:9637–9641
6. Soriano P, Montgomery C, Geske R, Bradley A (1991) Targeted disruption of the c-src proto-oncogene leads to osteopetrosis in mice. Cell 64:693–702
7. Grigoriadis HE, Wang RO, Cecchini MG, Hofstetter W, Felix R, Fleish HA, Wagner EF (1994) C-fos: a key regulator of osteoclast-macrophage lineage determination and bone remodelling. Science 266:443–448
8. Mundy GR (1992) Cytokines and local factors which affect osteoclast function. Int Cell Cloning 10:215–222

9. Roodman GD (1992) Interleukin-6: An osteotropic factor? J Bone Miner Res 7:475–478

10. Lerner UH, Ohlin A (1993) Tumor necrosis factor alpha and beta can stimulate bone resorption in cultured mouse calvariae by a prostaglandin-independent mechanism. J Bone Miner Res 8:147–155

11. Passeri G, Girasole G, Manolagas SC (1994) Endogenous production of tumor necrosis factor by primary cultures of murine calvaria cells: Influence on IL-6 production and osteoclast development. Bone Miner 24:109–226

12. Yin T, Taga T, Tsang ML, Yasukawa K, Kishimoto T, Yang YC (1993) Involvement of IL-6 signal trasducer gp130 in IL-11 mediated signal transduction. J Immunol 151:2551–2561

13. Tamura T, Udagawa N, Takahashi N, Miyaura C, Tanaka S, Yamada Y, Koishihara Y, Ohsugi Y, Kumaki K, Taga T, Kishimoto T, Suda T (1993). Soluble interleukin-6 receptor triggers osteoclast formation by interleukin-6. Proc Natl Acad Sci USA 90:11924–11928

14. Girasole G, Passeri G, Jilka RL, Manolagas SC (1994) Interleukin-11: a new cytokine critical for osteoclast development. J Clin Invest 93:1516–1524

15. Udagawa N, Takahashi N, Akatsu T, Tanaka H, Sasaki T, Nishihara T, Koga T, Martin TJ, Suda T (1990) Origin of osteoclasts: mature monocytes and macrophages are capable of differentiating into osteoclasts under a suitable microenvironment prepared by bone marrow-derived stromal cells. Proc Natl Acad Sci USA 87:7260–7264

16. Perkins SL, Teitelbaum SL (1991) 1,25-Dihydroxyvitamin D3 modulates colony stimulating factor-1 receptor binding by murine bone marrow macrophage precursors. Endocrinology 128:303–311

17. Hough S, Avioli LV, Muir H, Gelderblom D, Jenkins G, Kurasi H, Slatopolsky E, Bergfeld MA, Teitelbaum SL (1988) Effects of hypervitaminosis A on the bone and mineral metabolism of the rat. Endocrinology 122:2933–2939

18. Colucci S, Grano M, Mori G, Scotlandi K, Mastrogiacomo M, Mori C, Zambonin Zallone A (1996) Retinoic acid induces cell proliferation and modulates gelatinases activity in human osteoclast-like cell lines. Biochem Biophys Res Commun 2227:47–52

19. Merke J, Klaus G, Hugel U, Waldherr R, Rits E (1986) No 1,25-dihydroxyvitamin D3 receptors on osteoclasts of calcium deficient chicken despite demonstrable receptors on circulating monocytes. J Clin Invest 77:312–314

20. Bellido T, Girasole G, Passeri G, Yu XP, Mocharla A, Jilka RL, Notides A, Manolagas SC (1993) Demonstration of estrogen and vitamin D receptors in bone marrow derived stromal cells: upregulation of the estrogen receptor by 1,25-dihydroxyvitamin D3. Endocrinology 133:553–562

21. Kitazawa R, Kimble RB, Vannice JL, Kung VT, Pacifici R (1994) Interleukin-1 receptor antagonist and tumor necrosis factor binding protein decrease osteoclast formation and bone resorption in ovariectomized mice. J Clin Invest 94:2397–2406

22. Nicholson GC, Moseley JM, Sexton PM, Mendelsohn FAO, Martin TJ (1984)

Abundant calcitonin receptors in isolated rat osteoclasts. J Clin Invest 78:335–360

23. Sago K, Ross FP, Martin J, Li C-F, Chappel J, Mimura H, Reichardt LF, Venstrom K, Teitelbaum SL, Cao X (1993) Expression of the integrin avb5 on avian osteoclast precursors is regulated transcriptionally by retinoic acid. J Bone Miner Res 8:S121

24. Teti A (1993) Biology of osteoclasts and molecular mechanisms of bone resorption. Ital J Min Electr Metab 7:123–133

25. Teitelbaum SL, Abu-Amer J, Ross FP (1995) Molecular mechanism of bone resorption. J Cell Biochem 59:1–10

26. Malone JD, Teitelbaum SL, Griffen GL, Senior MR, Kahn AJ (1982) Recruitment of osteoclast precursor by purified bone matrix constituents. J Cell Biol 92:227–230

27. Mundy GR, Poser JW (1983) Chemotactic activity of the gamma-carboxyglutamic acid containing protein in bone. Calcif Tissue Res 35:164–169

28. Grano M, Colucci S, De Bellis, Zigrino P, Argentino L, Zambonin G, Serra M, Scotlandi K, Teti A, Zambonin Zallone A (1994) New model for bone resorption study in vitro: human osteoclast-like cells from giant cell tumors of bone. J Bone Miner Res 9:1013–1020

29. Grano M, Zigrino P, Zambonin G, Trusolino L, Zambonin G, Serra M, Baldinin N, Teti, A Marchisio PC, Zambonin Zallone A (1990) Adhesion properties and integrin expression of cultured human osteoclast-like cells. Exp Cell Res 212:209–218

30. Chenu C, Colucci S, Grano M, Zigrino P, Barattolo R, Zambonin G, Baldini N, Vergnaud P, Delmas PD, Zambonin Zallone A (1994) Osteocalcin induces chemotaxis, secretion of matrix proteins and calcium-mediated intracellular signaling in human osteoclast-like cells. J Cell Biol 4:1149–1158

31. Paniccia R, Colucci S, Grano M, Serra S, Zambonin Zallone A, Teti A (1993) Immediate cell signal by bone-related peptides in human osteoclast-like cells. Am J Physio 265:C1289–C1297

32. Pellettier AJ, Kunicki T, Quaranta V (1996) Activation of the integrin $\alpha_v\beta_3$ involves a discrete cation-binding site that regulates conformation. J Biol Chem 271:1364–1370

33. Baron R, Neff L, Brown W, Courtoy PJ, Louvard D, Farquar MJ (1988) Polarized secretion of lysosomal enzymes: codistribution of cation-independent mannose-6-phosphate receptors and lysosomal enzymes along the osteoclast exocytic pathway. J Cell Biol 106:1863–1872

34. Lakkakorpi P, Tuukkanen J, Huntunen T, Jarvelin K, Vaananen HK (1989) Organization of osteoclast microfilaments during the attachment to bone surfaces in vitro. J Bone Miner Res 4:817–825

35. Lakkakorpi P, Vaananen HK (1991) Kinetics of the osteoclast cytoskeleton during the resorption cycle in vitro. J Bone Miner Res 6:817–826

36. Kanehisa J, Jamanaka T, Doi S, Heersche JNM (1990) A band of F-actin containing podosomes is involved in bone resorption by osteoclast. J Bone Miner Res 5:287–293

37. Marchisio PC, Naldinin L, Cirillo D, Primavera MV, Teti A, Zambonin Zallone A (1984) Cell-substratum interaction of cultured avian osteoclasts is mediated by specific adhesion structures. J Cell Biol 99:1696–1705
38. Marchisio PC, Cirillo D, Zambonin Zallone A, Tarone G (1987) Rous sarcoma virus transformed fibroblasts and cells of monocytic origin display a peculiar dot-like organization of cytoskeletal proteins involved in microfilament-membrane interactions. Exp Cell Res 169:202–214
39. Zambonin Zallone A, Teti A, Grano M, Rubinacci M, Abbadinin M, Gaboli M, Marchisio PC (1989) Immunocytochemical distribution of extracellular matrix receptors in human osteclast. A β_3 integrin is colocalized with vinculin in the podosomes of osteclastoma giant cells. Exp Cell Res 182:645–652
40. Mattsson JP, Schlesinger PH, Keeling DJ, Teitelbaum SL, Stone DK, Xie X-S (1994) Isolation and reconstruction of a vacuolar-type proton pump of osteoclast membranes. J Biol Chem 269:24979–24982
41. Blair HC, Teitelbaum SL, Grosso LE, Lacey DL, Tan H-L, McCourt DW, Jeffrey JJ (1993) Extracellular matrix degradation at acid pH: avian osteoclast acid collagenase isolation and characterization. Biochem J 290:873–884
42. Sasaki T, Ueno-Matsuda E (1993) Cystein proteinase localization in osteoclasts: an immunocytochemical study. Cell Tissue Res 271:177–179
43. Teti A, Blair HC, Schlesinger PH, Grano M, Zambonin Zallone A, Kahn AJ, Teitelbaum SL, Hruska KA (1989) Extracellular protons acidify osteoclasts, reduce cytosolic calcium and promote expression of cell-matrix attachment structures. J Clin Invest 84:773–780
44. Teti A, Blair HC, Zambonin Zallone A, Schlesinger PH, Kahn AJ, Teitelbaum SL (1989) Cytoplasmic pH regulation in chloride-bicarbonate exchange in avian osteoclasts. J Clin Invest 83:227–233
45. Blair HC, Teitelbaum SL, Tan H-L, Koziol CM, Schlesinger PH (1991) Passive chloride permeability charge coupled to H+-ATPase of avian osteoclast ruffled membrane. Am J Physiol 260:C1315–1324
46. Horne WC, Neff L, Chatterjee D, Lomri A, Levy JB, Baron L (1992) Osteoclasts express high levels of pp60$^{c\text{-}}$*src* in association with intracellular membranes. J Cell Biol 119:1003–1113
47. Salo JJ, Metsikko K, Palokangas H, Lehenkari P, Vaananen HK (1996). J Cell Sci 109:301–308
48. Salo JJ, Lehenkari P, Mulari M, Metsikko K, Vaananen HK (1997) Removal of osteoclast bone resorption products by transcytosis. Science 276:270–273
49. Nesbitt SA, Horton MA (1997) Trafficking of matrix collagens through bone-resorbing osteoclasts. Science 276:266–269
50. Malgaroli A, Meldolesi J, Zambonin Zallone A, Teti A (1989) A control cytosolic free calcium in rat and chicken osteoclasts: the role of extracellular calcium and calcitonin. J Biol Chem 264:14343–14347
51. Zaidi M, Datta HK, Patchell A, Moonga BS, MacIntyre I (1989) "Calcium activated" intracellular calcium elevation: a novel mechanism of osteoclast regulation. Biochem Biophys Res Comm 163:907–912

52. Zaidi M, Shankar VS, Adebanjo OA, Lai PF, Pazianas M, Sunavala G, Spielman AI, Rifkin BR (1996) Regulation of extracellular calcium sensing in rat osteoclasts by fentomolar calcitonin concentations. Am J Physiol 271:F637–F644

53. Fried RM, Tashjian AM Jr (1986) Unusual sensititvity of cytosolic free Ca++ to changes in extracellular Ca++ in rat C cells. J Biol Chem 261:7669–7674

54. Nemeth EF, Scarpa A (1987) Rapid mobilization of cellular Ca2+ in bovine parathyroid cells evoked by extracellular covalent cations. J Biol Chem 262:5188–5193

55. Grano M, Faccio R, Colucci S, Paniccia R, Baldinin R, Zambonin Zallone A, Teti A (1994) Extracellular Ca2+ sensing is modulated by pH in human osteoclast-like cells in vitro. Am J Physiol 36:C961–C968

56. Zaida M, Shankar VS, Tunwell R, Adebanjo J, MacKrill J, Pazianas M, O'Connel D, Simon BJ, Rifkin BR, Venkitaran AR, Huang CLH, Lai FA (1995) A ryanodine receptor-like molecule expressed in the osteoclast plasma membrane functions in extracellular Ca2+ sensing. J Clin Invest 96:1582–1590

57. Rodan GA, Martin TJ (1981) Role of osteoblasts in hormonal control of bone resorption. A hypothesis. Calcif Tissue Int 33:249–351

58. Pfeilschifter J, Seyeedin SM, Mundy GR (1988) Transforming growth factor beta inhibits bone resorption in fetal long bone cultures. J Clin Invest 82:680–685

59. Chenu C, Pfeilschifter J, Mundy GR, Roodman GD (1988) Transforming growth factor beta inhibits formation of osteoclast-like cells in long term bone marrow cultures. Proc Natl Acad Sci USA 85:5683–5687

60. Oreffo ROC, Mundy GR, Seyendin S, Bonewald L (1989) Activation of the bone-derived latent TGF β complex by isolated osteoclasts. Biophys Res Commun 158:817–823

61. Nakamura T, Nishizawa T, Hagiya M, Seki T, Shimonishi M, Sugimura A, Tashiro K, Shimizu S (1989) Molecular cloning and expression of human hepatocyte growth factor. Nature 342:440–443

62. Giordano S, Ponzetto C, De Renzo MR, Cooper CS, Comoglio PM (1989) Tyrosine kinase receptor indistinguishable from the c-met protein. Nature 339:155–156

63. Grano M, Galimi F, Zambonin G, Colucci S, Cottone E, Zambonin Zallone A, Comoglio P (1996) Hepatocyte growth factor is a coupling factor for osteoclasts and osteoblasts in vitro. Proc Natl Acad Sci USA: 93:7644–7648

64. Bussolino F, Di Renzuo MF, Ziche M, Boccietto E, Olivero M, Naldini L, Gaudino G, Bardelli A, Tamagnone M, Coffer A, Comoglio PM (1992) Hepatocyte growth factor is a potent angiogenic factor which stimulates endothelial cell motility and growth. J Cell Biol 119:629–641

65. Canalis E (1993) Regulation of bone remodeling. In: Favus MJ (ed) Primer on the metabolic bone diseases and disorders of mineral metabolism. Raven, New York, pp 22–37

66. Pacifici R (1996) Interleukins and their receptors in osteoporosis. Curr Op Orthop 5:16–22

6 Biochemical Markers of Bone Turnover

K. Ziambaras and R. Civitelli

Introduction

The bone turnover (remodeling) cycle is characterized by two opposite but finely coupled processes, bone formation and resorption. In adult normal bone these two processes represent not only the physiological response of the skeleton to injuries, but they also provide the mechanism for renewal of aging bone and remodeling of the skeletal architecture to maximize its flexibility to stress and resistance to load. Most metabolic bone diseases, including osteoporosis, are the consequence of an unbalanced bone turnover.

Although the status of bone turnover is not pathognomonic of any particular disorder, estimation of the processes of bone formation and resorption may add information about the prognosis of the disease and aid in some decision-making circumstances. As detailed in Chap. 10, histomorphometry of the iliac crest allows a precise assessment of bone remodeling at the cell and tissue level and represents the gold standard for estimating the status of bone turnover. However, bone biopsy is not part of the routine evaluation of osteoporotic patients because it is an invasive and expensive procedure. In addition, assessment of bone turnover is limited to a small area of the cancellous and cortical bone which may not always reflect the remodeling process at other skeletal sites [1].

More readily available to the general practitioner and to the specialty physician who manages patients with metabolic bone diseases are some biochemical tests performed on blood or urine samples, which mirror the ongoing bone remodeling processes [2–4]. These biochemical markers are based on the measurement of either an enzymatic activity characteristic of the bone forming or resorbing cells, such as alkaline and acid phosphatase, or bone matrix components released into the circulation during bone apposition or resorption. Markers of bone formation are:
- Serum alkaline phosphatase
- Serum osteocalcin (BGP)
    - Serum type I collagen propeptides
    - C-terminal propeptide (PICP)
    - N-terminal propeptide (PINP)

Markers of bone resorption are:
- Urine hydroxyproline
- Serum tartrate-resistant acid phosphatase

- Urine hydroxylysine glycosides
- Pyridinoline cross-links
  - Urine N-terminal-to-helix cross-links (NTX)
  - Urine C-terminal-to-helix cross-links (CTX)
  - Serum C-terminal-to-helix cross-links (ICTP)

Although this classification of markers implies that each parameter is an indicator of either formation or resorption, this phase-specificity should not be assumed very strictly. Because of the coupling between bone formation and resorption, which is maintained in most pathological conditions, whenever bone turnover is increased, both processes are accelerated and thus markers of both phases are increased. In addition, matrix products can be released into the circulation during both their synthesis (bone formation) or breakdown (bone resorption). Thus in most cases each biochemical marker must be considered as being prevalently associated with either bone formation or resorption.

Some general limitations to the clinical application of these biochemical parameters must be kept in mind. Biochemical markers cannot discriminate whether changes in remodeling rates are the result of focal bone diseases or reflect systemic conditions. These indexes give an estimation of remodeling activity in the whole skeleton, or represent a dilution of the marker produced at extremely high rates by focal disorders (e. g., Paget's disease of bone). By the same token, because bone histomorphometry provides information on a limited area of bone tissue, it may not necessarily be representative of the entire skeleton. Consequently finding bad correlations between biochemical and histomorphometric parameters of bone remodeling does not necessarily imply a failure of a certain index to predict a certain phase of bone remodeling, as it may only reflect a sampling bias. It is also important to consider that biochemical markers do not provide quantitative assessment of bone resorption or formation rates. The unequal specificity, sensitivity, and normality ranges of each marker preclude any such quantitative comparisons. Finally, circulating levels of these markers can be influenced by factors other than bone turnover. Depending on the parameter considered, liver uptake and metabolism, renal excretion, trapping in the bone tissue or uptake by osteoblasts may significantly affect the results. Therefore careful clinical correlations are required for a correct interpretation of these tests.

Parameters of Bone Formation

Serum Alkaline Phosphatase

Human alkaline phosphatase (AP) constitutes a system of enzymes that hydrolyze a phosphoric ester bond from organic and inorganic substrates at an alkaline pH optimum. In human serum three isoenzymes have been identified, including tissue-nonspecific (liver, bone, and kidney), intestinal, and placental AP [5, 6]. A fourth isoenzyme, so-called placenta-like AP, with structure and properties similar but not identical to those of placental AP, has also been identified in small amounts in thymus and testis [7]. Although the isoenzymes from liver, bone, and kidney are products of a single gene [8], post-translational modifications result in altered electrophoretic mobility as well as altered stability to heat and urea [9–11], thus conferring "secondary" tissue specificity [8]. Among the several tissues containing AP, the liver and the bone isoenzymes are the major contributors to serum levels, each accounting for about 50% of the total circulating enzyme activity [12]. The intestinal isoenzyme becomes a significant source of serum AP in diseases of the digestive tract [13] and the liver, such as cirrhosis [14]. In bone AP is localized on the plasma membrane of osteoblasts and is released into the circulation after cleavage by phospholipases.

Total AP activity is measured in plasma or serum using a colorimetric assay, based on the ability of the enzyme to hydrolyze inorganic phosphate substrates. In an attempt to improve the specificity and the sensitivity of serum AP as a marker of bone turnover, techniques have been developed to identify the bone isoenzyme, such as heat inactivation [15], urea denaturation [13], amino acids inhibition (phenylalanine) [16], and separation by either agarose–gel electrophoresis [17] or liver specific antibodies [18, 19]. Heat inactivation is the simplest method used to separate the bone and liver isoenzymes and is based on the higher heat lability of the bone isoform than the liver species. A residual activity of less than 20% after 10 min incubation at 56°C suggests that the specimen originally contained predominantly bone AP [11]. However, the sensitivity of this method is poor, and precise quantitation is virtually impossible due to the high dependency of the assay on substrate concentration, pH [20], temperature [21], and serum protein content. On the other hand, biochemical techniques for identifying bone-derived AP are time consuming and their long-term precision is somewhat variable. Immunoassays based on antibodies specific for the bone isoenzyme have been successfully used in bone-specific AP (BSAP) assays [18, 22, 23]. Cross-reactivity with the liver isoenzyme is usually low because of the much greater affinity of the antibodies for the circulating bone isoform [18, 19].

As do all the other biochemical markers, circulating AP changes with age and menopause. BSAP increases linearly with age in both men and women [24–26] and is correlated well with total AP [19]. In actively growing children the enzyme activity is two- to threefold higher than in adults [11]. Between the second and fourth decades of life circulating AP is higher in men than in women, whereas in the fifth and sixth decades it is higher in women than in men, in association with a postmenopausal increase in bone turnover [19, 27]. As one would expect, the effect of menopause is greater on BSAP than on total enzyme activity; the bone isoenzyme can increase up to 75% in women within 10 years after menopause whereas total AP increases by only 25% [19]. After the sixth decade of life, sex differences disappear, and the enzyme activity follows a slow and gradual increase with aging [12, 19, 25]. Unlike osteocalcin (see below), BSAP levels are unaffected by glomerular filtration rate, a useful feature in patients with impaired renal function [26].

The assumption that AP activity reflects mainly bone formation rather than resorption is based on the fact that the enzyme is expressed as a constitutive protein by osteoblasts, cells that are pivotal to bone formation. Indeed, clinical studies have demonstrated good correlations of the enzyme activity with kinetic and histological parameters of bone formation, but mainly in diseases characterized by extremely elevated bone turnover such as Paget's disease of bone and primary hyperparathyroidism [28, 29]. In contrast, the narrow range of bone turnover rates and the low sensitivity of the assay makes total AP of little diagnostic help in osteoporosis. Finally, it is important to consider that certain drugs, including gold salts, nonsteroidal anti-inflammatory agents, allopurinol, and oral hypoglycemic agents, can elevate circulating AP levels without affecting bone metabolism.

Serum Osteocalcin
(Bone Gla Protein)

Osteocalcin, also referred to as bone Gla-protein (BGP), is a small, noncollagenous protein almost exclusively present in bone and dentin [30]. Mature BGP is a small 49 amino acid peptide, with characteristic residues of gamma-carboxyglutamic acid (Gla), generated by posttranslational carboxylation of three glutamic acid residues in the polypeptide chain. This is a critical step since in the presence of calcium the Gla residues allow specific conformational changes and promote BGP binding to hydroxyapatite and subsequent accumulation in bone matrix [31]. A fraction of BGP, however, remains undercarboxylated, and thus does not bind to hydroxyapatite. This fraction increases with aging [32]. Gamma-carboxylation is a vitamin K dependent process [30], analogous to carboxylation of some clotting factors containing Gla residues, with which BGP shares structural homology. Animal studies have in fact demonstrated that vitamin K deficient diets result in a substantial decrease in BGP, whereas vitamin K supplementation increases BGP concentration in bone. Gamma-carboxylation is sensitive to warfarin [33], although the synthesis of the protein is not. Although prolonged treatment with warfarin does not appear to significantly impair bone formation in adults, exposure of the fetus to sodium warfarin during the first trimester may result in infants born with a hypoplastic saddle nose, punctuate calcifications in distal phalanges and vertebrae, and stubby fingers. Despite its very high affinity to calcium ions [34], the physiological role of BGP is still not totally clear. The recent development of transgenic mice lacking the BGP genes indicate that BGP functions as an inhibitor, rather than a stimulator of calcification [35].

BGP is synthesized predominantly by mature osteoblasts [36, 37] and is incorporated into the extracellular matrix of bone. About 10%–25% of newly synthesized BGP is released into the circulation [34]. Circulating BGP has a short half-life and is almost entirely cleared by the kidneys [38]. When renal function is severely impaired, circulating BGP increases dramatically, commensurate with serum creatinine [39]. However, this is not observed until the glomerular filtration rate drops 70%–80% below the normal level [39]. Nevertheless, when serum values can be adequately corrected for renal function, BGP is a significantly better predictor of bone mineralization than AP in renal insufficiency. Finally, serum BGP is not cleared by hemodialysis [40]; therefore no changes in serum BGP should be expected after hemodialysis.

Intact BGP represents about one-third of the immunoreactivity in the adult serum, while another one-third is represented by several small fragments derived from matrix breakdown during the resorptive process [41]. The remaining one-third is constituted by a large N-terminal midmolecule fragment generated by proteolytic cleavage of the intact molecule in the serum [42]. It is the intact molecule and the longer fragments that are recognized by the antibodies employed in immunoassays for BGP. Although some antibodies may also recognize BGP fragments, their contribution to total BGP is believed to be modest, and for this reason it is reasonable to consider serum BGP a very reliable index of bone formation [43].

Diurnal variations of serum BGP are normal in both sexes, with a 5% to 25% variation between peak at 4 A.M. and nadir, usually occurring around 5 P.M. [44]. Oscillations also occur during the menstrual cycle, with a peak at the end of the luteal phase, when BGP is on average 20% higher than in the follicular phase [45]. BGP levels decline in the first trimester of pregnancy, rise again toward the end of the third trimester, and remain elevated in the postpartum period [46]. Ethnic differences also exist, with lower BGP levels in African-Americans than in whites [47]. As with AP, BGP levels vary with age, reflecting the changes in bone turnover at different times in life. In the neonatal period, BGP concentration ranges 20–40 ng/ml [48], but it is heavily affected by feeding practices. Breast-fed infants have higher circulating BGP than infants fed cow milk [49]. BGP slightly declines during infancy and it remains relatively constant, ranging between 15 and 25 ng/ml, until onset of puberty [50]. During adolescence, a period of active bone growth, serum BGP is markedly increased, reaching levels that are higher than adults, with a peak around the pubertal age for both sexes [51, 52]. After puberty BGP declines to 2–12 ng/ml [50]. In women serum BGP gradually increases around the fourth decade whereas in men aged 30–60 years it remains relatively constant [53]. Around the fifth or sixth decade a significant twofold rise occurs in women superimposed on the age-related pattern [54]. This increase is linked strictly to the menopausal ovarian failure [55, 56], is reproduced by oophorectomy [57], and is reversed by estrogen therapy [58]. This wide physiological variability should be always borne in mind when interpreting serum BGP, especially if the measurement is used to verify changes from previous conditions or to monitor the efficacy of treatment. The menopausal increase in serum BGP is associated with a wider range of individual values observed in subjects with osteoporosis than in normal peers, reflecting the heterogeneity of bone turnover in these patients. On the other hand, the under-carboxylated fraction of BGP, i.e., the fraction which does not bind to hydroxyapatite, increases consistently with age, reaching its highest levels (approx. 20% of total) in the seventh and eight decades of life, probably as the consequence of an age-dependent impairment of gamma-carboxylation [32].

Serum BGP is correlated with static and dynamic indexes of bone formation. Histomorphometry and calcium kinetic studies have demonstrated that in most pathological conditions serum BGP is a valid marker of bone turnover when resorption and formation are coupled, i.e., postmenopausal osteoporosis [56], primary hyperparathyroidism [59], hyperthyroidism [59], and chronic renal failure [60]. When the two remodeling phases are uncoupled, such as in multiple myeloma [61], chronic use of corticosteroids [59], and tumor-associated hypercalcemia [62] serum BGP is closely correlated with bone formation. Therefore BGP provides a reliable, specific index of bone formation.

Serum Type I Procollagen Propeptide

Type I collagen constitutes more than 90% of the organic matrix of bone [63]. During the extracellular processing of type I procollagen molecules, and before collagen is assembled into fibrils, both the N- and C-terminal ends of the propeptide are proteolytically cleaved by specific endopeptidases [64, 65]. The resulting cleavage products, referred to as procollagen type I carboxyl- (PICP) and amino-terminal (PINP) propeptides, are then released into the extracellular fluid. Unlike PICP, a fraction of PINP may be incorporated into the bone matrix where it is released during bone resorption [65, 66]. Nevertheless, the presence of both these collagen fragments in the circulation is directly related to deposition of new type I collagen, thereby representing a potential specific marker of bone formation. Although type I collagen is not exclusively produced in bone, the contribution of soft tissues to circulating PICP is quite small.

PICP is a large, globular glycoprotein, consisting of three polypeptide chains, connected by both intra- and interchain disulfide bonds [67]. These disulfide bonds stabilize the molecule and may allow it to circulate as a single structure after enzymatic cleavage [65]. Because of its large molecular weight (approx. 100 000), PICP cannot be filtered by the renal glomeruli [67]. Metabolism of this peptide in humans is not entirely clear, although studies in rats suggest that most of the circulating PICP is taken up by the hepatic endothelial cells [68]. On the other hand, PINP is an elongated triple-helical peptide smaller than PICP. Having only intrachain disulfide bonds, it is also more unstable than PICP, and it is probably the major substrate of the many smaller circulating monomeric procollagen fragments [64, 69]. PINP is also cleared from the circulation by the endothelial cells of the liver through the scavenger receptor. Because their catabolism occurs in the liver, these peptides can be safely used in patients with renal failure, a slight advantage over BGP. Although the relationship between serum PICP and liver function is still unknown, prudence would discourage the use of this parameter in liver diseases [70].

Radioimmunoassays using antibodies directed against human or synthetic PICP or PINP fragments have been developed. Although both markers should in theory be produced in equal amounts during procollagen processing, PINP assays usually yield circulating levels of the peptide significantly higher than those obtained using PICP assays [71,72]. This apparent difference probably reflects differences in the stability or rate of plasma clearance of the two peptides. Fragments of PINP incorporated into bone and released during bone resorption may also represent an additional source of peptide.

Serum PICP peaks around puberty in girls and declines after age 14–15 years [71]. A slow but progressive age-related increase then ensues, and PICP levels can be up to 40% higher at age 90 than at age 20, but they never reach the adolescent level [71]. Menopause induces an approx. 20% increase in serum PICP concentration [73], which is reversed by hormonal replacement therapy [70,71]. Surprisingly, similar age-related changes have not been detected for PINP [71]. PICP is more sensitive than PINP in detecting deviations from normal in patients with metabolic bone diseases [71, 74] and is better correlated with the calcium kinetics or bone histomorphometry [70, 75]. Unfortunately, the degree of PICP variation in pathological conditions is not as large as that of BGP and AP [71]. Although the reason for this relative insensitivity of the serum procollagen assays may rest on technical problems (e.g., the antigen recognized by the commercial PICP assay may differ immunologically from the native, circulating form of PICP), these markers offer no clear advantage over AP or BGP in routine clinical applications. Precise characterization of the circulating immunoreactive forms of type I procollagen may improve the sensitivity and specificity of these assays.

Parameters of Bone Resorption

Fasting urinary calcium measured on a morning sample and corrected for creatinine excretion is the cheapest assay of bone resorption. This test has been utilized under the assumption that during bone resorption calcium is released from the bone, and if not reutilized by the osteoblasts for new bone formation, the excess calcium enters the circulation and is cleared by the kidney. Therefore an increased bone turnover would lead to an increased urinary calcium output. However, not only is urinary calcium not immune from the effect of calciotropic hormones, but it can only provide a rough estimate of bone remodeling.

Urine Hydroxyproline

One of the early steps in the posttranslational processing of procollagen chains is the hydroxylation of proline and lysine residues. This metabolic pathway is peculiar to collagen and essential for the protein to acquire its characteristic helix conformation. Hydroxyproline is therefore found almost exclusively in collagen, representing about 13% of the amino acid content of the molecule [76]. Free hydroxyproline released into the circulation during collagen degradation cannot be reutilized for synthesis of collagen, and therefore it is excreted into the urine. Since half of human collagen resides in bone, where its turnover is probably faster than in soft tissues, excretion of hydroxyproline in the urine should be correlated to bone resorption [77]. Unfortunately, the contribution of other tissues, most importantly, the C1q component of complement, can be as high as 40% of the total urinary hydroxyproline in normal adults [78,79]. Furthermore, hydroxyproline may also derive as a byproduct of collagen synthesis, either from the breakdown of the procollagen N-terminal peptides (see above) or from intracellular degradation of newly synthesized collagen molecules that are not incorporated into the matrix [80,81].

About 90% of hydroxyproline derived from the breakdown of collagen in the tissues is released into the circulation as free amino acid, which is filtered and almost entirely reabsorbed by the kidney for final catabolism in the liver [82]. The remaining 10% circulates in a peptide-bound form, and is filtered and excreted in the urine without any further metabolism. Thus, total urinary hydroxyproline represents only about 10% of total collagen catabolism and is constituted by three moieties; the free amino acid, small dialyzable hydroxyproline-containing peptides, which account for 90% of total urinary excretion (*dialyzable* hydroxyproline), and nondialyzable hydroxyproline-containing polypeptides (*nondialyzable* hydroxyproline) [76]. The dialyzable form is believed to originate from collagen degradation, thus representing the real bone resorption marker, whereas the nondialyzable form probably derives from newly synthesized collagen fragments that are not incorporated into the matrix. As such it reflects bone formation. Although in theory fractionation of hydroxyproline by dialysis could provide information on both formation and resorption processes, this time-consuming and cumbersome method has never gained widespread enthusiasm. Total urinary hydroxyproline is in fact well correlated with kinetic parameters of bone resorption.

Hydroxyproline is measured using a colorimetric assay after complete hydrolysis to free amino acid. Since urinary hydroxyproline depends directly on the glomerular filtration rate, the results are usually corrected by urinary creatinine excretion or clearance. Other correction factors have also been used, such as body weight, body surface area, and bone mass of the radius [83]. The excretion of hydroxyproline in a 24-h urine sample is heavily dependent on dietary collagen. Therefore the patient must be instructed to follow a collagen-free diet for at least 2 days before urine collection. Although this procedure can be easily complied with, it represents an additional burden for the applicability of the test. Alternatively, hydroxyproline can be measured in a 2-h urine collection and corrected for creatinine after an overnight fast. The latter method seems to offer the same diagnostic value as the 24-h sample, with the advantage of being quicker and less sensitive to dietary collagen.

As a consequence of the physiological coupling between bone resorption and formation, urinary hydroxyproline, as most of the other markers, is sensitive to age- and sex-related changes of bone turnover throughout life. Accordingly, this urinary amino acid is higher in growing children than in adults, reaching a peak around the pubertal age and decreasing thereafter. Hydroxyproline excretion is almost five times higher in children aged 2–15 years than in adults [84]. Although the absolute amount of hydroxyproline in the urine decreases with age, probably reflecting a reduced bone mass; renal function also decreases. Consequently the urinary hydroxyproline/creatinine ratio increases slightly with age. A further postmenopausal increase in total hydroxyproline also occurs.

Urine Hydroxylysine Glycosides

Hydroxylysine is another amino acid unique to collagen and proteins containing collagenlike sequences. As mentioned above, lysine and proline residues are hydroxylated during the post-translational processing of collagen chains. Hydroxylysine residues are then glycosylated forming either -1-galactosyl-hydroxylysine (GHL), or -1,2-glycosyl-galactosyl-hydroxylysine (GGHL). As with hydroxyproline, glycosylated hydroxylysine is not reutilized for collagen biosynthesis, and although it is much less abundant than hydroxyproline it also reflects bone matrix breakdown [79]. Theoretically, measuring this amino acid in the urine should provide a more selective index of bone resorption than hydroxyproline because hydroxylysine glycosides are entirely excreted into the urine [79].

Glycosylation of lysine residues during collagen processing is to a certain extent tissue specific. Accordingly, GHL is a prevalent product of bone collagen, whereas GGHL is more specific of skin collagen [85]. In fact the GGHL/GHL ratio could provide an index reflecting the metabolic activity of either bone or skin [85]. Indeed, in high bone turnover conditions such as Paget's disease of bone levels of GHL are increased, whereas burn patients with extensive skin damage and therefore increased skin metabolism have increased levels of GGHL [79]. However, treatment with salmon calcitonin decreases both GHL and GGHL, suggesting that either "abnormal" glycosylation profiles exist [79], or that some urinary GGHL originates from synthesis of other types of collagen (perhaps type III collagen) which is not incorporated into the extracellular bone matrix [86].

Aging is associated with increments in urinary GHL in both sexes, similar to those observed for hydroxyproline, but the increase is more marked in women than in men [87]. Men and women excrete practically the same amounts of GHL between 30 and 80 years of age. A peak of GHL occurs in women in their fifth decade of life (i. e., just after the menopause), reflecting the high rate of bone resorption after the menopause. Similarly, urine GHL excretion is higher in elderly men than in young men, and it is inversely correlated with bone density [87]. Unfortunately, the pattern of glycosylated hydroxylysine excretion in normal subjects and in patients with Paget's bone disease is not entirely consistent with an exclusive bone origin (see below). Considering also the complexity of the method for measuring hydroxylysine glycosides, which requires HPLC, the application of this marker for routine clinical settings is still very limited.

Plasma Tartrate-Resistant Acid Phosphatase

Acid phosphatase is a lysosomal enzyme present in bone, prostate, platelets, erythrocytes, and spleen. Its enzymatic properties are similar to those of AP except that its pH optimum is acidic. The different isoenzymes can be separated by electrophoretic methods, which are unsuitable for routine clinical applications. The bone isoenzyme is characteristically expressed by osteoclasts [88, 89], although minor enzyme activity is also present in osteoblasts and osteocytes [90]. Thus acid phosphatase is released into the circulation during bone resorption [89]. Among the acid phosphatases detected in serum by gel electrophoresis, only the bone derived enzyme is resistant to L(+)-tartrate [91]. This allows distinguishing the bone isoform from the prostatic isoenzyme, the other major moiety present in the circulation in normal individuals. Circulating acid phosphatase activity is higher in serum than in plasma because of the contribution of platelet phosphatase activity released during the clotting process.

Tartrate resistant acid phosphatase (TRAP) in the circulation varies with sex and hormonal status. Its serum levels do not significantly change until menopause, when the enzyme activity increases to a maximum within 12 months [92], and declines thereafter [93]. A good correlation has been observed between TRAP and urinary hydroxyproline after oophorectomy [93] and in patients with vertebral osteoporosis [94]. Although a negative correlation has been reported between TRAP and bone mineral density in osteoporotic patients [95], the instability of TRAP activity in frozen plasma samples and the presence of enzyme inhibitors in serum are potential drawbacks which have limited the diffusion of this marker in clinical applications. New immunoassays using monoclonal antibodies which specifically recognize the bone isoenzyme of TRAP [96] should help define the diagnostic value of this marker for osteoclast activity [97].

Urine Pyridinoline Cross-Links

Collagen fibrils are stabilized in their characteristic trimeric structure by specific covalent cross-links, formed within the triple helical chains and between adjacent trimeric assemblies. This posttranslational cross-linking is initially formed between amino acid residues, mostly lysine, hydroxylysine, and histidine. In bone, cross-linking involves lysine and hydroxylysine, whereas in the skin, histidine is the major residue to be cross-linked [98]. This tissue specificity offers the basis for the use of collagen cross-links as markers of bone turnover. As the post-translational cross-linking proceeds, the aldehydric bonds are converted to mature nonreducible compounds [99, 100]. Two major cross-links are present in the matrix of bone and cartilage, hydroxylysyl-pyridinoline and lysyl-pyridinoline, also known as pyridinoline (Pyr), and deoxypyridinoline (D-Pyr), respectively. Thus Pyr and D-Pyr cross-links bind adjacent collagen molecules via three hydroxylysine residues (or 2 hydroxylysine and 1 lysine in the case of D-Pyr), two of them originating from the short, terminal, nonhelical sequences and one from the helicoidal domain of the collagen molecule.

The concentration of Pyr and D-Pyr in connective tissues is very low and varies among tissue types [101, 102]. D-Pyr is present in relatively high concentrations in bone and dentin, where it constitutes about 22% of total hydroxypyridinoline cross-links [102]. It is also present, although at much lower concentrations, in the aorta, human tendon (6%), and articular cartilage (2%), but it is absent from the skin [102, 103]. Pyr is also present in articular cartilage, where it reaches its highest concentration, bone, tendon, and most other connective tissues except skin [98, 102, 103]. Since bone is by far the most abundant source of collagen matrix, and its turnover rate is markedly higher than that of other connective tissues, Pyr and D-Pyr present in biological fluids could be considered as deriving predominantly from bone. Both collagen cross-link metabolites are released from bone matrix during collagen degradation into the circulation and are finally excreted into the urine. The ratio of Pyr to D-Pyr existing in the bone matrix is maintained in the urine [104, 105] and is affected by neither bone turnover rate nor sex [106]. Pyr and D-Pyr are not metabolized in vivo, and they cannot be reutilized [101, 103]. Therefore they are excreted in the urine unchanged either as free (approx. 40%) or as peptide-bound forms (approx. 60%). Pyridinoline cross-links have generated enthusiasm among the investigators in this field as markers of bone resorption. Their advantages over urinary hydroxyproline stem from their complete urinary excretion, their absence in immature and skin collagen, and their insensitivity to dietary gelatin [107].

Measurements are commonly performed in a 24-h urine sample. A fasting 2-h urine collection has also been proposed, although it should be considered that an early morning urine sample after an overnight fast yields higher values of both Pyr and D-Pyr than 24-h urine samples [108]. This is the consequence of the bone resorption occurring more rapidly during the night than during daytime. As seen for BGP, a circadian rhythm of pyridinoline excretion has been observed in both normal and osteoporotic women, with peak in the early morning and nadir in the evening [109]. Daily variations in urinary pyridinoline cross-links are more pronounced than for any other marker, with values that can oscillate up to 100% from peak to nadir during a 24-h period [109, 110]. Similar to other markers, urinary Pyr and D-Pyr change with age [106, 111]. Thus, circulating levels are many-fold higher in children than in adults, decline progressively in late puberty and during adolescence, then fall within the normal adult range around age 15–17 years [51, 112, 113]. Menopause is followed by a two- to threefold increase in circulating cross-links [108], which rapidly return to premenopausal levels after estrogen treatment [108]. Pyr and especially D-Pyr, are correlated with bone turnover measured by calcium kinetics [114] and bone histomorphometry [115].

Total pyrydinoline cross-link concentration can be measured by fluorometric methods after separation by reverse-phase HPLC, utilizing their natural fluorescence [102, 116]. This assay is considered the gold standard for measuring cross-links, but it is inconveniently complex and time consuming. Various immunoassays, more suitable for routine use, have been recently developed using antibodies which recognize either Pyr or D-Pyr free fractions, or epitopes in the cross-linked domains of type I collagen. The N-telopeptide-to-helix (NTX) end of the collagen molecule (i.e., the part of the collagen molecule that includes the N-telopeptide and the helicoidal part) presumably is the source of almost 60% of the D-Pyr in human bone collagen, as opposed to a 40% contributed by the C-telopeptide-to-helix (CTX) end [117]. Furthermore, at this end of the collagen molecule, pyridinoline cross-links are formed between either α_1 (I) or α_2 (I) and α_2 (I) chains, which differ from other tissue type I collagen cross-links. On the contrary, only an α_1 (I) to α_1 (I) cross-link can be formed at the C-telopeptide end, resulting in a fragment that is produced by all tissues in which type I collagen is cross-linked by pyridinoline [118]. Collagen telopeptides are highly immunogenic [119], and the considerable variability between the different collagen types provides the opportunity for developing collagen type-specific immunoassays.

Free Pyr or D-Pyr concentration in the urine measured by the Pyrilink and Pyrilink-D assays, respectively, are correlated well with total pyridinoline excretion measured by HPLC. Both parameters increase significantly after menopause and in patients with active Paget's disease of bone [106, 120, 121]. Direct measurement of peptide-bound cross-links demonstrated that when bone turnover increases, the abundance of the peptide-bound moiety of cross-links is higher relative to free Pyr and D-Pyr, although both fractions increase in absolute terms [122]. This is probably the result of a faster metabolic clearance of the free cross-links than peptide-bound cross-links, and perhaps a preferential release of the peptide-bound forms during bone resorption [97].

The monoclonal antibody used in the Osteomark NTX assay recognizes epitopes in the NTX cross-linking domain of human bone type I collagen [117]. As mentioned above, in theory the participation of α_2 (I) collagen chains to the cross-linking at the N-terminus of the molecule should confer a higher bone specificity to NTX than to CTX assays. Immunoaffinity chromatography has demonstrated that all the epitopes recognized by the monoclonal antibody used in this assay derive from the α_2 (I) NTX cross-linking domain of human type I collagen, whereas free Pyr is not recognized by this monoclonal antibody [117]. Urine NTX concentration measured by this quite specific assay is markedly increased after menopause and in patients with hyperthyroidism or Paget's disease of bone [117].

The antibody used in the Crosslaps assay is raised against a synthetic octapeptide corresponding to a fragment of the C-telopeptide sequence of α_1 (I) collagen chain, in which one lysine residue is involved in the cross-linking [123, 124]. This should ensure minimal cross-reactivity with other types of collagen. Urine CTX levels are increased after menopause in almost one-third of all postmenopausal women [123], consistent with the notion that about one-third of all women experience accelerated bone loss after menopause [125]. As with NTX, urine CTX is also increased in patients with Paget's disease of bone, hyperparathyroidism and hyperthyroidism [126], and are correlated well with hydroxyproline [123, 127] and free D-Pyr [128].

An immunoassay that measures type I collagen C-telopeptides (ICTP) in the serum has been recently tested [129]. As noted above, the helical part of the α-chains is strongly conserved among different types of collagen. Therefore, the specificity of this assay in reflecting bone resorption may not be the best, and degradation products of collagen type II and/or III may cross-react with this antibody [123, 130]. Nonetheless, serum ICTP levels are correlated with histomorphometric measurements of bone turnover in iliac crest biopsies [130,131]. As one would anticipate, the concentration of circulating ICTP is subject to significant diurnal oscillations, with mean values 20%–25% higher at night than in the afternoon [125,132]. Furthermore, a severely decreased glomerular filtration rate increases ICTP [133]. While this index is increased in patients with bone metastases [128,134], it is surprisingly not high in Paget's disease of bone, nor does hormonal replacement therapy significantly alter serum ICTP [130]. On the contrary, anabolic steroids that presumably decrease bone resorption and increase collagen synthesis can increase serum ICTP concentration [130]. Consequently serum ICTP can be considered a good index of collagen turnover but a less sensitive marker of bone resorption [130].

Clinical Applications

Diagnostic Value in Osteoporosis

Great efforts have been expended in the past few years to define the potential clinical usefulness of biomarkers of bone turnover in the management of patients with osteoporosis. Indeed the ability to predict bone loss and more importantly the risk of new fractures by a simple biochemical test would simplify the diagnostic process in these patients with significant cost savings. As discussed in more detail herein, there is clear evidence that patients with more accelerated remodeling rates experience faster bone loss and respond better to antiresorptive therapy than subjects with normal or reduced bone turnover. The improved sensitivity and precision of biochemical markers and, in particular, the newly developed assays for bone resorption can provide reliable detection of such diversity of bone remodeling rates in osteoporotic populations. Notwithstanding the recent enthusiasm and plethora of publications, major limitations to the application of these biochemical parameters to critical diagnostic and therapeutic decisions in osteoporosis still exist. These stem from the inadequacy of a single biochemical test to reliably predict bone loss and fracture risk in individual patients, the relatively high day-to-day variability, and ultimately the cost and availability of the test itself. Whereas these theoretical considerations may prove insurmountable for the applicability of bone turnover markers to estimation of bone loss and fracture risk, it seems likely that a lower cost and perhaps the inclusion of one of these parameters in automated analyzers would immediately expand the use of bone remodeling markers to other clinical questions that can be effectively addressed by the use of these tests. These include, but are not limited to, monitoring patient compliance and short-term response to therapy.

Prediction of Bone Loss and Fracture Risk

With age bone turnover slowly but gradually increases in both sexes. In women a postmenopausal transient is overimposed upon the age-related increase. Accordingly, menopause is followed by significant changes in the levels of almost all biochemical markers of bone turnover. Detectable increases in AP (total and bone specific isoenzyme), BGP and PICP occur in the transition from pre- to postmenopause [135]. Similar changes have been observed for all bone resorption markers, with different degrees of sensitivity [105]. There is a wide individual variability in the magnitude of the postmenopausal increase in bone turnover, depending upon the individual genetic background and life-style habits, and this variability translates into a similar histological heterogeneity [136, 137]. However, because of the postmenopausal increase in bone turnover average remodeling rates are higher than normal in unselected osteoporotic populations [137, 138]. A number of studies have reported negative correlations between markers of bone turnover and bone density, a correlation that becomes stronger with aging [139–141]. However, when the contribution of bone turnover was estimated in women within 10 years of menopause, the rate of remodeling – assessed by a battery of biochemical markers – accounted for only 10% of bone density [97]. Although the weight of bone remodeling on bone density may increase with higher menopausal age [97], these observations exemplify the limitations of a single determination of bone turnover to reliably predict bone density unless bone is rapidly being lost. This notion becomes rather obvious if one considers that a biochemical marker reflects the cellular activity at that particular moment in time, whereas bone mass is the result of a life-long process of modeling and remodeling. Better correlations have been observed between biochemical markers and *rates* of bone loss. Thus higher serum BGP levels are associated with more rapid bone loss at the distal radius and the lumbar spine in both perimenopausal and early postmenopausal women [58, 138]. A single measurement of D-Pyr has been shown to be correlated – albeit weakly – with the subsequent rate of bone loss measured during 2 years in a small group of recently menopausal women [108]. Again, the low correlation coefficients and the high standard errors of estimate preclude extrapolation of these results to individual patients.

Combination of different markers, such as fasting Pyr or D-Pyr, urinary hydroxyproline, and serum BGP, increase the predictive value for subsequent bone loss in postmenopausal women over that of a single parameter, with a correlation coefficient high enough to allow consideration for a potential clinical use [108, 142]. A similar approach has been taken by another group to construct an algorithm based on multiple markers and bone density measurements that could be applied as a screening procedure to diagnose osteoporosis and estimate future bone loss [125]. Based on this method postmenopausal women can be classified as "fast losers" if the predicted bone loss is greater than 3% per annum or as "slow losers" if less than this level. A 12-year follow-up of a relatively large group of postmenopausal women indicated that despite identical bone mass at baseline, "fast losers" lost 50% more bone than those identified as "slow losers" [143]. These observations are encouraging, and although such results need to be confirmed in larger populations, combining one baseline bone mass measurement with a battery of bone turnover markers is a plausible approach to estimate the rate of bone loss and thus identify those menopausal women who are at highest risk of developing osteoporosis [144].

Another probably less critical limitation to the clinical application of biochemical markers is the day-to-day variability that may reflect short-term changes in bone turnover occurring during a lifetime. Although indices of bone formation and resorption may fluctuate randomly in osteoporotic patients, subjects with high-turnover forms of osteoporosis generally continue in this category [145]. Furthermore, repeated measurements of bone formation and resorption markers for several months in osteoporotic women yield relatively low individual long-term coefficients of variation [146]. Thus with the refinement of the technical aspects of the biochemical assays it is reasonable to expect that this source of variability may be controlled in the near future.

The possibility of using biochemical markers of bone turnover to predict the risk of hip fracture represents the ultimate standard for assessing the validity of these parameters as diagnostic tool in osteoporosis. As one would anticipate, solid and consistent data are not available to this end. One study found urinary Pyr cross-links measured immediately after a hip fracture event – thus before a reactive increase in bone resorption could in theory have occurred – to be higher than in a random sample of healthy individuals [147]. Although the authors concluded that increased bone resorption may have contributed to the low bone mass detected in these patients, the lack of good controls and the cross-sectional nature of this study limit its significance. In more recent longitudinal study on a large number of postmenopausal women, higher baseline values of urinary CTX and free D-Pyr were observed in subjects who sustained a hip fracture in the following 2 years than in age-matched women who did not experienced hip fractures [148]. Interestingly, only these two bone resorption markers were significantly elevated in this cohort, as NTX and bone formation markers (BGP, BSAP) did not differ between cases and controls. Furthermore, only women in the highest quartile for CTX had a twofold relative risk of hip fractures, independently of bone density and physical performance.

Elderly institutionalized women who sustained a hip fracture during a 18-month follow up study revealed a significantly higher circulating level of under-carboxylated BGP at baseline than control subjects without fractured [149]. This puzzling observation may reflect a vitamin K deficiency, which is not uncommon in elderly patients with hip fracture [150]. Thus the combined subclinical deficiency of vitamin K and vitamin D, also relatively prevalent at this age, represents a rather unfavorable condition that may be conducive to increased risk for bone loss and fractures in elderly persons. These results are rather appealing, but it remains to be seen how the additional information provided by biochemical markers can be translated into decision-making differences compared to measurement of bone density only.

Selection of Treatment

Because patients with accelerated bone turnover tend to lose bone at a faster rate than those with normal turnover [125, 138], theoretically they should be the best candidates for antiresorptive therapy. This hypothesis was first demonstrated in a study from our group on a series of postmenopausal osteoporotic women treated with subcutaneous salmon calcitonin [132]. Patients with high-turnover osteoporosis responded to this therapy with significant gains in vertebral bone density, as opposed to no changes observed in individuals with normal bone remodeling [132]. Similar results have been later reported by other investigators who were able to predict the response to calcitonin therapy in terms of changes in bone density by baseline measurements of biochemical markers of bone turnover [151]. Response to estrogen has also been found to be correlated to levels of bone turnover markers at the initiation of treatment in at least two studies using calcitonin and transdermal estrogen [152, 153]. The relevance of these studies is immediately obvious, but the clinical impact of effective screening methods to identify subjects that would better respond to antiresorptive therapy relies entirely upon our ability to precisely predict bone loss by a single assessment of bone turnover, an issue that is far from being settled, as discussed above. Moreover, because antiresorptive therapies depress bone remodeling, prediction of response to these type of medications is by definition limited to short-term changes, certainly not longer than 1 year after initiation of treatment. The current lack of valid alternatives to antiresorptive medications for the treatment of osteoporosis further reduces the clinical relevance of screening programs based on bone turnover for decision making on osteoporosis therapy. However, this conclusion may change in the near future with the introduction of anabolic agents that may uncouple the remodeling cycle by stimulating bone formation.

Monitoring Treatment Compliance and Efficacy

Hormone replacement therapy decreases both resorption and formation markers, which reach premenopausal levels within 3–6 months of therapy [97]. Even more rapid responses have been obtained with bisphosphonates. Treatment with alendronate dose-dependently decreases serum BGP and urinary Pyr after only 6 weeks of treatment [154]. Interestingly, resorption markers decrease earlier than formation markers on alendronate therapy [146]. This reflects a positive though transient uncoupling of the remodeling cycle, the basis for the therapeutic effect of these drugs. Thus biochemical markers can rapidly report changes in bone turnover in response to antiresorptive therapy. After withdrawal of hormonal replacement therapy bone turnover markers return to pretreatment values within 3 months, the same time that is necessary to detect a decrease following initiation of therapy [155]. Considering the relatively low compliance to hormone replacement therapy, the potential clinical utility of these parameters in this context is rather obvious. If the current costs can be lowered, it is very likely that physicians will find biochemical markers of bone turnover very useful in monitoring compliance to bone active medications.

On the other hand, using bone turnover markers to predict response to treatment is still very controversial. A significant, although rather weak correlation has been recently reported between percentage change in biochemical markers at 3 months and spinal bone mineral density after 24 months of treatment with estrogen [146]. A very recent study also reported a weak correlation between changes in one bone resorption marker, NTX, and changes in bone density after 12 months of estrogen replacement, with a 2.2-fold higher likelihood of gaining bone density in 1 year of treatment in those subjects who experienced a 30% decline of NTX than in those who exhibited lesser or no changes [156]. However, 57% of the treated patients with less than 30% decrease in NTX still improved or maintained bone density. Furthermore, the predictive value of NTX was significant only for vertebral and not proximal femur bone density [156].

Although these data are of extreme importance and significance, they should not be construed to suggest that two serial measurements of a bone turnover marker at baseline and 3–6 months into treatment would yield the same information about the efficacy of antiresorptive therapy as can be obtained by measuring bone density in 1–2 years. Such a spectacular conclusion would be ill-advised, not only because of the shortcomings of these particular results – poor correlations, high standard errors of estimates – but also for some obvious theoretical considerations. In the vast majority of postmenopausal women, values of bone turnover markers fall within the normal range. In fact only a minority of subjects experience high bone turnover and "fast" bone loss [137, 138, 143]. Because the precision error of the currently used biochemical markers of resorption, especially those measured in the urine [95, 109], exceeds the magnitude of the change that occurs during treatment, in most cases it is impossible to distinguish between treatment effect and day-to-day individual variability. Averaging more than one measurement may reduce this variability, but the problem remains that individual responses cannot be inferred by group behaviors, and in the clinical setting, it is the individual patient that is assessed.

Diagnostic Value in Other Metabolic Bone Diseases

Biochemical estimation of bone turnover is the procedure of choice for the follow-up of patients with Paget's bone disease, and it can be useful in decisions about therapeutic interventions. To date the best and most used marker remains AP activity [28]. Total AP is well correlated with the extent of bone involvement in Paget's bone disease, and as expected, the enzymatic activity in the circulation of these patients is accounted for almost exclusively by the bone isoform [19]. Treatment with bone resorption inhibitors, i.e., calcitonin or bisphosphonates, rapidly decreases serum AP, and the degree of change is commonly used to assess the magnitude of response. Thus a 50% decline after 3–4 months of therapy is considered an indication of therapeutic effectiveness. Evidence for relapse and further decision about treatment is heavily based on AP levels, in addition to the symptoms. Although BSAP is more sensitive to antiresorptive treatment than total enzyme activity [19], in most cases total AP is adequate. Other bone formation and resorption markers are also increased as the consequence of the extremely fast remodeling and the conserved coupling between the resorptive and formative processes in this disorder. Thus any marker could be used in Paget's disease with the exception of BGP. Perhaps because of the extremely high degree of the cellular activity in the areas affected, the osteoblasts may actually reaccumulate some of the released BGP and reuse it in the rapidly remodeling pagetic bone. Thus the amount of BGP entering the circulation may not be sufficient to cause a detectable increase, which may explain the surprisingly low BGP levels reported in some patients [157, 158]. Therefore this marker is not a good diagnostic tool in this condition. The more recent bone resorption markers are more sensitive to the effect of therapy in Paget's bone disease. For example, both Pyr and D-Pyr decline within 2 days of treatment with bisphosphonates [106], well before any decrease in AP or urine hydroxyproline occur [106]. Likewise, urine NTX measured before and after a short period of treatment with a bisphosphonate (about 10 days) may be sufficient to predict the therapeutic outcome [159].

In primary hyperparathyroidism serum AP and BGP increase along with serum calcium and parathyroid hormone and their serum levels are correlated with the weight of the parathyroid adenoma [62]. Serum BGP returns to normal within 2–6 months after removal of the tumor, suggesting that this parameter reflects increased turnover at the tissue level more than a direct effect of PTH on BGP production by osteoblasts. Furthermore, in patients with mild hypercalcemia due to asymptomatic primary hyperparathyroidism BGP can be elevated even in the presence of normal PTH levels, implying that measurement of BGP might be a useful ancillary test in such cases [62]. Markers of bone resorption are all typically increased in primary hyperparathyroidism, including urinary hydroxyproline, TRAP, and Pyr and D-Pyr [95, 160, 161]. There is a close association between bone resorption and formation markers in primary hyperparathyroidism, a reflection of the conserved coupling between bone formation and resorption. The decrease in bone resorption markers following surgical removal of the parathyroid adenoma usually precedes the reduction of AP [161]. Serum TRAP or urine Pyr and D-Pyr normalize earlier than urine hydroxyproline, confirming their higher sensitivity and specificity. Nonetheless, the clinical usefulness of bone turnover markers in this disease is minimal, if any.

In contrast to primary hyperparathyroidism, BGP levels are subnormal in hypercalcemia of malignancy and bone metastasis, the consequence of an uncoupling of the bone remodeling cycle [62]. It has been suggested that the simultaneous assessment of serum BGP and urinary hydroxyproline could be useful in the differential diagnosis of hypercalcemia [162]. If both markers are increased, primary hyperparathyroidism is more likely, a condition in which resorption and formation remain coupled. If hydroxyproline is elevated with normal or low serum BGP, hypercalcemia of malignancy is more likely since the bone remodeling cycle is uncoupled. Obviously these should be considered only ancillary findings in such conditions. Interestingly, urine Pyr and D-Pyr, which increase two- to threefold in patients with hypercalcemia of malignancy, decrease less than urine calcium after bisphosphonate therapy, suggesting that the effect of this treatment on bone mineral and organic matrix is dissociated [163].

Patients with multiple myeloma have depressed bone formation, reflected by low BGP levels, and increased resorption mediated by local factors active on bone present in the marrow of myeloma [61,164]. In fact complete response to chemotherapy alone has been associated with a significant increase in BGP levels. On the other hand, long-term treatment with corticosteroids results in subnormal BGP levels [1]. The decline in serum BGP, which reflects the inhibition of osteoblastic activity induced by corticosteroids, occurs within a few days after initiation of corticosteroid therapy, and it is correlated with the daily dose of the drug, thus representing a good index of the degree of steroid-induced suppression of bone formation.

Moreover, urinary Pyr excretion is increased in osteomalacia, in hyperthyroidism, in acromegaly, and after treatment with growth hormone [165, 166]. A decrease in bone resorption markers in these conditions indicates an improvement in the resorptive process and can be used to follow the response to treatment.

Future Directions

Despite the noteworthy efforts expended in the last few years and the improved sensitivity and precision of biochemical markers of bone turnover, controversy still exists as far as their real clinical usefulness. While BGP and BSAP currently represent the most specific markers of bone formation, there are still plenty of indications for continuing to use the less sensitive, but simple and inexpensive total AP, especially in very high bone-turnover conditions. The increasing knowledge of the structure and regulation of other noncollagenous bone matrix proteins, such as bone sialoprotein and proteoglycans, all synthetic products of osteoblasts, will direct the future development of bone formation markers. Because of the potential clinical usefulness in therapeutic decisions involving bone resorption inhibitors most recent efforts in this field have focused on bone resorption markers. The development of assays for measurement of pyridinoline crosslinks represents the most important step in this direction and has provided a valuable marker whose clinical use will certainly increase in the near future.

Although markers of bone turnover most likely will never supplant bone densitometry as the standard diagnostic tool for the diagnosis and management of osteoporosis, it is possible that with the improved sensitivity, precision, and availability of the biochemical assays they will become part of the diagnostic approach to the osteoporotic patient. Defining the most appropriate therapeutic intervention and monitoring treatment effectiveness are two critically important niches for the use of biochemical markers on bone turnover in this condition. It is foreseeable that with the increasing available therapeutic options and the mounting prevalence of osteoporosis in elderly populations these two niches will expand in the near future.

References

1. Delmas PD (1988) Biochemical markers of bone turnover in osteoporosis. In: Riggs BL, Melton LJ III (eds) Osteoporosis: etiology, diagnosis, and management. Raven, New York, pp 297–316
2. Calvo MS, Eyre DR, Gundberg CM (1996) Molecular basis and clinical application of biological markers of bone turnover. Endocr Rev 17:333–368
3. Akesson K (1995) Biochemical markers of bone turnover. Acta Orthop Scand 66:376–386
4. Eriksen EF, Brixen K, Charles P (1995) New markers of bone metabolism: clinical use in metabolic bone disease. Eur J Endocrinol 132:251–263
5. Seargeant LE, Stinson RA (1979) Evidence that three structural genes code for human alkaline phosphatase. Nature 281:152–154
6. Harris H (1989) The human alkaline phosphatases: what we know and what we don't know. Clin Chim Acta 180:177–188
7. Goldstein DJ, Rogers C, Harris H (1982) A search for trace expression of placental-like alkaline phosphatase in non-malignant human tissues: demonstration of its occurence in lung, cervix, testis and thymus. Clin Chim Acta 125:63–75
8. Weiss MJ, Henthorn PS, Lafferty MA, Slaughter C, Raducha M, Harris H (1986) Isolation and characterization of a cDNA encoding a human liver/bone/kidney-type alkaline phosphatase. Proc Natl Acad Sci USA 83:7182–7186
9. Petitclerc C (1976) Quantitative fractionation of alkaline phosphatase isoenzymes according to their thermostability. Clin Chem 22:42–48
10. Rosalki SB, Foo AY (1984) Two new methods for separating and quantifying bone and liver alkaline phosphatase isoenzymes in plasma. Clin Chem 30:1182–1186
11. Moss DW (1982) Alkaline phosphatase isoenzymes. Clin Chem 28:2007–2016
12. Van Hoof VO, Hoylarts MS, Geryl H, Van Mullem M, Lepoutre LG, Broe ME (1990) Age and sex distribution of alkaline phosphatase isoenzymes by electrophoresis. Clin Chem 36:875–878
13. Dent CE, Norris TSM, Smith R, Sutton RAL, Temperley JM (1968) Steatorrhea with striking increase of plasma alkaline phosphatase of intestinal origin. Lancet 1:1333–1336
14. Stolbach LL, Krant MJ, Inglis NR, Fishmann WH (1967) Correlation of serum L-phenylalanine sensitive alkaline phosphatase derived from intestine with ABO blood group of cirrhotics. Gastroenterology 52:819–827
15. Harris SS, Dawson-Hughes B (1994) Caffeine and bone loss in healthy postmenopausal women. Am J Clin Nutr 60:573–578
16. Komoda T, Hokari S, Somoda M, Sakagishi Y, Tamara T (1982) L-Phenylala-

nine inhibition of human alkaline phosphatase with p-nitrophenylphosphate as substrate. Clin Chem 28:2426–2428

17. Onica D, Sundblad L, Waldenlind L (1986) Affinity electrophoresis of human isoenzymes in agarose gel containing lectin. Clin Chem 155:285–294

18. Hill GS, Wolfert RL (1989) The preparation of monoclonal antibodies which react preferentially with human bone alkaline phosphatase and not with liver alkaline phosphatase. Clin Chim Acta 186:315–320

19. Garnero P, Delmas PD (1993) Assessment of the serum levels of bone alkaline phosphatase with a new immunoradiometric assay in patients with metabolic bone disease. J Clin Endocrinol Metab 77:1046–1053

20. Moss DW, Shakespeare MJ, Thomas DM (1972) Observations on the heat-stability of alkaline phosphatase isoenzymes in serum. Clin Chim Acta 40:35–41

21. Whitby LG, Moss DW (1975) Analysis of heat inactivation curves of alkaline phosphatase isoenzymes in serum. Clin Chim Acta 59:361–367

22. Lawson GM, Katzmann JA, Kimlinger TK, O'Brien JF (1985) Isolation and preliminary characterization of a monoclonal antibody that interacts preferentially with the liver isoenzyme of human alkaline phospatase. Clin Chem 31:381–385

23. Bailyes EM, Seabrook RN, Calvin J (1987) The preparation of monoclonal antibodies to human bone and liver alkaline phosphatases and their use in immunoaffinity purification and in studying these enzymes when present in serum. Biochem J 244:725–733

24. Schiele F, Henny J, Hitz S, Petitclerc C, Gueguen R, Siest G (1983) Total, bone and liver alkaline phosphatases in plasma: biological variation and reference limits. Clin Chem 23:634–641

25. Kuwana T, Sugita O, Yakata M (1988) Reference limits of bone and liver alkaline phosphatase isoenzymes in the serum of healthy subjects according to age and sex as determined by wheat germ lectin affinity electrophoresis. Clin Chim Acta 173:273–280

26. Duda RJ, O'Brien JF, Katzmann JA, Peterson JM, Mann KG, Riggs BL (1988) Concurrent assays of circulating bone Gla protein and bone alkaline phosphatase: effects of sex, age, and metabolic bone disease. J Clin Endocrinol Metab 66:951–957

27. Crilly RG, Jones MM, Horsman A, Nordin BEC (1980) Rise in plasma alkaline phosphatase at the menopause. Clin Sci 58:341–342

28. Meunier PJ, Salson C, Mathieu L (1987) Skeletal distribution and biochemical parameters of Paget's disease. Clin Orthop 217:37–44

29. Podenphant J, Johansen JS, Thomsen K (1987) Bone turnover in spinal osteoporosis. J Bone Miner Res 2:497–503

30. Price PA (1987) Vitamin K-dependent bone proteins. In: Cohn DV, Martin TJ, Meunier PJ (eds) Calcium regulation and bone metabolism: basic and clinical aspects. Elsevier Science, Amsterdam, pp 419–426

31. Hauschka PV, Carr SA (1982) Calcium-dependent α-helical structure in osteocalcin. Biochemistry 21:638

32. Plantalech L, Guillaumont M, Leclercq M, Delmas PD (1991) Impaired carboxylation of serum osteocalcin in elderly women. J Bone Miner Res 6:1211–1216

33. Levy RJ, Lian JB (1979) Gamma-carboxyglutamate excretion and warfarin therapy. Clin Pharmacol Ther 25:562–570

34. Price PA (1985) Vitamin K-dependent formation of bone Gla protein (osteocalcin) and its function. Vitam Horm 42:65–108

35. Ducy P, Desbois C, Boyce BF, Pinero G, Story B, Dunstan C, Smith E, Bonadio J, Glodstein S, Gundberg CM, Bradley A, Karsenty G (1996) Increased bone formation in osteocalcin-deficient mice. Nature 382:448–452

36. Rodan GA, Rodan SB (1987) Expression of the osteoblast phenotype. In: Peck WA (ed) Bone and mineral research. Elsevier/North Holland, Amsterdam, pp 244–286

37. Gerstenfeld LC, Chipman JJ, Glowacki J, Lian JB (1987) Expression of differential function in mineralizing cultures of chicken osteoblasts. Dev Biol 122:49–60

38. Price PA, Williamson M, Lothringer JW (1981) Origin of vitamin K-dependent bone protein found in plasma and its clearance by kidney and bone. J Biol Chem 256:12760–12766

39. Delmas PD, Wilson DM, Mann KG, Riggs BL (1983) Effect of renal function on plasma levels of bone Gla-protein. J Clin Endocrinol Metab 57:1028–1030

40. Epstein S, Traberg H, Raja R, Poser JW (1985) Serum and dialysate osteocalcin levels in hemodialysis and peritoneal dialysis patients after renal transplantation. J Clin Endocrinol Metab 60:1253–1256

41. Taylor AK, Linkart S, Mohan S, Chrinstenson RA, Singer FR, Baylink D (1990) Multiple osteocalcin fragments in human urine and serum as detected by a midmolecule osteocalcin radioimmunoassay. J Clin Endocrinol Metab 70:467–472

42. Garnero P, Grimaux M, Seguin P, Delmas PD (1994) Characterization of immunoreactive forms of human osteocalcin generated in vivo and in vitro. J Bone Miner Res 9:255–264

43. Deftos LJ, Parthermore JG, Price PA (1980) New biochemical marker for bone metabolism: measurement by radioimmunoassay of bone GLA protein in the plasma of normal subjects and in patients with bone disease. J Clin Invest 66:878–883

44. Nielsen HK, Brixen K, Mosekilde L (1990) Diurnal rhythm and 24-hour integrated concentrations of serum osteocalcin in normals: influence of age, sex, season, and smoking habits. Calcif Tissue Int 47:284–290

45. Nielsen HK, Brixen K, Bouillon R, Mosekilde L (1990) Changes in biochemical markers of osteoblastic activity during the menstrual cycle. J Clin Endocrinol Metab 70:1431–1437

46. Cole DEC, Gundberg CM, Stirk LJ, Atkinson SA, Hanley DA, Ayer LM, Baldwin LS (1987) Changing osteocalcin concentrations during pregnancy and lactation: implications for maternal mineral metabolism. J Clin Endocrinol Metab 65:290–294

47. Bell NH, Greene A, Epstein RS, Oexmann MJ, Shaw S, Shary J (1985) Evidence for alteration of the vitamin D-endocrine system in blacks. J Clin Invest 76:470–473

48. Shima M, Seino Y, Tanaka H, Yabuuchi H, Tsutsumi C, Moriuchi S (1986) Bone gamma-carboxyglutamic acid containing protein in the perinatal period. Acta Paed Scand 74:674–677

49. Lichtenstein P, Gormley C, Martinez R, Poser JW, Specker BL, Tsang RC (1983) Elevated serum Gla-protein in infancy: higher values in breast milk vs. cow milk formula feeding. Pediatr Res 17:292–293

50. Gundberg CM, Lian JB, Gallop PM (1983) Measurements of gamma-carboxyglutamate and circulation osteocalcin in normal adults and children. Clin Chim Acta 128:1–8

51. Johansen JS, Giwereman A, Hartwell D, Nelsen CT, Price PA, Christiansen C, Skakkebaek NE (1988) Serum bone GLA-protein as a marker of bone growth in children and adolescents: correlation with age, height, serum insulin-like growth factor I, and serum testosterone. J Clin Endocrinol Metab 67:273–278

52. Modrowski D, del Pozo E, Miravet L (1992) Dynamics of circulating osteo-calcin in rats during growth and under experimental conditions. Horm Metab Res 24:474–477

53. Delmas PD, Steiner D, Wahner HW, Mann KG, Riggs BL (1983) Serum bone Gla-protein increases with aging in normal women: implications for the mechanism of age-related bone loss. J Clin Invest 71:1316–1321

54. Delmas PD, Stenner D, Wahner HW, Mann KG, Riggs BL (1983) Increase in serum bone gamma-carboxyglutamic acid protein with aging in women. J Clin Invest 71:1316–1321

55. Delmas PD, Wahner HW, Mann KG, Riggs BL (1983) Assessment of bone turnover in postmenopausal osteoporosis by measurement of serum bone Gla-protein. J Lab Clin Med 102:470–476

56. Brown JP, Delmas PD, Malaval L, Edouard C, Chapuy MC, Meunier PJ (1984) Serum bone Gla-protein: a specific marker for bone formation in post-menopausal osteoporosis. Lancet 1:1091–1093

57. Dannucci GA, Martin BR, Patterson-Buckendahl P (1987) Ovariectomy and trabecular bone remodeling in the dog. Calcif Tissue Int 40:194

58. Johansen JS, Riss BJ, Delmas PD (1988) Plasma BGP: an indicator of sponta-neous bone loss and effect of estrogen treatment in postmenopausal women. Eur J Clin Invest 18:191–195

59. Delmas PD, Malaval L, Arlot ME, Meunier PJ (1985) Serum bone Gla-protein compared to bone histomorphometry in endocrine diseases. Bone 6:339–341

60. Malluche HH, Faugere MC, Fanti P, Price PA (1984) Plasma levels of bone Gla protein reflect bone formation in patients on chronic maintenance dialysis. Kidney Int 26:869–874

61. Bataille R, Delmas PD, Sany J (1987) Serum bone Gla-protein in multiple myeloma. Cancer 59:329–334

62. Delmas PD, Demiaux B, Malaval L, Chapuy MC, Edouard C, Meunier PJ (1986) Serum bone gamma carboxyglutamic acid-containing protein in primary hyperparathyroidism and in malignant hypercalcemia. J Clin Invest 77:985–991

63. Robey PG, Fisher LW, Young MF, Termine JD (1988) The biochemistry of bone. In: Riggs BL, Melton LJ III (eds) Osteoporosis: etiology, diagnosis and management. Raven, New York, pp 95–109

64. Fessler JH, Fessler LI (1978) Biosynthesis of procollagen. Annu Rev Biochem 47:129–162

65. Golderg B, Sherr CJ (1973) Secretion and extracellular processing of procollagen by cultured human fibroblasts. Proc Natl Acad Sci USA 70:361–365

66. Fleischmajer R, Timpl R, Tuderman L, Raisher L, Wiestner M, Perlish JS, Graves PN (1981) Ultrastructural identification of extension amino-propeptides of type I and III procollagens in human skin. Proc Natl Acad Sci USA 78:7360–7364

67. Prockop DJ, Kivirikko KI, Tuderman L, Guzman NA (1979) The biosynthesis of collagen and its disorders. (first of two parts) N Engl J Med 301:13–23

68. Smedsrod B, Melkko J, Risteli L, Risteli J (1990) Circulating C-terminal propeptide of type I procollagen is cleared mainly via the mannose receptor in liver endothelial cells. Biochem J 271:345–350

69. Prockop DJ, Kivirikko KI, Tuderman L, Guzman NA (1979) The biosynthesis of collagen and its disorders. (second of two parts) N Engl J Med 70:361–365

70. Parfitt AM, Simon LS, Villanueva AR, Krane SM (1987) Procollagen type I carboxy-terminal extension peptide in serum as a marker of collagen biosynthesis in bone. Correlation with iliac bone formation rates and comparison with total alkaline phosphatase. J Bone Miner Res 2:427–436

71. Ebeling PR, Peterson JM, Riggs BL (1992) Utility of type I procollagen propeptide assay for assessing abnormalities in metabolic bone diseases. J Bone Miner Res 7:1243–1250

72. Melkko J, Niemi S, Risteli J (1990) Radioimmunoassay of the carboxy terminal propeptide of human type I procollagen. Clin Chem 36:1328–1332

73. Hassager C, Fabbri-Mabelli G, Christiansen C (1993) The effect of the menopause and hormone replacement therapy on serum carboxyterminal propeptide of type I collagen. Osteoporosis Int 3:50–52

74. Simon LS, Krane SM, Wortman PD, Krane IM, Kovitz KL (1984) Serum levels of type I and III procollagen fragments in Paget's disease of bone. J Clin Endocrinol Metab 58:110–120

75. Eriksen EF (1986) Normal and pathological remodeling of human trabecular bone: three dimensional reconstruction of the remodeling sequence in normal and in metabolic bone disease. Endocr Rev 7:739–409

76. Prockop OJ, Kivirikko KI (1968) Hydroxyproline and the metabolism of collagen. In: Gould BS (ed) Treatise on collagen. Academic, New York, pp 215–246

77. Prockop OJ, Kivirikko KI, Tuderman K (1979) The biosynthesis of collagen and its disorders. N Engl J Med 301:13–23

78. Nimni ME (1974) Collagen: its structure and function in normal and pathological connective tissues. Semin Arthritis Rheum 4:95–150

79. Krane SM, Kantrowitz FG, Byrne M, Pinnel SR, Singer FR (1977) Urinary excretion of hydroxylysine and its glycosides as an index of collagen degradation. J Clin Invest 59:819–827

80. Gallagher JA, Guenther HL, Fleish HA (1982) Rapid intracellular degradation of newly synthesized collagen by bone cells. Effect of dichloromethylenebisphosphonate. Biochem Biophys Acta 719:349–355

81. Prockop DJ (1964) Isotopic studies on collagen degradation and the urine excretion of hydroxyproline. J Clin Invest 43:453–460

82. Kivirikko KI (1983) Excretion of urinary hydroxyproline peptide in the assessment of bone collagen deposition and resorption. In: Frame B, Potts JTJ (eds) Clinical disorders of bone and mineral metabolism. Excerpta Medica, Amsterdam, pp 105–107

83. Pødenphant J, Larsen NE, Christiansen C (1984) An easy and reliable method for determination of urinary hydroxyproline. Clin Chim Acta 142:145–148

84. Jasin HE, Fink CW, Wise W, Ziff M (1962) Relationship between urinary hydroxyproline and growth. J Clin Invest 41:1928–1935

85. Segrest JP, Cunningham LW (1970) Variations in the human urinary o-hydroxylysyl glycoside and their relationship to collagen metabolism. J Clin Invest 49:1497–1509

86. Askenasi R, DeBacker M, Devos A (1976) The origin of urinary hydroxylysyl glycosides in Paget's disease of bone and in primary hyperparathyroidism. Calcif Tissue Int 22:35

87. Moro L, Mucelli RS, Gazzarrini C, Modricky C, Marotti F, De Bernard B (1988) Urinary -1-galactosyl-o-hydroxylysine (GH) as a marker of collagen turnover of bone. Calcif Tissue Int 42:87–90

88. Hammarstrom LE, Hanker JS, Toverud SU (1971) Cellular differences in acid phosphatase isoenzymes in bone and teeth. Clin Orthop 78:151–167

89. Minkin C (1982) Bone acid phosphatase: tartrate-resistant acid phosphatase as a marker of osteoclast function. Calcif Tissue Int 34:285–290

90. Bianco P, Ballanti P, Bonucci E (1988) Tartrate resistant acid phosphatase activity in rat osteoblasts and osteocytes. Calcif Tissue Int 43:167–171

91. Li CY, Chuda RA, Lam WKW (1973) Acid phosphatase in human plasma. J Lab Clin Med 82:446–460

92. Schiele F, Artur Y, Floch AY, Siest G (1988) Total, tartrate-resistant, and tartrate-inhibited acid phosphatases in serum: biological variations and reference limits. Clin Chem 34:685–690

93. Stepán JJ, Pospícal J, Presl J, Pacovsky V (1987) Bone loss and biochemical indices of bone remodeling in surgically induced postmenopausal women. Bone 8:279–284

94. Piedra C, Torres R, Rapado A (1989) Serum tartrate resistant acid phosphatase and bone mineral content in postmenopausal osteoporosis. Calcif Tissue Int 45:58–60

95. Popp-Snijders C, Lips P, Netelenbos JC (1996) Intra-individual variation in bone resorption markers in urine. Ann Clin Biochem 33:347–348

96. Kraenzlin M, Lau KHW, Liang L (1990) Development of an immunoassay for human serum osteoclastic tartrate-resistant acid phosphatase. J Clin Endocrinol Metab 71:442–451

97. Delmas PD, Garnero P (1996) Utility of biochemical markers of bone turnover in osteoporosis. In: Marcus R, Feldman D, Kelsey J (eds) Osteoporosis. Academic, New York, pp 1075–1088

98. Eyre DR, Paz MA, Galop PM (1984) Cross linking in collagen and elastin. Annu Rev Biochem 53:717–748

99. Fujimoto D, Morigachi T, Ishida T, Hayasi H (1978) The structure of pyridinoline, a collagen crosslink. Biochem Biophys Res Commun 84:52–57

100. Eyre DR (1984) Crosslink maturation in bone collagen. In: Veis A (ed) The chemistry and biology of mineralized connective tissues. Elsevier, Amsterdam, pp 51–55

101. Eyre DR (1987) Collagen crosslinking amino-acids. Methods Enzymol 144:115–139

102. Eyre DR, Koob TJ, Van Ness KP (1984) Quantification of hydroxypyridinium crosslinks in collagen by high-performance liquid chromatography. Anal Biochem 137:380–388

103. Eyre DR, Dickson IR, Van Ness KP (1988) Collagen crosslinking in human bone and articular cartilage. Age-related changes in the content of mature hydroxypyridinium residues. Biochem J 252:495–500

104. Seibel M, Duncan A, Robins SP (1989) Urinary hydroxy-pyridinium crosslinks provide indices of cartilage, bone involvement in arthritic diseases. J Rheumatol 16:964–970

105. Beardsworth LJ, Eyre DR, Dickson IR (1990) Changes with age in urinary excretion of lysyl- and hydroxylysyl pyridinoline, two new markers of bone collagen turnover. J Bone Miner Res 5:671–676

106. Delmas PD, Gineyts E, Bertholin A, Garnero P, Marchand F (1993) Immunoassay of pyridinoline crosslink excretion in normal adults and in Paget's disease. J Bone Miner Res 8:643–648

107. Colwell A, Eastell R, Assiri AMA, Russell RGG (1990) Effect of diet on deoxypyrinoline excretion. In: Christiansen C, Overgaard K (eds) Osteoporosis. Osteopress, Aalborg, pp 520–591

108. Uebelhart D, Schlemmer A, Johansen JS, Gineyts E, Christiansen C, Delmas PD (1991) Effect of menopause and hormone replacement therapy on the urinary excretion of pyridinium cross-links. J Clin Endocrinol Metab 72:367–373

109. Schlemmer A, Hassager C, Jensen SB, Christiansen C (1992) Marked diurnal variation in urinary excretion of pyridinium cross-links in premenopausal women. J Clin Endocrinol Metab 74:476–480

110. Blumsohn A, Herrington K, Hannon RA, Shao P, Eyre DR, Eastell R (1994) The effect of calcium supplementation on the circadian rhythm of bone resorption. J Clin Endocrinol Metab 79:730–735

111. Eastell R, Delmas PD, Hodgson SF, Eriksen EF, Mann KG, Riggs BL (1988) Bone formation rate in older normal women: concurrent assessment with bone histomorphometry, calcium kinetics and biochemical markers. J Clin Endocrinol Metab 67:741–748

112. Marowska J, Kobylinska M, Lukaszkiewicz J, Talajko A, Rymkiewicz-Kluczynska B, Lorenc RS (1996) Pyridinium crosslinks of collagen as a marker of bone resorption rates in children and adolescents: normal values and clinical application. Bone 19:669–677

113. Blumsohn A, Hannon KS, Wrate R, Barton J, Al-Dehaimi AW, Colwell A, Eastell R (1994) Biochemical markers of bone turnover in girls during puberty. Clin Endocrinol 40:663–670

114. Eastell R, Hampton L, Colwell A (1990) Urinary collagen crosslinks are highly correlated with radio isotopic measurements of bone resorption. In: Christiansen C, Overgaard K (eds) Proceedings of the 3rd International Symposium on Osteoporosis. Osteopress, Aalborg, pp 469–470

115. Delmas PD, Schlemmer A, Gineyts E, Riis BJ, Christiansen C (1991) Urinary excretion of pyridinoline crosslinks correlates with bone turnover measured on iliac crest biopsy in patients with vertebral osteoporosis. J Bone Miner Res 6:639–644

116. Black DM, Dunkan A, Robins SP (1988) Quantitative analysis of the pyridinium crosslinks of collagen in urine using ion-paired reversed-phase high-performance liquid chromatography. Anal Biochem 169:197–203

117. Hanson DA, Weis MA, Bollen AM, Maslan SL, Singer FR, Eyre DR (1992) A specific immunoassay for monitoring human bone resorption: quantitation of type I collagen cross-linked N-telopeptides in urine. J Bone Miner Res 7:1251–1258

118. Bernard MP, Myers JC, Chu ML, Ramirez F, Eikenberry EF, Prockop DJ (1983) Structure of a cDNA for the proα$_2$ chain of human type I procollagen. Comparison with chick cDNA for pro $_2$(I) identifies structural conserved features of the protein and the gene. Biochemistry 22:1139–1145

119. Timpl R (1976) Immunological studies on collagen. In: Ramachandran GN, Reddi AH (eds) Biochemistry of collagen. Plenum, New York, pp 319–375

120. Robins SP, Woitge H, Hesley R, Ju J, Seyedin SM, Seibel MJ (1994) Direct, enzyme-linked immunoassay for urinary deoxypyridinolin as a specific marker for measuring bone resorption. J Bone Miner Res 1643–1649

121. Eyre DR, Ericsson L, Simon L, Krane S (1988) Identification of urinary peptides derived from cross-linking sites in bone collagen in Paget's disease. J Bone Miner Res 3:S210

122. Garnero P, Gineyts E, Arbault P, Christiansen C, Delmas PD (1995) Different effects of bisphosphonate and estrogen therapy on free and peptide-bound bone cross-links excretion. J Bone Miner Res 10:641–649

123. Bonde M, Qvist P, Fledelius C, Riis BJ, Christiansen C (1994) Immunoassay for quantifying type I collagen degradation products in urine evaluated. Clin Chem 40:2022–2025

124. Kuhn K (1982) Chemical properties of collagen. In: Furthmayr H (ed) Immuno-
     chemistry of the extracellular matrix. CRC, Boca Raton, pp 1–30
125. Christiansen C, Riis BJ, Rødbro P (1987) Prediction of rapid bone loss in post-
     menopausal women. Lancet 1:1105–1108
126. Garnero P, Gineyts E, Riou J, Delmas PD (1994) Assessment of bone resorp-
     tion with a new marker of collagen degradation in patients with metabolic
     bone disease. J Clin Endocrinol Metab 79:780–785
127. Partridge NC, Alcorn D, Michelangeli VP, Kemp BE, Ryan GB, Martin TJ
     (1981) Functional properties of hormonally responsive cultured normal and
     malignant rat osteoblastic cells. Endocrinology 108:213–219
128. Uebelhart D, Gineyts E, Chapuy MC, Delmas PD (1990) Urinary excretion of
     pyridinium cross-links: a new marker of bone resorption in metabolic bone
     disease. Bone Miner 8:87–96
129. Risteli J, Niemi S, Elomaa I, Risteli L (1991) Bone resorption assay based on
     a peptide liberated during type I collagen degradation. J Bone Miner Res 6
     [Suppl 1]:S251
130. Hassager C, Jensen FT, Podenphant J, Thomsen K, Christiansen C (1994) The
     carboxy-terminal pyridinoline cross-linked telopeptide of type I collagen
     in serum as a marker of bone resorption: the effect of nandrolone decanoate
     and hormone replacement therapy. Calcif Tissue Int 54:30–33
131. Eriksen EF, Charles P, Melsen F, Mosekilde L, Risteli L, Risteli J (1993) Serum
     markers of type I procollagen formation and degradation in metabolic
     bone disease: correlation to bone histomorphometry. J Bone Miner Res
     8:127–132
132. Hassager C, Risteli J, Risteli L, Jensen SB, Christiansen C (1992) Diurnal vari-
     ation in serum markers of type I collagen synthesis and degradation in
     healthy premenopausal women. J Bone Miner Res 66:337–341
133. Risteli J, Elomaa I, Niemi S, Novamo A, Risteli L (1993) Radioimmunoassay
     for the pyridinoline cross-linked carboxyl-terminal telopeptide of type I col-
     lagen: a new serum marker of bone collagen degradation. Clin Chem 39:635–
     640
134. Elomaa I, Virkkunen P, Risteli L, Risteli J (1992) Serum concentrations of the
     cross-linked carboxyterminal telopeptide of type I collagen (ICTP) is a use-
     ful prognosis indicator in multiple myeloma. Br J Cancer 66:337–341
135. Kushida K, Takahashi M, Kawana K, Inoue T (1995) Comparison of markers
     for bone formation and resorption in premenopausal and postmenopausal
     subjects and osteoporosis patients. J Clin Endocrinol Metab 80:2447–2450
136. Whyte MP, Bergfeld MA, Murphy WA, Avioli LV, Teitelbaum SL (1982) Post-
     menopausal osteoporosis: a heterogeneous disorder as assessed by histo-
     morphometric analysis of iliac crest bone from untreated patients. Am J Med
     72:193–202
137. Civitelli R, Gonnelli S, Zacchei F, Bigazzi S, Vattimo A, Avioli LV, Gennari C
     (1988) Bone turnover in postmenopausal osteoporosis: effect of calcitonin
     treatment. J Clin Invest 82:1268–1274

138. Slemenda CW, Hui SL, Longcope C, Johnston CC Jr (1987) Sex steroids and bone mass. A study of changes about the time of menopause. J Clin Invest 80:1261–1269

139. Ebeling PR, Atley LM, Guthrie JR, Burger HG, Dennerstein L, Hopper JL, Wark JD (1996) Bone turnover markers and bone density across the menopausal transition. J Clin Endocrinol Metab 81:3366–3371

140. Ravn P, Fledelius C, Rosenquist C, Overgaard K, Christiansen C (1996) High bone turnover is associated with low bone mass in both pre- and post-menopausal women. Bone 19:291–298

141. Cosman F, Nieves J, Wilkinson C, Schnering D, Shen V, Lindsay R (1996) Bone density change and biochemical indices of skeletal turnover. Calcif Tissue Int 58:236–243

142. Garnero P, Sornay-Rendu E, Delmas PD (1996) Classification of post-menopausal women with markers of bone turnover (MK): a longitudinal study. J Bone Miner Res 11 [Suppl 1]:S157

143. Hansen MA, Kirsten O, Riss BJ, Christiansen C (1991) Role of peak bone mass and bone loss in postmenopausal osteoporosis: a 12 year study. BMJ 303:961–964

144. Sowers MF, Jannausch M, Russell-Aulet M, Crutchfield M (1996) Predicting "fast" bone loss with osteocalcin and bone mineral density measurements. J Bone Miner Res 11 [Suppl 1]:S154

145. Arlot ME, Bradbeer JN, Edouard C, Green JR, Hesp R, Roux J, Meunier PJ, Reeve J (1993) Temporal variations in iliac trabecular bone formation in vertebral osteoporosis. Calcif Tissue Int 52:10–15

146. Garnero P, Shih WJ, Gineyts E, Karpf DB, Delmas PD (1994) Comparison of new biochemical markers of bone turnover in late postmenopausal osteoporotic women in response to alendronate treatment. J Clin Endocrinol Metab 79:1693–1700

147. Akesson K, Vergnaud P, Gineyts E, Delmas PD, Obrant K (1993) Impairment of bone turnover in elderly women with hip fracture. Calcif Tissue Int 53:162–169

148. Garnero P, Hausherr M, Chapuy MC (1995) Can markers of bone turnover predict hip fractures in elderly women? The EPIDOS study. J Bone Miner Res 10 [Suppl 1]:S140

149. Szulc P, Chapuy MC, Meunier PJ, Delmas PD (1993) Serum undercarboxylated osteocalcin is a marker of the risk of hip fracture in elderly women. J Clin Invest 91:1769–1774

150. Hodges SJ, Pilkington MJ, Stam TCB, Catterall A, Sheraer MJ, Bitensky L, Chayen J (1991) Depressed levels of circulating menaquinones in patients with osteoporotic fractures of the spine and femoral neck. Bone 12:387–389

151. Overgaard K, Hansen MA, Nielsen VA, Riis BJ, Christiansen C (1990) Discontinuous calcitonin treatment of established osteoporosis - effects of withdrawal of treatment. Am J Med 89:1–6

152. Overgaard K, Riis BJ, Christiansen C, Podenphant J, Johansen JS (1989) Nasal

calcitonin for treatment of established osteoporosis. Clin Endocrinol 30:435–442

153. Lufkin EG, Wahner HW, O'Fallon WM, Hodgson SF, Kotowicz MA, Lane AW, Judd HL, Caplan RH, Riggs BL (1992) Treatment of postmenopausal osteoporosis with transdermal estrogen. Ann Intern Med 117:1–9

154. Harris ET, Gertz BJ, Genant HK (1993) The effect of short term treatment with alendronate on vertebral density and biochemical markers of bone remodeling in early postmenopausal women. J Clin Endocrinol Metab 76:1399–1403

155. Prestwood KM, Pilbeam CC, Burleson JA, Woodiel FL, Delmas PD, Deftos LJ, Raisz LG (1994) The short term effects of conjugated estrogen on bone turnover in older women. J Clin Endocrinol Metab 79:366–371

156. Chesnut CH, III, Bell NH, Clark GS, Drinkwater BL, English SC, Johnston CC Jr, Notelovitz M, Rosen CJ, Cain DF, Flessland KA, Mallinak NJS (1997) Hormone replacement therapy in postmenopausal women: urinary N-telopeptide of type I collagen monitors therapeutic effect and predicts response of bone mineral density. Am J Med 102:29–37

157. Delmas PD, Demiaux B, Malaval L, Chapuy MC, Meunier PJ (1986) Serum bone Gla-protein is not a sensitive marker of bone turnover in Paget's disease of bone. Calcif Tissue Int 38:60–61

158. Wilkinson MR, Wagstaffe C, Delbridge L, Wiseman J, Posen S (1986) Serum osteocalcin concentrations in Paget's disease of bone. Arch Intern Med 146:268

159. Papapoulos SE, Frolich M (1996) Prediction of the outcome of treatment of Paget's disease of bone with bisphosphonates from short-term changes in the rate of bone resorption. J Clin Endocrinol Metab 81:3993–3997

160. Stepán JJ, Silinkova-Malkova E, Havranek T, Formankova J, Zichova M, Lachmanova J, Strakova M, Broulik P, Pacovsky V (1983) Relationship of plasma tartrate resistant acid phosphatase to the bone isoenzyme of serum alkaline phosphatase in hyperparathyroidism. Clin Chim Acta 133:189–200

161. Seibel M, Gartenberg F, Silverberg SJ, Ratcliffe A, Robins SP, Bilezikian JP (1992) Urinary hydroxypyridinium cross-links of collagen in primary hyperparathyroidism. J Clin Endocrinol Metab 74:481–486

162. De La Piedra C, Toural V, Rapado A (1987) Osteocalcin and urinary hydroxyproline/creatinine ratio in the differential diagnosis of primary hyperparathyroidism and hypercalcemia of malignancy. Scand J Clin Lab Invest 47:587–592

163. Body J, Delmas PD (1992) Urinary pyridinium cross-links as markers of bone resorption in tumor-associated hypercalcemia. J Clin Endocrinol Metab 74:471–475

164. Valentin-Opran A, Charhon SA, Meunier PJ, Edouard CM, Arlot ME (1982) Quantitative histology of myeloma-induced bone changes. Br J Haematol 52:601–610

165. Robins SP, Black DM, Paterson CR, Reid DM, Duncan A, Seibel M (1991) Evaluation of urinary hydroxypyridinium crosslink measurements as resorption markers in metabolic bone disease. Eur J Clin Invest 21:310–315

166. Harvey D, McHardy KC, Reid IW, Paterson F, Bewsher PD, Duncan A, Robins SP (1991) Measurements of bone collagen degradation in hyperthyroidism and during thyroxine replacement therapy using pyridinium cross-links as specific urinary markers. J Clin Endocrinol Metab 72:1189–1194

7 Determinants of Bone Loss

S. Adami and V. Braga

Introduction

The loss of bone mass and of its microarchitectural integrity is a slow process which remains asymptomatic until the appearance of the typical low trauma fracture. In order to effectively prevent the osteoporotic fractures methods of identifying individuals at risk earlier in the disease are needed. There are several different categories of risk factors for osteoporotic fractures. They may be related to the determinants of bone mineral density (BMD), to propensity for falling, and to skeletal fragility independently of BMD. The risk factors for the latter are relatively uncommon and poorly understood mainly because bone "quality" cannot be properly assessed in vivo. In some cases the risk factors can be generally defined as independent of BMD. This is the case for previous fractures, which are associated with an approximate doubling of fracture risk after correction for BMD (Ross et al. 1991), for the length of the head of the femur or for the thickness of the fat tissue overlying the hip (Reid et al. 1994b; Cummings 1995). In other cases the risk for fractures are linked to a greater liability to falls (poor visual acuity, neuromuscular impairment, inadequate lighting, use of benzodiazepines, age per se, etc.; Cooper et al. 1988; Meyer et al. 1995; Cummings et al. 1995)

Currently the best available predictor of osteoporotic fractures is BMD as measured by dual-energy X-ray absortiometry (DXA) (Cummings et al. 1995).

In the last decade a number of cross-sectional and longitudinal studies have identified a series of conditions characterized by a lower peak bone mass and accelerated bone loss in the middle-aged and senile population. The identification of these risk factors may be relevant for osteoporosis prevention and to target for further investigation by DXA only those women at greatest risk of osteoporosis.

In this chapter we review principally the relevant "life-style" determinants of the rate of bone loss: genetic factors, estrogen deficiency, body weight and fat mass, smoking, nutrition, caffeine, and physical exercise. The secondary causes of osteoporosis (osteopenic diseases and drugs) and the other determinants of osteoporotic fracture risk are discussed in separate chapters of this book. The data discussed here refer mostly to women. The determinants of bone loss in men have not been extensively investigated, but it is plausible that most of them do not differ substantially to those identified in women (Glynn et al. 1995).

Genetic Factors

Family and twin studies indicate that there is a genetic component of bone density and the development of osteoporosis (Krall and Dawson-Hughes 1993; Christian et al. 1989). There is some evidence that the genotype influences both the peak
bone mass and the rate of bone loss (Krall et al. 1995) although the gene polymorphism implicated is controversial. Vitamin D receptor gene polymorphisms have
been found to be correlated with bone turnover and the rate of bone loss in some
studies (Krall et al. 1995) but not in others (Garnero et al. 1996a). The controversy may be related to the multifactorial genetic control of bone mass. Indeed collagen 1α gene and IL1 polymorphism have recently been associated with bone
density.

The relative contribution of genetic and noncongenital factors on the rate of
bone loss varies individually but that of each is still poorly defined. If the rate of
bone loss were genetically determined one would expect bone mass to be distributed bimodally among the elderly, but this has never been found at any age. A relevant genetic control of the rate of bone loss also implies that having a given rate
of bone loss would be permanent and that the "congenital" fast-loser should be
treated as soon as identified. In two studies, patients classified by the rate of bone
loss at a given time were reevaluated in a subsequent period. Only 20%–40% of
the patients classified as fast losers retained their first classification (Pouillès et
al. 1996; Hui et al. 1990). These data emphasise the importance of life-style factors which also interact with genetic determinants. Thus the less favorable genotype polymorphism for vitamin D receptor is associated with a more favorable
response to higher calcium intake and physical activity (Ferrari et al. 1995; Salamone et al. 1996).

African women are at lower risk of osteoporosis than white women (Nelson
et al. 1988), and this is due largely to the attainment of greater peak bone mass by
early adulthood. However, slower rate of bone loss in the early postmenopausal
period has also been found to contribute to the higher bone density of older black
women (Luckey et al. 1996).

Age

Data collected from cross-sectional studies suggest that bone loss does not occur
in the elderly, or if it does then at a very much more attenuated rate than that after
menopause. However, all these studies failed to take into account several factors
that underestimate the rate of bone loss with age (Adami and Kanis 1995). Prospective studies in the elderly suggest that bone loss occurs at rates comparable to those
at menopause at least at the cortical level (Jones et al. 1994; Orwoll et al. 1990),
with bone density of the femoral neck declining at an increasing rate both in
elderly men and women. Biochemical indices of bone turnover consistently show
an increase with age (Delmas et al. 1983; Garnero et al. 1996b). It is not clear to
what extent this acceleration of the rate of bone loss is an effect of age itself or is

secondary to factors such as malnutrition, vascular or hormonal deficits, decrease in muscle mass, and decrease in physical activity. Adjustment of bone mass for muscle mass almost completely eliminates the apparent loss, suggesting that skeletal mass remains somewhat appropriate for muscle mass (Thomsen et al. 1986). In any case these observations emphasize the greater attention that should be paid to the management of osteoporosis in the elderly. Indeed, because older subjects have an increasing rate of bone loss and the greatest risk of fracture, treatment of the very elderly may be the most cost effective.

Estrogen Deficiency

Immediately after menopause trabecular bone is lost at high rate. This finding led to increased support for a preventive strategy beginning as soon as possible after menopause, but it also generated confusion regarding the relative importance of menopausal status and aging on the development of osteoporosis in women.

The interaction of estrogen deficiency and aging on the rate of bone loss is nowadays reasonably defined. The rate of bone loss is suddenly raised at menopause by accelerated bone turnover, with a consequent increase in the so-called remodeling space. This bone loss is potentially reversible, and its extent is the same irrespective of the age at which menopause occurs, but it does depend on the severity of estrogen deficiency (Seeman et al. 1988). This bone loss should be distinguished from irreversible age-related bone loss, which is due to an uncoupling of resorption and formation within the individual bone metabolic unit, and which may start some time before menopause, around the fourth decade of life.

After menopause the rate of bone loss is maintained above the premenopausal levels as a consequence of both increased bone turnover due to estrogen deficiency

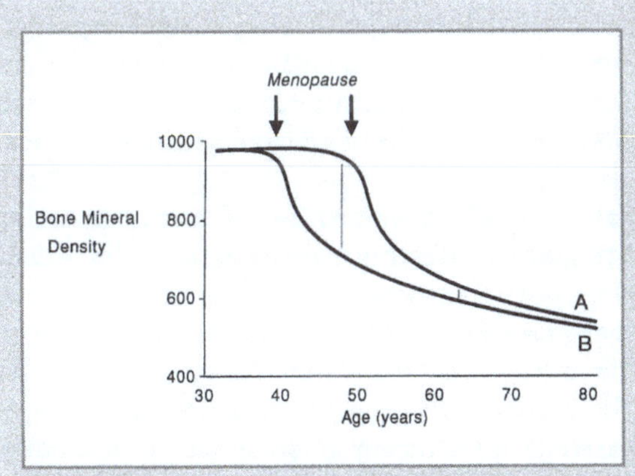

Fig. 7-1 Hypothetical life-long values of BMD in two women of the same age but who became menopausal at 40 years (patient B), and at 50 years (patient A) respectively. The BMD difference is the highest when the women are 45–50 years old, but it is negligible 20 years later

and negative bone balance due to an effect of aging. Thus estrogen deficiency accelerates the bone-loss process, but it is not the primary cause of bone loss at the level of the remodeling unit. In this hypothetical schema an early menopause raises the risk of osteoporosis by anticipating the amplification of the age-related bone loss, but its responsibility for the appearance of osteoporosis decreases with advancing age (Luisetto et al. 1995). Thus the difference in bone mass between two groups of women of the same age but who experience menopause by the age of 40 or 50 years old, respectively, is the highest around the age of 50 but hardly appreciable 20 years later (Fig. 7-1).

This conceptual model is consistent with the accentuation of bone losses that occurs in disorders in which the activation of bone turnover is increased, such as hyperparathyroidism and hyperthyroidism.

Body Weight

Various measures of body size have been associated with increased bone density. This association may depend on a combination of factors, including decreased peripheral production of estrogens and decreased weight on the skeleton.

In large persons the areal measurement of BMD (g/cm^2) overestimates the volumetric bone density (Adami and Kanis 1995), and this explains the almost invariable correlation observed between body weight and BMD as measured by DXA. In a cross-sectional study including a large number of white men and women, Edelstein and Barrett-Connor (1993) showed that all measures of body size [total weight, body mass index (BMI), lean mass, fat mass, height] were better markers of BMD in weight-bearing sites than in non-weight-bearing sites. These differences were also significant when the body weight was corrected for height (BMI, kg/m^2). Therefore it seems that the relationship between BMD and body mass may reflect not simply the higher BMD values expected in taller individuals but also the mechanical effect of body weight on weight-bearing skeletal segments.

Weight alone explains 15%–30% of the variance in BMD, and percentage of fat explains 20%–40%. Percentage of fat has been found to be substantially better than any index derived from a combination of qualitative risk factors (Gunnes et al. 1996; Michaelsson et al. 1996).

Fat mass is more closely related to BMD in women than in men, supporting the proposed importance of fat tissue derived estrogen in regulation of bone density (Edelstein and Barrett-Connor 1993). This hypothesis has also been confirmed in longitudinal studies (Reid et al. 1994a; Slemenda et al. 1996; Tremollieres et al. 1993). In overweight women the rate of bone loss is significantly lower than in women of normal weight, and this is apparently related to higher plasma estrogen concentration, reflecting increased peripheral conversion of dehydroepiandrosterone to estrogen. In this way the adipose tissue plays an important role in determining the time of menopause, postmenopausal circulating levels of estradiol, control of bone turnover, and perhaps bone mass (Heiss et al. 1995; Pedersen et al. 1995).

Lower BMI has been shown to be a risk factor for hip fracture also (Johnell et al. 1995; Meyer et al. 1995), possibly as a reflection of the mechanical protection during fall by the larger fat pad overlaying the hip joint.

The intra-individual variance of BMI may also reflect differences in nutrition. Thus it has been ascertained that voluntary weight loss in obese women is accompanied by proportional bone losses (Jensen et al. 1994), and that weight loss between 50 years and old age is associated with increased risk of hip fracture (Langlois et al. 1996).

High BMI values may arise from either increased lean or fat mass. In a cross-sectional study BMD was found to be better related to lean mass than to fat mass, and this appears to be associated with factors such as exercise, life-style, and estrogen levels (Salamone et al. 1995). Lean body mass may be the result also of genetic factors (Krall et al. 1995) regulating by common mechanisms both lean and bone cortical mass, whereas fat mass may be more closely related to bone turnover and thereby to bone trabecular volumetric density (Khosla et al. 1996).

Smoking

There are a number of indications that smoking during adulthood is associated with decreased hip (Hollenbach et al. 1993) and lumbar spine (Egger et al. 1996) bone density later in life both in men and in women; however, smoking cessation, at whatever age, limits bone loss (Hollenbach et al. 1993). An elegant demonstration of the effect of tobacco use comes from a study of 41 pairs of twins discordant for smoking by at least 5 pack-years. The twins who smoked more heavily had BMD values 5% and 10% lower at femoral neck and lumbar spine, respectively, for each 20 pack-years difference (Hopper et al. 1994). It was suggested that smoking increases catabolism and decreases secretion of estrogens, leading to early menopause, increased bone resorption, and higher rate of bone loss. The risk of osteoporosis may also be related to the fact that smokers are generally thinner than their nonsmoking counterparts. The associations between heavy smoking and osteoporosis are:
- Hormonal consequences
  - Accelerated menopause
  - Accelerated metabolism of endogenous estrogens
  - Accelerated metabolism of exogenous estrogens
- Decreased BMI and fat mass
  - Decreased peripheral production of estrogens
  - Decreased resistance to falls
  - Decreased weight on skeleton
  - Association with alcohol consumption and other life-style factors

The observed differences in BMD are considered sufficient to increase the risk of fracture, and smoking is indeed associated with an increased risk for hip fracture (Forsen et al. 1994). This may be related to other concomitant factors which decrease bone mass (lack of physical activity, poorer health associated with smoking). However, the relative risk of hip fracture associated with smoking has been shown to remain significant after adjusting for BMD (Cummings et al. 1995).

Alcohol

Chronic alcoholism decreases the formation and increases the resorption of bone, perhaps by a direct toxic effect (Diamond et al. 1989; Diez et al. 1994). The associated lower BMD (Peris et al. 1995) may also be related in postmenopausal women to the effect of ethanol on the clearance of estradiol.

In a large proportion of alcoholics an elevated fracture incidence (or prevalence of vertebral fractures) is associated with normal or modestly reduced BMD (Peris et al. 1995), and alcoholism, after adjusting for BMD, is only a moderately low risk factor for hip fracture in women (Cummings et al. 1995). This suggests that trauma or undefined alterations in bone structure may also play an important role in fractures. It should also be recalled that chronic severe alcoholism is associated with dietary disturbances such as protein malnutrition, other changes in life-style, liver disease, and a decrease in testosterone which may have additional effects.

Nutrition

Regular nutrition plays a crucial role in both the attainment of the peak bone mass and its maintenance. Several nutritional disturbances have been related to osteoporosis, but for only a few of them are proper clinical data available:
- Important
    - Low calcium diet
    - Low intake of vitamin D
    - Malnutrition
    - High intake of alcohol
    - Deficiency of vitamin C, B_6, and B_{12}
    - Vitamin K deficiency
- Uncertain
    - High protein or phosphate diet
    - Low intake of fluoride
    - Zinc and boron deficiency
    - Caffeine
    - High sodium diet

Calcium

The relationship between calcium intake and bone mass has been described in several studies. It seems to play a critical role in the attainment of bone mass (Adami 1994) ant its maintenance (Matkovich et al. 1979; Holbrock et al. 1995). The issue remains highly controversial since the differences in calcium nutrition around the world cannot explain differences in the risk of fractures between communities (Kanis and Passmore 1989).

A distinction should be made between severe calcium deficiency (and/or hypovitaminosis D) and changes in calcium intake ranging from low-normal to very high. The minimum "normal" allowance of calcium has not been precisely defined, and it may depend on a number of factors: calcium absorption, values for calcitriol, target tissue resistance to calcitriol, and menopausal status. Thus the recommended daily allowance is estimated as 1000 mg in premenopausal and 1500 mg in postmenopausal women (Riggs 1986). However, for others the daily allowance may be lower, and objections have been raised against the methods used for assessing it (Kanis 1991). The controversy can be in part solved by considering separately the consequences of a very low calcium intake, marginal deficits, and large excess. A very low calcium intake is frequently associated with secondary hyperparathyroidism (McKane et al. 1996; Chapuy et al. 1996), in which the bone losses are determined by focal mineralization defects and by secondary increases in bone turnover. For calcium intake above the minimum allowance (i.e., not associated with secondary hyperparathyroidism) the relationship with bone mass and the rate of bone loss are related exclusively to suppression of PTH production and that of bone turnover. Any change in bone turnover alters the so-called remodeling space, and this may affect the skeletal loss due to focal imbalance between bone resorption and formation associated with aging or estrogen deficiency. This explains why to a certain extent the higher the calcium intake is, the greater the bone mass. Obviously all the changes in bone mass related to lower remodeling space are transient and rapidly reversible.

Vitamin D

Prolonged vitamin D deficiency induces osteomalacia and secondary hyperparathyroidism, which complicate and accelerate the development of osteoporosis. Subtle and seasonal vitamin D deficiency are extremely frequent in the elderly and in institutions and geriatric hospitals where exposure to sunlight is low and nutrition (animal fat) may be inadequate (Holick 1986; Van der Wielen et al. 1995; Chapuy et al. 1996; Stein et al. 1996). Vitamin D levels are correlated with BMD at proximal femur and vertebrae in both elderly and younger women with a variable vitamin D status (Orwol and Meier 1986; Khaw et al. 1992; Villareal et al. 1991). In vitamin D deficiency the low serum concentrations of 25-hydroxyvitamin D lead to a low 1,25-dihydroxyvitamin D concentration and then to higher serum parathyroid hormone concentrations. Histologically the increased parathyroid activity is associated with high bone turnover, leading to cortical bone loss and low density bone (Lips et al. 1982).

Disturbances in the activation of vitamin D (1α hydroxylase activity) have been found after the menopause and with advancing age (Slovik et al. 1981; Tsai et al. 1984). This provides the basis for the use of calcitriol in osteoporotic subjects. However, the observed changes in vitamin D metabolism are a consequence of osteoporosis rather then a contributing factor. If the renal function is reasonably preserved (Gallagher et al. 1979), there is no evidence of declining vitamin D activation with advancing age.

Vitamin D insufficiency is often associated with some degree of proximal myopathy, which may increase the propensity of falling particularly in the elderly.

Protein and Phosphate

Several studies have suggested that a high animal protein and/or phosphate consumption induce hypercalciuria and increase the risk of osteoporotic fractures (Feskanich et al. 1996). The real clinical relevance of this observation remains uncertain and confined to populations with unusually high intake of proteins. Protein malnutrition is more frequent in the elderly, and this is associated with low bone mass and high risk of fractures (Cooper et al. 1996). Protein malnutrition induces bone loss per se but frequently is also an aspect of a general malnutrition, including inadequate intake of calories vitamin D and calcium. Malnutrition is often reported in the elderly, and in patients with hip fractures improved nutrition during the hospital stay decreases the risk of complications and mortality (Delmi et al. 1990).

Caffeine

Large quantities of coffee can increase the urinary excretion of calcium and have been associated with decreasing bone density and higher incidence of osteoporotic fractures (Heaney and Recker 1982). The clinical significance of these observations is uncertain. The apparent negative effect of coffee is easily offset by daily milk consumption and is not shared by tea which also contains caffeine and the use of which is, on the contrary, associated with a decrease in hip fracture incidence (Barrett-Connor et al. 1994).

Sodium Intake

High sodium diets increase urinary excretion of calcium, and this is associated with higher bone turnover. This is due to a decrease in tubular reabsorption of calcium, marginal decrease in serum calcium and stimulation of PTH secretion (Nordin et al. 1993). The magnitude of these effects in humans has not been properly assessed in terms of bone mass and osteoporotic fractures. The protective effect on BMD preservation of chronic use of thiazide (Herings et al. 1996) shares the opposite pathophysiological mechanism, i.e., increased tubular reabsorption of calcium at proximal tubule due to decreases of extracellular volumes.

Physical Exercise

Limb paralysis through peripheral nerve section is one of the most effective models of experimental osteoporosis. The homeostatic regulation of bone mass is largely dependent upon weight bearing and on the number and amplitude of episodic strains. The overall number of the latter are likely to be expressed by muscle mass and bone loading, and bone strains are likely to be the regulators of bone mass distribution. This conceptual model of bone mass homeostasis is based on a large number of experimental and clinical observations: forced bed rest, prolonged space flight, hemiplegia, etc.

Surprisingly, the ability of extensive physical exercises to counteract age-related bone loss has never been addressed in controlled prospective studies, but there is evidence that muscle mass strength and mass are strictly related to BMD of adjacent skeletal segments (Vico et al. 1995; Burckardt 1996) with 10%–20% of the variance in BMD being accounted for by physical activity. When life-style factors related to BMD were examined in the elderly, tobacco use, calcium intake, and physical activity were of primary importance (Nguyen et al. 1994).

Conclusions

Osteoporotic fractures are associated with considerable morbidity, mortality, and cost (Chrischilles et al. 1994), and they can be prevented by intervening early in the disease process. Therefore there is a need for an early identification of the individuals at risk. BMD evaluation is currently considered the best available prediction of osteoporotic fractures, but the technique may be considered too expensive for screening the entire population at regular age intervals. It has been suggested that identifiable risk factors may provide the basis to target women at greatest risk of osteoporosis. Taking into account all these risk factors, the proportion of variation in bone mineral density predicted ranges from 15% to 40% (Table 7-1). It is therefore clear that they cannot be used as a surrogate for bone

Table 7-1 Predictive values (percentage of variance explained) of risk factor models for bone mineral density in postmenopausal women

Reference	n	Lumbar spine	Femoral neck	Proximal radius
Stevenson et al. 1989	248	33	24	–
Kleerkoper et al. 1989	417			37
Slemenda et al. 1990	84	35	17	47
Ribot et al. 1992	1565	25		
Bauer et al. 1993	5400			28
Melton et al. 1993	304	43		
Nguyen et al. 1994	1080	15	31	
Tuppurainen et al. 1995	1605	18	27	
Weighted average		22.4	26.9	28.9

mass measurements nor for excluding a priori individual patients from having a bone measurement. The poor prediction of the models adopted may be explained in part by genetic factors which are important determinants of bone mass. These were not included in the analysis (Table 1), but they may be more precisely identified in the near future. In any case the identification of the above risk factors, together with BMD evaluation, remains of critical importance in assessing the prognosis of osteoporosis, its management, and pharmacological treatment threshold.

References

Adami S (1994) Optimizing peak bone mass: what are the therapeutic possibilities? Osteoporosis Int 1:S27–30

Adami S, Kanis JA (1995) Assessment of involutional bone loss: methodological and conceptual problems. J Bone Miner Res 10:511–517

Barrett-Connor E, Chang JC, Edelstein SL (1994) Coffee-associated osteoporosis offset by daily milk consumption. The Rancho Bernardo Study. JAMA 271:280–283

Bauer BC, Browner WS, Cauley JA et al (1993) Factors associated with appendicular bone mass in older women. Ann Intern Med 118:657–665

Burckardt P (1996) Are hip fractures preventable with nutritional measure and exercise in the elderly? Osteoporosis Int 3 [Suppl]:S56–S59

Chapuy MC, Schott AM, Garnero P, Hans D, Delmas PD, Meunier PJ, EPIDOS study group (1996) Healthy elderly French women living at home have secondary hyperparathyroidism and high turnover in winter. J Clin Endocrinol Metab 81:1129–1133

Christian JC, Yu F-L, Slemenda CW, Johnston CC JR (1989) Heritability of bone mass: a longitudinal study in aging male twins. Am J Hum Genet 44:429–433

Chrischilles E, Shireman T, Wallace R (1994) Costs and health effects of osteoporotic fractures. Bone 15:377–386

Cooper C, Barker DJ, Wickam C (1988) Physical activity, muscle strength and calcium intake in fracture of the proximal femur in Britain. BMJ 297:1443–1446

Cooper C, Shah S, Hand DJ (1991) Screening for vertebral osteoporosis using individual risk factors. Osteoporosis Int 2:48–253

Cooper C, Atkinson EJ, Hensrud DD, Wahner HW, O'Fallon WM, Riggs BL, Melton LJ III (1996) Dietary intake and bone mass in women. Calcif Tissue Int 58:320–325

Cummings SR (1995) Bone mass measurements and risk of fracture in Caucasian women: a review of findings from prospective studies. Am J Med 98 [Suppl 2A]:24S–28S

Cummings SR, Nevitt MC, Browner WS et al (1995) Risk factors for hip fracture in white women. N Engl J Med 332:767–773

Daniell HW (1983) Postmenopausal tooth loss: contribution to edentulism by osteoporosis and cigarette smoking. Arch Intern Med 143:1678–1682

Delmas PD, Stenner D, Wahner HW, Mann KG, Riggs BL (1983) Serum bone Gla-protein increases with aging in normal women: implication for the mechanism of age-related bone loss. J Clin Invest 71:1316–1321

Delmi M, Rapin Ch, Begoa JM, Delmas PD, Varsey H, Bonjour JP (1990) Dietary supplementation in elderly patients with fractured neck of the femur. Lancet 335:1013–1016

Diamond T, Stiel G, Posen S (1989) Osteoporosis in hemochromatosis: iron excess, gonadal deficiency or other factors? Ann Intern Med 110:430–436

Diez A, Puig J, Serrano S, Marinosa M-L, Bosch J, Marrogat J, Mellibovsky L, Nogucs X, Knobel H, Aubia J (1994) Alcohol-induced bone disease in the absence of severe chronic liver damage. J Bone Miner Res 9:825–831

Edelstein SL, Barrett-Connor E (1993) Relation between body size and bone mineral density in elderly men and women. Am J Epidemiol 138:160–169

Egger P, Dugglkeby S, Hobbs R, Fall C, Cooper C (1996) Cigarette smoking and bone mineral density in the elderly. J Epidemiol Community Health 50:47–50

Ferrari S, Rizzoli R, Chevalley T, Slosman D, Eisman JA, Bonjour JP (1995) Vitamin D receptor-gene polymorphisms and change in lumbar spine bone mineral density. Lancet 345:423–424

Feskanich D, Willett WC, Stampfer MJ, Colditz GA (1996) Protein consumption and bone fractures in women. Am J Epidemiol 143:472–479

Forsen L, Bjørndal A, Bjartveit K, Edna T-H, Holmen J, Jessen V, Westberg J.(1994) Interaction between current smoking, leanness, and physical inactivity in the prevention of hip fracture. J Bone Miner Res 9:1671–1678

Gallagher JC, Riggs BL, Eisman J, Hamstra A, Arnaud SB, DeLuca HF (1979) Intestinal calcium absorption and serum vitamin D metabolites in normal subjects and osteoporotic patients: effect of age and dietary calcium. J Clin Invest 64:729–736

Garnero P, Borel O, Sornay-Rendu E, Arlot ME, Delmas PD, (1996a) Vitamin D receptor gene polymorphisms are not related to bone turnover, rate of bone loss, and bone mass in postmenopausal women: the OFELY study. J Bone Miner Res 11:827–834

Garnero P, Sornay-Rendu E, Chapuy M-C, Delmas PD, (1996b) Increased bone turnover in late postmenopausal women is a major determinant of osteoporosis. J Bone Miner Res 11:337–349

Ginsburg ES, Walsh BW, Shea BF, Gao XG, Gleason RE, Barbieri RL (1995) The effects of ethanol on the clearance of estradiol in postmenopausal women. Fertil Steril 63:1227–1230

Glynn NW, Milahn EN, Charron M, Anderson SJ, Kuller LH, Cauley JA (1995) Determinants of bone mineral density in older men. J Bone Min Res 10:1769–1777

Gunnes M, Lehmann EH, Mellstrom D, Johnell O (1996) The relationship between anthropometric measurements and fractures in women. Bone 19:407–413

Heany RP, Recker RR (1982) Effect of nitrogen phosphorus and caffeine on calcium balance in women. J Lab Clin Med 99:46–55

Heiss CJ, Sanborn CF, Nichols DL, Bonnick SL, Alford BB (1995) Associations of body fat distribution, circulating sex hormones, and bone density in postmenopausal women. J Clin Endocrinol Metab 80:1591–1596

Herings RMC, Stricker BHC, de Boer A, Bakker A, Jurmans F, Stergachis A (1996) Current use of thiazide diuretics and prevention of hip fracture. J Clin Endocrinol Metab 49:115–119

Holbrook TL, Barrett-Connor E (1995) An 18-year prospective study on dietary calcium and bone mineral density in the hip. Calcif Tissue Int 56:364–367

Holick MF (1986) Vitamin D requirements for the elderly. Clin Nutr 5:121–129

Hollenbach KA, Barrett-Connor E, Edelstein SL, Holbrook T (1993) Cigarette smoking and bone mineral density in older men and women. Am J Public Health 83:1265–1270

Hopper JL, Seeman E, Austin Hosp (1994) The bone density of female twins discordant for tobacco use. N Engl J Med 330:387–392

Hui SL, Slemenda CW, Johnston CC (1990) The contribution of bone loss to postmenopausal osteoporosis. Osteoporosis Int 1:30–34

Jensen LB, Quaade F, Sorensen OH (1994) Bone loss accompanying voluntary weight loss in obese humans. J Bone Miner Res 9:459–463

Johnell O, Gullberg B, Kanis J A, Allander E, Elffors L, Dequeker J, Dilsen G, Gennari C, Lopes Vaz A, Lyritis G, Mazzuoli G, Miravet L, Passeri M, Cano RP, Rapado A, Ribot C (1995) Risk factors for hip fracture in European women: the MEDOS study. J Bone Miner Res 10:1802–1815

Jones G, Nguyen T, Sambrook P, Eisman JA (1994) Progressive loss of bone in the femoral neck in elderly people: longitudinal findings from the Dubbo osteoporosis epidemiology study. BMJ 309:691–695

Kanis JA, Passmore R (1989) Calcium supplementation of the diet. BMJ 298:137–140, 205–208, 673–674

Kanis JA (1991) Calcium requirements for optimal skeletal health in women. Calcif Tissue Int 49 [Suppl]:S33–S41

Khaw KT, Sneyd MJ, Compston J (1992) Bone density, parathyroid hormone and 25-hydroxyvitamin D concentrations in middle aged women. BMJ 305:2273–2276

Khosla S, Atkinson EJ, Riggs BL, Melton LJ III, (1996) Relationship between body composition and bone mass in women. J Bone Miner Res 11:857–863

Kleerekoper M, Peterson E, Nelson D (1989) Identification of women at risk for developing postmenopausal osteoporosis with vertebral fractures: role of history and single photon absortiometry. Bone Mineral 7:171–186

Krall EA, Dawson-Hughes B (1993) Heritable and life-style determinants of bone mineral density. J Bone Miner Res 8:1–9

Krall EA, Parry P, Lichter JB, Dawson-Hughes B (1995) Vitamin D receptor alleles and rates of bone loss: influence of years since menopause and calcium intake. J Bone Min Res 10:978–984

Langlois JA, Harris T, Looker AC, Madans J (1996) Weight changes between 50 years and old age is associated with risk of hip fracture in white women aged 67 years and older. Arch Intern Med 156:989–994

Lips P, Netelenbos JC, Jongen MJ, van Ginkel FC, Althuis AL, van Schaik CL (1982) Histomorphometric profile and vitamin D status in patients with femoral neck fracture. Metab Bone Dis Relat Res 4:85–93

Luckey MM, Wallenstein S, Lapinski R, Meier DE (1996) A prospective study of bone loss in African-American and white women-a clinical research center study. J Clin Endocrinol Metab 81:2948–2956

Luisetto G, Zangari M, Bottega F, Peccolo F, Galuppo P, Nardi A, Ziliotto D (1995) Different rates of forearm bone loss in healthy women with early or late menopause. Osteoporosis Int 5:54–62

Matkovic V, Kostial K, Simonovic I, Buzina R, Broderec A, Nordin BEC (1979) Bone status and fracture rates in two regions of Yugoslavia. Am J Clin Nutr 32:540–549

McKane WR, Khola S, Egan KS, Robins SP, Burritt MF, Rigg BL (1996) Role of calcium intake in modulating age-related increases in parathyroid function and bone resorption. J Clin Endocrinol Metab 81:1699–703

Melton III LJ, Bryant SC, Wahner HW (1993) Influence of breastfeeding and other reproductive factors on bone mass later in life. Osteoporosis Int 3:76–83

Meyer HE, Henriksen C, Falch JA, Pedersen JI, Tverdal A (1995) Risk factors for hip fracture in a high incidence area: a case-control study from Oslo, Norway. Osteoporosis Int 5:239–246

Michaelsson K, Bergstrom R, Mallmin H, Holmberg L, Wolk A, Ljunghall S (1996) Screening for osteopenia and osteoporosis: selection by body composition. Osteoporosis Int 6:120–126

Nelson DA, Kleerekoper M, Parfitt AM (1988) Bone mass, skin color and body size among black and white women. Bone Miner 4:257–264

Nguyen TV, Kelly PJ, Sambrook PN, Gilbert C, Poock NA, Eisman JA (1994) Lifestyle factors and bone density in the elderly: implications for osteoporosis prevention. J Bone Min Res 9:1339–1344

Nordin BEC, Horowitz M, Need A, Morris HA (1994) Renal leak of calcium in postmenopausal osteoporosis. Clin Endocrinol 41:41–45

Orwol ES, Meier DE (1986) Alterations in calcium, vitamin D, and parathyroid hormone physiology in normal men with aging: relationship to the development of senile osteopenia. J Clin Endocrinol Metab 63:1262–1269

Orwoll ES, Oviatt SK, Mann T (1990) The impact of osteophytic and vascular calcifications on vertebral mineral density measurements in men. J Clin Endocrinol Metab 70:1202–1207

Pedersen SB, Borglum JD, Brixen K, Richelsen B (1995) Relationship between sex hormones, body composition and metabolic risk parameters in premenopausal women. Eur J Endocrinol 133:200–206

Pouillès JM, Tremollieres F, Ribot C, CHU Purpan, Toulouse (1996) Variability of vertebral and femoral postmenopausal bone loss: a longitudinal study. Osteoporosis Int 6:320–324

Reid IR, Ames RW, Evans MC, Sharpe SJ, Gamble GD (1994) Determinants of the rate of bone loss in normal postmenopausal women. J Clin Endocrinol Metab 79:950–954

Reid IR, Chin K, Evans MC, Jones JG (1994) Relation beteween increases in length of hip axis in older women between 1950s and 1990s and increase in age specific rates of hip fracture. BMJ 309:508–509

Ribot C, Pouillès JM, Bonneu M, Trémolières F (1992) Assessment of the risk of postmenopausal osteoporosis using clinical risk factors. Clin Endocrinol 36:225–228

Ribot C. Trémolières F, Pouillés JM (1995) Can we detect women with low bone mass using clinical risk factors? Am J Med 98 [Suppl 2A]:52–53

Riggs BL (1986) Involutional osteoporosis. N Engl J Med 314:1676–86

Ross PD, Davis JW, Wasnich RD (1991) Pre-existing fractures and bone mass predict vertebral fracture incidence in women. Ann Intern Med 114:919–923

Salamone LM, Glynn N, Black D, Epstein RS, Palermo L, Meilahn E, Kuller LH, Cauley JA (1995) Body composition and bone mineral density in premenopausal and early perimenopausal women. J Bone Min Res 10:1762–1768

Salamone LM, Glynn NW, Black DM, Ferrell RE, Palermo L, Epstein RS, Kuller LH, Cauley JA (1996) Determinants of premenopausal bone mineral density: the interplay of genetic and lifestyle factors. J Bone Min Res 11:1557–1565

Seeman E, Cooper M, Hopper JL, Parkinson E, McKay J, Jerumus G (1988) Effect of early menopause on bone mass in normal women and paients with osteoporosis. Am J Med 85:213–216

Slemenda C, Longcope C, Peacock M, Hui S, Johnston CC (1996) Sex steroids, bone mass, and bone loss. A prospective study of pre-, peri-, and postmenopausal women. J Clin Invest 97:14–21

Slemenda CW, Hui SL, Langcope C, Wellman H, Johnston CC (1990) Predictor of bone mass in perimenopausal women: a prospective study of clinical data using photon absortiometry. Ann Intern Med 112:96–101

Slovik DM, Adams JM, Neer RM, Holick MF, Potts JT jr.(1981) Deficient production of 1,25-dihydroxyvitamn D in elderly patients. N Engl J Med 305:372–374

Stein MS, Scherer SC, Walton SL, Gilbert RE, Ebeling PR, Flicker L, Wark JD (1996) Risk factors for secondary hyperprathyroidism in a nursing home population. Clin Endocrinol 44:375–383

Stevenson JC, Lees B, Devenport M Cust MP, Ganger KF (1989) Determinants of bone density in normal women: risk factors for future osteoporosis? BMJ 298:924–8

Thomsen K, Gotfredsen A, Christiansen C (1986) Is postmenopausal bone loss an age-related phenomenon? Calcif Tissue Int 39:123–127

Tremollieres FA, Pouilles J-M, Ribot C, CHU Purpan (1993) Vertebral postmenopausal bone loss is reduced in overweight women: a longitudinal study in 155 early postmenopausal women. J Clin Endocrinol Metab 77:683–686

Tsai KS, Health H III, Kumar R, Riggs BL (1984) Impaired vitamin D metabolism with aging in women: possible role in pathogenesis of senile osteoporosis. J Clin Invest 73:1668–1672

Tuppurainen M, Kroger H, Saarikoski S, Honkanen R, Alhava E (1995) The effect of gynecological risk factors on lumbar and femoral bone mineral density in peri- and postmenopausal women. Maturitas 21:137–145

Van der Wielen RP, Löwick MRH, Van der Berg H, L CPMG de Groot, Haller J, Moreiras O, van Staveren WA (1995) Serum vitamin D concentrations among elderly people in Europe. Lancet 346:207–210

Vico L, Pouget JF, Calmels P, Chatard JC, Rehailia M, Minaire P (1995) The relations between physical ability and bone mass in women aged over 65 years. J Bone Min Res 10:374–383

Villareal DT, Civitelli R, Chines A, Avioli LV.(1991) Subclinical vitamin D deficiency in postmenopausal women with low vertebral bone mass. J Clin Endocrinol Metab 72:628–634

8   Biomechanical Properties of Bone

J. L. Ferretti

What Are Bones Made For?

There is no scientific answer to this teleological question. Bones may be either regarded as "serving" to protect bone marrow from cosmic radiation and to store quantities of electrolytes that are essential for life, or merely to act as columns or levers to support the body and allow locomotion and work, and so on.

Undoubtedly, natural selection must have contributed to develop dense, electrolyte-rich, and rigid skeletal structures; otherwise no vertebrate species could have existed. However, no blood illness deriving from an insufficient armour of the bone marrow is known, nor is any disturbance of the internal milieu induced by an electrolyte scarcity in the skeletal bank. Instead, extensive libraries have been written on "skeletal dysfunctions" that produce bone deformities and fractures, pain, disability, poor quality of life, and food for thought for specialists in rheumatology and orthopedics.

It can be concluded therefore that there is at least one bone property that has not yet been completed by evolution, that of the "supporting function" of the skeleton. In fact, apart from dental tissues, bone is the stiffest biological tissue produced by nature [12]. From the clinical point of view, bones are important because of their undesirable tendency to fail to behave as rigid structures, and that problem is discussed here.

Why Be Stiff?

When any solid, fixed structure becomes loaded, it undergoes a certain degree of strain (change in size and shape in different directions and locations). Figure 8-1 shows the changes in shape produced by a bending load on a tubular structure. The shortening in the concave side of the structure leads to a certain degree of compression stress of its constitutive material. The lengthening in the convex side induces some traction stress in it.

Depending on material strength or toughness, microfractures are more or less easily produced in the loaded structure. If the structure is weaker in traction than in compression (as a bone is) [9], microfractures tend to appear on the convex side. Once microfractures occur, and provided that sufficient load is exerted on the structure, the microfracture traces progress easily and eventually determine its complete fracture (separation into two or more pieces).

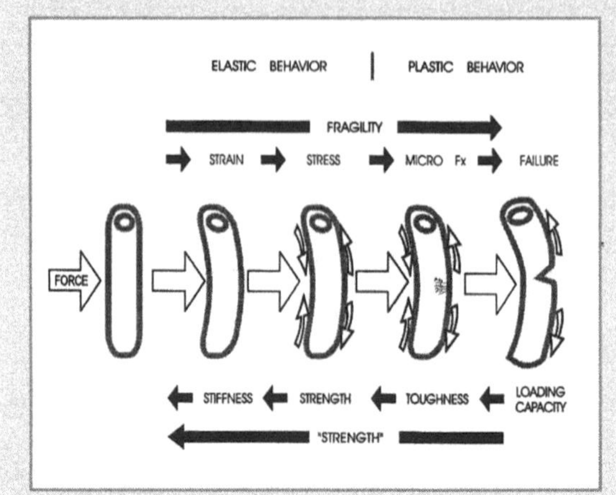

Fig. 8-1 Diagram of the action of a bending force upon a solid, tubular structure

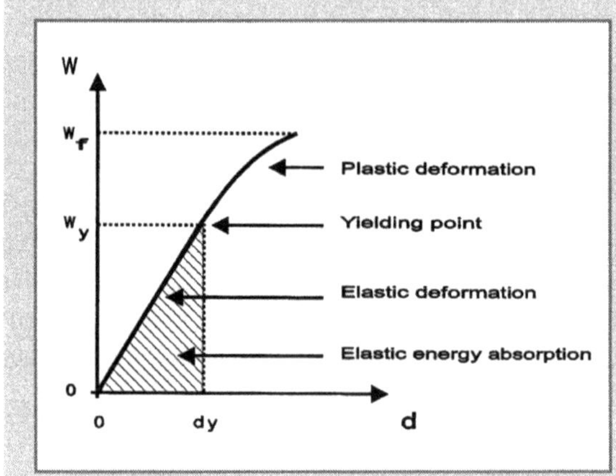

Fig. 8-2 Classic load/deformation curve resulting from a three-point bending test of a long bone

In some cases the load initially determines what is called a linearly elastic strain (i. e., constantly proportional to load, and reversible) until a critical accumulation of microfractures takes place [44]. Microfractures determine a different behavior of the structure, which is called plastic deformation (i.e., not linearly proportional to load, and nonreversible) [9]. This biphasic behavior defines the "elastic-plastic" structures (of which bones are examples) and may be experimentally described by load/deformation curves as shown in Fig. 8-2.

A typical sequence in the mechanism of production of a bone fracture would therefore be: load→elastic strain (stress without microfractures)→plastic strain (stress-derived microfractures)→fracture (no more stress). The induction of bone strain is always the first step in the mechanism of production of any fracture (Fig. 8-1). In fact, there is no known solid structure that can fail without previously showing a deformation that generates the necessary stress. Therefore the achievement of an acceptable degree of resistance to strain (stiffness) confers a reasonable resistance to stress and fracture (strength) to the structure. This positive interrelation between stiffness and strength is true (and generally linear) for young, adult, and elderly bone structures, but only within certain limits [46]. Highly deformable bones sometimes resist fracture better than normal ones, such as in children. On the other hand, an extreme stiffness should facilitate the progression of fracture traces and enhance the brittleness of bone structure, as observed in osteopetrosis.

It is therefore reasonable to acknowledge that the selective "sense" of the evolution of bone structures, if any, should have focused on the achievement of an optimal degree of stiffness, i.e., resistance to strain [13], which is the chief determinant of the stress of the structure that may cause it to fracture.

How To Achieve Stiffness?

Being biological structures, living bones are able to grow rigid by themselves. Since fractures are relatively rare events in a bone's life, some mechanism should "govern" bone growth, modeling or remodeling in such a way that the chance of suffering a fracture be minimal. This means that bones should be permanently controlled by a system that maintains their stiffness and strength within "adequate" values. The question then is, what is actually controlled, stiffness or strength, and how much is "adequate"?

Strikingly, the propensity to fracture cannot be "sensed" by any biological structure. In fact, there is no apparent way in which a bone can "measure" any variable that directly defines its strength. Instead there is increasing evidence that the true "structural" bone cells (osteocytes and lining cells) are able to sense bone strain [33]. Either as a change in length of cell prolongations, a shift in the piezo-electrical environment, a variation in the extracellular ionic flow, or any other suitably "measurable" phenomenon at cellular level, osteocytes or lining cells seem to be able directionally to detect bone strain and "qualify" it as compression or traction induced.

If strain direction and magnitude can actually be sensed at the cellular level, a regulating mechanism based on the control of a "strain-signal error" by bone cells is a certain possibility [33]. We know that it is not body mass (impossible to be measured at cellular level) but appetite (as related to metabolite concentrations in blood) that is actually controlled. Analogously, it is not bone strength but bone stiffness that is under biological regulation [17, 21].

It is clear that bones behave as if they "need" to be stiff in order to be strong; however, it is less obvious (yet equally true) that they do not need to be massive to grow stiff.

Why Not Just Be Massive?

It may seem obvious that the more massive the structure, the stronger it should be. In fact, massiveness may be convenient but certainly is not a necessary condition. The mechanical effectiveness of a solid body strongly depends on (a) the intrinsic mechanical quality of its constitutive substance (material properties) and (b) the amount ("mass") and the spatial distribution of that substance concerning the mode of action of the deforming force (macroarchitecture, or geometry) [4, 45] (Fig. 8-3).

Concerning the kind of substance that the structure is made of, what generally matters is its "intrinsic stiffness," as described by Young's "modulus of elasticity" [9]. The modulus of elasticity of a given material is proportional to its specific resistance to strain, irrespective of size and shape of the piece considered, in relation to a given mode of action of the deforming force.

The modulus of elasticity of bone tissue depends largely on the amount of mineral in it (i.e., the "true," volumetric mineral density of the solid bone) [14] and also on many other microstructural factors (arrangement of crystal and collagen fibers, composition of collagen and ground substance, microfractures, etc) [7,36]. The three-dimensional directionality of most of these factors determines that the mechanical behavior of bone material depends on the mode of action of the deforming force (bone material anisotropy) [1, 3, 9].

Bone material quality is genetically determined, and it therefore varies relatively little in different skeletal regions of the same individual [9]. However, it may change noticeably over time as a function of the remodeling rate [14]. Bone remodeling results from the coupled bone resorption/formation that replaces tiny pieces of bone (bone structural units) on trabecular surfaces and within cortical bone. This mechanism, the only one known to induce bone loss [25, 27], may affect cor-

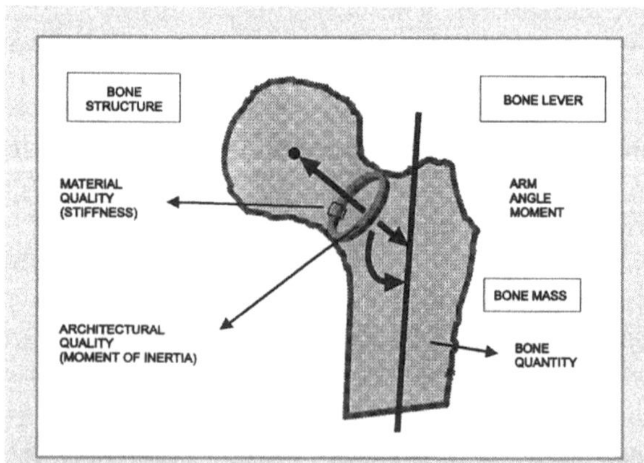

Fig. 8-3 Didactic representation of mass, mechanical quality, and distribution of bone material as determinants of the mechanical properties of a whole bone

tical bone material quality by reducing its volumetric bone mineral density (BMD) because of an excessive haversianization. It may, conversely, be beneficial because, apart from being essential for maintaining Ca-P homeostasis, it is also the only mechanism known to repair bone microfractures [26].

Macroarchitecture (or simply "architecture") is also a strong determinant of the mechanical ability of any structure [4]. When the load is exerted in uniaxial compression (i.e., along the central axis of the structure), it does not generate any bending or torsional strain on it. In this case the more significant feature from the mechanical point of view may be just how much material is supporting the load, and not how well is it distributed over a cross-section of the structure. However, this may completely describe the compression strength only in solid, homogeneous structures. In more complicated frames as vertebral bodies other conditions become significant, namely, the vertical and horizontal disposition of trabecular struts and the intertrabecular connectivity, which are independent of bone mass itself. This points out that other, mass-unrelated factors such as the distribution of the hard material also play very important roles in determining bone stiffness and strength [38, 39].

The crucial role of all these factors is especially evident when a certain degree of bending or torsional strain is induced (a very common situation for long bones in normal life and when a trauma induces a bone fracture). In these conditions massiveness by itself does not describe the structure's stiffness or strength. If the bone tends to become bent or torsioned by the load, its stiffness (and hence its strength) depends chiefly on the spatial disposition of its constitutive material

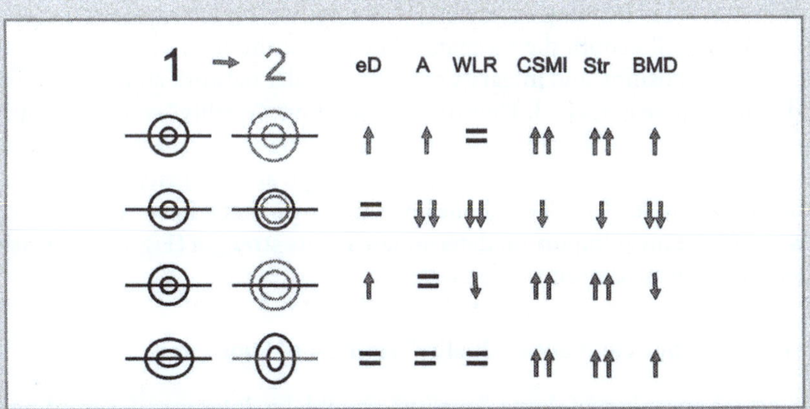

Fig. 8-4 Changes in cross-sectional moment of inertia (CSMI) and bending strength (Str) of a tubular bone in bending on passing from size/shape 1 to 2, as related to modifications of its external diameter (eD), cross-sectional area (A), and wall-to-lumen ratio (WLR). The bending axis is represented horizontally in every case. First row, enhancement of eD and A with no change in WLR; second row, increase in internal diameter with no change in eD; third row, increase in internal and external diameters without change in A; fouth row, 90° rotation of the (elliptically shaped) section with respect to the bending axis. In all cases bone strength varies closely to CSMI, and this reflects the distance from cortical bone to the reference axis, regardless of the changes in the other geometric parameters

throughout its cross-section with respect to the bending or torsional axis in question. Two tubular structures made of the same material and showing a similar cross-sectional area are similarly stiff and strong in compression. However, the one with a larger external diameter (i.e., with thinner walls) shows higher stiffness and strength than the other in bending or torsion [46]. In tubular structures a variable that expresses the mechanical significance of both the mass and the spatial distribution of the resistive material is the cross-sectional moment of inertia (CSMI) with reference to a bending or torsion axis [46] (Fig. 8-4).

Concerning bones, macroarchitecture or geometry results chiefly (in addition to growth in length) from bone modeling. Bone modeling is determined by the uncoupled periosteal and peritrabecular apposition and trabecular or endosteal resorption that occurs in any bone during youth and adulthood (peritrabecular apposition occurs also in the elderly). Apart from bone growth in length, this is the only known process that determines bone size and shape, improves CSMI during aging, and provides any kind of bone mass gain [25, 27]. Bone remodeling may also affect bone macroarchitecture when it determines a sufficiently large material loss in the region.

What Is Necessary To Be Strong?

As is noted above, bone stiffness and strength generally depend not only on bone mass but also on bone material quality and distribution (architecture). Engineers usually calculate the flexural or torsional stiffness and strength of tubular structures as functions of merely the product of the material's modulus of elasticity and the bending or torsional CSMI. The same applies to tubular bones that are usually stressed in bending or torsion [3]. Similarly, for the compression analysis of vertebral bodies, both the mechanical quality of the solid bone material and the spatial disposition and integrity of the trabecular network should be considered besides bone mass [37]. Thus the (whole-) bone "quality" concept comprises no less than three different aspects, namely, massiveness, intrinsic stiffness (bone "material quality"), and architectural design and integrity.

In addition to the length of a bone lever, the angle that it forms in certain cases is one of the most important determinants of its strength (Fig. 8-3), at least as crucial as bone mass itself [15, 29].

Are Bone Strength and Bone "Quality" Equivalent Concepts?

The actual meaning of bone "quality" should be interpreted according to mechanical concepts [5]. Determination of bone biomechanical parameters has recently been incorporated into the United States Food and Drug Administration (FDA) Guidelines as a requisite for studies aimed to support registration of new drugs for treatment of bone-weakening diseases [19].

Moreover, this also concerns bone anisotropy and regional differences. A bone should show a good mechanical "quality" regarding each possible kind of fracture. That is to say, a good, healthy bone must show both a high mechanical quality of its constitutive material (modulus of elasticity of solid bone) and an adequate amount and spatial distribution of the material concerning different ways of action of the deforming forces (different types of fractures). Bone "quality" is then a directional, "vectorial" property that should be defined concerning all the possible instances in which bone stiffness and strength are important.

How Do Bones Acquire an Optimal Mechanical Quality?

Let us assume that bone modeling and remodeling are the only known mechanisms that, in addition to longitudinal growth, provide adaptational changes in bone structure to cope with mechanical usage throughout life [23]. Let us also suppose that any feedback mechanism controlling bone mechanical quality should measure bone strain at cellular level and take care of it at tissue and organ levels [33]. Bone cells should then be regarded as the central pieces in the regulatory process [33], a version of which can be sketched following the theoretical background of Frost's "mechanostat" [22] as shown in Fig. 8-5.

The strain induced at organ/tissue levels by mechanical usage would be sensed by osteocytes or lining cells and defined as coming from compression or traction on a given region of the structure. Any amount of unusual strain should be taken as a "signal error." This would determine a certain spatial orientation of the releasing of cell factors that locally stimulate or inhibit uncoupled (modeling) or coupled (remodeling) bone formation or resorption by cells that are actually extrinsic to the resistive bone structure (osteoblasts and osteoclasts). The effects of these cell-cell interactions would result in changes of not only bone mass but also either bone material quality or distribution, or both (Fig. 8-6).

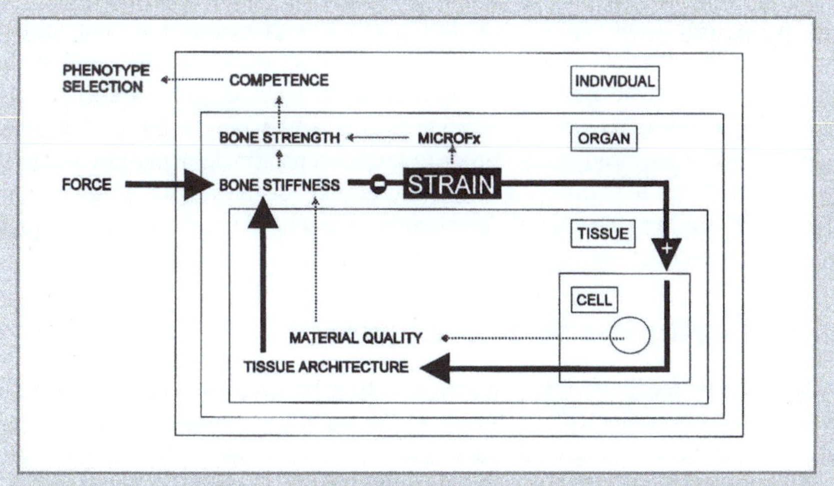

Fig. 8-5 Diagram of bone mechanostat according to the levels of biological complexity of the structures involved

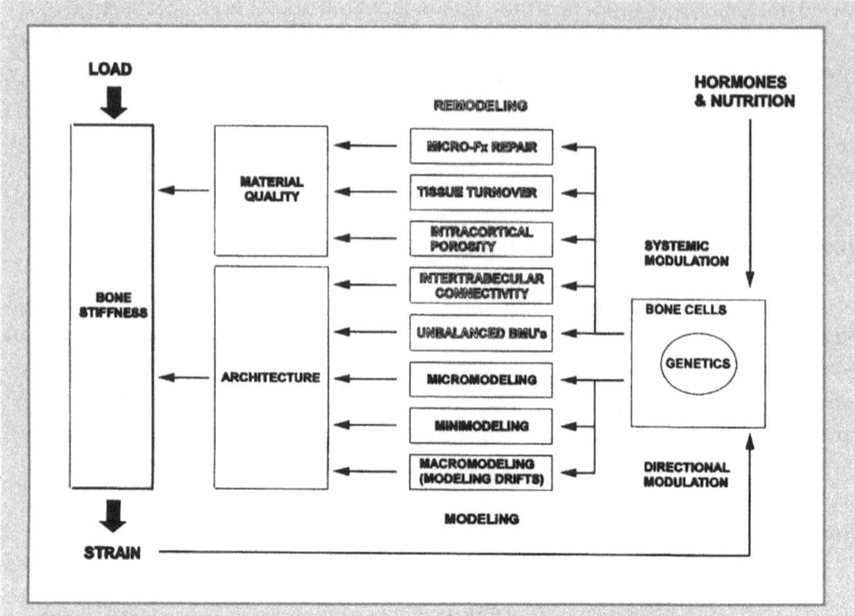

Fig. 8-6 Diagram of bone mechanostat according to the role of bone modeling and remodeling in the production of the structural changes

These changes would "optimize" bone structure in mechanical terms in order to minimize the signal error (local strain) for the next instance [28,33]. Optimization of bone strain signals as related to customary mechanical usage provides adequate protection against the production and accumulation of microfractures over the natural tissue repairing ability [5, 26]. Therefore bones do not control their mass in order to become adequately strong; they actually control the mechanical quality of their structure in order to grow adequately stiff [17, 21]. This in turn indirectly optimizes bone mechanical strength because heavier loads should be required in the future to induce a plastic deformation and provoke a fracture in the region (Fig. 8-5). It has already been shown that the regional muscle strength is the chief determinant of the whole-bone mechanical quality, independently of sex, age, and body habitus [42].

Are Bones No More Than "Mechanical Structures"?

Reasonably, all feedback mechanisms affecting bones and dealing with bone marrow protection, electrolyte storage and availability, compensation for metabolic disturbances, mechanical usage, etc., should have been selected in parallel by all vertebrates [13]. Therefore bones should behave as mechanical structures and function as required by any other mechanism essential for life at the same time.

However, the resisting structure which is contained within bones behaves exactly as if the challenge to cope with mechanical usage were something inherent, native to it [40]. When so interpreted, the hard bone structure seems to accomplish its mechanical function despite the existence of the other, endocrine-metabolic feedback systems that are focused to control different signal errors such as metabolite concentrations in blood or hormone production by mother glands. In fact, the huge losses of bone mass (and structural mechanical efficiency) induced by complete immobilization or weightlessness occur despite the normal, healthy condition of all those systems. Conversely, any disturbance of endocrine-metabolic systems may affect bone structure without any commitment to amend the deteriorations eventually induced in its mechanical efficiency. There is no feedback loop mutually governing the integrity of bone structure and the efficiency of the endocrine-metabolic system (Fig. 8-7).

This means that although an endocrine-metabolic equilibrium is essential for normal skeletal development and structural integrity, endocrine-metabolic imbalances usually act as disturbers of the mechanostatic feedback mechanism, with no chance of any autocontrol of the situation at the individual level of organization. Only when the mechanostat is able to keep control and deal with the structural problem induced, should skeletal "quality" be maintained; otherwise it would not [20].

In this regard there is evidence that regional muscle force is the main determinant of the mechanical efficiency of bone structure [23, 42]. However, no positive results of exercise programs are to be expected if the endocrine equilibrium of the patient is so altered as to throw the mechanostat permanently out of control. Conversely, no mechanical improvement can be expected from the administration of hormones that are under normal equilibrium in the subject, nor from any

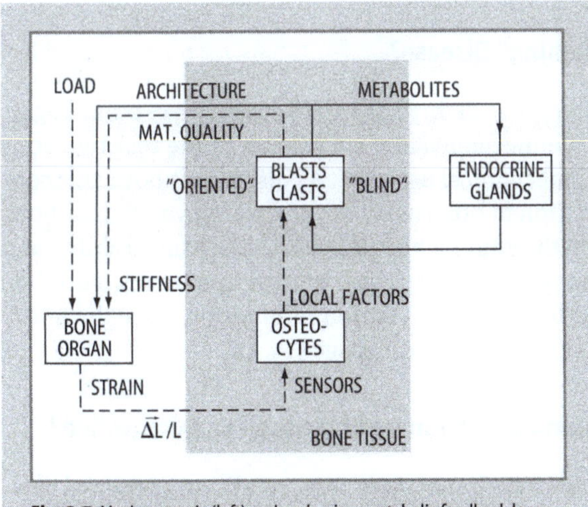

Fig. 8-7 Mechanostatic (left) and endocrine-metabolic feedback loops (right) affecting bone structure

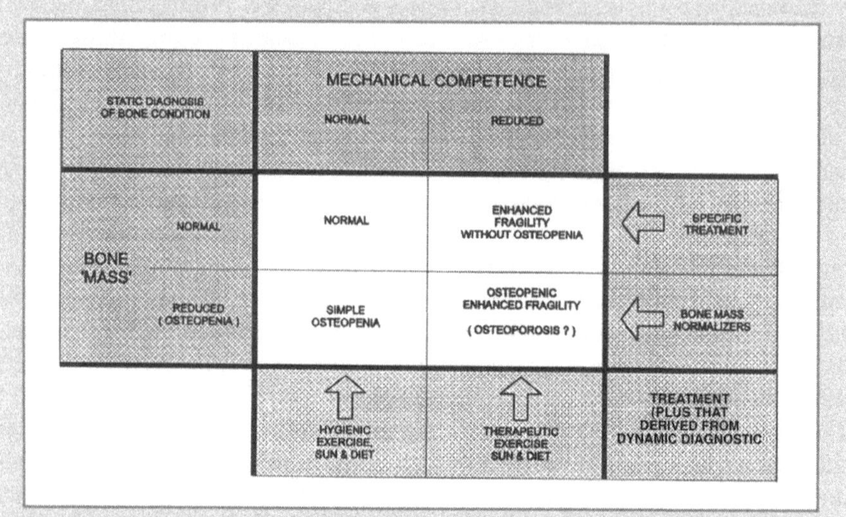

Fig. 8-8 Independent and complementary evaluations of bone mass and mechanical competence in the diagnosis of a bone-weakening disease

hormonal, nutritional, or pharmacological manipulation if bones are not adequately stressed by mechanical usage [27, 28]. For the same reasons, exercise plans are usually not effective in improving bone mass in normal conditions, but they are highly efficient in avoiding or recovering disuse-induced bone losses.

In other words, bones are not actually pure "mechanical structures" at organ level, but the hard structure contained within bones behaves as a primarily mechanical apparatus [12, 13].

What Then Is a "Bone-Weakening" Disease?

A bone-weakening disease should be defined as an enhancement of bone fragility derived from an inadequate mechanostatic adaptation of the resistive bone structure to customary, local mechanical usage [5]. As discussed above, this concept may be related to a reduction in bone mass, but again it may not, since bone "quality" depends not only on the amount but also on the mechanical ability and the spatial distribution of bone material [38, 39]. It must also be related to the condition of the subject and to the skeletal region in question since the above definition is related to customary mechanical usage [23, 42].

How Should a Bone-Weakening Condition Be Diagnosed and Controlled?

It follows that to properly diagnose a bone-weakening condition a regional deterioration of both bone mass and bone material quality and/or spatial distribution should be demonstrated, in relation to customary mechanical use [5, 23].

However, this is not all. "Fracture risk" is an epidemiological concept related to the probability of a fracture occurring during a given time. It involves not only bone health and robusticity but also a number of anatomical and physiological factors which contribute to bone protection against trauma and trauma circumstances.

As our interest is focused on bone health, we may disregard the analysis of trauma-associated factors. We may also ignore mechanical use until suitable diagnostic resources and standardized data are available. The remaining problem depends on our ability noninvasively to measure bone mass, bone material quality, and gross bone architecture in suitable, mechanically meaningful terms [15, 31] (Fig. 8-8). However, we must not forget that what actually matters is not just a bone, but the human owner of that bone and his or her particular type of activity and environment.

How Can Bone Absorptiometry Assess Bone Quality?

Bone Mass Measurements

Undoubtedly the best known procedure to measure bone "mass" (i.e., how much mineralized bone tissue is within a bone organ or region) with acceptable accuracy and precision is standard bone densitometry [single-photon absorptiometry, dual-photon absorptiometry, dual-beam X-ray absorptiometry (DXA)], especially if the data are expressed as bone mineral content (BMC) in mass units [15, 31]. This determination has repeatedly been shown to be significantly correlated with the actual, mechanically assessed bone strength [15, 29, 31].

However, the correlation coefficients obtained have generally been poor because of a high dispersion of the data and frequent overlap between values from fractured and unfractured subjects [11]. This implies that the determining power of these correlations is rather low, and therefore they should not be invoked to infer causal interrelationships between BMC and bone strength. In other words, the assumption that "the better the BMC, the higher (i.e., not the lower) the strength" may be taken as a reliable description of a tendency for the whole population; however, the predictive power of a DXA determination of BMC or BMD to estimate actual bone strength of a given individual is relatively poor. Therefore DXA-assessed BMC or BMD, expressed either in absolute or Z or T score values, should be regarded only as excellent indicators of osteopenic (not osteoporotic) conditions (Fig. 8-8), because of their inability to express bone material quality and spatial distribution [27, 38, 39]. In some bones, for example, the vertebral bodies, BMC values obtained either by DXA or axial quantitative computed tomography (QCT) have been shown to be reasonably well correlated with compression strength [15, 29, 31]. This can be explained because bone mass is more closely (and causally) associated to compression than to other kinds of bone stress. In these cases BMC values may be regarded as appropriate estimates of bone strength until we have better methods to approach it.

Bone Material Quality Determinations

The intrinsic stiffness (modulus of elasticity) of bone material has been shown to be linearly or exponentially associated to its volumetric mineral density (vBMD) [8, 14]. Unfortunately, standard densitometry does not provide any data on the vBMD of bone material. In fact, in bones with similar levels of vBMD the areal BMD measures merely bone size. Furthermore, different levels of vBMD would be blunted to densitometry by the spatial distribution of bone material (Fig. 8-4). Instead, vBMD determinations by axial or peripheral QCT (pQCT) may approach the mineralization-related component of bone material quality [16, 29, 30, 32, 34, 41, 42].

However, bone material quality is actually determined not only by vBMD but also by a number of mineralization-unrelated factors, such as the composition of ground substance and collagen, arrangement of collagen fibers and crystals, density of microfractures, etc. [1, 3, 4, 9, 14, 36, 46], which are beyond the scope of any kind of absorptiometric procedure. This restricts the application of vBMD determinations to estimate bone material quality in mechanical terms only to those conditions in which a relative invariance of all the other significant factors can be assumed. Otherwise, the indirect assessment of bone material quality as related to vBMD should be taken carefully.

Other technologies such as ultrasound measurements may provide more integral determinations of bone material quality (referred to as "stiffness" by manufacturers). This is undoubtedly a promising fact, yet the true correlations of ultrasound data with the directly measured bone material properties and their corresponding determining powers must still be defined.

Bone Macroarchitecture Assessment

There are two classical examples of the biomechanical meaningfulness of this aspect of bone quality, namely, the horizontal/vertical disposition and integrity of bone trabeculae inside vertebral bodies, and the cross-sectional distribution of cortical tissue in long bones with reference to given bending or torsion axes (CSMI).

No resource appears to exist for noninvasively assessing the trabecular network arrangement or integrity. Standard densitometry is obviously out of the question. A significant enhancement in resolution of current axial tomography may offer some possibility. Interesting approaches may come from sophisticated procedures such as fractal analysis, but we are far from obtaining a reliable, standardized method to cope with this problem. In the meanwhile we depend on invasive techniques such as bone histomorphometry, which are obviously restricted to very special indications.

Cross-sectional analysis of long bones poses quite a different matter. In long bones, cortical bone seems to be the most significant type of structure providing resistance against fracture production [44]. In effect, diaphyseal or metaphyseal fractures usually begin in the outer bone surface, never in the internal trabecular network. Therefore cortical (not trabecular) stiffness and strength are essential for preventing a fracture trace from starting.

No information on cortical bone architecture can be provided by standard densitometry. However, it can easily be analyzed in cross-sectional QCT or, better, pQCT scans [2, 10, 16, 29–31, 35, 41–44] from which not only the cortical area but also the flexural (rectangular) and torsional (polar) CSMIs can be determined. These are calculated automatically as the integral sum of the products of each cortical bone pixel area and its squared distance to the reference, bending, or torsion axes [16, 42].

Noninvasive Estimations of Whole-Bone Quality

The solution to this problem depends on the skeletal region selected for study. In general, there are two typically different kinds of regions in this regard, namely, vertebral bodies and long bones.

The estimation of compression strength of vertebral bodies is currently restricted only to that provided by BMC determinations made by axial QCT or, alternatively, by DXA measurements in lateral projections. In fact, bone "mass" alone may deal with a high proportion of whole-bone quality in these compression-stressed regions [15, 29, 31]. However, a significant contribution to strength also comes from the mechanical ability of the trabecular network [30, 32, 37, 43, 44], which is neglected by merely measuring BMC. We will remain unable to accurately assess vertebral bodies' strength until we can properly evaluate the mechanical efficiency of the trabecular network structure.

Noninvasive assessment of long-bone strength seems to be an easier problem. As noted above, calculation of the CSMIs of the cortical region from pQCT scans of long bones takes into account both bone tissue "mass" (pixel areas or voxel volumes) and distribution (distances from each pixel or voxel to the reference axes; Fig. 8-3) [16, 42]. Therefore the CSMI's are especially convenient for noninvasively estimating the whole-bone quality in mechanical terms when combined with suitable indicators of bone material quality as the pQCT determined vBMD. This concept provided the basis for the development of what I called bone strength indices (BSI), which are given by the product of a CSMI and the vBMD of cortical bone of the cross-section. One such BSI has been validated as a pQCT-determined indicator of bending strength in rat femurs [18, 21]. It was correlated linearly and very closely with the actual breaking force of a number of bones within a large range of values of CSMI and vBMD, independently of the animal condition (Fig. 8-9a). This correlation was stronger than those obtained between breaking force and any of the two components of the BSI alone (CSMI, vBMD), or the DXA-assessed, areal BMD of the mechanically tested portion of the bones (Fig. 8-9b). The success of combining "material" (cortical vBMD) and "architectural" (CSMI) variables into a single index for achieving a precise and accurate estimation of bone strength is not surprising, as they are inversely interrelated by

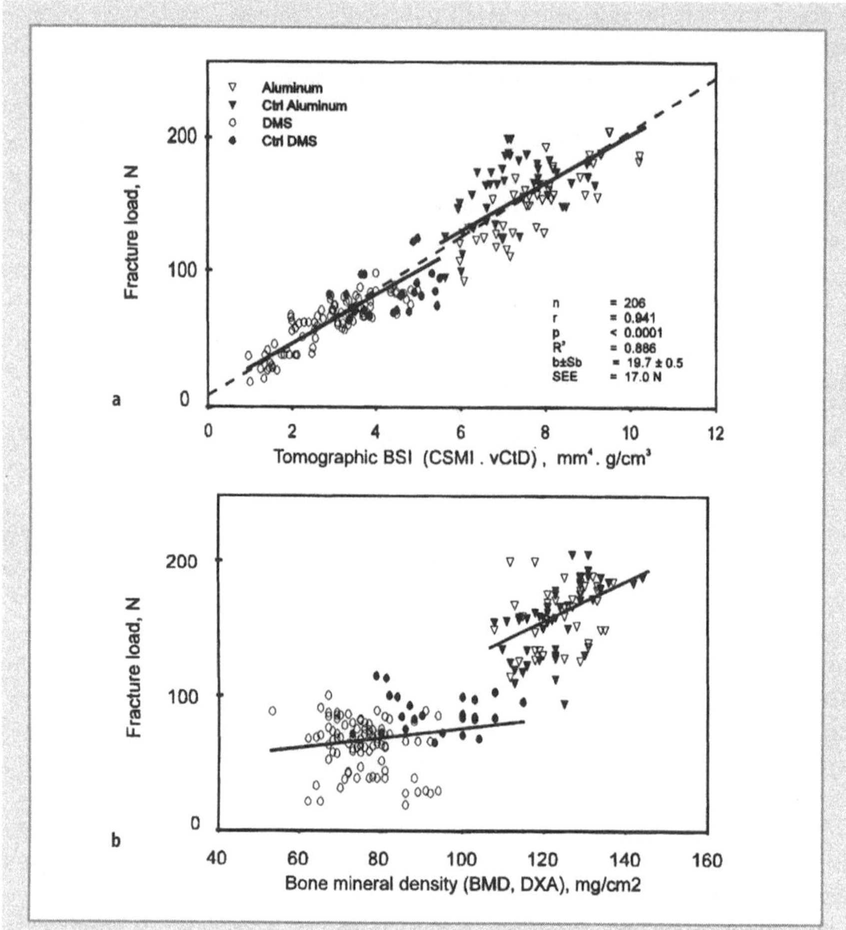

Fig. 8-9 Correlations between the measured breaking bending strength of femurs from young and adult rats treated with high doses of dexamethasone or intoxicated with aluminum [18] and the pQCT-determined bone strength index of the middiaphyseal scans (a) or the DXA-assayed BMD of the mechanically tested segments (b) of the same bones

the mechanostat "in order to" provide adequate bone strength for mechanical usage [16, 21, 22, 24, 28]. A convenient feature of the BSI is that it can be determined in anesthesized animals in either cross-sectional or longitudinal in vivo studies.

The new FDA Guidelines to basic and clinical research recommend performing combined, tomographic-biomechanical determinations to provide experimental support to drug registration for treatment of bone-weakening diseases [19]. We have performed a number of such studies employing pQCT and three-point bending tests in long bones from small animals. These were aimed at developing new, noninvasive methods for not only determining bone strength but also

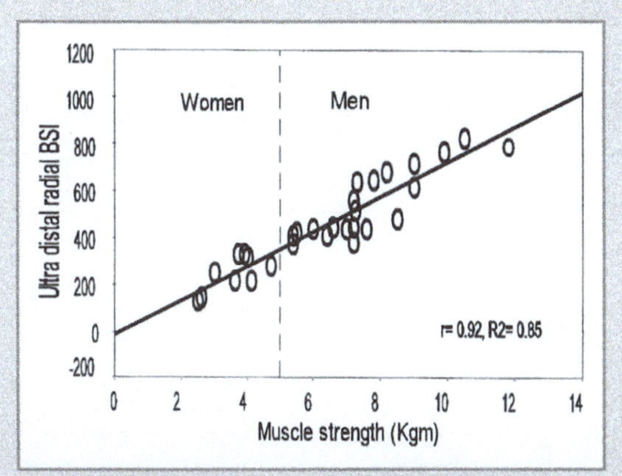

Fig. 8-10 Correlation between the measured maximal muscle force (arm/forearm flexor moment) and a tomographic (pQCT) bone strength index *(BSI)* calculated for the distal radius in normal men and women aged 16–76 years [42]

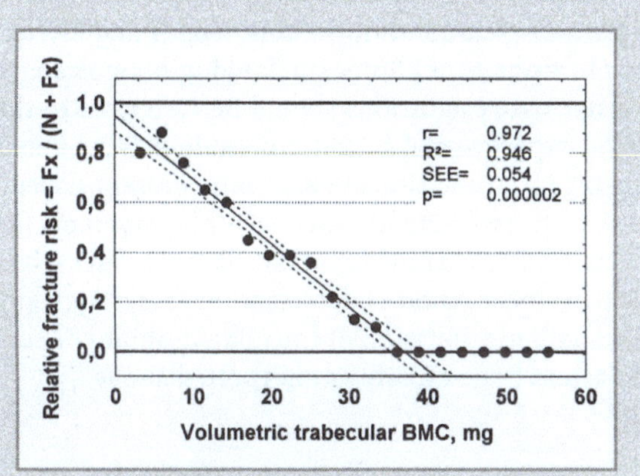

Fig. 8-11 Correlation between the realtive risk to have a Colles' fracture (RFR=Fx/(Fx+N) cases) calculated for 20 consecutive intervals of trabecular vBMC values measured in pQCT scans of the distal radius in a sample of 270 age-paired, normal *(N)* or fractured *(Fx)* men and women [43]

for analyzing the mechanostatic interrelationships between architectural and material properties of cortical bone in different conditions [16].

We have also shown that similar BSIs can estimate the strength of human long bones in comparable conditions. One such BSI calculated from scans at the ultra-distal radius was correlated very closely with the maximal muscle force of the forearm [28, 42] (Fig. 8-10) and with the relative risk to have a Colles' fracture [43] in large samples of healthy and wrist-fractured men and women. The relative Colles' fracture risk was also approached very closely by the pQCT measured trabecular vBMC (an easy-to-measure indicator of changes in cortical bone; Fig. 8-11) and

Table 8-1 Relative ability of current noninvasive techniques to assess bone quality

		Biomechanical determinations		
Method	Mineral mass	Material quality	Architecture	Strength
In vertebral bodies				
DXA	+++	–	–	++
QCT	++++	++	–	+++
In long bones				
DXA	++++	–	–	+
Ultrasound	++	+++	–	++
pQCT	+++	++	++++	+++

cortical bone area of the same region. An excellent correlation between the cross-sectional geometry and the mechanically assessed bone strength was also reported by others in cadaveric human radiuses [2].

Consideration of other mechanical factors related to bone size or shape affecting bone function as a lever in physiological conditions (bone length, angles, etc.) could further improve the predicting power of BSIs or similar long-bone strength indicators [15]. However, the proposed applications should be restricted to the skeletal region, type of bone, and experimental conditions studied. It is biomechanical nonsense to assimilate the interpretation of data from different skeletal regions, however they be statistically associated. Bone anisotropy compels the mechanical analysis to differ according to (a) the regional characteristics within each particular bone [28] and (b) the method of deformation assayed [15, 45].

Table 8-1 shows a rough personal interpretation of the relative ability of current noninvasive techniques to assess bone quality as interpreted above.

References

1. Ascenzi A, Bell GH (1972) Bone as a mechanical engineering problem. In: Bourne GH (ed) The biochemistry and physiology of bone, 2nd edn. Academic, New York, pp 311–352
2. Augat P, Reeb H, Claes L (1995) Second moment of inertia of the distal radius predicts the stability of the radius and the femoral neck. Calcif Tissue Int 56:453
3. Baker JL, Haugh CG (1989) Mechanical properties of bone. A review. Trans Am Soc Agr Eng 22:678–687
4. Burr DB (1980) The relationships among physical, geometrical and mechanical properties of bone, with a note on the properties of nonhuman primate bone. Yearb Phys Anthropol 23:109–146
5. Burr DB, Martin RB (1989) Errors in bone remodeling: toward a unified theory of metabolic bone disease. Am J Anat 186:186–216

6. Burr DB, Martin RB, Schaffler MB, Radin EL (1985) Bone remodeling in response to in vivo fatigue microdamage. J Biomech 18:189–200

7. Burstein AH, Zilka JM, Heiple KG, Klein L (1975) Contribution of collagen and mineral to the elastic-plastic properties of bone. J Bone Joint Surg Am 57:956–960

8. Carter DR, Hayes WC (1977) The compressive behavior of bone as a two-phase porous structure. J Bone Joint Surg Am 59:954–962

9. Carter DR, Spengler DM (1978) Mechanical properties and composition of cortical bone. Clin Orthop Relat Res 135:192–217

10. Corcoran TA, Sandler RB, Myers ER, Lebowitz HH, Hayes WC (1994) Calculation of cross-sectional geometry of bone from CT images with application in postmenopausal women. J Comput Assist Tomogr 18:626–633

11. Cummings GR, Marcus R, Palermo L et al (1994) Does estimating volumetric bone density of the femoral neck improve the prediction of hip fracture? A prospective study. J Bone Miner Res 9:1429–1432

12. Currey JD (1981) What is bone for? Property-function relationships in bone. In: Cowin SC (ed) Mechanical properties of bone. ASME, New York, pp 13–26

13. Currey JD (1984) What should bones be designed to do? Calcif Tissue Int 36 (S1):S7–S10

14. Currey JD (1988) The effects of porosity and mineral content on the Young's modulus of elasticity of compact bone. J Biomech 21:131–140

15. Faulkner KG, Glüer CC, Majumdar S, Lang P, Engelke K, Genant HK (1991) Noninvasive measurements of bone mass, structure, and strength. Current methods and experimental techniques. Am J Roentgenol 157:1229–1237

16. Ferretti JL (1995) Perspectives of pQCT technology associated to biomechanical studies in skeletal research employing rat models. Bone 17(4S):353S–364S

17. Ferretti JL, Capozza RF, Mondelo N, Zanchetta JR (1993) Interrelationships between densitometrical, geometric and mechanical properties of rat femurs. Inferences concerning mechanical regulation of bone modeling. J Bone Miner Res 8:1389–1396

18. Ferretti JL, Capozza RF, Zanchetta JR (1996) Mechanical validation of a tomographic (pQCT) index for noninvasive estimation of rat femur bending strength. Bone 18:97–102

19. Ferretti JL, Frost HM, Gasser J, High W, Je WSS, Jerome C, Mosekilde L, Thompson DD (1995) Perspectives on osteoporosis research: its focus and some insights from a new paradigm. Calcif Tissue Int 57:399–404

20. Ferretti JL, Gaffuri O, Capozza R, Cointry G, Bozzini C, Olivera M, Zanchetta JR, Bozzini CE (1995) Dexamethasone effects on mechanical, geometric and densitometric properties of rat femur diaphyses as described by peripheral quantitative computerized tomography and bending tests. Bone 16:119–124

21. Ferretti JL, Spiaggi EP, Capozza R, Cointry G, Zanchetta JR (1992) Interrelationships between geometric and mechanical properties of long bones from three rodent species with very different biomass. Phylogenetic implications. J Bone Miner Res 7(S2):S423–S425

22. Frost HM (1987) Bone "mass" and the "mechanostat": a proposal. Anat Rec 219:1–9
23. Frost HM (1989) Mechanical usage, bone mass, bone fragility. A brief overview. In: Kleerekoper M, Krane SM (eds) Clinical disorders of bone and mineral metabolism. Liebert, New York, pp 15–42
24. Frost HM (1990) Skeletal structural adaptations to mechanical usage (SAT-MU). I. Redefining Wolff's Law: the bone modeling problem. Anat Rec 226:403–413
25. Frost HM (1990) Skeletal structural adaptations to mechanical usage (SAT-MU). II. Redefining Wolff's Law: The remodeling problem. Anat Rec 226:414–422
26. Frost HM (1991) Some ABC's of skeletal pathophysiology. 5. Microdamage physiology. Calcif Tissue Int 49:229–231
27. Frost HM (1996) Introduction to a new skeletal physiology, vol I. Pajaro Group, Pueblo
28. Frost HM, Ferretti JL, Jee WSS (1997) On the roles of mechanical usage (MU), muscle strength and the mechanostat in skeletal physiology, disease and future research. Calcif Tissue Int (in press)
29. Genant HK, Engelke K, Fuerst T, Glüer CC, Grampp S, Harris ST, Jergas M, Lang T, Lu Y, Majumdar S, Mathur A, Takada M (1996) Noninvasive assessment of bone mineral and structure. State of the art. J Bone Miner Res 11:707–730
30. Gordon CL, Webber CE, Adami JD, Christoforou N (1996) In vivo assessment of trabecular bone structure at the distal radius from high-resolution computed tomography images. Phys Med Biol 41:495–508
31. Hayes WC, Piazza SJ, Zysser PK (1991) Biomechanics of fracture risk prediction of the hip and spine by quantitative computed tomography. Radiol Clin North Am 29:1–18
32. Lang T, Keyak J, Heitz M, Augat P, Genant HK (1996) A 3D anatomic coordinate system for hip QCT. Osteoporosis Int 6 (Suppl 1): 203
33. Lanyon LE, Rubin CT, Raisz LE, Marotti G, Lees H (1993) Osteocytes, strain detection, bone modeling and remodeling. Calcif Tissue Int 53 (S1):S102–S107
34. Lotz JC, Hayes WC (1990) The use of quantitative computed tomography to estimate risk of fracture of the hip from falls. J Bone Joint Surg A-72:689–700
35. Louis O, Willnecker J, Soykens S, van den Winkel P, Osteaux M (1995) Cortical thickness assessed by peripheral quantitative computed tomography. Accuracy evaluated on radius specimens. Osteoporosis Int 5:446–449
36. Martin RB (1991) Determinants of the mechanical properties of bone. J Biomech 24(S1):79–88
37. Mosekilde L (1995) Assessing bone quality. Animal models in preclinical osteoporosis research. Bone 17(4S):343S–352S
38. Ott SM, Parfitt AM, Raisz LG, Biewener J (1993) When bone mass fails to predict bone failure. Calcif Tissue Int 53 (S1):S7–S13
39. Recker RR (1989) Low bone mass may not be the only cause of skeletal fragility in osteoporosis. Proc Soc Exp Biol Med 191:272–274

40. Rubin CT, McLeod KJ (1996) Inhibition of osteopenia by biophysical intervention. In: Marcus R (ed) Osteoporosis. Academic, New York, pp 351–371
41. Rüegsegger P (1994) The use of peripheral QCT in the evaluation of bone remodelling. Endocrinologist 4:167–176
42. Schiessl H, Ferretti JL, Tysarczyk-Niemeyer G, Willnecker J (1996) Noninvasive bone strength index as analyzed by peripheral quantitative computed tomography. In: Schönau E (ed) Paediatric osteology: new developments in diagnostics and therapy. Elsevier, Amsterdam, pp 141–146
43. Schneider P, Ferretti JL, Capozza RF, Braun M, Reiners C (1996) Bone densitometric and biomechanical properties of the distal radius by noninvasive assessment. Osteoporosis Int 6 (S1):176
44. Spadaro JA, Werner FW, Brenner RA, Fortino MD, Fay LA, Edwards WT (1994) Cortical and trabecular bone contribute strength to the osteopenic distal radius. J Orthop Relat Res 126:211–218
45. Turner CH, Burr DB (1993) Basic biomechanical measurements of bone. A tutorial. Bone 14:595–608
46. Wainwright SA, Biggs WD, Currey JD, Gossline JM (1976) Mechanical design in organisms. Arnold, London

9 Risk Factors for Osteoporosis Fractures

O. Johnell

Risk Factors for Osteoporosis Fractures

The major risk factor for osteoporosis fractures is low bone mass, which is a subject discussed in other chapters of this volume. Also, risks may be indicated by biochemical markers. In the literature there are several studies on risk factors and osteoporosis. In a Medline search the osteoporosis field has increased substantially from 1980 to 1995, as has the number of papers on bone mineral density (BMD). However, the increase in studies on other risk factors has increased 112 times (Table 9-1). I discuss some of the risk factors identified in the literature and their possible clinical usefulness.

Table 9-1 Studies on risk factors for osteoporosis fractures

Year	Total in Medline	Osteo-porosis	Risk factors	BMD	Osteo-porosis % of total	% Risk factors of total Medline	% BMD of total Medline
1980	263 281	255	1	85	0.097	0.000	0.032
1981	265 390	260	1	122	0.098	0.000	0.046
1982	275 325	337	4	135	0.122	0.001	0.049
1983	287 635	298	3	144	0.104	0.001	0.050
1984	297 292	370	6	150	0.124	0.002	0.050
1985	307 587	424	5	180	0.138	0.002	0.059
1986	320 503	450	3	206	0.140	0.001	0.064
1987	337 144	550	22	261	0.163	0.007	0.077
1988	354 135	563	62	335	0.159	0.018	0.095
1989	369 394	726	87	399	0.197	0.024	0.108
1990	376 618	808	104	460	0.215	0.028	0.123
1991	375 749	830	107	518	0.221	0.028	0.138
1992	377 251	826	132	575	0.219	0.035	0.152
1993	381 932	1035	188	715	0.271	0.049	0.187
1994	386 079	1089	181	804	0.282	0.047	0.208
1995	367 221	1067	157	815	0.291	0.043	0.222
			Difference 1995/1980		3.000	112.562	6.874

Anthropometric Measurements

Height

Hip Fractures

Meyer et al. (1995a) examined the relationship between anthropometric measurements and fatal hip fractures in a 16-year follow-up study of 674 000 Norwegian men and women. They found that for a 10-cm increase in height in men the relative risk for a later hip fracture was 1.08 (1.01–1.16) and in women 1.10 (1.04–1.16). In the SOF study Cummings et al. (1995) found a significant effect of height at age 25; in a multivariate model for every 6-cm increase the relative risk was 1.3 (1.1–1.5). Cumming and Klineberg (1994a) found an effect of height at age 20 years when they compared the highest quintile with the lowest, a relative risk of 2.1 (1.0–4.4), and for current age 1.9 (0.8–4.4). In MEDOS (Johnell et al. 1995) low height (below 149 cm) had a significantly reduced risk of hip fractures. In a case-control study of 30 000 Norwegian women Gunnes et al. (1996) found for an increase in height of 5.6 cm a relative risk of 1.22 (1.13–1.31). For height at age 25 years the relative risk for an increase of 5.4 cm was 1.35 (1.24–1.47) and for loss of height the lowest quartile (>3 cm loss) as compared with the second quartile (2 cm loss) had a relative risk of 0.81 (0.59–1.10), for the third quartile (approximately 1 cm loss) 0.56 (0.39–0.79), and for the fourth quartile (no loss) 0.78 (0.58–1.05). Another indirect measure of height is the femoral neck length, which has been found to be a strong predictor of hip fractures (Faulkner et al. 1993).

Other Fractures

Gunnes et al. (1996) also studied the relationship between height and other fractures and found a significant relationship between present height and fracture of the distal end of the radius (relative risk 1.07) for a 1 SD change (5.6 cm) and for height at age 25 years a significant relationship for spine (relative risk 1.14), and all fragility fractures (relative risk 1.16) for a 1 SD change (5.4 cm). Height loss was significantly related to all fractures, especially clinical spine fractures.

There are some studies indicating the opposite relationship between BMD and height: increasing BMD with increasing height (Bauer et al. 1993).

In most studies there is a significant relationship between hip fractures, other fractures and body height, approximately a relative risk of 1.3 per 5 cm change. This corresponds to a difference in hip BMD of 4%. This risk factor is weak in itself and can be used only for selection of individuals in conjunction with other risk factors. However height loss is stronger; a difference of −2 cm has a relative risk of 1.3.

From an ecological point of view it is interesting to notice that persons are taller in the geographical areas where hip fractures are most common.

Body Weight

Hip Fractures

In several studies increasing weight has been found to be associated with a decreasing risk of hip fracture. In a case-control study Cumming and Klineberg (1994a) compared the highest quintile of body weight with the lowest; the relative risk at age 25 was 2.1, but not significant. At current age the similar difference carried a relative risk of 0.4 (0.2–0.9), indicating that increasing weight is protective. The difference between the cutoff points in weight between the quintiles was 15 kg. In the MEDOS (Johnell et al. 1995) the relative risk ratio between the third, fourth or fifth quintile compared with the lowest was approximately 0.5. The cutoff point for the lowest quintile was 50 kg and for the third quintile 59 kg. In the case-control study by Gunnes et al. (1996) for a 11 kg increase in weight the relative risk was 0.82 (0.75–0.89). There was no significant relationship for weight at age 25 years. In addition, there was also a relationship between weight changes since the age of 25 and hip fractures. There was a similar effect on the highest three quintiles (mean +4.1, +9.3, +19 kg) with a relative risk of approximately 0.5 compared with the lowest ("highest loss" mean –4.8 kg).

Other studies have also found that a change in weight is important for hip fractures. In the SOF study Cummings et al. (1995) found that an increase in weight after age 25 per 20% change the relative risk was 0.8 (0.6–0.9). Langlois et al. (1996) observed that a weight loss of 10% or more beginning at age 50 is associated with an increased risk of hip fractures, relative risk 2.9 (2.4–4.1), and was more pronounced in women in the lowest and middle thirtiles of body mass index. In the thinnest women a loss of more than 5% is associated with an increased risk of hip fractures, relative risk 2.3 (1.0–5.2), whereas a weight gain of 10% or more has a relative risk of 0.7 (0.4–1.0). Meyer et al. (1995b) studied 21 000 women and 21 000 men and found, compared with the mean (+1.3 kg), that women who lose more than 3 kg have a relative risk of 2.6. Surprisingly, those who gain more than 5–6 kg also have a relative risk of 2.3. For men the correponding figures were 2.12 and 1.67.

Other Fractures

Gunnes et al. (1996) found that for a 11 kg increase in body weight spine fractures had a relative risk of 0.92 (0.88–0.96), humerus fractures 0.82 (0.75–0.89), whereas fracture of the distal end of the radius was not significantly related to weight. Weight at age 25 was unrelated to fracture risk. Weight changes were also related to other fractures, but less than hip fractures, in quartiles 2, 3, and 4 the risk was 0.7 compared with the lowest quartile. There was no significant relationship except for in the fourth quartile for fracture of the distal end of the radius (relative risk 0.86).

It seems as if the risk is associated merely with the very low body weight, and that increasing body weight is not protective. Whether hip fracture could be prevented if these subjects increased their weight is unknown since there has been no prospective, randomized trial. If a weight difference of 11 kg between two women had a relative risk of hip fracture of 0.82 this would correspond to a difference in hip bone density of 3%, unadjusted for bone mass the relative risk was 0.6, which corresponds to a bone mass difference of 8%.

Body Mass Index

Hip Fractures
Since decreasing weight is a substantial risk factor as well as increasing height, it is obvious that body mass index (BMI, kg/m^2) is a substantial risk factor. Moreover, the effect of BMI may even be underestimated since height may be reduced by the spine fractures, several hip fracture patients have had spine fractures. Also, with age increasing kyphosis reduces the height. Height loss greater than 3 cm may indicate osteoporosis. Several of the above-mentioned studies also demonstrated relationships between BMI and hip fracture. Meyer et al. (1995a) compared the three highest quartiles of BMI with the lowest; the relative risk was 0.68 (0.63–0.72). Cummings et al. (1995) found for BMI of current age a relative risk of 0.3 when comparing the highest and lowest quintiles. In MEDOS for each unit decrease in BMI the hip fracture risk increased by 7.4% and for –1 SD (–4.7) by 35%. The relationship between BMI and hip fracture was not linear but decreased until a BMI of 26 and then remained unchanged. Gunnes et al. (1996) found for a change in BMI of 3.9 U a relative risk of 0.72 (0.66–0.79) and when comparing the quartiles the greatest difference was between the lowest quartile and the rest. The cutoff point for the lowest was 18.8 and for the second 20.2. In the NHANES study Farmer et al. (1989) comparing those at 25th percentile with those at the 75th percentile in a multivariate analysis found a relative risk of 2.6 (1.8–3.9). In black women (Grisso et al. 1994) there was a relative risk of 5.6 when comparing those below a BMI of 22.6 with those above 31.6 – similar to that among white women. The cutoff point for intervention may be BMI 20, 21, 22, or 23. However, at present there is no study proving that this selects women suitable for therapy or prevention.

Also, the residents of countries with the highest number of osteoporosis fractures have the lowest BMI. However, this difference can explain only part of the differences in hip fracture incidence.

Other Fractures
Gunnes et al. (1996) found that BMI is significantly related to most fragility fractures. For a 3.9-U difference the relative risk of spine fractures was 0.84, radius fractures 0.88 and humerus fracures 0.98.

Previous Fractures

Previous fractures seem to be a clinically important risk factor, and the advantage is that these patients are already in the health care system since almost all are seeing a physician for their fracture (except some vertebral fractures/deformities).

Hip Fractures
Wolinski and Fitzgerald (1994a) followed 368 hip fractures in a longitudinal study and found that 27 of these had a subsequent hip fracture with a rate of 1 per every 338 person-years. In Rochester, Minnesota (Melton et al. 1982), the 5-year recurrency rate was 8%. In men and women with a wrist fracture (Bengnér and Johnell 1985) the risk of having a hip fracture was doubled. In a cohort with fracture of the distal end of the radius followed over 24 years Mallmin et al. (1993) found a relative risk of 1.54 in women and 2.27 in men for having a subsequent hip fracture. Lauritzen et al. (1993) found that women age 60–79 with a wrist fracture had a relative risk of sustaining a hip fracture of 1.9; for those with a fracture of the proximal end of the humerus the relative risk was 2.5.

Other Fractures
Gärdsell et al. (1989) found that in subjects age 40–49 years with a previous wrist fracture the relative risk was 2.67 for having a later fragility fracture, 7.2 for a previous cervical hip fracture. In the age group 50–59 the risk ratio for previous wrist fracture was 2.32 and for previous clinical vertebral fracture 3.68. A previous vertebral fracture had a relative risk of 7.4 for having a later vertebral fracture, thus being an independent risk factor (Ross et al. 1993). Similar findings were observed in the SOF study by Cummings et al. (1995); a woman who had had a fracture after age 50, had a relative risk of 1.5 (1.1–2.0) adjusted for bone mass for a later hip fracture.

A previous fracture seems to be one of the clinically most useful risk factors. Almost all patients with a fracture attend the health care system. Patients with osteoporosis fracture, i.e., a fracture caused by a low energy trauma (fall in the same level), especially a vertebral fracture or a fracture of the upper end of the humerus, should be offered further examination for osteoporosis. For wrist fractures the relationship is less obvious. However, also wrist fracture patients should be offered further examination, especially if they have additional risk factors such as low body weight. Since there seems to be a strong relationship with later hip fractures for previous fractures independently of bone mass, in the future this might serve as a guideline for intervention, for example, three or four vertebral fractures. It has been shown that treatment is effective in these cases (Black et al. 1996).

Falling Tendency

Hip Fractures
The EPIDOS (Dargent-Molina et al. 1996) is a prospective study of 7500 women, aged 75 or more with a 1.9-year follow-up period. Fall-related factors were in a multivariate analysis of predictors of hip fracture. Slower gait speed had a rela-

tive risk of 1.4 for a 1 SD decrease, difficulties in doing a tandem walk relative risk 1.2 for one point difficult score, reduced visual acuity relative risk 2.0 for acuity less than 2/10, and small calf circumference 1.5. In women classified as high-risk patients because of both fall risk factor and low bone mineral mass the hip fracture risk was 29 per 1000 women-years, as compared with 11 per 1000 women-years in those classified as high risks by only one of these factors. In women classified as low risks by both criteria the rate was only 5 per 1000 women-years. The SOF study (Cummings et al. 1995) identified independent risk factors for falls: current use of long-acting benzodiazepines (relative risk 1.6), inability to rise from a chair (relative risk 2.1), lowest quartile for distant depth perception (relative risk 1.5), and poor contrast sensitivity for a 1 SD decrease (relative risk 1.2), also indicating that risk factors for fall are important.

The Framingham study (Felson et al. 1989) demonstrated that with poor or moderately impaired vision the relative risk was 1.96 in women but not in men (0.79). Cataract was the most common cause of fracture-related visual impairment. In a longitudinal study Wolinsky and Fitzgerald (1994b) found that a history of falling during the year prior to baseline had a relative risk of 1.5 for a later hip fracture. Lau and Donnan (1990) examined risk factors for hip fractures in Hong Kong Chinese and identified a history of falls the previous year as a risk factor, with a relative risk of 1.8 (1.3–2.5). Grisso et al. (1991) also identified several risk factors, for example, neurological conditions, barbiturate use, and visual impairment. Cumming and Klineberg (1994b) showed that women with a fall in the past year had an increased risk for a later hip fracture. For one fall during the past year the relative risk in women was 1.54, for more than four falls 4.4. In men the values were higher. In a case-control study Lichtenstein et al. (1994) showed that several risk factors were associated with hip fractures; impaired vision (odds ratio 2.0), confusion presently (odds ratio 2.5), psychotropic drugs, antidepressants, and benzodiazepines – the relative risk was greater than 2; with an earlier fall in hospital the relative risk was 2.7.

Other Fractures

Nguyen et al. (1993) found in a prospective study that body sway was an independent risk factor, even when adjusted for BMD for a fracture. For a 1 SD change the relative risk was 2.23 in men. In women the corresponding figure was 1.90. In a prospective study Gärdsell et al. (1989) found that falls without a fracture had a high risk of having a later fracture with a high relative risk of 4.6 at the age 40–49 and one of 4.0 after the age of 70.

Thus falls and fall tendency are important predictors for hip fractures. The first step should be an intervention. Balance may be improved by training programs. However, there are no prospective studies suggesting that hip fractures will decrease. At present no convincing proof exists that bone mineral measurements are useful in falls. Should pharmacological interventions be undertaken in these high-risk individuals? There are no randomized trials that have selected subjects in this way. The question thus remains unanswered. Lauritzen et al. (1993) published a randomized trial demonstrating that hip protectors were useful in nursing home patients.

Physical Activity

Hip Fractures
Continuing physical activity reduces the risk of hip fractures. In the SOF study (Cummings et al. 1995) women who walked for exercise had a relative risk of 0.7 for a later hip fracture. A similar effect was observed by Cumming and Klineberg (1994a). In the MEDOS (Johnell et al. 1995) women with recreational physical activity had a relative risk of 0.76 and with a nonsedentary job 0.62. In a case-control study Jaglal et al. (1995) found that 20 years in a moderate to heavy activity job had a relative risk of 0.53. Other significant risk factors in that study were past and recent leisure time activity, estrogen use, and previous fractures.

Low physical activity is a risk factor best compensated by increased physical activity. There are, however, few prospective randomized studies to show that this intervention reduces the number of hip fractures. Individuals with a low physical activity should be examined with regard to osteoporosis.

Other risk factors include smoking, high alcohol intake, previous diseases, and treatment with drugs such as glucocorticoids etc. are imortant in selectory patients for evaluation of osteoporosis.

Risk Factors in Men

Seeman et al. (1983) studied risk factors for vertebral fractures in men and found an increased risk in those who smoked cigarettes (relative risk 2.3), drank alcoholic a beverages (relative risk 2.4), or had a medical condition known to affect calcium or bone metabolism (relative risk 5.5). Obesity was protective. Nguyen et al. (1996) studied risk factors for osteoporotics fractures in elderly men. Several risk factors were identified in a univariate model; femoral neck, BMD, quadriceps weakness, body sway, falls in the preceding 12 months, a history of fractures in the previous 5 years, low body weight, and short current height. Use of thiazide diuretics, higher physical activity, and moderate alcohol intake were protective against fractures. In a multivariate model the odds ratio was 1.45 per 0.12 g/cm^2 BMD, for quadriceps strength 1.43 and for body sway 1.25 per 5.15 cm^2. The MEDOS also showed that low body weight and low physical activity were related to hip fractures.

Poor et al. (1995) studied risk factors for hip fracture in men. Risk factors were secondary osteoporosis and falling tendency. Hemenway et al. (1994) examined risk factors for hip fractures in United States men, aged 40–75 – 50 000 were followed prospectively. They found that BMI, smoking, and alcohol consumption were not associated with hip fractures, but that age and height were.

It seems that risk factors for men are fairly similar to those for women, may be more pronounced and thus until further data are available the same indications for evaluation and intervention against osteoporosis based on risk factors should be applied as for women.

Combination of Risk Factors for Prediction of Hip Fractures

Several studies have indicated that risk factors should be combined with BMD to decide who should have an intervention, thus identifying the high-risk patient for later hip fractures. In the SOF study Cummings et al. (1995) found that the risk was not only dependent on BMD but also on a number of other risk factors. For example, women in the highest third of BMD and with no more than two risk factors had a rate of hip fractures of 1.1 per 1000 women-years, those in the middle third 1.1, and those in the lowest third 2.6, whereas for those with more than five risk factors the corresponding numbers were 9.4, 14.7, and 27.3. This suggests the concept that it is important to create an index with risk factors and BMD to detect the high-risk group.

Similar relationships were observed in the EPIDOS where addition of fall-related factors made the prediction much better than using BMD alone. Most of the quoted studies are on elderly women; few are from menopause. It is still hard to draw safe conclusions about perimenopausal risk factors since long-term follow-up studies are lacking. From a practical point of view, a risk factor of 1.3 corresponds to a difference in BMD between two women of 4%. The bone density deviation is 6% for a risk ratio of 1.5, 11% for 2, for 14% 2.5, and 17% for 3. In some studies the risk factors have been adjusted for BMD, for example, if the risk factor is 1.3, a woman has the same risk of having a later fracture if she also has a 4% higher BMD than a woman without that risk factor.

References

Bauer DC, Browner WS, Cauley JA, Orwoll ES, Scott JC, Black DM, Tao JL, Cummings SR, the Study of Osteoporotic Fractures Research Group (1993) Factors associated with appendicular bone mass in older women. Ann Intern Med 118:657–665

Bengnér U, Johnell O (1985) Increasing incidence of forearm fractures. Acta Orthop Scand 56:158–160

Black DM, Cummings SR, Karpf DB, Cauley JA, Thompson DE, Nevitt MC, Bauer DC, Genant HK, Haskell WL, Marcus R, Ott SM, Torner JC, Quandt SA, Reiss TF, Ensrud KE, the Fracture Intervention Trial Research Group (1996) Randomised trial of effect of alendronate on risk of fracture in women with existing vertebral fractures. Lancet 348:1535–1541

Cumming RG, Klineberg RJ (1994a) Case-control study of risk factors for hip fractures in the elderly. Am J Epidemiol 139:493–503

Cumming RG, Klineberg RJ (1994b) Fall frequency and characteristics and the risk of hip fractures. J Am Geriatr Soc 42:774–778

Cummings SR, Nevitt MC, Browner WS, Stone K, Fox KM, Ensrud KE, Cauley J,

Black D, Vogt TM, the Study of Osteoporotic Fractures Research Group (1995) Risk factors for hip fracture in white women. N Engl J Med 332:767–773

Dargent-Molina P, Favier F, Grandjean H, Baudoin C, Schott AM, Hausherr E, Meunier PJ, Bréart G, the EPIDOS Group (1996) Fall-related factors and risk of hip fractures: the EPIDOS prospective study. Lancet 348:145–149

Farmer ME, Harris T, Madans JH, Wallace RB, Cornoni-Huntley J, White LR (1989) Anthropometric indicators and hip fracture. J Am Geriatr Soc 37:9–16

Faulkner KG, Cummings SR, Black D, Palermo L, Glüer CC, Genant HK (1993) Simple measurement of femoral geometry predicts hip fracture: the study of osteoporotic fractures. J Bone Miner Res 8:1211–1217

Felson DT, Anderson JJ, Hannan MT, Milton RC, Wilson PWF, Kiel DP (1989) Impaired vision and hip fracture. J Am Geriatr Soc 37:495–500

Gärdsell P, Johnell O, Nilsson BE, Nilsson JÅ (1989) The predictive value of fracture, disease, and falling tendency for fragility fractures in women. Calcif Tissue Int 45:327–330

Grisso JA, Kelsey JL, Strom BL, Chiu GY, Maislin G, O'Brian LA, Hoffman S, Kaplan F, the Northeast Hip Fracture Study Group (1991) Risk factors for falls as a cause of hip fracture in women. N Engl J Med 324:1326–1331

Grisso JA, Kelsey JL, Strom BL, O'Brien LA, Maislin G, LaPann K, Samelson L, Hoffman S, the Northeast Hip Fracture Study Group (1994) Risk factors for hip fracture in black women. N Engl J Med 330:1555–1559

Gunnes M, Lehmann EH, Mellström D, Johnell O (1996) The relationship between anthropometric measurements and fractures in women. Bone 19:407–413

Hemenway D, Azrael DR, Rimm EB, Feskanich D, Willett WC (1994) Risk factors for hip fracture in US men aged 40 through 75 years. Am J Publ Health 84:1843–1845

Jaglal SB, Kreiger N, Darlington GA (1995) Lifetime occupational physical activity and risk of hip fracture in women. Ann Epidemiol 5:321–324

Johnell O, Gullberg B, Kanis JA, Allander E, Elffors L, Dequeker J, Dilsen G, Gennari C, Lopes Vaz A, Lyritis G, Mazzuoli G, Miravet L, Passeri M, Perez Cano R, Rapado A, Ribot C (1995) Risk factors for hip fracture in European women: the MEDOS study. J Bone Miner Res 10:1802–1815

Langlois JA, Harris T, Looker AC, Madans J (1996) Weight change between age 50 years and old age is associated with risk of hip fracture in white women aged 67 years and older. Arch Intern Med 156:989–994

Lau EMC, Donnan SPB (1990) Falls and hip fracture in Hong Kong Chinese. Publ Health 104:117–121

Lauritzen JB, Schwarz P, McNair P, Lund B, Transbøl I (1993) Radial and humeral fractures as predictors of subsequent hip, radial or humeral fractures in women, and their seasonal variation. Osteoporosis Int 3:133–137

Lichtenstein MJ, Griffin MR, Cornell JE, Malcolm E, Ray WA (1994) Risk factors for hip fractures occurring in the hospital. Am J Epidemiol 140:830–838

Mallmin H, Ljunghall S, Persson I, Naessén T, Krusemo U-B, Bergström R (1993) Fracture of the distal forearm as a forecaster of subsequent hip fracture: a pop-

ulation-based cohort study with 24 years of follow-up. Calcif Tissue Int
52:269–272

Melton LJ III, Ilstrup DM, Beckenbaugh R, Riggs BL (1982) Hip fracture recurrence. A population-based study. Clin Orthop 167:131–138

Meyer KE, Tverdal A, Falch JA (1995a) Body height, body mass index, and fatal hip fractures: 16 years' follow-up of 674,000 Norwegian women and men. Epidemiology 6:299–305

Meyer KE, Tverdal A, Falch JA (1995b) Changes in body weight and incidence of hip fracture among middle aged Norwegians. BMJ 311:91–92

Nguyen T, Sambrook P, Kelly P, Jones G, Lord S, Freund J, Eisman J (1993) Prediction of osteoporotic fractures by postural instability and bone density. BMJ 307:1111–1115

Nguyen TV, Eisman JA, Kelly PJ, Sambrook PN (1996) Risk factors for osteoporotic fractures in elderly men. Am J Epidemiol 144:255–263

Poor G, Atkinson EJ, O'Fallon WM, Melton LJ III (1995) Predictors of hip fractures in elderly men. J Bone Miner Res 10:1900–1907

Ross PD, Genant HK, Davis JW, Milder PD, Wasnich RD (1993) Predicting vertebral fracture incidence from prevalent fractures and bone density among non-black, osteoporotic women. Osteoporosis Int 3:120–126

Seeman E, Melton LJ III, O'Fallon WM, Riggs BL (1983) Risk factors for spinal osteoporosis in men. Am J Med 75:977–983

Wolinski FD, Fitzgerald JF (1994a) Subsequent hip fracture among older adults. Am J Publ Health 84:1316–1318

Wolinski FD, Fitzgerald JF (1994b) The risk of hip fracture among noninstitutionalized older adults. J Gerontol 49:S165–S175

10 Bone Biopsy in Metabolic Bone Disease

E. Bonucci

Introduction

The morphological study of bone tissue is a necessary complement to clinical investigations that aim to diagnose metabolic bone disease. A number of reviews have stressed the important diagnostic role of histological, histochemical, ultrastructural, and biophysical studies that can be carried out on bone specimens (Faugere and Malluche 1983; Girasole and Passeri 1994; Jowsey 1977; Weinstein 1992). In the past these studies were limited to skeletal segments taken at the autopsy or after surgery. The discovery that specimens suitable for microscopic investigations can be obtained by safe and relatively painless needle biopsies of the iliac crest (Bordier et al. 1964; Ellis et al. 1964) has provided a new tool for the diagnosis of metabolic bone disease, and for the monitoring of its evolution during and after therapeutic treatments.

The Bone Biopsy

A needle bone biopsy is currently carried out in the iliac crest about 2 cm behind the anterior superior spine. The ideal needle should be a trephine with an inner diameter of about 8 mm because below this value the bioptic cylinder would be too thin for quantitative histomorphometric measurement. However, if the biopsy is intended for a qualitative evaluation alone, trephines with diameters below 8 mm can be used. Both transversal (transiliac) and vertical biopsies are suitable; the former are preferred because they are less uncomfortable for the patient, and they allow the inner and outer cortical bone to be studied, as well as spongy bone.

The processing of a bone biopsy routinely includes fixation, embedding and sectioning. The bone cylinder is fixed soon after removal from the trephine. It is left in the fixative (usually 4% formaldehyde or 2% glutaraldehyde, buffered at pH 7.2) for about 2 h. It is then treated according to the various methods of microscopic study. If intended for paraffin embedding, the bone specimen is decalcified by treatment with an acid solution (1% formic acid or other acid solutions) or with EDTA until it becomes soft and easily deformable (usually 12 h for a 6-mm-thick cylinder). This procedure, which is suitable for simple morphological studies, should be avoided for histochemical and histomorphometric analysis because decalcification induces the extraction of several organic compounds and often causes shrinkage and distortion in cells and matrix. An undecalcified specimen is usually embedded in resins because their hardness and elasticity, similar to those of bone, allow suitable sections to be obtained even from fully calcified specimens. Various types of resins can be used: epoxy (Araldite, Epon), polyester (westopal W), methacrylic (methacrylates), water-miscible (glycol methacrylate, Lowicryls, Durcupan, LR white), or a mixture of these (see Hayat 1989). Sections of variable thickness can be obtained from undecalcified bone: thin sections (1–2 µm thick) for light microscopy, ultrathin sections (about 75 nm) for electron microscopy, and thick sections (about 5 µm thick) for examination in UV light.

On the basis of the aim of the biopsy, several staining methods and treatments, single or in combination, can be used. Those most often used are: hematoxylin-eosin and Goldner's method for routine examination or histomorphometry; azure II–methylene blue for undecalcified thin sections; von Kossa method for calcium phosphate; PAS, Alcian blue, colloidal iron for glycoproteins and proteoglycans; Burstone's method for alkaline and acid phosphatases, preferably after glycol methacrylate embedding; peroxydase, avidin-biotin, alkaline phosphatase, immunogold for immunohistochemical demonstration of special antigens. Some of these and other methods, based on the use of heavy metals, can be applied to transmission electron microscopy (Hayat 1989). Several types of biophysical examination and microanalysis can also be carried out (Arsenault 1990; Lewinson and Silbermann 1990). Tetracycline fluorescence (see below) attains greatest visibility in unstained, thick sections.

Without considering their use in the diagnosis of hematological disorders, bone biopsies can have a variety of aims: histological diagnosis of bone diseases concerning single patients or groups of patients; histochemical, immunohistochemical, and ultrastructural evaluations of bone composition and organization; biophysical examination (including microradiography) of the mineral substance; quantitative histomorphometric evaluation (static and dynamic) of bone turnover; the longitudinal or transversal study of groups of patients; and the monitoring of therapeutic treatments.

The Microscopic Structure of Bone

Even if some bone biopsies are transiliac, so that cortical bone is present at both their ends, most morphological studies examine trabecular bone, because this is metabolically more active and more susceptible to pathological changes than compact bone. For this reason this review refers mainly to the spongy bone of adults.

Because of the complexity of the bone biology (reviewed by Marks and Popoff 1988), several parameters must be considered when an iliac crest biopsy is examined: the bone cells (osteoblasts, osteoclasts, osteocytes, lining cells), the structure, organization, composition and degree of calcification of the bone matrix, the morphology of bone trabeculae, and, above all, their microarchitecture (referred to as "connectivity").

The osteocyte is the true cell of the bone tissue, but very little is known about its function, activity, or pathology (see Bonucci 1990a; Marotti 1990). For this reason it is often neglected in the study of metabolic bone disease, although it has a leading role in maintaining the integrity of the tissue (Aarden et al. 1994), and in transmitting mechanical stimulations (Klein-Nulend et al. 1995; Lanyon 1993).

So-called lining cells are very frequent in the adult skeleton. These are very flat, endothelial-like elements which line the endosteal surface of the trabeculae (Fig. 10-1a) and divide the bone marrow compartment from that of bone matrix (Miller et al. 1989; Parfitt 1989). They have no osteogenic activity and are not engaged in bone resorption, so that the bone tissue is defined as "inert" or "resting" when lined by these cells alone. More than 70% of the whole endosteal surface is covered by lining cells in the adult skeleton; as a result the corresponding bone is considered to be resting.

The osteoblast is the cell which synthesizes the bone matrix. Its morphology (Fig. 10-1b) and ultrastructure are well known (reviewed by Scherft and Groot 1990), and it is not commented on further here. Histochemistry can be valuable in recognizing it. Osteoblasts are in fact characterized by a strong alkaline phosphatase activity. The enzyme is present chiefly along the outer surface of the cell membrane, from which it is transported into the uncalcified matrix of the

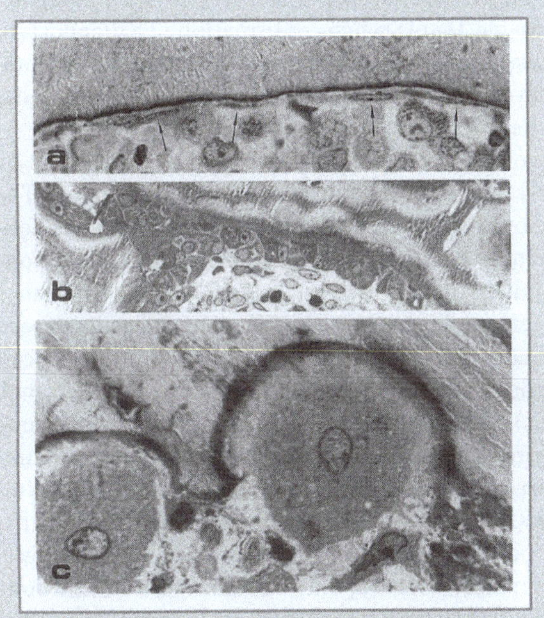

Fig. 10-1 a Part of a trabecula: the bone matrix (above) is lined by a thin osteoid border (black) and by lining cells, only the nuclei of which are recognizable (arrows). A few cells of the bone marrow are visible (below). **b** Area of ossification with osteoblasts along the border of the osseous trabecula. **c** Osteoclasts within Howship's lacunae. ×1100

osteoid tissue (Bonucci et al. 1992). The reaction product is visible along the osteoblast peripheral membrane, among collagen fibrils of the uncalcified matrix, and around matrix vesicles (Bernard 1978; Bonucci et al. 1992).

The osteoclast is the cell which resorbs the calcified bone matrix (Fig. 10-1c; reviewed by Marks and Popoff 1990). Histochemically a strong tartrate-resistant acid phosphatase (TRAP) activity is demonstrable in its cytoplasm (Akisaka et al. 1989; Andersson and Ek-Rylander 1995; Fukushima et al. 1991; Van de Wijngaert and Burger 1986). A carbonic anhydrase activity is also present, mainly at the resorbing side of the cell. This enzyme is probably involved in the proton transport needed for the acidification of the resorbing area and for the dissolution of the inorganic substance (Guillemin et al. 1995; Hall et al. 1991; Hunter et al. 1991). Several reviews are available on the mechanism of osteoclastic bone resorption (Doty 1991; Holtrop 1991; Marks and Popoff 1990; Teti 1993). The comparative study of alkaline phosphatase- and TRAP-positive cells present on endosteal surfaces can be useful for the diagnosis of metabolic bone disease (Bianco and Bonucci 1991).

The ultrastructure of bone cells has often been studied (for review see McKee and Nanci 1993). Although the electron microscopic investigation of the bone biopsy has provided many important morphological, histochemical, and immunohistochemical findings, this technique is usually not adopted when a bone biopsy is examined for diagnostic purposes. However, in at least one case ultrastructural study is almost indispensable, that is, when confirmation of a diagnosis of Paget's disease of bone is required. In fact, the characteristic viral inclusions present in the nuclei and cytoplasm of pagetic osteoclasts are recognizable only under the electron microscope (see below).

The bone matrix mainly consists of type I collagen fibrils, which may be arranged haphazardly (woven bone) or ordered in lamellae (lamellar bone). The presence of woven bone in a bone biopsy usually points to a high turnover condition, such as that found in hyperparathyroidism. Differing amounts of noncollagenous proteins are present in different types of bone, where they appear as interfibrillary patches (Bonucci and Silvestrini 1996). These proteins have been partially identified as osteopontin, bone sialoprotein, osteonectin, and osteocalcin (Bianco et al. 1993; Camarda et al. 1987; McKee and Nanci 1993; McKee et al. 1992, 1993; Riminucci et al. 1995). Moreover, within areas of calcification the bone matrix contains lipids that correspond to acidic phospholipids and/or calcium-phospholipid-phosphate complexes (Boyan et al. 1989; Wuthier 1973). In the fully calcified bone matrix, lipids are so closely related to the mineral substance that they remain in the "anorganic bone" (Shapiro 1970a) even when all organic material is removed. For the same reason, they can only be removed from the bone matrix after this has been decalcified (Boyan et al. 1989; Shapiro 1970b). Also alkaline phosphatase is present in the calcified bone matrix, where it can be demonstrated by immunohistochemistry (de Bernard et al. 1986) and not by histochemistry. This means that, although it is present in the bone matrix, it is inactive, probably because it is trapped and made inactive by the inorganic substance during calcification (Bonucci et al. 1992). Another noncollagenous protein present in the bone matrix is the bone morphogenetic protein (Cook and Rueger 1996; Reddi and Cunningham 1993; Riley et al. 1996; Urist 1994; Wozney et al. 1990). Other growth factors and cytokines seem to be present, too (Mundi and Bonewald 1992; Seyedin and Rosen 1992).

The degree of calcification of bone matrix, which may be altered in several pathological conditions, could be evaluated by microradiography. However, this technique can only be carried out in thick sections (ground sections) and is usually not adopted in bone biopsy studies. The calcification process of the bone matrix can be indirectly evaluated on the basis of the tetracycline uptake. It is known that the deposition of tetracyclines only occurs in areas of bone mineralization (Teitelbaum and Nichols 1977), where they remain till they are removed by osteoclast resorption. Because tetracyclines are fluorescent under ultraviolet light, their presence in bone is easy to demonstrate. A time-spaced, double administration of tetracyclines induces two linear fluorescent markers in the ossification areas. Obviously the two markers define the area of bone that has been deposited and calcified during the time that has elapsed between the first and second tetracycline administration (Frost 1969). Thus measurement of the interval between the markers indicates the amount of bone synthesized by osteoblasts in that period. The finding can be used to calculate the bone formation rate (for histomorphometric nomenclature, see Parfitt et al. 1987).

The bone trabeculae of the spongy bone are thin and wide laminae, which are interconnected to form a frame in which they are arranged according to the the orientation and architecture which best resist the mechanical load. The complex of trabeculae forming this frame is known as "connectivity" (Goldstein et al. 1993; Hahn et al. 1992; Mosekilde 1993). The measurement of connectivity is a rather difficult and time-consuming task. Several direct and indirect methods have been proposed (Croucher et al. 1996; Delling et al. 1995; Engelke et al. 1996; Mosekilde 1988).

Bone Remodeling

In the adult skeleton osteoblasts and osteoclasts are only found in areas where bone remodeling is active. They are collected in the so-called basic multicellular units (BMUs). These are transitory complexes of bone cells which initially induce the removal of microscopic portions of bone matrix and then regenerate the removed matrix to such an extent as to leave the same amount of bone at the end of the process as there was at its beginning (reviewed by Bonucci 1990b). This apparently useless process has two extremely important functions (reviewed by Baron et al. 1983; Huffer 1988; Parfitt 1988); one is metabolic (contribution to the regulation of calcemia) and the other is mechanical (modification of the bone structure induced by variations of mechanical loads).

As far as calcemia is concerned, resorption of the bone matrix leads to the release of hydroxyapatite calcium phosphate and to the solubilization of calcium ions which can be introduced into the circulating calcium pool. Although the amount of ions produced by each BMU is small, that produced by the whole BMU system is large enough to lead to a significant increase in the calcium concentration in the blood. On the other hand, the BMU-induced bone resorption does not reduce bone strength, because the width and depth of each BMU are very small, and because however frequent BMUs may be, they are scattered over a wide endosteal surface (practically, the endosteal surface of the whole skeleton), most of which remains in a resting phase. The bone remodeling induced by the decrease in calcemia is promoted and regulated by a complex of systemic [parathyroid hormone (PTH), $1,25(OH)_2D_3$, estrogens, calcitonin, etc.] and local factors (cytokines, growth factors), whose "synarchic" (Baron et al. 1983) interaction leads to the formation of BMUs.

The bone remodeling induced by mechanical forces (or by their absence) occurs through a complex, poorly known process of cellular interactions, which Frost has tried to rationalize in a concept called "mechanostat" (Frost 1987, 1996). This appears to assign a leading role to osteocytes and their processes (Aarden et al. 1994; Klein-Nulend et al. 1995; Lanyon 1993; Marotti et al. 1994).

The short life of BMUs begins with the recruitment and activation of osteoclasts (activation phase). Osteoclasts can reach the bone matrix only after this has been partially uncovered by the shrinkage of bone lining cells, probably induced by PTH (Chambers and Fuller 1985; Jones and Boyde 1976). At the same time the lining cells produce collagenase. This digests the thin osteoid border which by covering the bone surface would stop osteoclasts adhering to the calcified matrix (Heath et al. 1984). In the following phase (resorption phase), osteoclasts resorb a microscopic portion of bone and produce a resorption lacuna (or Howship's lacuna; Fig. 10-1c). Osteoclasts then disappear, leaving space for the so-called "intermediate" or postosteoclastic cells, which seem to have both osteoclastic and osteoblastic properties (Baron et al. 1983; Tran Van et al. 1982). Their presence characterizes the so-called reversal phase, after which the intermediate cells disappear, leaving space for osteoblasts and the final osteogenic phase. During this phase osteoblasts synthesize as much new bone matrix as it is required for the reconstitution of the original shape and volume of bone. After this final stage osteoblasts disappear, and the new bone surface is again covered by lining cells. The quantitative equilibrium which occurs in the BMU between bone resorption and bone formation is called "osteoclast-osteoblast coupling."

Bone Biopsy in Metabolic Bone Diseases

The morphological study of a bone biopsy is a subsidiary method of investigation in diagnosing metabolic bone disease. For obvious reasons noninvasive methods are preferred in achieving this aim. Even so, a bone biopsy is often needed to identify not only the type of disease but also its evolution, the severity of bone involvement, and any association with other pathologies or changes induced by therapies.

Bone biopsy appears especially useful in osteoporosis, although it is rarely used in this disease probably because it is hard to convince patients, who are generally healthy subjects, to undergo an invasive, not completely painless technique. The histomorphometric measurement of trabecular bone volume, which provides the degree of osteopenia and the evaluation of connectivity, can be very useful in assessing precise criteria of therapy and prognosis in osteoporosis.

Trabecular bone volume is the histomorphometric variable which is most frequently altered in osteoporosis. This variable, which has a value of about 25% during the third decade, declines progressively with age until the very low values which are attained in the osteopenia of senescence (Ballanti and Bonucci 1988; Ballanti et al.1990; Ellis and Peart 1972; Hoikka and Arnala 1981; Malluche et al.1982; Melsen et al.1978; Merz and Schenk 1970; Vedi et al.1982). A condition of manifest osteoporosis is reached when the value of the trabecular bone volume falls below 16%, and vertebral fractures become almost inevitable below the threshold value of 10% (Meunier 1995; Meunier et al.1976).

Although it is important, trabecular bone volume alone is not enough to allow predictions of the probability of fracture in osteoporosis. Recent investigations have shown that the resistance of spongy bone to mechanical loads depends not only on the bone volume of the trabeculae but also, and primarily, on their architecture or connectivity. A number of papers have recently been published on this important topic (Compston et al. 1987, 1989; Hahn et al. 1992; Kinney et al. 1995; Kleerekoper et al. 1985; Parisien et al. 1995). All of them conclude that the reduction in bone volume occurs together with perforation and discontinuity of trabecular laminae (Fig. 10-2a), so that those which remain are overloaded, suffer fatigue damage, and fracture easily (Kleerekoper et al. 1985; Parfitt 1987; Recker 1993). The loss of connectivity is also of significance for therapy because it is possible to increase trabecular thickness, but it is highly unlikely that the lost trabeculae can ever be restored (Weinstein and Hutson 1987).

The study of bone biopsies has provided important information about the pathogenesis of osteoporosis. Obviously the fall in bone volume which characterizes this disease is due to an uncoupling between osteoclast and osteoblast activity. Some of the therapies used in osteoporosis (calcitonin, bisphosphonates, ipriflavone, calcium supplementation) are based on the assumption that the disease is due mainly to an increase in osteoclast activity. This possibility is supported by several clinical and metabolic data, especially in the menopause period (Blumsohn and Eastell 1995). On the other hand, it is poorly supported by morphological data: in fact, the endosteal surfaces found in the biopsies of patients with established involutional osteoporosis do not show morphological signs of increased bone resorption, and most of them appear as smooth bone surfaces covered by lining cells (see above). This picture, and the fact that the histomorphometric parameters of bone formation and bone resorption are similar to those of normal adult subjects, i.e., are characterized by very low values (Ballanti and Bonucci 1988), suggest that the fall in bone volume is not due to an increase in osteoclastic resorption.

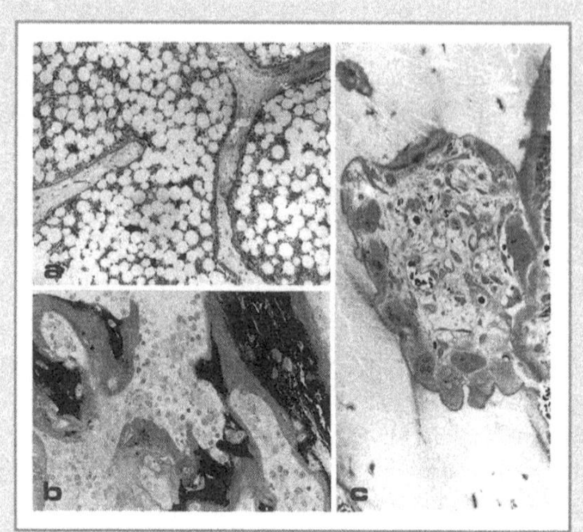

Fig. 10-2 a The osteoporotic bone is characterized by thin and frequently interrupted trabeculae. ×45   **b** Osteomalacic bone: the trabeculae mainly consist of osteoid tissue (gray); the calcified matrix (black) appears as small irregular islands within the osteoid. ×280   **c** Area of lacunar resorption such as those which are present in severe hyperparathyroidism: note the numerous osteoclasts along the resorption front. ×1000

Static histomorphometry is probably incapable of solving this problem, because the factor(s) which induce(s) the uncoupling between osteoblast and osteoclast activities may be of such a limited degree as only to produce an effect on bone over a number of years. Because of its negligible extent this effect may be undetectable by static histomorphometry. However, if dynamic histomorphometric methods are adopted, two types of osteoporosis can be distinguished, a "high turnover" or "active" osteoporosis, and a "low turnover" or "inactive" osteoporosis (discussed by Meunier 1995), the former characterized by increased bone resorption. As reported above, there is a period of unknown length during which the menopause is associated with increased bone turnover (Blumsohn and Eastell 1995). Moreover, studies of bone tissue carried out soon after ovariectomy show a net increase in bone resorption (Ballanti et al. 1993; Beaudreuil et al. 1995; Bonucci et al. 1995; Faugere et al. 1990; Miller et al. 1991; Nakamuta et al. 1993; Wronski and Yen 1991). Thus these data and the occurrence of high turnover cases of osteoporosis suggest that estrogen withdrawal due to spontaneous or surgical menopause induces transitory episodes of higher osteoclastic bone resorption (high turnover osteoporosis) followed by long-lasting osteoblastic insufficiency and lower levels of bone formation (inactive osteoporosis; Fiore et al. 1987; Rosso et al. 1995).

Bone biopsy is very valuable in the study of osteomalacia (Fig. 10-2b). This bone disorder is characterized by the presence of variable amounts of uncalcified osteoid matrix. Because this is not recognizable either by X-ray examination of the skeleton or by bone densitometry, and because the clinical parameters are not predictive of the osteomalacic condition (Hruska et al. 1978), a bone biopsy is often the only technique which allows a well-grounded diagnosis.

The need for bone biopsy is even greater in cases of osteoporomalacia. This condition, which represents an additional impairment for the osteoporotic skeleton and needs a specific therapy, is more frequent than is usually supposed (Ballanti and Bonucci 1988; Sorensen et al. 1977; Vignon et al. 1970) and is hard to identify with noninvasive methods (Sorensen et al. 1977). The presence of calcification defects as complicating factors in osteoporosis explains the good results that are sometimes obtained by therapy with vitamin D or its metabolites.

Bone biopsy is also recommended in primary or secondary hyperparathyroidism to establish the degree of bone involvement, presence of hyperosteoidosis or osteomalacia, development of bone marrow fibrosis, and rate of osteoclasia and osteogenesis (reviewed by Habener and Potts 1990). Further diagnostic advantages can be produced by histochemical (Bianco and Bonucci 1991) and ultrastructural (Bonucci et al. 1978) studies on the bone specimen. A frequent use of bone biopsy has been made in cases of renal osteodystrophy (reviewed by Slatopolsky and Coburn 1990). This secondary hyperparathyroidism can show various morphological patterns, on the basis of which it can be divided into three types (Delling 1977):

- Type I: osteoclastic bone resorption and bone marrow fibrosis are the dominant aspects of the disease (Fig. 10-2c)
- Type II: characterized by the presence of severe calcification defects, with development of osteomalacia
- Type III: a combination of the changes present in type I and II (Bonucci et al. 1990)

Moreover, the histochemical staining of the bone biopsy with aluminon has demonstrated the accumulation of aluminum in bone in dialysis patients, especially if treated with aluminum hydroxyde as a phosphate chelator (Andress et al. 1986; Boyce et al. 1982; Malluche et al. 1991; Parkinson et al. 1981; Rodriguez et al. 1989; Sedman et al. 1987). The morphological study of bone biopsies has also helped to define the role of aluminum in the development of osteomalacia (Ballanti et al. 1989; Ellis et al. 1979), its interference with parathyroid activity (Pun et al. 1990; Slatopolsky 1987), and the therapeutic effect of deferoxamine (Coburn and Norris 1986; Jablonski et al. 1996; Molitoris et al. 1987). The biopsy studies carried out over a number of years have also shown that the special form of renal osteodystrophy called "aplastic" or "adynamic bone disease" (Malluche and Faugere 1990; Parisien et al. 1988) is independent of aluminum intoxication (Ballanti et al. 1996; Cohen-Solal et al. 1992; Fournier et al. 1991). The therapeutic effects of diets and drugs on renal osteodystrophy have often been assessed by histological investigations, with or without histomorphometry (Malluche and Monier-Faugere 1991).

A diagnosis of Paget's disease of bone should always be confirmed by the morphological investigation of a bone biopsy and, above all, by electron microscopy.

This shows the most characteristic finding of the disease – the presence of paracrystalline inclusions in the nuclei and cytoplasm of pagetic osteoclasts (Gherardi et al. 1980; Rebel et al. 1975, 1980; Singer and Mills 1983). These inclusions behave as viruses (Abe et al. 1995) and may correspond to the viral nucleocapsids of paramixovirus, probably the measles virus (Reddy et al. 1995; Singer and Mills 1983). A distemper virus has also been implicated (Gordon et al. 1991). Therefore Paget's disease of bone could have a viral etiology, although similar paracrystalline inclusions have been found in giant cells in cases of primary oxalosis (Bianco et al. 1992), osteopetrosis (Mills et al. 1988), giant cell tumor of bone (Abelanet et al. 1986; Schajowicz et al. 1985), and pycnodysostosis (Beneton et al. 1987).

Conclusions

Bone biopsy is strongly indicated in all metabolic bone diseases and, although invasive and slightly painful, it should be recommended to the patient because its advantages outweigh the discomfort. A bone biopsy is mandatory when osteomalacia, osteoporomalacia, Paget's disease of bone, or hematological disorders are suspected. The histological study of the biopsy can be completed by histochemical, ultrastructural, and electron microscopic research. Moreover, static and dynamic histomorphometry permit a quantification of the changes in bone. These auxiliary techniques are only rarely required for a pathological diagnosis, which must be based on the histological changes in the bone tissue. They may be helpful in obtaining further morphologic elements in doubtful cases and in supporting the pathologist's decision in difficult ones. Moreover, histomorphometry is particularly valuable in comparing groups of patients, following the course of diseases, and assessing the modifications induced by therapy. Close collaboration between the clinician and the pathologist may be necessary to determine the best way to process and examine a bone biopsy.

Acknowledgements. The personal investigations mentioned in this paper have been supported by grants of the Italian National Research Council (CNR), the Ministry of University and Scientific and Technological Research (MURST), and La Sapienza University of Rome.

References

Aarden EM, Burger EH, Nijweide PJ (1994) Function of osteocytes in bone. J Cell Biochem 55:287–299

Abe S, Ohno T, Park P, Higaki S, Unno K, Takeishi A (1995) Viral behaviour of paracrystalline inclusions in osteoclasts of Paget's disease of bone. Ultrastruct Pathol 19:455–461

Abelanet R, Daudet-Monsac M, Laoussadi S, Forest M, Vacher-Lavenu M-C (1986) Frequency and diagnostic value of the virus-like filamentous intranuclear inclusions in giant cell tumor of bone, not associated with Paget's disease. Virchows Arch [A] Pathol Anat 410:65–68

Akisaka T, Subita GP, Kawaguchi H, Shinegawa Y (1989) Different tartrate sensitivity and pH optimum for two isoenzymes of acid phosphatase in osteoclasts. An electron-microscopic enzyme-cytochemical study. Cell Tissue Res 255:69–76

Andersson G, Ek-Rylander B (1995) The tartrate-resistant purple acid phosphatase of bone osteoclasts – a protein phosphatase with multivalent substrate specificity and regulation. Acta Orthop Scand 66 [Suppl 266]:189–194

Andress DL, Maloney NA, Endres DB, Sherrard DJ (1986) Aluminum-associated bone disease in chronic renal failure: high prevalence in a long-term dialysis population. J Bone Miner Res 1:391–398

Arsenault AL (1990) The ultrastructure of calcified tissues: methods and technical problems. In: Bonucci E, Motta PM (eds) Ultrastructure of skeletal tissues. Kluwer Academic, Boston, pp 1–18

Ballanti P, Bonucci E (1988) Histomorphometric aspects of bone in involutive osteoporosis. Giorn It Metab Min Elettrol 2:203–216

Ballanti P, Bonucci E, Della Rocca C, Milani S, Lo Cascio V, Imbimbo B (1990) Bone histomorphometric reference values in 88 normal Italian subjects. Bone Miner 11:187–197

Ballanti P, Martelli A, Mereto E, Bonucci E (1993) Ovariectomized rats as experimental model of postmenopausal osteoporosis: critical considerations. It J Miner Electrol Metab 7:243–248

Ballanti P, Martin Wedard B, Bonucci E (1996) Frequency of adynamic bone disease and aluminium storage in Italian uraemic patients – retrospective analysis of 1429 iliac crest biopsies. Nephrol Dial Transplant 11:663–667

Ballanti P, Mocetti P, Della Rocca C, Bonucci E, Costantini S, Giordano R, Ioppolo A, Mantovani A (1989) Experimental aluminum intoxication and parathormone: effects on the mineralization process. Miner Electrol Metab 15:233–240

Baron R, Vignery A, Horowitz M (1983) Lymphocytes, macrophages and the regulation of bone remodeling. In: Peck WA (Ed) Bone and mineral research, annual 2. Elsevier Science, Amsterdam, pp 175–243

Beaudreuil J, Mbalaviele G, Cohen-Solal M, Morieux C, De Vernejoul C, Orcel P (1995) Short-term local injections of transforming growth factor-β_1 decrease ovariectomy-stimulated osteoclastic resorption in vivo in rats. J Bone Miner Res 10:971–977

Beneton MNC, Harris S, Kanis JA (1987) Paramixovirus-like inclusions in two cases of pycnodysostosis. Bone 8:211–217

Bernard GW (1978) Ultrastructural localization of alkaline phosphatase in initial intramembranous osteogenesis. Clin Orthop 135:218–225

Bianco P, Bonucci E (1991) Endosteal surfaces in hyperparathyroidism: an enzyme cytochemical study on low-temperature-processed, glycol-methacrylate-embedded bone biopsies. Virchows Arch [A] Pathol Anat 419:425–431

Bianco P, Silvestrini G, Ballanti P, Bonucci E (1992) Paramixovirus-like inclusions identical to those of Paget's disease of bone detected in giant cells of primary oxalosis. Virchows Arch [A] Pathol Anat 421:427–433

Bianco P, Riminucci M, Silvestrini G, Bonucci E, Termine JD, Fisher LW, Robey PG (1993) Localization of bone sialoprotein (BSP) to Golgi and post-Golgi secretory structures in osteoblasts and to discrete sites in early bone matrix. J Histochem Cytochem 41:193–203

Blumsohn A, Eastell R (1995) Age-related factors. In: Riggs BL, Melton LJ (eds) Osteoporosis: etiology, diagnosis, and management. Raven, New York, pp 161–182

Bonucci E (1990a) The ultrastructure of the osteocyte. In: Bonucci E, Motta PM (eds) Ultrastructure of skeletal tissues. Kluwer Academic, Boston, pp 223–237

Bonucci E (1990b) The basic multicellular unit of bone. It J Miner Electrol Metab 4:115–125

Bonucci E, Silvestrini G (1996) Ultrastructure of the organic matrix of embryonic avian bone after en bloc reaction with various electron-dense 'stains.' Acta Anat 156:22–33

Bonucci E, Lo Cascio V, Adami S, Cominacini L, Galvanini G, Scuro A (1978) The ultrastructure of bone cells and bone matrix in human primary hyperparathyroidism. Virchows Arch [A] Pathol Anat Histol 379:11–23

Bonucci E, Ballanti P, Mocetti P (1990) Histological types of renal osteodystrophy and their meaning. Contrib Nephrol 77:187–193

Bonucci E, Silvestrini G, Bianco P (1992) Extracellular alkaline phosphatase activity in mineralizing matrices of cartilage and bone: ultrastructural localization using a cerium-based method. Histochemistry 97:323–327

Bonucci E, Ballanti P, Ramires PA, Richardson JL, Benedetti LM (1995) Prevention of ovariectomy osteopenia in rats after vaginal administration of Hyaff 11 microspheres containing salmon calcitonin. Calcif Tissue Int 56:274–279

Bordier P, Matrajt H, Miravet L, Hioco D (1964) Mesure histologique de la masse et de la résorption des travées osseuses. Pathol Biol 12:1238–1243

Boyan BD, Schwartz Z, Swain LD, Khare A (1989) Role of lipids in calcification of cartilage. Anat Rec 224:211–219

Boyce BF, Fell GS, Elder HY, Junor BJ, Elliot HL, Beastall G, Fogelman I, Boyle IT (1982) Hypercalcaemic osteomalacia due to aluminium toxicity. Lancet 2:1009–1013

Camarda AJ, Butler WT, Finkelman RD, Nanci A (1987) Immunocytochemical localization of γ-carboxyglutamic acid-containing proteins (osteocalcin) in rat bone and dentine. Calcif Tissue Int 40:349–355

Chambers TJ, Fuller K (1985) Bone cells predispose bone surfaces to resorption by exposure of mineral to osteoclast contact. J Cell Sci 76:155–165

Coburn JW, Norris KC (1986) Diagnosis of aluminum-related bone disease and treatment of aluminum toxicity with deferoxamine. Semin Nephrol 6 [Suppl 1]:12–21

Cohen-Solal ME, Sebert JL, Boudailliez B, Westeel PF, Morinière PH, Marie A, Garabedian M, Fournier A (1992) Non-aluminic adynamic bone disease in non-dialyzed uremic patients: a new type of osteopathy due to overtreatment? Bone 13:1–5

Compston JE, Mellish RWE, Garrahan NJ (1987) Age-related changes in iliac crest trabecular microanatomic bone structure in man. Bone 8:289–292

Compston JE, Mellish RWE, Croucher P, Newcombe R, Garrahan NJ (1989) Structural mechanisms of trabecular bone loss in man. Bone Miner 6:339–350

Cook SD, Rueger DC (1996) Osteogenic protein 1. Biology and applications. Clin Orthop 324:29–38

Croucher PI, Garrahan NJ, Compston JE (1996) Assessment of cancellous bone structure: comparison of strut analysis, trabecular bone pattern factor, and marrow space star volume. J Bone Miner Res 11:955–961

De Bernard B, Bianco P, Bonucci E, Costantini M, Lunazzi GC, Martinuzzi P, Modricky C, Moro L, Panfili E, Pollesello P, Stagni N, Vittur F (1986) Biochemical and immunohistochemical evidence that in cartilage an alkaline phosphatase is a Ca^{2+}-binding glycoprotein. J Cell Biol 103:1615–1623

Delling G, Hahn M, Bonse U, Busch F, Günnewig O, Beckmann F, Uebbing H, Graeff W (1995) Neue Möglichkeiten der Strukturanalyse von Knochenbiopsien bei Anwendung der Microcomputertomographie (µCT). Pathologe 16:342–347

Delling GR (1977) Bone cells as well as bone remodelling surfaces in renal bone disorders and their changes after therapy – a quantitative analysis. In: Norman AW, Schaefer K, Coburn JW, DeLuca HF, Fraser D, Grigoleit HG, von Herrath D (eds) Vitamin D: biochemical, chemical and clinical aspects related to calcium metabolism. De Gruyter, Berlin, pp 359–368

Doty SB (1991) Histochemistry and enzymology of osteoclasts. In: Hall BK (ed) Bone, vol 2. CRC, Boca Raton, pp 61–85

Ellis HA, Peart KM (1972) Quantitative observations on mineralized and non-mineralized bone in the iliac crest. J Clin Pathol 25:277–286

Ellis LD, Jensen WN, Westerman MP (1964) Needle biopsy of bone and marrow. An experience with 1,455 biopsies. Arch Intern Med 114:213–221

Ellis HA, McCarthy JH, Herrington J (1979) Bone aluminium in haemodialysed patients and in rats injected with aluminium chloride: relationship to impaired bone mineralisation. J Clin Pathol 32:832–844

Engelke K, Song SM, Glüer CC, Genant HK (1996) A digital model of trabecular bone. J Bone Miner Res 11:480–489

Faugere M-C, Friedler RM, Fanti P, Malluche HH (1990) Bone changes occurring early after cessation of ovarian function in beagle dogs: a histomorphometric study employing sequential biopsies. J Bone Miner Res 5:263–272

Faugere MC, Malluche HH (1983) Comparison of different bone-biopsy techniques for qualitative and quantitative diagnosis of metabolic bone diseases. J Bone Joint Surg Am 65:1314–1320

Fiore CE, Falcidia E, Foti R, Caschetto S, Grimaldi DR (1987) Postoophorectomy bone loss is associated with reduced bone Gla-protein serum levels: a possible effect of osteoblastic insufficiency. Calcif Tissue Int 41:303–306

Fournier A, Morinière P, Cohen Solal ME, Boudaillliez B, Achard JM, Marie A, Sebert JL (1991) Adynamic bone disease in uremia: may it be idiopathic? Is it an actual disease? Nephron 58:1–12

Frost HM (1969) Tetracycline-based histological analysis of bone remodeling. Calcif Tissue Res 3:211–237

Frost HM (1987) Bone "mass" and the "mechanostat": a proposal. Anat Rec219:1–9

Frost HM (1996) Perspectives: a proposed general model of the "mechanostat" (suggestions from a new skeletal-biologic paradigm). Anat Rec 244:139–147

Fukushima O, Bekker PJ, Gay CV (1991) Ultrastructural localization of tartrate-resistant acid phosphatase (purple acid phosphatase) activity in chicken cartilage and bone. Am J Anat 191:228–236

Gherardi G, Lo Cascio V, Bonucci E (1980) Fine structure of nuclei and cytoplasm of osteoclasts in Paget's disease of bone. Histopathology 4:63–70

Girasole G, Passeri G (1994) Local factors, bone remodeling and skeletal disorders. It J Miner Electr Metab 8:153–165

Goldstein SA, Goulet R, McCubbrey D (1993) Measurement and significance of three-dimensional architecture to the mechanical integrity of trabecular bone. Calcif Tissue Int 53 [Suppl 1]:S127–133

Gordon MT, Anderson DC, Sharpe PT (1991) Canine distemper virus localised in bone cells of patients with Paget's disease. Bone 12:195–201

Guillemin G, Hunter SJ, Gay CV (1995) Resorption of natural calcium carbonate by avian osteoclasts in vitro. Cells Mater 5:157–165

Habener JF, Potts JT Jr (1990) Primary hyperparathyroidism. In: Avioli LV, Krane SM (eds) Metabolic bone disease and clinically related disorders, 2nd edn. Saunders, Philadelphia, pp 475–545

Hahn M, Vogel M, Pompesius-Kempa M, Delling G (1992) Trabecular bone pattern factor – a new parameter for simple quantification of bone microarchitecture. Bone 13:327–330

Hall TJ, Higgins W, Tardif C, Chambers TJ (1991) A comparison of the effects of inhibitors of carbonic anhydrase on osteoclastic bone resorption and purified carbonic anhydrase isozyme II. Calcif Tissue Int 49:328–332

Hayat MA (1989) Principles and techniques of electron microscopy. Biological applications, 3rd edn. McMillan, Houndmills

Heath JK, Atkinson SJ, Meikle MC, Reynolds JJ (1984) Mouse osteoblasts synthesize collagenase in response to bone resorbing agents. Biochim Biophys Acta 802:151–154

Hoikka V, Arnala I (1981) Histomorphometric normal values of the iliac crest cancellous bone in a Finnish autopsy series. Ann Clin Res 13:383–386

Holtrop ME (1991) Light and electronmicroscopic structure of osteoclasts. In: Hall BK (ed) Bone, vol 2. CRC, Boca Raton, pp 1–29

Hruska KA, Teitelbaum SL, Kopelman R, Richardson CA, Miller P, Debman J, Martin K, Slatopolsky E (1978) The predictability of the histological features of uremic bone disease by non-invasive techniques. Metab Bone Dis Relat Res 1:39–44

Huffer WE (1988) Morphology and biochemistry of bone remodeling: possible control by vitamin D, parathyroid hormone, and other substances. Lab Invest 59:418–442

Hunter SJ, Rosen CJ, Gay V (1991) In vitro resorptive avtivity of isolated chick osteoclasts: effects of carbonic anhydrase inhibition. J Bone Miner Res 6:61–66

Jablonski G, Klem KH, Danielsen CC, Mosekilde L, Gordeladze JO (1996) Aluminium-induced bone disease in uremic rats: effect of deferoxamine. Biosci Rep 16:49–63

Jones SJ, Boyde A (1976) Experimental study of changes in osteoblastic shape induced by calcitonin and parathyroid extract in an organ culture system. Cell Tissue Res 169:449–465

Jowsey J (1977) The bone biopsy. In: Avioli LV (ed) Topics in bone and mineral disorders. Plenum Medical, New York

Kinney JH, Lane NE, Haupt DL (1995) In vivo, three-dimensional microscopy of trabecular bone. J Bone Miner Res 10:264–270

Kleerekoper M, Villanueva AR, Stanciu J, Sudhaker Rao J, Parfitt AM (1985) The role of three-dimensional trabecular microstructure in the pathogenesis of vertebral compression fractures. Calcif Tissue Int 37:594–597

Klein-Nulend J, Van Der Plas A, Semeins CM, Ajubi NE, Frangos JA, Nijweide PJ, Burger EH (1995) Sensitivity of osteocytes to biomechanical stress in vitro. FASEB J 9:441–445

Lanyon LE (1993) Osteocytes, strain detection, bone modeling and remodeling Calcif Tissue Int 53 [Suppl 1]:S102–S107

Lewinson D, Silbermann M (1990) Ultrastructural localization of calcium in normal and pathologic cartilage. In: Bonucci E, Motta PM (eds) Ultrastructure of skeletal tissues. Kluwer Academic, Boston, pp 129–152

Malluche H, Faugere M-C (1990) Renal bone disease 1990: an unmet challenge for the nephrologist. Kidney Int 38:193–211

Malluche HH, Sherman D, Meyer W, Massry SG (1982) Quantitative bone histology in 84 normal American subjects. Calcif Tissue Int 34:499–455

Malluche HH, Monier-Faugere M-C (1991) Uremic bone disease: current knowledge, controversial issues, and new horizons. Miner Electrol Metab 17:281–296

Marks SC Jr, Popoff SN (1988) Bone cell biology: the regulation of development, structure, and function in the skeleton. Am J Anat 183:1–44

Marks SC Jr, Popoff SN (1990) Ultrastructural biology and pathology of the osteoclast. In: Bonucci E, Motta PM (eds) Ultrastructure of skeletal tissues. Kluwer Academic, Boston, pp 239–252

Marotti G (1990) The original contributions of the scanning electron microscope to the knowledge of bone structure. In: Bonucci E, Motta PM (eds) Ultrastructure of skeletal tissues. Kluwer Academic, Boston, pp 19–39

Marotti G, Muglia MA, Palumbo C, Zaffe D (1994) The microscopic determinants of bone mechanical properties. It J Miner Electr Metab 8:167–175

McKee MD, Nanci A (1993) Ultrastructural, cytochemical and immunocytochemical studies of bone and its interface. Cells Mater 3:219–243

McKee MD, Glimcher MJ, Nanci A (1992) High-resolution immunolocalization of osteopontin and osteocalcin in bone and cartilage during endochondral ossification in the chicken tibia. Anat Rec 234:479–492

McKee MD, Farach-Carson MC, Butler WT, Hauschka PV, Nanci A (1993) Ultrastructural immunolocalization of noncollagenous (osteopontin and osteocalcin) and plasma (albumin and α_2HS-glycoprotein) proteins in rat bone. J Bone Miner Res 8:485–496

Melsen F, Melsen B, Mosekilde L, Bergmann S (1978) Histomorphometric analysis of normal bone from the iliac crest. Acta Pathol Microbiol Scand [A] 86:70–81

Merz WA, Schenk RK (1970) A quantitative histological study on bone formation in human cancellous bone. Acta Anat 75:54–66

Meunier PJ (1995) Bone histomorphometry. In: Riggs BL, Melton LJ (eds) Osteoporosis: etiology, diagnosis, and management. Raven, New York, pp 299–318

Meunier P, Courpron P, Giroux JM, Edouard C, Bernard J, Vignon G (1976) Bone histomorphometry as applied to research on osteoporosis and to diagnosis of "hyperosteoidosis states." Calcif Tissue Res 21 [Suppl]:354–360

Miller SC, de Saint-Georges L, Bowman BM, Jee WSS (1989) Bone lining cells: structure and function. Scann Microsc 3:953–961

Miller SC, Bowman BM, Miller MA, Bagi CM (1991) Calcium absorption and osseous organ-, tissue-, and envelope-specific changes following ovariectomy in rats. Bone 12:439–446

Mills BG, Yabe H, Singer FR (1988) Osteoclasts in human osteopetrosis contain viral-nucleocapsid-like nuclear inclusions. J Bone Miner Res 3:101–106

Molitoris BA, Alfrey PS, Miller NL, Hasbargen JA, Kaehney WD, Alfrey AC, Smith BJ (1987) Efficacy of intramuscular and intraperitoneal deferoxamine for aluminum chelation. Kidney Int 31:986–991

Mosekilde L (1988) Age-related changes in vertebral trabecular bone architecture – assessed by a new method. Bone 9:247–250

Mosekilde L (1993) Vertebral structure and strength in vivo and in vitro. Calcif Tissue Int 53 [Suppl 1]:S121–126

Mundy GR, Bonewald LF (1992) Transforming growth factor beta. In: Gowen M (ed) Cytokines and bone metabolism. CRC, Boca Raton, pp 93–107

Nakamuta H, Sasaki M, Ichikawa M, Koida M (1993) An acute and focal osteopenia model using ovariectomized rats: a rapid detection of the protective effect of salmon calcitonin. Biol Pharmacol Bull 16:325–327

Parfitt AM (1987) Trabecular bone architecture in the pathogenesis and prevention of fracture. Am J Med 82 [Suppl 1B]:68–72

Parfitt AM (1988) Bone remodeling: relationship to the amount and structure of bone, and the pathogenesis and prevention of fractures. In: Riggs BL, Melton LJ (eds) Osteoporosis: etiology, diagnosis, and management. Raven, New York, pp 45–93

Parfitt AM (1989) Plasma calcium control at quiescent bone surfaces: a new approach to the homeostatic function of bone lining cells. Bone 10:87–88

Parfitt AM, Drezner MK, Glorieux FH, Kanis JA, Malluche H, Meunier PJ, Ott SM, Recker RR (1987) Bone histomorphometry: standardization of nomenclature, symbols, and units. J Bone Miner Res 2:595–610

Parisien M, Charhon SA, Arlot M, Mainetti E, Chavassieux P, Chapuy MC, Meunier PJ (1988) Evidence for a toxic effect of aluminum on osteoblasts: a histomorphometric study in hemodialysis patients with aplastic bone disease. J Bone Miner Res 3:259–267

Parisien M, Cosman F, Mellish RWE, Schnitzer M, Nieves J, Silverberg SJ, Shane E, Kimmel D, Recker RR, Bilezikian JP, Lindsay R, Dempster DW (1995) Bone structure in postmenopausal hyperparathyroid, osteoporotic, and normal women. J Bone Miner Res 10:1393–1399

Parkinson IS, Ward MK, Kerr DNS (1981) Dialysis encephalopathy, bone disease and anemia: the aluminium intoxication syndrome during regular haemodialysis. J Clin Pathol 34:1285–1294

Pun KK, Ho PWW, Lau P (1990) Effects of aluminum on the parathyroid hormone receptors of bone and kidney. Kidney Int 37:72–78

Rebel A, Bregeon C, Basle M, Malkani K (1975) Les inclusions des ostéoclastes dans la maladie osseuse de Paget. Rev Rhumat 42:637–641

Rebel A, Basle M, Pouplard A, Malkani K, Filmon R, Lepatezour A (1980) Bone tissue in Paget's disease of bone. Ultrastructure and immunocytology. Arthritis Rheum 23:1104–1114

Recker RR (1993) Architecture and vertebral fracture. Calcif Tissue Int 53 [Suppl 1]:S319–142

Reddi AH, Cunningham NS (1993) Initiation and promotion of bone differentiation by bone morphogenetic protein. J Bone Miner Res 8 [Suppl 2]:S499–502

Reddy SV, Singer FR, Roodman GD (1995) Bone marrow mononuclear cells from patients with Paget's disease contain measles virus nucleocapsid messenger ribonucleic acid that has mutations in a specific region of the sequence. J Clin Endocrinol Metab 80:2108–2111

Riley EH, Lane JM, Urist MR, Lyons KM, Lieberman JR (1996) Bone morphogenetic protein–2. Biology and applications. Clin Orthop 324:39–46

Riminucci M, Silvestrini G, Bonucci E, Fisher LW, Gehron Robey P, Bianco P (1995) The anatomy of bone sialoprotein immunoreactive sites in bone as revealed by combined ultrastructural histochemistry and immunohistochemistry. Calcif Tissue Int 57:277–284

Rodriguez M, Felsenfeld AJ, Llach F (1989) The evolution of osteomalacia in the rat with acute aluminum toxicity. J Bone Miner Res 4:687–696

Rosso R, Minisola S, Scarda A, Pacitti MT, Carnevale V, Romagnoli E, Mazzuoli GF (1995) Temporal relationship between bone loss and increased bone turnover: a longitudinal study following natural menopause. J Endocrinol Invest 18:723–728

Schajowicz F, Ubios AM, Santini Araujo E, Cabrini RL (1985) Virus-like intranuclear inclusions in giant cell tumor of bone. Clin Orthop 201:247–250

Scherft JP, Groot CG (1990) The electron microscopic structure of the osteoblast In: Bonucci E, Motta PM (eds) Ultrastructure of skeletal tissues. Kluwer Academic, Boston, pp 209–222

Sedman AB, Alfrey AC, Miller NL, Goodman WG (1987) Tissue and cellular basis for impaired bone formation in aluminum-related osteomalacia in the pig. J Clin Invest 79:86–92

Seyedin SM, Rosen DM (1992) Unique bone-derived cytokines. In: Gowen M (ed) Cytokines and bone metabolism. CRC, Boca Raton, pp 109–113

Shapiro IM (1970a) The association of phospholipids with anorganic bone. Calcif Tissue Res 5:13–20

Shapiro IM (1970b) The phospholipids of mineralized tissues I. Mammalian compact bone. Calcif Tissue Res 5:21–29

Singer FR, Mills BG (1983) Evidence for a viral etiology of Paget's disease of bone. Clin Orthop 178:245–251

Slatopolsky E (1987) The interaction of parathyroid hormone and aluminum in renal osteodystrophy. Kidney Int 31:842–854

Slatopolsky E, Coburn JW (1990) Renal osteodystrophy. In: Avioli LV, Krane SM (eds) Metabolic bone disease and clinically related disorders, 2nd edn. Saunders, Philadelphia, pp 452–474

Sorensen OH, Andersen RB, Christensen MS, Friis T, Hjorth L, Jorgensen FS, Lund B, Melsen F, Mosekilde L (1977) Treatment of senile osteoporosis with 1α-hydroxyvitamin D_3. Clin Endocrinol 7 [Suppl]:169S–175S

Teitelbaum SL, Nichols SH (1977) Tetracycline-based morphometric analysis of trabecular bone kinetics. In: Meunier PJ (ed) Bone histomorphometry. Armour Montagu, Paris, pp 311–319

Teti A (1993) Biology of osteoclasts and molecular mechanisms of bone resorption. It J Miner Electrol Metab 7:123–133

Tran Van P, Vignery A, Baron R (1982) An electron microscopic study of the bone remodeling sequence in the rat. Cell Tissue Res 225:283–292

Urist MR (1994) The search for and the discovery of bone morphogenetic protein (BMP). In: Urist MR, O'Conner BT, Burwell RG (eds) Bone grafts, derivatives and substitutes. Butterworth Heinemann, London, pp 315–362

Van de Wijngaert FP, Burger EH (1986) Demonstration of tartrate-resistant acid phosphatase in un-decalcified, glycolmethacrylate-embedded mouse bone: a possible marker for (pre)osteoclast identification. J Histochem Cytochem 34:1317–1323

Vedi S, Compston JE, Webb A, Tighe JR (1982) Histomorphometric analysis of bone biopsies from the iliac crest of normal British subjects. Metab Bone Dis Relat Res 4:231–236

Vignon G, Meunier P, Pansu D, Bernard J (1970) Enquêt clinique et anatomique sur l'étiopathogénie de l'ostéoporose sénile. Rev Rhumat 37:615–627

Weinstein RS (1992) Clinical use of bone biopsy. In: Coe FL, Murray JF (eds) Disorders of bone and mineral metabolism. Raven, New York, pp 455–474

Weinstein RS, Hutson MS (1987) Decreased trabecular width and increased trabecular spacing contribute to bone loss with aging. Bone 8:137–142

Wozney JM, Rosen V, Byrne M, Celeste AJ, Moutsatsos I, Wang EA (1990) Growth factors influencing bone development. J Cell Sci 13 [Suppl]:149–156

Wronski TJ, Yen C-F (1991) The ovariectomized rat as an animal model for post-menopausal bone loss. Cells Mater [Suppl] 1:69–74
Wuthier RE (1973) The role of phospholipids in biological calcification: distribution of phospholipase activity in calcifying epiphyseal cartilage. Clin Orthop 90:191–200

11 Radiology of Osteoporosis

M. Jergas

Introduction

The term osteoporosis is widely used clinically to mean generalized loss of bone, or osteopenia, accompanied by relatively atraumatic fractures of the spine, wrist, hips, or ribs. Because of uncertainties of specific radiological interpretation, the term osteopenia ("poverty of bone") has been used as a generic designation for radiographic signs of decreased bone density. Radiographic findings suggestive of osteopenia and osteoporosis are frequently encountered in daily medical practice and can result from a wide spectrum of diseases ranging from highly prevalent causes such as postmenopausal and involutional osteoporosis to very rare endocrinological and hereditary or acquired disorders. The value of conventional radiographs for detecting and quantifying osteopenia and osteoporosis has raised scientific interest for many years.

With the advent of highly accurate and precise quantitative techniques such as single- and dual-photon absorptiometry (SPA, DPA), single and dual X-ray absorptiometry (SXA, DXA) and quantitative computed tomography (QCT) the status of conventional radiography for the diagnosis and follow-up of osteoporosis has changed [60, 89]. Nevertheless, conventional radiography is widely available, and it remains useful for the detection of specific alterations in certain instances (e.g., subperiosteal resorption in hyperparathyroidism). Alone and in conjunction with modern imaging techniques such as bone scinitigraphy and magnetic resonance imaging, conventional radiography is still widely used for the detection of complications of osteopenia, such as fractures, for the differential diagnosis of osteopenia, and for follow-up examinations in specific clinical settings (progression of soft tissue calcifications or signs of secondary hyperparathyroidism and osteomalacia in renal osteodystrophy).

Principal Radiographic Findings in Osteopenia and Osteoporosis

A knowledge of both the physical nature of X-ray absorption by biological tissues and the histopathological changes leading to osteopenia and osteoporosis is required to understand the resulting radiographic findings. The absorption of X-rays by a tissue depends on the quality of the X-ray beam, the character of the atoms composing the tissue, the physical density of the tissue, and the thickness of the penetrated structure. The amount of X-ray absorption defines the density of the X-ray shadow that a tissue casts on the film. Because the absorption raises with the third power of the atomic number [196], and because calcium has a high atomic number, it is primarily the amount of calcium that affects the X-ray absorption of bone. The amount of calcium per unit of mineralized bone volume in osteoporosis remains constant at about 35% [3, 4, 21, 109], and therefore a decrease in the mineralized bone volume results in decreased total bone calcium and decreased absorption of the X-ray beam. On the X-ray film this phenomenon is referred to as increased radiolucency.

At the same time as bone mass is lost, changes in the bone structure occur, and these can be observed radiographically (Fig. 11-1). Bone is composed of two compartments: cortical bone and trabecular bone. The structural changes seen in cortical bone represent bone resorption at different sites (e.g., inner and outer surfaces of the cortex, or within the cortex in the Haversian and Volkmann channels). These three sites (endosteal, intracortical, and periosteal) react differently to distinct metabolic stimuli, and careful investigation of the cortices may be of value in the differential diagnosis of metabolic disease affecting the skeleton.

Cortical bone remodeling typically occurs in the endosteal "envelope," and thus the interpretation of subtle changes in this layer may be difficult at times.

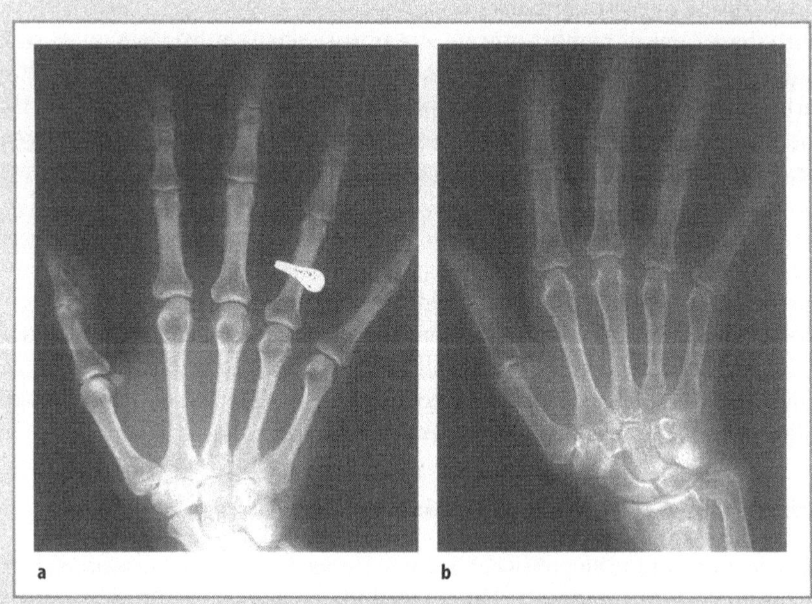

Fig. 11-1 Radiographs of the hand of a healthy woman **a** and a woman with osteoporosis. There is an overall increased radiolucency as well as cortical thinning and widening of the marrow canal in the osteoporotic hand, primarily resulting from endosteal bone resorption.

With increasing age there is a widening of the marrow canal due to an imbalance of endosteal bone formation and resorption that leads to a "trabeculization" of the inner surface of the cortex. Endosteal scalloping due to resorption of the inner bone surface can be seen in high bone turnover states such as reflex sympathetic dystrophy.

Intracortical bone resorption may cause longitudinal striation or tunneling, predominantly in the subendosteal zone. These changes are seen in various high turnover metabolic diseases affecting the bone such as hyperparathyroidism, osteomalacia, renal osteodystrohy, and acute osteoporosis from disuse or the reflex sympathetic dystrophy syndrome but also postmenopausal osteoporosis. Intracortical tunneling is a hallmark of rapid bone turnover. It is usually not apparent in disease states with relatively low bone turnover such as senile osteoporosis. Accelerated endosteal and intracortical resorption with intracortical tunneling and indistinct border of the inner cortical surface is best depicted with high-resolution radiographic techniques. Intracortical tunneling must be distinguished from nutritional foraminae, which are isolated and present with an oblique orientation. Intracortical resorption is also a sign of bone viability and is not seen in necrotic or allograft bone.

Subperiosteal bone resorption is associated with an irregular definition of the outer bone surface. This finding is pronounced in diseases with a high bone turnover, principally primary and secondary hyperparathyroidism (see also below). However, rarely it is also present in other diseases. Cortical thinning with expansion of the medullary cavity occurs as endosteal bone resorption exceeds periosteal bone apposition in most adults. In the late stages of osteoporosis the cortices appear paper thin with the endosteal surface usually being smooth.

The trabecular bone has greater surface and responds more rapidly to metabolic changes than does cortical bone. It is metabolically eight times more active than cortical bone [48]. Trabecular bone changes are most prominent in the axial skeleton and in the ends of the long and tubular bones of the appendicular skeleton (juxta-articular), for example, proximal femur, distal radius. These are sites with a relatively great proportion of trabecular bone. Loss of trabecular bone (in cases of low rates of loss) occurs in a predictable pattern. Non-weight-bearing trabeculae are resorbed first. This leads to a relative prominence of the weight-bearing trabeculae. The remaining trabeculae may even become thicker, which can result in a distinct radiographic trabecular pattern. For example, early changes of osteopenia in the lumbar spine typically include a rarefication of the horizontal trabeculae accompanied by a relative accentuation of the vertical trabeculae (Fig. 11-2). This may lead to an appearance of vertical striation of the bone. With decreasing density of the trabecular bone the cortical rim of the vertebrae are more accentuated, and the vertebrae may have a "picture-frame" appearance. In addition to the changes in the trabecular bone, thinning of the cortical bone occurs. Changes of the bone structure at distinct skeletal sites are assessed for the differential diagnosis of various skeletal conditions. For the evaluation of very

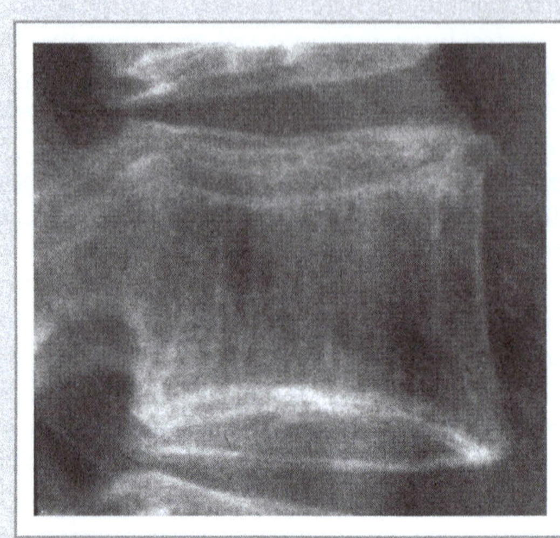

Fig. 11-2 Radiograph of a single vertebra displaying characteristic features of osteoporosis including an overall increased radiolucency as well as 'verticalization' of the trabeculae.

subtle changes, such as different forms of bone resorption, high-resolution radiographic techniques with optical or geometric magification may be may be required [58, 59, 113].

The anatomic distribution of the osteopenia or osteoporosis depends on the underlying cause. Osteopenia can be generalized, affecting the whole skeleton, or regional, affecting only a part of the skeleton, usually in the appendicular skeleton. Typical examples of generalized osteopenias are involutional and postmenopausal osteoporosis and osteoporosis caused by endocrine disorders such as hyperparathyroidism, hyperthyroidism, osteomalacia, and hypogonadism. Regional forms of osteoporosis result from factors affecting only parts of the appendicular skeleton such as disuse, reflex sympathetic syndrome, and transient osteoporosis of large joints. The distribution of osteopenia may vary considerably between different diseases and be suggestive of a specific diagnosis. Focal osteopenia reflects primarily the underlying cause such as inflammation, fracture, or tumor and is not the subject of this chapter.

Thus it seems that a number of characteristic features of conventional radiography make the diagnosis of osteopenia or osteoporosis possible. However, the detection of osteopenia by conventional radiography is inaccurate since it is influenced by many technical factors. These include [82]:

- Radiation source
  - Exposure time
  - Film-focus distance
  - Anode characteristics

- Voltage
- Beam filtration
- Object
  - Thickness of bone
  - Bone mineral content
  - Soft tissue composition
  - Scattering
- Film and screen
  - Film granularity
  - Emulsion of film
  - Film speed
  - Screen properties
- Film processing
  - Developing time
  - Temperature of developer
  - Type of developer
  - Type of fixer
  - Type of processing (automated vs. manual)

It has been estimated that as much as 20%–40% of bone mass must be lost before a decrease in bone density can be seen in lateral radiographs of the thoracic and lumbar spine [108, 191]. Finally, the diagnosis of osteopenia from conventional radiographs is also dependent on the experiences of the reader and his/her subjective interpretation [45]. Therefore the sensitivity of conventional radiography to detect early bone loss based on the increased radiolucency is generally considered to be low [39, 45, 195].

In summary, a radiograph may reflect the amount of bone mass, histology and gross morphology of the skeletal part examined. The principal findings of osteopenia are increased radiolucency, changes in bone microstructure, for example, rarefication of trabeculae, thinning of the cortices, eventually resulting in changes of the gross bone morphology, i. e., changes in the shape of the bone and fractures. Further characteristics of osteopenic and osteoporotic disease conditions and specific techniques for their radiological assessment are described in greater detail below.

Diseases Characterized by Generalized Osteopenia

Involutional Osteoporosis

Involutional osteoporosis is the most common generalized skeletal disease. Cases can be classified as a type I or postmenopausal osteoporosis and a type II or senile osteoporosis [3, 151]. Gallagher added a third type, secondary osteoporosis (Tables 11-1, 11-2) [49]. Although the importance of estrogen deficiency for

Table 11-1 Classification of osteoporosis: types (after [3, 49, 151, adapted from [50])

	Type I, postmeno-pausal	Type II, senile	Type III, secondary
Age	55–70	75–90	Any age
Years past menopause	5–15	25–40	–
Sex ratio (Female:male)	20:1	2:1	1:1

Table 11-2 Classification of osteoporosis: fracture sites (after [3, 49, 151, adapted from [50])

	Spine	Hip, spine, pelvis, humerus	Spine, hip, peripheral skeleton
Bone loss			
Trabecular	+++	++	+++
Cortical	+	++	+++
Contributing factor			
Menopause	+++	++	++
Age	+	+++	++

postmenopausal osteoporosis has been established, the distinction between the first two types of osteoporosis is not generally accepted. Distinctions between postmenopausal and senile osteoporosis may sometimes be arbitrary, and the assignment of fracture sites to the different types of osteoporosis is uncertain.

The radiographic appearance of the skeleton in involutional osteoporosis may include all of the above characteristics for generalized osteoporosis. The high prevalence of involutional osteoporosis with its typical radiographic manifestations has lead to numerous attempts to diagnose and quantify osteoporosis based on its radiographic characteristics.

Osteopenia and Osteoporosis of the Axial Skeleton

The radiographic manifestations of osteopenia of the axial skeleton include increased radiolucency of the vertebrae, which may assume the radiographic density of the intervertebral disk space, vertical striation of the vertebrae, framed appearance of the vertebrae (picture framing), and increased biconcavity of the vertebral endplates. A classification of these characteristics is provided by the Saville index [164]:

o Normal bone density
1 Minimal loss of density; endplates begin to stand out giving a stencilled effect
2 Vertical striation is more obvious; endplates are thinner

3 More severe loss of bone density than grade 2; endplates becoming less visible

4 Ghostlike vertebral bodies; density is no greater than soft tissue; no trabecular pattern is visible

This index, however, has never gained wide acceptance because it is prone to great subjectivity and experience of the reader. Doyle and colleagues found that none of the above signs of osteopenia reliably reflect the bone mineral status of an individual and therefore cannot be used for follow-up of osteopenic patients [38]. Thus bone density measurements using specific densitometric methods have widely replaced the subjective analysis of bone density from conventional radiographs. Densitometric results may suggest osteopenia even if the bone loss is not detectable on a spine radiograph [91]. Nevertheless, the above radiographic signs of osteoporosis have been found to be significantly related to measured bone density, and normal bone densitometry measurements may sometimes have to be considered false if the radiograph shows clear characteristic changes of osteopenia [54, 91].

Vertebral Fractures and Their Diagnosis

Vertebral fractures are the hallmarks of osteoporosis, and although one may argue that osteopenia per se cannot be diagnosed reliably from spinal radiographs, spinal radiography continues to be a substantial aid in diagnosing and following vertebral fractures [98, 132]. Changes in the gross morphology of the vertebral body have a wide range of appearances, from increased concavity of the endplates to a complete destruction of the vertebral anatomy in vertebral crush fractures (Figs. 11-3, 11-4) In clinical practice conventional radiographs of the thoracolumbar region in lateral projection are analyzed qualitatively by radiologists or experienced clinicians to identify vertebral deformities or fractures. For an experienced radiologist this assessment generally is uncomplicated, and it can be aided by additional radiographic projections such as anteroposterior and oblique views or by complimentary examinations such as bone scintigraphy, computed tomography, and even magnetic resonance imaging. Further detailed information on the assessment of vertebral fractures in the context of epidemiological studies and clinical drug trials is given in Chap. 12.

Osteopenia and Osteoporosis at Other Skeletal Sites

The axial skeleton is not the only site where characteristic changes of osteopenia and osteoporosis can be depicted radiographically. Changes in the trabecular and cortical bone can also be seen in the appendicular skeleton, and methods to quantitate these changes have been proposed and also clinically applied.

Urist and colleagues reported that in women with hip fracture the principal compressive trabeculae in the proximal femur become more prominent while other groups of trabeculae are resorbed [188]. Based on this observation in women

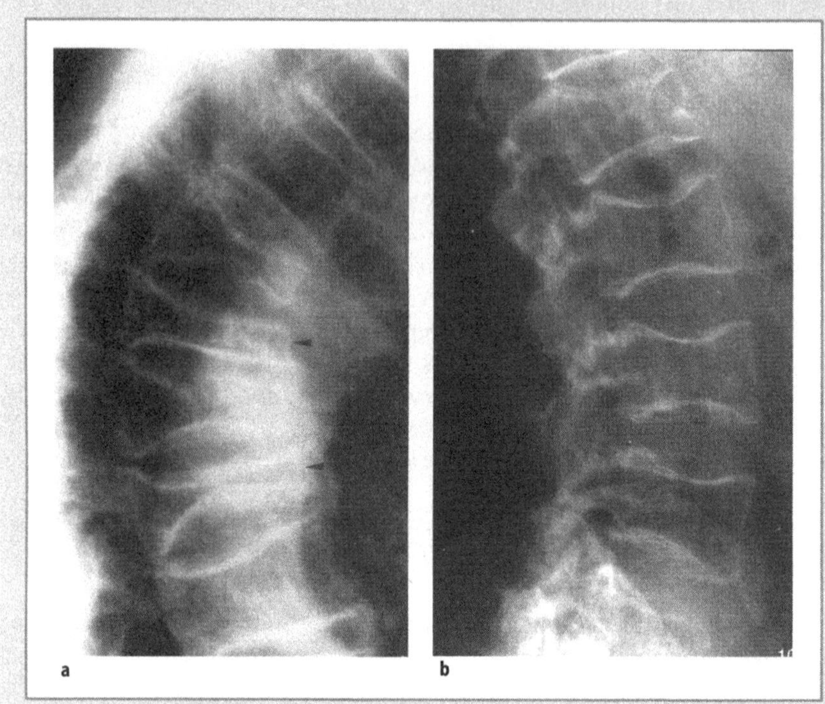

Fig. 11-3 Involutional osteoporosis presents with multiple fractures in the thoracic **a** and in the lumbar spine **b**. The types of fractures shown here are wedge and compression fractures as well as endplate fractures presenting as biconcavities of the vertebral bodies.

with advanced osteoporosis Singh et al. proposed a femoral index for the diagnosis of osteoporosis in 1970 based on the assumption that the trabeculae in the proximal femur disappear in a predictable sequence depending on their original thickness (Fig. 11-5) [171]. The authors considered that the thickness and spacing of trabeculae in the various trajectorial groups (principal compressive, secondary compressive, greater trochanter, principal tensile, and secondary tensile group) depend on the intensity of stresses normally carried by these trabeculae, and with advancing bone loss trabeculae that are thinner become invisible first on the radiograph. Singh and coworkers introduced a classification ranging from grade VI (normal, all trabecular groups visible) to grade I (markedly reduced reduction in even the principal compressive trabeculae) according to the degree of bone loss. Singh et al. later added a grade VII to their scale for individuals with dense bone, as the Ward's triangle (an area on radiographs of the proximal femur enclosed by the principle and secondary compressive, and the tensile groups) contained trabeculae that were as dense as the other surrounding trabeculae [170].

The authors reported a relatively good discrimination of individuals with and without vertebral fractures. A range of interobserver variation has been report-

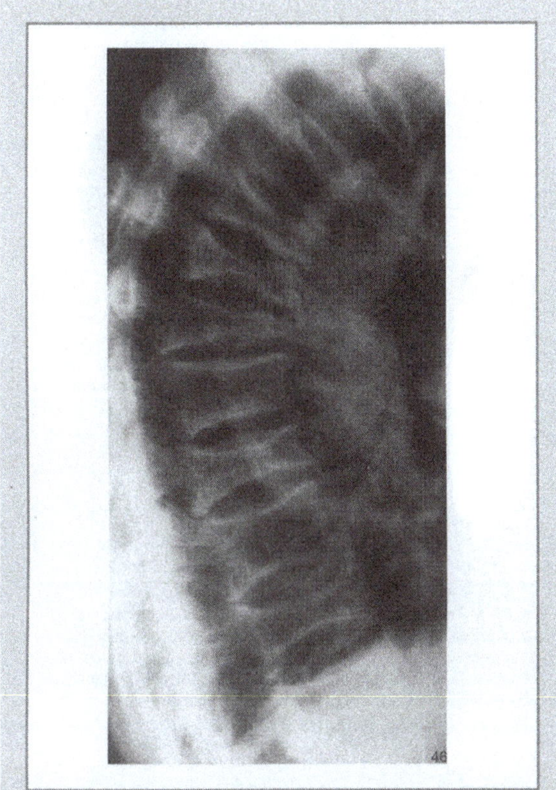

Fig. 11-4 Advanced involutional osteoporosis presenting with multiple vertebral fractures of various degrees of severity. The radiograph demonstrates substantial kyphosis of the thoracic spine. Thickened and sclerotic trabeculae indicate preceding fluoride therapy.

ed for the Singh index with the variability being influenced strongly by the quality of the radiographs, the degree of osteoporosis, with moderate changes being harder to agree on than the extremes, and the experience of the observer [22, 32, 114, 194]. Right-left comparisons of the Singh index show a concordance on the order of 80% [22, 103]. The Singh index has been applied since in a number of studies showing varying results in the relationship to bone mass and vertebral appearance [22, 37, 103]. A more recent study indicates that the underlying assumption of the Singh index, the organized sequential loss of trabeculae, may be false, and a generalized loss of bone mineral in both the tensile and compressive occurs [160].

Radiogrammetry is the simple measurement of cortical thickness potentially applied in virtually every long bone (Fig. 11-6). It is easy to perform with a caliper or graduated magnifying glass. Simple cortical measurements may be represented in several ways. For example, one method involves summing the thick-

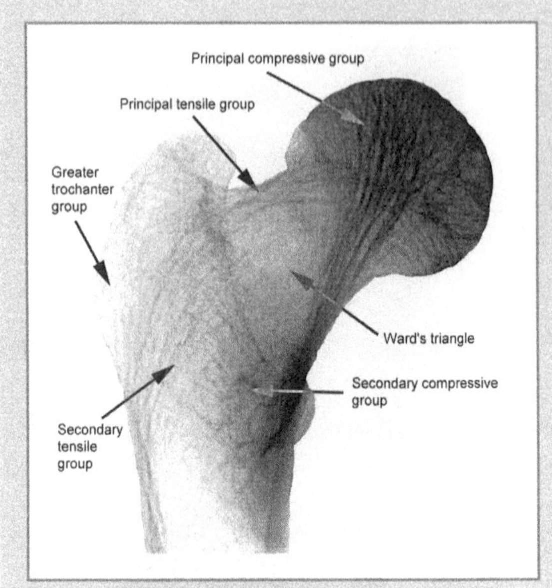

Fig. 11-5 The Singh index is based on the assumption that the trabeculae in the proximal femur disappear in a predictable sequence. This figure shows a schematic representation of the five normal groups of trabeculae. Ward's triangle is an area enclosed by the principal and secondary compressive and the principal tensile groups.

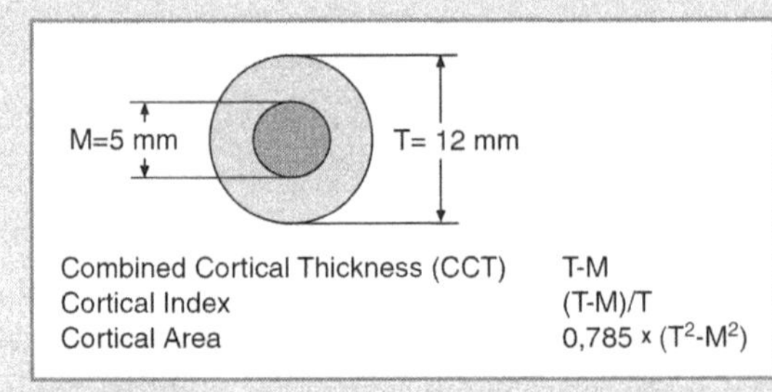

Fig. 11-6 Schematic representation of a cross-section of a tubular bone, showing several parameters that may be determined using radiogrammetry.

ness of both cortices as an index of bone mass; another uses the combined cortical thickness divided by the total bone width as a measure of density; finally, a circular cross-section of bone is taken as a given with the measurements of bone width and cortical thickness converted to cortical area that more closely parallels actual physical mass. These methods have proven to be reproducible within 5%–10% depending on the specific site that is measured [31, 52, 95, 150, 192]. Radiogrammetry is applied most often to the metacarpal bones. Systematic errors are introduced by variations in soft tissue thickness and in radiographic geometry.

As a consequence of these inaccuracies and the imprecision of the measurements, the values for compact bone area derived from radiogrammetry at different skeletal locations are only moderately correlated ($r=0.5-0.7$), whereas the correlation between right- and left-sided bones is higher ($r=0.75-0.9$) [11, 80]. While Meema and Meindok reported a good correlation between radiogrammetric measurements and DPA of the spine, other studies suggested only a poor to moderate correlation with other methods of bone mineral measurements, such as SPA and DPA at various sites [65, 124, 155]. Simple cortical measurements, particularly when obtained at several anatomic sites, provide information that is more useful in clinical research than in individual patient management. For example, extensive data on metacarpal changes in populations show a loss with aging of compact bone on the order of 0.9% per year in women and of 0.4% in men in the age range from 50–80 years [31, 41, 53, 65]. Falch and Sandvik described a premenopausal annual decrease in the combined cortical width of 0.4% compared to a postmenopausal annual decrease of 1.3% postmenopausal [42]. Comparable results were given by Genant et al. who reported an annual decrease in the combined cortical thickness of 1.45% in untreated women after oophorectomy [57]. In women who received conjugated estrogen in a dose of 0.6 mg/day after oophorectomy, the decrease in the combined cortical thickness was only 0.5%. Meema found radiogrammetry to be a good discriminator between postmenopausal women with and without vertebral fractures [121, 123], and a prospective study by Jergas et al. found radiogrammetry to be predictive of future hip fractures to a similar extent as was radial bone density [90].

Studies of patients with primary hyperparathyroidism, rheumatoid arthritis, and systemic lupus erythematosus have revealed substantial reductions of the combined cortical thickness compared to normal controls [61, 94]. One major limitation leading to the potential insensitivity of radiogrammetry is related to the failure to measure intracortical resorption or porosity and irregular endosteal scalloping or erosion. As intracortical resorption and trabecular bone resorption are important indicators of high bone turnover states, the fact that they are not measured by this technique is significant. Despite its shortcomings when applied to individual patients, radiogrammetry remains an important research tool to study changes in cortical bone [28, 51, 64].

Other sites of the appendicular skeleton such as the radius, calcaneus, and mandibula are also affected by osteoporosis, and they may bear characteristic signs of this disease [92, 157]. However, as of yet reports on characteristic changes at these sites or their usefulness for the clinical diagnosis of osteoporosis are relatively scarce. For the study of osteoporosis and related fractures, conventional radiography is the basis for a number of recent studies exploring new aspects in conventional radiographs of the skeleton. The relatively clear depiction of trabecular microstructure, for example, led to a number of studies assessing structural changes in osteoporosis using sophisticated image analysis procedures such as fractal analysis or fast Fourier transforms [9,16,63,157,161]. Other groups have focused on new high-resolution imaging techniques based on computed tomography and magnetic resonance imaging to evaluate bone structure [18,20,88,115–118,134]. This scientific field is relatively young, and first clinical results appear to be promising. Larger systematic studies are to be expected.

Another example for rather recent developments are the measurements of geometric properties of the proximal femur which were found to be associated with the risk of hip fractures [66]. The association of four measures derived from pelvic radiographs, cortical thickness of the femoral shaft, cortical thickness of the femoral neck, number of tensile trabeculae and width of the trochanteric region, with hip fractures was comparable to that of bone density with hip fracture. Similarly, hip axis length, as measured with a DXA densitometer, is associated with hip fracture, independently of bone density [24, 43, 44, 138].

Other Causes of Generalized Osteoporosis

Aside from senile and postmenopausal states leading to a generalized osteoporosis, there are various other conditions that may be accompanied by generalized osteoporosis. While most of the previously mentioned radiographic characteristics are shared by a variety of conditions, there are some differences in the appearance of osteoporosis compared to involutional osteoporosis.

Endocrine Disorders Associated with Osteoporosis

Increased serum concentrations of the parathyroid hormone in hyperparathyroidism may result from autonomous hypersecretion by a parathyroid adenoma or diffuse hyperplasia of the parathyroid glands (primary hyperparathyroidism). A long sustained hypocalcemic stimulus may result in hyperplasia of all parathyroid glands and secondary hyperparathyroidism. The cause of hypocalcemia usually is chronic renal failure or rarely malabsorption states. Patients with long-standing hyperparathyroidism may develop autonomous function and hypercalcemia (tertiary hyperparathyroidism). While it is the increase in serum parathyroid hormone and calcium that establishes the diagnosis, radiographs document the severity and the course of the disease. Hyperparathyroidism leads to both increased bone resorption and bone formation. In fact, the skeletal changes and their radiographic appearance induced by hyperparathyroidism are quite complex [61, 62]. Bone resorption can affect all bone surfaces, including subperiosteal, intracortical, endosteal, subchondral, subepiphyseal, subligamentous and subtendinous, and trabecular bone.

Subperiosteal bone resorption is the most characteristic radiographic feature of hyperparathyroidism (Fig. 11-7) [17]. It is especially prominent in the hand, wrist, and foot but may also be seen other sites. Radiographically the outer margin of the bone becomes indistinct [77]. Scalloping and spiculations of the cortex may occur in later stages. A distinctive type of acro-osteolysis may also be

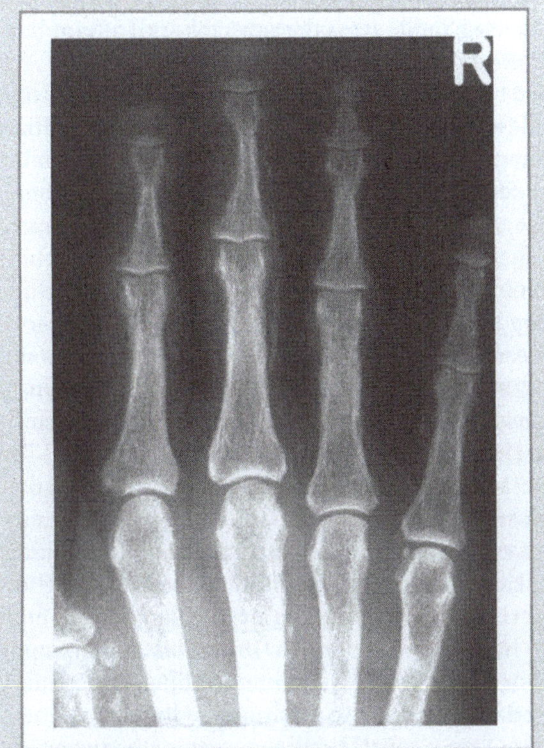

Fig. 11-7 Radiograph of the hand in secondary hyperparathyroidism showing subperiosteal resorption with scalloping and spiculations of the outer cor-tex, endosteal tunneling, acro-osteolyses, and soft tissue calcifications.

observed [147]. Intracortical resorption results in longitudinally oriented linear striations within the cortex, and endosteal bone resorption leads to scalloping of the inner cortex, cortical thinning, and widening of the medullary canal [122,147].

Subchondral bone resorption is another common manifestaion of hyperparathyroidism that most frequently affects the joints of the axial skeleton [36, 144]. For example, it may mimic widening of the sacroiliac joint space leading to "pseudowidening" of the joint [77]. The osseous surface may collapse, and thus may simulate subchondral lesions of inflammatory disease. Osteopenia occurs frequently in hyperparathyroidism and may be observed throughout the skeleton [149].

Other radiographic signs of hyperparathyroidism include focal bone lesions ("brown tumors"), cartilage calcification and also bone sclerosis [46, 176]. Increased amounts of trabecular bone leading to bone sclerosis may occur especially in patients with renal osteodystrophy and secondary hyperparathyroidism [23, 29, 56]. Increased bone density may occur, preferably in the axial skeleton, and lead to deposition of bone in subchondral areas of the vertebral body, resulting in an appearance of radiodense bands across the superior and inferior border and normal or decreased density of the center (rugger-jersey spine).

While osteoporosis is defined by a reduction in regularly mineralized osteoid, findings in osteomalacia include an abnormally high amount of nonmineralized osteoid, and a reduction in mineralized bone volume. Thus radiographic abnormalities in osteomalacia include osteopenia (reduction in mineralized bone), coarsened, indistinct trabeculae, and unclear delineation of cortical bone (excessive apposition of nonmineralized osteoid), deformities, insufficiency fractures and true fractures (bone softening and weakening). The deformations include bowing and bending of the long bones, and biconcave deformities of the vertebrae. Pseudofractures, or Looser's zones, are diagnostic of osteomalacia and often occur bilaterally and symmetrically [110, 177, 178]. There are more than 50 different diseases that may cause osteomalacia of which chronic renal insufficiency, hemodialysis and renal transplantation are the most common [140]. The destruction of renal parenchyma impairs the metabolism of calcium, phosphorus, and vitamin D, which is essential for the normal development of bone mineral. A decrease in this vitamin and reduced responsiveness in chronic renal insufficiency results in osteomalacia and rickets. The additional secondary hyperparathyroidism leads to a superimposition of radiographic changes from both osteomalacia and secondary hyperparathyroidism [181]. This radiographic appearance is termed renal osteodystrophy. A common finding in secondary hyperparathyroidism associated with renal osteodystrophy is the osteosclerosis resulting in typical appearance of the vertebral bodies as seen in the rugger-jersey spine (Figs. 11-8, 11-9) [140, 141]. Several other radiographic abnormalities may be frequently seen in renal osteodystrophy including amyloid deposits, destructive spondylarthropathy, inflammatory changes, and avascular necrosis, soft tissue calcification, and arteriosclerosis [97, 104, 130, 183].

Hyperthyroidism is a high-turnover disease, and it is associated with an increase in both bone resorption and bone formation [129]. Since bone resorption exceeds bone formation rapid bone loss may occur and result in generalized osteoporosis [40, 106]. This effect is especially pronounced in patients with thyrotoxicosis, or with a history of thyrotoxicosis [105, 112, 186]. Thyrotropin-suppressive doses of thyroid hormone have been reported to decrease, or have no effect on bone density [105]. Radiological findings of hyperthyroidism-induced osteoporosis are those that are commonly seen in involutional or senile osteoporosis, including generalized osteopenia and cortical thinning and tunneling [19]. The fractures associated with this condition affect the spine, hip, and distal radius [25, 174].

Medication-Induced Osteoporosis

Hypercortisolism is probably the most common cause of medication-induced generalized osteoporosis while the endogenous form of hypercortisolism, Cushing's disease, is relatively rare [1, 13, 71–74, 87, 107, 139, 159, 165]. This is why this

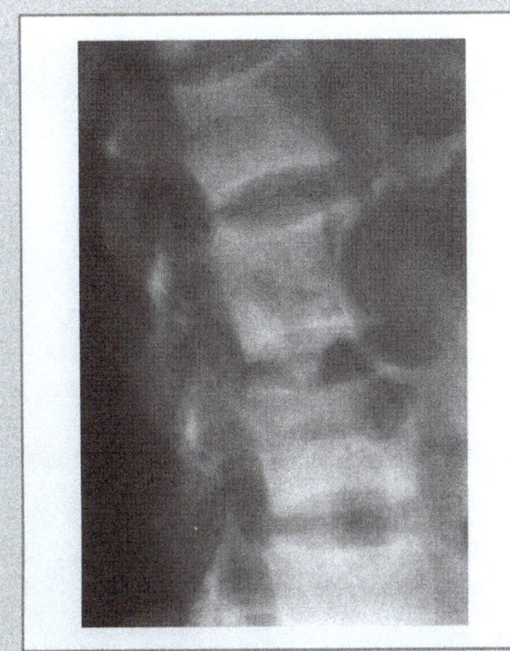

Fig. 11-8 Renal osteodystrophy usually is a combination of osteomalacia and secondary hyperparathyroidism, resulting in the 'rugger-jersey' appearance of the spine with sclerosis of the endplates.

form of osteoporosis is considered here under medication-induced osteoporosis. Decreased bone formation and increased bone resorption have been observed in hypercortisolism. This has been attributed to inhibition of osteoblast formation, either direct stimulation of osteoclast activity or increased secretion of parathyroid hormone. The typical radiographic appearance of steroid-induced osteoporosis comprises generalized osteoporosis, at predominantly trabecular sites, with decreased (Fig. 11-10) bone density and fractures of the axial but also of the appendicular skeleton. A characteristic finding in steroid-induced osteoporosis is the marginal condensation of the vertebral bodies resulting from exuberant callus formation. Osteonecrosis is another complication of hypercortisolism, most frequently involving the femoral head and to a lesser extent the humeral head and the femoral condyles [79, 145]

Generalized osteoporosis has been observed in patients receiving high-dose heparin therapy [7, 68, 156, 175]. The radiological features of heparin-induced osteoporosis include generalized osteopenia and vertebral compression fractures (Fig. 11-11) [158]. The pathomechanism of heparin-induced osteoporosis is not completely clear, and the changes may be reversible with cessation of therapy [131, 166, 184].

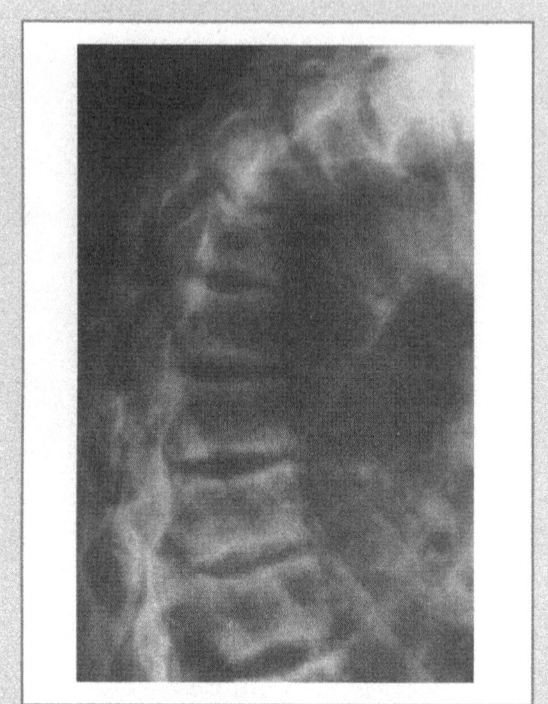

Fig. 11-9 Renal osteodystrophy with sclerosis of the vertebral end-plates and vertebral fractures, resulting in extreme kyphosis.

Miscellaneous Causes of Generalized Osteoporosis

Other causes of generalized osteoporosis include malnutrition, chronic alcoholism (if associated with malnutrition), smoking and caffein intake, Marfan's syndrome, and (rather uncommonly) pregnancy [8, 10, 27, 34, 76, 81, 83, 100, 163, 168, 173]. Marrow abnormalities associated with osteoporosis are anemias (sickle cell anemia, thalassemia), plasma cell myeloma, leukemia, Gaucher's disease and glycogen storage disease (Fig. 11-12, 11-13) [5, 15, 35, 67, 125, 142, 143, 169]. This list is certainly far from complete, but it presents some of the major causes of osteoporosis. Additional imaging techniques such as computed tomography, magnetic resonance tomography, and bone scintigraphy as well as clinical information may be helpful in differential diagnosis of the various conditions associated with osteoporosis [84].

There are some conditions of the juvenile skeleton that result in generalized osteoporosis. Rickets is characterized by inadequate mineralization of the bone matrix. and some of its radiographic appearance may resemble that of osteomalacia [128, 137, 178]. Widening of the growth plates, cupping of the metaphysis, and decreased density and irregularities of the metaphyseal margins may be present

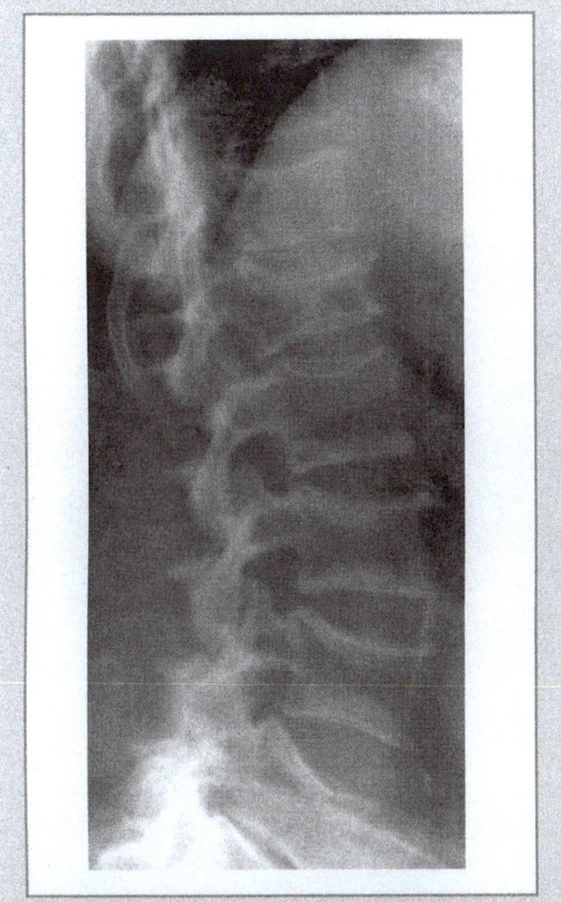

Fig. 11-10 Secondary osteoporosis induced by corticosteroids. The lateral radiograph of the lumbar spine shows multiple biconcave deformities and typi-cal radiodense endplates due to exuberant callus formation.

[141, 193]. Epiphyseal ossification centers may show delayed ossification and unclear borders [177]. Overgrowth of the hyaline cartilage may lead to prominence of costochondral junctions of the ribs (rachitic rosary). The child's age at the onset of the disease determines the pattern of bone deformity, with bowing of the long bones being more pronounced in infancy and early childhood, and vertebral deformities and scoliosis in older children [136]. Further deformities that may be observed in rickets include pseudofractures, basilar invagination, and triradiate configuration of the pelvis [154]. Idiopathic juvenile osteoporosis is a self-limited disease of childhood with recovery occurring as puberty progresses [30, 85, 119, 172]. A typical feature of this condition is the increased vulnerability of the metaphyses, often resulting in metaphyseal injuries of the knees

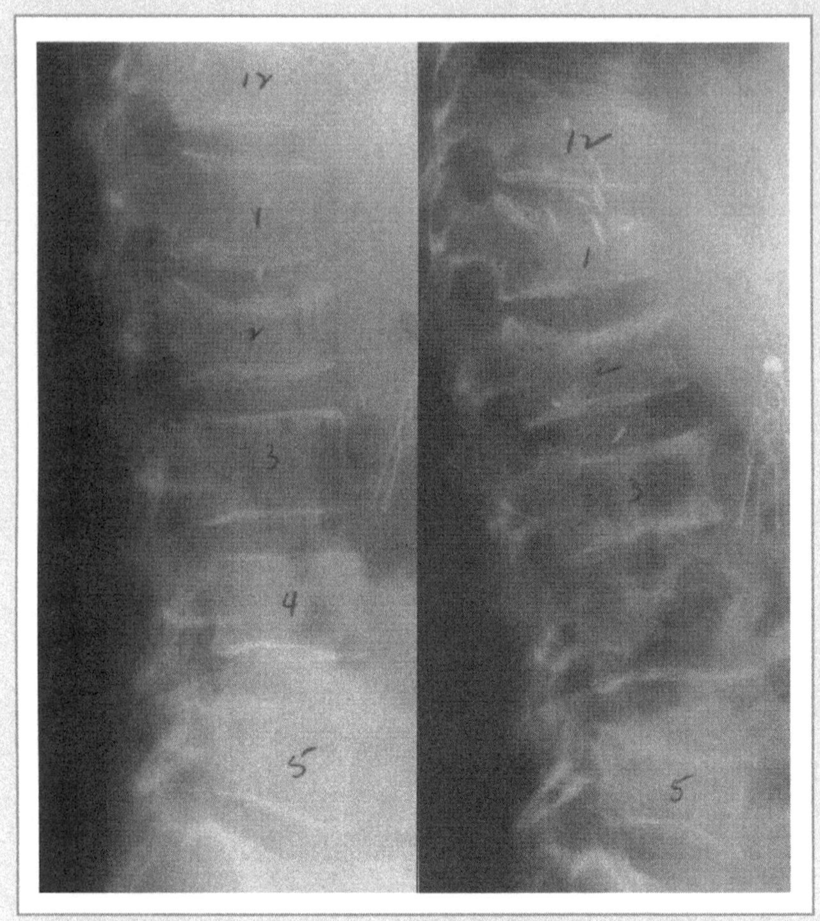

Fig. 11-11 Serial radiographs in heparin-induced osteoporosis. The follow-up radiograph on the right reveals multiple new fractures. Note vena cava filter.

and ankles. Idiopathic juvenile osteoporosis must be distinguished from osteogenesis imperfecta, another disease often presenting with radiographic signs of generalized osteoporosis [197]. Osteogenesis imperfecta is divided into four major types, and the degree of osteoporosis in osteogenesis imperfecta depends strongly on the type of disease. Patients with type III disease have a significantly decreased bone density presenting with generalized osteopenia, thinned cortices, fractures of long bones and ribs, exuberant callus formation and bone deformation [14, 75, 190]. The degree of osteopenia is highly variable, however, and at the mild end of the spectrum some patients do not have any radiographic signs of osteopenia [152].

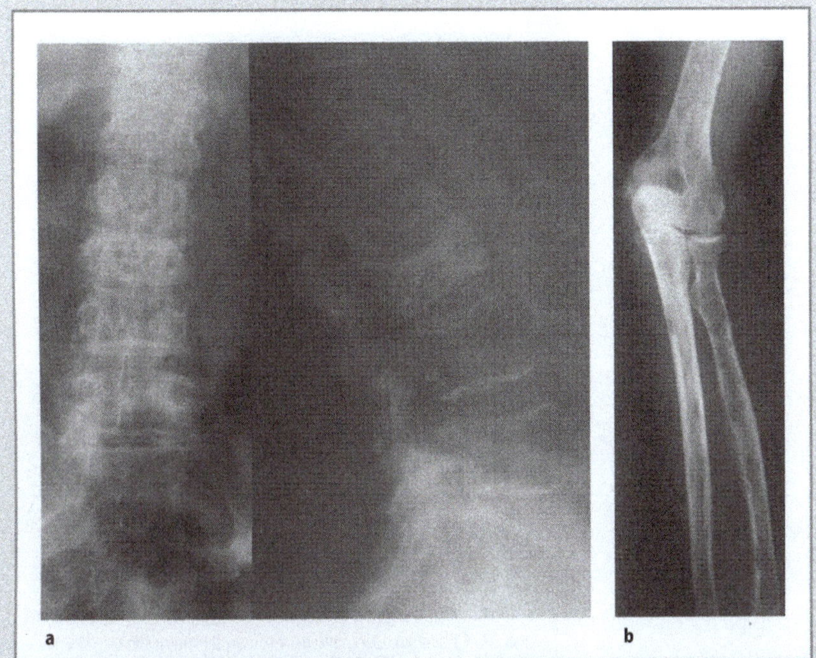

Fig. 11-12 Changes in the spine in multiple myeloma (A), here presenting with increased radiolucency and vertebral deformities, may easily be confused with osteoporotic changes. However, additional typical lesions at other sites (besides clinical features and relatively typical laboratory values) may reveal the nature of the underlying disease. In this example, multiple osteolytic lesions in the forearm (B) support the diagnosis of multiple myeloma.

Regional Osteoporosis

Osteoporosis may also be confined to only a segment of the body. This type of osteoporosis is called regional osteoporosis, and it is commonly caused by some disorder of the appendicular skeleton. Osteoporosis due to immobilization or disuse, characteristically occurs in the immobilized regions of patients with fractures, motor paralysis due to central nervous system disease or trauma, and bone and joint inflammation [99]. Chronic and acute disease may vary in their radiographic appearance somewhat showing diffuse osteopenia, linear radiolucent bands, speckled radiolucent areas, and cortical bone resorption (Fig. 11-14) [6, 93, 96].

Reflex sympathetic dystrophy, sometimes also termed Sudeck's atrophy or algodystrophy, has the radiographic appearance of a high-turnover process [126,167]. It most often occurs in patients with trauma, such as Colles' fracture, but also in patients with any neurally related musculoskeletal, neurological, or vascular condition such as hemiplegia or myocardial infarction [2, 55, 101, 127, 135, 162, 180]. This condition is probably related to overactivity of the sympathetic nervous sys-

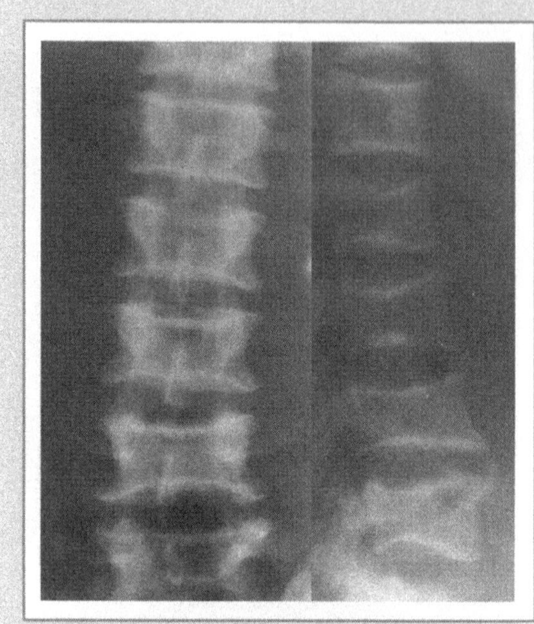

Fig. 11-13 Characteristic changes of sickle cell anemia in the lumbar spine of a young adult. Coarsened trabeculation due to marrow-hyperplasia and step-like endplate compression with a resulting biconcave appearance of the vertebrae. Substantial juxtacortical sclerosis.

tem with increased blood flow and increased intravenous oxygen saturation in the affected extremity [33, 126]. Its radiographic appearance includes soft tissue swelling and regional osteoporosis showing bandlike, patchy, or periarticular osteoporosis, subperiosteal bone resorption, introcortical tunneling, endosteal bone resorption with initial excavation and scalloping of the endosteal surface and subsequent remodeling and widening of the medullary canal, and subchondral and juxta-articular erosions [146]. Especially in the early stages of reflex sympathetic dystrophy bone scintigraphy may be helpful to establish the diagnosis [111, 179, 185].

Transient regional osteoporosis includes conditions that have in common the development of self-limited pain and radiographic osteopenia affecting one or several joints, most commonly the hip. Transient osteoporosis typically occurs in middle-aged men in and women during the third trimester of pregnancy [26, 86, 153, 182]. At the onset of clinical symptoms there may be normal radiographic findings, and within several weeks patients develop variable osteopenia of the hip, sometimes involving the acetabulum. Some patients later develop similar changes in the opposite hip or in other joints, in which case the term regional migratory osteoporosis may be used [70, 120]. No specific therapy is required, since all patients recover. The cause of transient regional osteoporosis is not known,

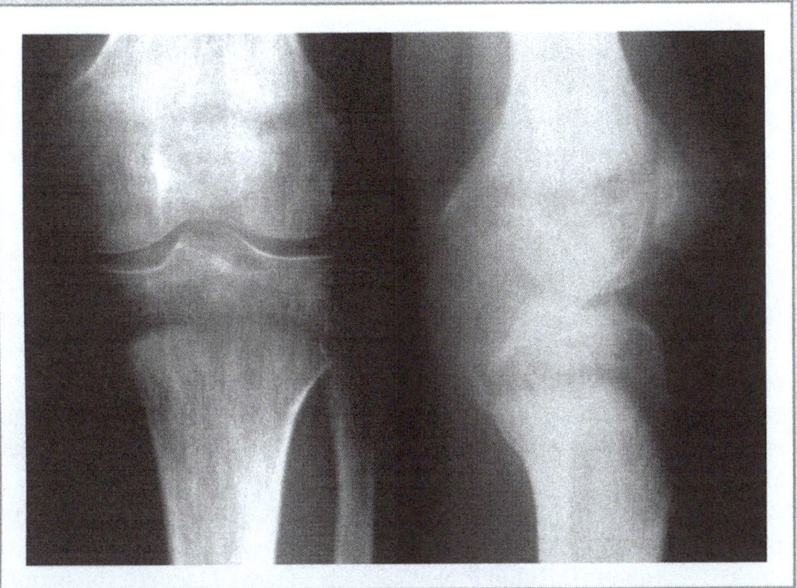

Fig. 11-14 Regional osteoporosis resulting from disuse of the knee following joint inflammation.

and it appears that it may be related to reflex sympathetic dystrophy. In some patients with clinically similar or identical manifestations, magnetic resonance imaging presents with transient regional bone marrow edema [12, 78]. Since not all patients with identical clinical symptoms and transient bone marrow edema develop regional osteoporosis, the sensitivity as to the detection of regional osteoporosis must be questioned as well as the interrelationship between transient regional osteoporosis and transient bone marrow edema. There also seems to be a relationship of transient bone marrow edema to ischemic necrosis of bone, and there is a need to define criteria for allowing differentiation of transient bone marrow edema and the edema pattern associated with osteonecrosis [47, 69, 102, 133, 148, 187, 189].

References

1.   Adachi JD, Bensen WG, Hodsman AB (1993) Corticosteroid-induced osteoporosis. Semin Arthritis Rheum 22:375–384
2.   Aisen PS, Aisen ML (1994) Shoulder-hand syndrome in cervical spinal cord injury. Paraplegia 32:588–592
3.   Albright F (1947) Osteoporosis. Ann Intern Med 27:861–882
4.   Albright F, Smith PH, Richardson AM (1941) Postmenopausal osteoporosis. Its clinical features. JAMA 116:2465–2474

5.   Amstutz HC, Carey EJ (1966) Skeletal manifestations and treatment of Gaucher's disease. Review of twenty cases. J Bone Joint Surg Am 48:670

6.   Arnstein AR (1972) Regional osteoporosis. Orthop Clin North Am 21:97–107

7.   Barbour LA, Kick SD, Steiner JF, LoVerde ME, Heddleston LN, Lear JL, Baron AE, Barton PL (1994) A prospective study of heparin-induced osteoporosis in pregnancy using bone densitometry. Am J Obstet Gynecol 170:862–869

8.   Bauer DC, Browner WS, Cauley JA, Orwoll ES, Scott JC, Black DM, Tao JL, Cummings SR (1993) Factors associated with appendicular bone mass in older women. Ann Intern Med 118:657–665

9.   Benhamou CL, Lespessailles E, Jacquet G, Harba R, Jennane R, Loussot T, Tourliere D, Ohley W (1994) Fractal organization of trabecular bone images on calcaneus radiographs. J Bone Miner Res 9:1909–1918

10. Blanch J, Pacifici R, Chines A (1994) Pregnancy-associated osteoporosis: report of two cases with long-term bone density follow-up. Br J Rheumatol 33:269–272

11. Bloom RA (1980) A comparative estimation of the combined cortical thickness of various bone sites. Skeletal Radiol 5:167–170

12. Boos S, Sigmund G, Huhle P, Nurbakhsch I (1993) Magnetresonanztomographie der sogenannten transitorischen Osteoporose. Primärdiagnostik und Verlaufskontrolle nach Therapie. Rofo Fortschr Geb Rontgenstr Neuen Bildgeb Verfahr 158:201–206

13. Brandli DW, Golde G, Greenwald M, Silverman SL (1991) Glucocorticoid-induced osteoporosis: a cross-sectional study. Steroids 56:518–523

14. Burchardt AJ, Wagner AA, Basse P (1994) Hyperplastic callus formation in osteogenesis imperfecta. A case report. Acta Radiol 35:426–428

15. Caffey J (1957) Cooley's anemia: a review of roentgenographic findings in the skeleton. Am J Radiol 78:381

16. Caligiuri P, Giger ML, Favus MJ, Jia H, Doi K, Dixon LB (1993) Computerized radiographic analysis of osteoporosis: preliminary evaluation. Radiology 186:471–474

17. Camp JD, Ochsner HC (1931) The osseous changes in hyperparathyroidism associated with parathyroid tumor: a roentgenologic study. Radiology 17:63

18. Chevalier F, Laval-Jeantet AM, Laval-Jeantet M, Bergot C (1992) CT image analysis of the vertebral trabecular network in vivo. Calcif Tissue Int 51:8–13

19. Chew FS (1991) Radiologic manifestations in the musculoskeletal system of miscellaneous endocrine disorders. Radiol Clin North Am 29:135–147

20. Chung HW, Wehrli FW, Williams JL, Kugelmass SD, Wehrli SL (1995) Quantitative analysis of trabecular microstructure by 400 MHz nuclear magnetic resonance imaging. J Bone Miner Res 10:803–811

21. Cooke AM (1955) Osteoporosis. Lancet 1:877–882

22. Cooper C, Barker DJP, Hall AJ (1986) Evaluation of the Singh index and femoral calcar width as epidemiological methods for measuring bone mass in the femoral neck. Clin Radiol 37:123–125

23. Crawford T, Dent CE, Lucas P (1954) Osteosclerosis associated with chronic renal failure. Lancet 2:981

24. Cummings SR, Cauley JA, Palermo L, Ross PD, Wasnich RD, Black D, Faulkner KG (1994) Racial differences in hip axis lengths might explain racial differences in rates of hip fractures. Osteoporosis Int 4:226–229

25. Cummings SR, Nevitt MC, Browner WS, Stone K, Fox K, Ensrud K, Cauley J, Black D, Vogt T (1995) Risk factors for hip fractures in white women. N Engl J Med 332:767–773

26. Curtiss PH, Kincaid WE (1959) Transitory demineralization of the hip in pregnancy. J Bone Joint Surg Am 41:1327–1333

27. Dalen N, Lamke B (1976) Bone mineral losses in alcoholics. Acta Orthop Scand 47:469–71

28. Danielsen CC, Mosekilde L, Svenstrup B (1993) Cortical bone mass, composition, and mechanical properties in female rats in relation to age, long-term ovariectomy, and estrogen substitution. Calcif Tissue Int 52:26–33

29. Davis JG (1953) Osseous radiographic findings of chronic renal insufficiency. Radiology 60:406

30. Dent CE, Friedman M (1965) Idiopathic juvenile osteoporosis. Q J Med 34:177

31. Dequeker J (1976) Quantitative radiology: radiogrammetry of cortical bone. Br J Radiol 49:912–920

32. Dequeker J, Gautama K, Roh YS (1974) Femoral trabecular patterns in asymptomatic spinal osteoporosis and femoral neck fracture. Clin Radiol 25:243–246

33. DeTakats G (1937) Reflex dystrophy of the extremities. Arch Surg 34:939

34. Diez A, Puig J, Serrano S, Marinoso M-L, Bosch J, Marrugat J (1994) Alcohol-induced bone disease in the absence of severe chronic liver damage. J Bone Miner Res 9:825–831

35. Diggs LW (1967) Bone and joint lesions in sickle-cell disease. Clin Orthop 52:119–143

36. Dihlmann W, Müller G (1973) Sacroiliacalbefunde beim Hyperparathyreoidismus. Radiologe 13:160

37. Disen A, Frey HM, Langholm R, Vagslid T (1979) Appearance of trabecular bone in the femoral neck (Singh index). Acta Radiol Diagn 20:372–378

38. Doyle FH, Gutteridge DH, Joplin GF, Fraser R (1967) An assessment of radiological criteria used in the study of spinal osteoporosis. Br J Radiol 40:241–250

39. Epstein DM, Dalinka MK, Kaplan FS, Aronchick JM, Marinelli DL, Kundel HL (1986) Observer variation in the detection of osteopenia. Skeletal Radiol 15:347–349

40. Eriksen EF (1986) Normal and pathological remodeling of human trabecular bone: three dimensional reconstruction of the remodeling sequence in normals and in metabolic bone disease. Endocr Rev 7:379–408

41. Evans RA, McDonell GD, Schieb M (1978) Metacarpal cortical area as an index of bone mass. Br J Radiol 51:428–431

42. Falch JA, Sandvik L (1990) Perimenopausal appendicular bone loss: a 10-year prospective study. Bone 11:425–428
43. Faulkner KG (1995) Hip axis length and osteoporotic fractures (letter to the editor). J Bone Miner Res 10:506–508
44. Faulkner KG, Cummings SR, Glüer CC, Palermo L, Black D, Genant HK (1993) Simple measurement of femoral geometry predicts hip fracture: the study of osteopotic fractures. J Bone Miner Res 8:1211–1217
45. Finsen V, Anda S (1988) Accuracy of visually estimated bone mineralization in routine radiographs of the lower extremity. Skeletal Radiol 17:270–275
46. Fordham CC, Williams TF (1963) Brown tumors and secondary hyperparathyroidism. N Engl J Med 269:129
47. Froberg PK, Braunstein EM, Buckwalter KA (1996) Osteonecrosis, transient osteoporosis, and transient bone marrow edema: current concepts. Radiol Clin North Am 34:273–291
48. Frost HM (1964) Dynamics of bone remodelling. In: Frost HM (ed) Bone biodynamics. Little Brown, Boston, pp 315–334
49. Gallagher JC (1990) The pathogenesis of osteoporosis. Bone Miner 9:215–227
50. Gallagher JC (1992) Pathophysiology of osteoporosis. Sem Nephrol 12:109–115
51. Gallagher JC, Kable WT, Goldgar D (1991) Effect of progestin therapy on cortical and trabecular bone: comparison with estrogen. Am J Med 90:171–178
52. Garn SM, Poznanski AK, Nagy JM (1971) Bone measurement in the differential diagnosis of osteopenia and osteoporosis. Radiology 100:509–518
53. Garn SM, Rohmann CG, Wagner B (1967) Bone loss as a general phenomenon of man. Fed Proc 26:1729–1736
54. Garton MJ, Robertson EM, Gilbert FJ, Gomersall L, Reid DM (1994) Can radiologists detect osteopenia on plain radiographs? Clin Radiol 49:118–122
55. Gellman H, Keenan MA, Stone L, Hardy SE, Waters RL, Stewart C (1992) Reflex sympathetic dystrophy in brain-injured patients. Pain 51:307–311
56. Genant HK, Baron JM, Straus FH, Paloyan E, Jowsey J (1975) Osteosclerosis in primary hyperparathyroidism. Am J Radiol 59:104–113
57. Genant HK, Cann CE, Ettinger B, Gordan GS (1982) Quantitative computed tomography of vertebral spongiosa: a sensitive method for detecting early bone loss after oophorectomy. Ann Intern Med 97:699–705
58. Genant HK, Doi K, Mall JC (1976) Comparison of non-screen techniques (medical vs. industrial film) for fine-detail skeletal radiography. Invest Radiol 11:486–500
59. Genant HK, Doi K, Mall JC, Sickles EA (1977) Direct radiographic magnification for skeletal radiology. Radiology 123:47–55
60. Genant HK, Engelke K, Fuerst T, Glüer C-C, Grampp S, Harris S, Jergas M, Lang T, Lu Y, Majumdar S, Mathur A, Takada M (1996) Noninvasive assessment of bone mineral and structure: state of the art. J Bone Miner Res 11:707–730
61. Genant HK, Heck LL, Lanzl LH, Rossmann K, Vander Horst J, Paloyan E (1973) Primary hyperparathyroidism. A comprehensive study of clinical, biochemical and radiographic manifestations. Radiology 109:513–519

62. Genant HK, Vander Horst J, Lanzl LH, Mall JC, Doi K (1974) Skeletal demineralization in primary hyperparathyroidism. In: Mazess RB (ed) Proceedings of international conference on bone mineral measurement. National Institute of Arthritis, Metabolism and Digestive Diseases, Washington, p 177

63. Geraets WGM, Van der Stelt PF, Elders PJM (1993) The radiographic trabecular bone pattern during menopause. Bone 14:859–864

64. Geusens P, Dequeker J, Nijs J, Verstraeten A, Bramm E (1991) Prevention and treatment of osteopenia in the ovariectomized rat: effect of combined therapy with estrogens, 1-alpha vitamin D, and prednisolone. Calcif Tissue Int 48:127–137

65. Geusens P, Dequeker J, Verstraeten A, Nijs J (1986) Age-, sex-, and menopause-related changes of vertebral and peripheral bone: population study using dual and single photon absorptiometry and radiogrammetry. J Nucl Med 27:1540–1549

66. Glüer CC, Cummings SR, Pressman A, Li J, Glüer K, Faulkner KG, Grampp S, Genant HK (1994) Prediction of hip fractures from pelvic radiographs: the study of osteoporotic fractures. J Bone Miner Res 9:671–677

67. Greenfield GB (1970) Bone changes in chronic adult Gaucher's disease. Am J Radiol 110:800–807

68. Griffith GC, Nichols G, Ashey JD, Flannagan B (1965) Heparin osteoporosis. JAMA 193:85–88

69. Guerra JJ, Steinberg ME (1995) Distinguishing transient osteoporosis from avascular necrosis of the hip. J Bone Joint Surg Am 77:616–624

70. Gupta RC, Popovtzer MM, Huffer WE, Smyth CJ (1973) Regional migratory osteoporosis. Arthritis Rheum 21:363–368

71. Hahn TJ (1978) Corticosteroid-induced osteopenia. Arch Intern Med 138:882–885

72. Hahn TJ, Bouisseau WV, Avioli LV (1974) Effect of chronic corticosteroid administration on diaphyseal and metaphyseal bone mass. J Clin Endocrinol Metab 39:274–81

73. Hall GM, Spector TD, Griffin AJ, Jawad AS, Hall ML, Doyle DV (1993) The effect of rheumatoid arthritis and steroid therapy on bone density in postmenopausal women. Arthritis Rheum 36:1510–1516

74. Hanania NA, Chapman KR, Sturtridge WC, Szalai JP, Kesten S (1995) Dose-related decrease in bone density among asthmatic patients treated with inhaled corticosteroids. J Allergy Clin Immunol 96:571–579

75. Hanscom DA, Winter RB, Lutter L, Lonstein JE, Bloom BA, Bradford DS (1992) Osteogenesis imperfecta. Radiographic classification, natural history, and treatment of spinal deformities. J Bone Joint Surg Am 74:598–616

76. Harding A, Dunlap J, Cook S, Mattalino A, Azar F, O'Brien M, Kester M (1988) Osteoporotic correlates of alcoholism in young males. Orthopedics 11:279–282

77. Hayes CW, Conway WF (1991) Hyperparathyroidism. Radiol Clin North Am 29:85–96

78. Hayes CW, Conway WF, Daniel WW (1993) MR imaging of bone marrow edema pattern: transient osteoporosis, transient bone marrow edema syndrome, or osteonecrosis. Radiographics 13:1001–1011

79. Heimann WG, Freiberger RH (1969) Avascular necrosis of the femoral and humeral heads after high-dosage corticosteroid therapy. N Engl J Med 263:672–674

80. Helela T, Virtama P (1970) Cortical thickness of long bones in different age groups. Symposium ossium. Livingstone, London, pp 238–240

81. Herzog W, Minne H, Deter C, Leidig G, Schellberg D, Wüster C, Gronwald R, Sarembe E, Kröger F, Bergmann G, Petzold E, Hahn P, Schepank H, Ziegler R (1993) Outcome of bone mineral density in anorexia nervosa patients 11.7 years after first admission. J Bone Miner Res 8:597–605

82. Heuck F, Schmidt E (1960) Die quantitative Bestimmung des Mineralgehaltes des Knochens aus dem Röntgenbild. Fortschr Rontgenstr 93:523–554

83. Hopper JL, Seeman E (1994) The bone density of twins discordant for tobacco use. N Engl J Med 330:387–392

84. Hosten N, Neumann K, Zwicker C, Schubeus P, Kirsch A, Huhn D, Felix R (1993) Diffuse Demineralisation der Lendenwirbelsaule. Magnetresonanztomographische Untersuchungen bei Osteoporose und Plasmozytom. Rofo Fortschr Geb Röntgenstr Neuen Bildgeb Verfahr 159:264–268

85. Hou JW, Wang TR (1995) Idiopathic juvenile osteoporosis: five-year case follow-up. J Formos Med Assoc 94:277–80

86. Hunder GG, Kelly PJ (1968) Roentgenologic transient osteoporosis of the hip. Ann Intern Med 68:539–552

87. Ip M, Lam K, Yam L, Kung A, Ng M (1994) Decreased bone mineral density in premenopausal asthma patients receiving long-term inhaled steroids (see comments). Chest 105:1722–1727

88. Ito M, Ohki M, Hayashi K, Yamada M, Uetani M, Nakamura T (1995) Trabecular texture analysis of CT images in the relationship with spinal fracture. Radiology 194:55–59

89. Jergas M, Genant HK (1993) Current methods and recent advances in the diagnosis of osteoporosis. Arthritis Rheum 36:1649–1662

90. Jergas M, San Valentin R, Black D, Nevitt M, Palermo L, Genant HK, Cummings SR (1995) Radiogrammetry of the metacarpals predicts future hip fractures. J Bone Miner Res 10:S371

91. Jergas M, Uffmann M, Escher H, Glüer CC, Young KC, Grampp S, Köster O, Genant HK (1994) Interobserver variation in the detection of osteopenia by radiography and comparison with dual X-ray absorptiometry (DXA) of the lumbar spine. Skeletal Radiol 23:195–199

92. Jhamaria NL, Lal KB, Udawat M, Banerji P, Kabra SG (1983) The trabecular pattern of the calcaneum as an index of osteoporosis. J Bone Joint Surg Br 65:195–198

93. Jones G (1969) Radiological appearance of disuse osteoporosis. Clin Radiol 20:345–353

94. Kalla AA, Kotze TJvW, Meyers OL (1992) Metacarpal bone mass in systemic lupus erythematosus. Clin Rheumatol 11:475–482

95. Kalla AA, Meyers OL, Parkyn ND, Kotze TJvW (1989) Osteoporosis screening – radiogrammetry revisited. Br J Rheumatol 28:511–517

96. Keats TE, Harrison RB (1978) A pattern of post-traumatic demineralization of bone simulating permeative neoplastic replacement: a potential source of misinterpretation. Skeletal Radiol 3:113

97. Kerr R, Bjorkengren A, Bielecki DK, Resnick D, Feinstein EI (1988) Destructive spondylarthropathy in hemodialysis: Report of four cases and prospective study. Skeletal Radiol 17:176–180

98. Kienböck R (1931) Die Krankheiten der Wirbelsäule im Röntgenbild. Wien Klin Wochenschr 44:232–234

99. Kiratli BJ (1996) Immobilization osteopenia. In: Marcus R, Feldman D, Kelsey J (eds) Osteoporosis. Academic, San Diego, pp 833–853

100. Kohlmeyer L, Gasner C, Marcus R (1993) Bone mineral status of women with Marfan syndrome. Am J Med 95:568–572

101. Kozin F (1992) Reflex sympathetic dystrophy syndrome: a review. Clin Exp Rheumatol 10:401–409

102. Kramer J, Hofmann S, Engel A, Leder K, Neuhold A, Imhof H (1993) Hüftkopfnekrose und Knochenmarksödemsyndrom in der Schwangerschaft. Rofo Fortschr Geb Rontgenstr Neuen Bildgeb Verfahr 159:126–131

103. Kranendonk DH, Jurist JM, Lee HG (1972) Femoral trabecular patterns and bone mineral content. J Bone Joint Surg Am 54:1472–1478

104. Kriegshauser JS, Swee RG, McCarthy JT, Hauser MF (1987) Aluminum toxicity in patients undergoing dialysis: Radiographic findings and prediction of bone biobsy results. Radiology 164:399–403

105. Krølner B, Jørgensen JV, Nielsen SP (1983) Spinal bone mineral content in myxoedema and thyrotoxicosis. Effects of thyroid hormone(s) and antithyroid treatment. Clin endocrinol 18:439–446

106. Kung AW, Lorentz T, Tam SC (1993) Thyroxine suppressive therapy decreases bone mineral density in post-menopausal women. Clin Endocrinol (Oxf) 39:535–540

107. Laan RF, Buijs WC, van Erning LJ, Lemmens JA, Corstens FH, Ruijs SH, van de Putte LB, van Riel PL (1993) Differential effects of glucocorticoids on cortical appendicular and cortical vertebral bone mineral content. Calcif Tissue Int 52:5–9

108. Lachmann E, Whelan M (1936) The roentgen diagnosis of osteoporosis and its limitations. Radiology 26:165–177

109. LeGeros RZ (1994) Biological and synthetic apatites. In: Brown PW, Constantz B (eds) Hydroxyapatite and related materials. CRC, Boca Raton, pp 3–28

110. Leicht E, Kramann B, Seitz G, Trentz O, Remberger K (1993) Oncogenic osteomalacia: imaging studies. Bildgebung 60:13–17

111. Leitha T, Staudenherz A, Korpan M, Fialka V (1996) Pattern recognition in five-phase bone scintigraphy: diagnostic patterns of reflex sympathetic dystrophy in adults. Eur J Nucl Med 23:256–262

112. Linde J, Friis T (1979) Osteoporosis in hyperthyroidism estimated by photon absorptiometry. Acta Endocrinol (Oxf) 91:437–448

113. Link TM, Rummeny EJ, Lenzen H, Reuter I, Roos N, Peters PE (1994) Artificial bone erosions: detection with magnification radiography versus conventional high resolution radiography. Radiology 192:861–864

114. Lips P, Taconis WK, Van Ginkel FC et al (1984) Radiographic morphometry in patients with femoral neck fractures and elderly control subjects. Clin Orthop 183:64–70

115. Majumdar S, Genant HK, Grampp S, Jergas M, Newitt D, Gies A (1994) Analysis of trabecular bone structure in the distal radius using high resolution MRI. Eur Radiol 4:517–524

116. Majumdar S, Genant HK, Grampp S, Newitt DC, Truong V-H, Lin JC, Mathur A (1997) Correlation of trabecular bone structure with age, bone mineral density, and osteoporotic status: in vivo studies in the distal radius using high resolution magnetic resonance imaging. J Bone Miner Res 12:111–118

117. Majumdar S, Newitt D, Mathur A, Osman D, Gies A, Chiu E, J. L, Kinney J, Genant HK (1996) Magnetic resonance imaging of trabecular bone structure in the distal radius: relationship with X-ray tmographic microscopy and biomechanics. Osteoporosis Int 6:376–385

118. Majumdar S, Weinstein RS, Prasad RR (1993) Application of fractal geometry techniques to the study of trabecular bone. Med Phys 20:1611–1619

119. Marhaug G (1993) Idiopathic juvenile osteoporosis. Scand J Rheumatol 22:45–47

120. McCord WC, Nies KM, Campion DS, Louie JS (1978) Regional migratory osteoporosis: an enervation disease. Arthritis Rheum 21:834–838

121. Meema HE (1991) Improved vertebral fracture threshold in postmenopausal osteoporosis by radiographic measurements: its usefulness in selection for preventative therapy. J Bone Miner Res 6:9–14

122. Meema HE, Meema S (1972) Microradioscopic and morphometric findings in the hand bones with densitometric findings in the proximal radius in thyrotoxicosis and in renal osteodystrophy. Invest Radiol 7:88

123. Meema HE, Meema S (1987) Postmenopausal osteoporosis: simple screening method for diagnosis before structural failure. Radiology 164:405–410

124. Meema HE, Meindok H (1992) Advantages of peripheral radiogrametry over dual-photon absorptiometry of the spine in the assessment of prevalence of osteoporotic vertebral fractures in women. J Bone Miner Res 7:897–903

125. Meszaros WT (1974) The many facets of multiple myeloma. Semin Roentgenol 9:219–228

126. Miller DS, DeTakats G (1942) Post-traumatic dystrophy of the extremities: Sudeck's atrophy. Surg Gynecol Obstet 75:558

127. Mitchell SW (1872) Gunshot wounds and other injuries. Lippincott, Philadelphia

128. Molpus WM, Pritchard RS, Walker CW, Fitzrandolph RL (1991) The radiographic spectrum of renal osteodystrophy. Am Fam Physician 43:151–158

129. Mosekilde L, Eriksen EF, Charles P (1990) Effects of thyroid hormones on bone and mineral metabolism. Endocrinol Metab Clin North Am 19:35–63

130. Murphey MD, Sartoris DJ, Quale JL, Pathria MN, Martin NL (1993) Musculoskeletal manifestations of chronic renal insufficiency. Radiographics 13:357–379

131. Mutoh S, Takeshita N, Yoshino T, Yamaguchi I (1993) Characterization of heparin-induced osteopenia in rats. Endocrinology 133:2743–2748

132. Nathanson L, Lewitan A (1941) Deformities and fractures of the vertebrae as a result of senile and presenile osteoporosis. Am J Roentgenol 46:197–202

133. Neuhold A, Hofmann S, Engel A, Leder K, Kramer J, Stiskal M, Plenk H, Wicke L (1993) Knochenmarködem – Frühform der Hüftkopfnekrose. Rofo Fortschr Geb Rontgenstr Neuen Bildgeb Verfahr 159:120–125

134. Ouyang X, Selby K, Lang P, Engelke K, Klifa C, Fan B, Zucconi F, Hottya G, Chen M, Majumdar S-H, Genant HK (1997) High resolution magnetic resonance imaging of the calcaneus: age-related changes in trabecular structure and comparison with dual X-ray absorptiometry measurements. Calcif Tissue Int 60:139–147

135. Oyen WJ, Arntz IE, Claessens RM, Van der Meer JW, Corstens FH, Goris RJ (1993) Reflex sympathetic dystrophy of the hand: an excessive inflammatory response? Pain 55:151–157

136. Park EA (1932) The Blackader lecture on some aspects of rickets. Can Med Assoc J 26:3

137. Park EA (1939) Observations on the pathology of rickets with particular reference to the changes at the cartilage-shaft junctions of growing bones. Bull NY Acad Med 15:495

138. Peacock M, Turner CH, Liu G, Manatunga AK, Timmerman L, Johnston CC Jr (1995) Better discrimination of hip fracture using bone density, geometry and architecture. Osteoporos Int 5:167–173

139. Peel NF, Moore DJ, Barrington NA, Bax DE, Eastell R (1995) Risk of vertebral fracture and relationship to bone mineral density in steroid treated rheumatoid arthritis. Ann Rheum Dis 54:801–806

140. Pitt MJ (1991) Rickets and osteomalacia are still around. Radiol Clin North Am 29:97–118

141. Pitt MJ (1995) Rickets and osteomalacia. In: Resnick D (ed) Diagnosis of bone and joint disorders 4. Saunders, Philadelphia, pp 1885–1922

142. Resnick D (1995) Hemoglobinopathies and other anemias. In: Resnick D (ed) Diagnosis of bone and joint disorders 4. Saunders, Philadelphia, pp 2107–2146

143. Resnick D (1995) Plasma cell dyscrasias and dysgammaglobulinemias. In: Resnick D (ed) Diagnosis of bone and joint disorders 4. Saunders, Philadelphia, pp 2147–2189

144. Resnick D, Niwayama G (1976) Subchondral resorption of bone in renal osteodystrophy. Radiology 118:315
145. Resnick D, Niwayama G (1995) Osteonecrosis: diagnostic techniques, specific situations, and complications. In: Resnick D (ed) Diagnosis of bone and joint disorders 5. Saunders, Philadelphia, pp 3495–3558
146. Resnick D, Niwayama G (1995) Osteoporosis. In: Resnick D (ed) Diagnosis of bone and joint disorders 4. Saunders, Philadelphia, pp 1783–1853
147. Resnick D, Niwayama G (1995) Parathyroid disorders and renal osteodystrophy. In: Resnick D (ed) Diagnosis of bone and joint disorders 4. Saunders, Philadelphia, pp 2012–2075
148. Richardson ML (1994) Can MR imaging distinguish between transient osteoporosis of the femoral head and osteonecrosis? AJR Am J Roentgenol 162:1244
149. Richardson ML, Pozzi-Mucelli RS, Kanter AS, Kolb FO, Ettinger B, Genant HK (1986) Bone mineral changes in primary hyperparathyroidism. Skeletal Radiol 15:85–95
150. Rico H, Hernandez ER (1989) Bone radiogrametry: caliper versus magnifying glass. Calcif Tissue Int 45:285–287
151. Riggs BL, Melton LJ (1983) Evidence for two distinct syndromes of involutional osteoporosis. Am J Med 75:899–901
152. Root L (1984) The treatment of osteogenesis imperfecta. Orthop Clin North Am 15:775
153. Rosen RA (1970) Transitory demineralization of the femoral head. Radiology 94:509–512
154. Rosenberg AE (1991) The pathology of metabolic bone disease. Radiol Clin North Am 29:19–35
155. Rosenthal DI, Gregg GA, Slovik DM, Neer RM (1987) A comparison of quantitative computed tomography to four techniques of upper extremity bone mass measurement. In: Genant HK (ed) Osteoporosis update 1987. Radiology Research and Education Foundation, San Francisco, pp 87–93
156. Rupp WM, McCarthy HB, Rohde TD, Blackshear PJ, Goldenberg FJ, Buchwald H (1982) Risk of osteoporosis in patients treated with long-term intravenous heparin therapy. Curr Surg 39:419–422
157. Ruttimann UE, Webber RL, Hazelrig JB (1992) Fractal dimension from radiographs of peridental alveolar bone. A possible diagnostic indicator of osteoporosis. Oral Surg Oral Med Oral Pathol 74:98–110
158. Sackler JP, Liu L (1973) Heparin-induced osteoporosis. Br J Radiol 46:548–550
159. Saito JK, Davis JW, Wasnich RD, Ross PD (1995) Users of low-dose glucocorticoids have increased bone loss rates: a longitudinal study. Calcif Tissue Int 57:115–119
160. Saitoh S, Nakatsuchi Y, Latta L, Milne E (1993) An absence of structural changes in the proximal femur with osteoporosis. Skeletal Radiol 22:425–431
161. Samarabandu J, Acharya R, Hausmann E, Allen K (1993) Analysis of bone X-rays using morphological fractals. IEEE Trans Med Imaging 12:466–470

162. Sarangi PP, Ward AJ, Smith EJ, Staddon GE, Atkins RM (1993) Algodystrophy and osteoporosis after tibial fractures. J Bone Joint Surg Br 75:450–452

163. Saville PD (1965) Changes in bone mass with age and alcoholism. J Bone Joint Surg Am 47:492–499

164. Saville PD (1967) A quantitative approach to simple radiographic diagnosis of osteoporosis: its application to the osteoporosis of rheumatoid arthritis. Arthritis Rheum 10:416–422

165. Schatz M, Dudl J, Zeiger RS, Harden K, Chilingar L, Forsythe A, Baylink DJ (1993) Osteoporosis in corticosteroid-treated asthmatic patients: clinical correlates. Allergy Proc 14:341–345

166. Schuster J, Meier-Ruge W, Egli F (1969) Zur Pathologie der Osteopathie nach Heparinbehandlung. Dtsch Med Wochenschr 94:2334

167. Schwartzman RJ, McLellan TL (1987) Reflex sympathetic dystrophy: a review. Arch Neurol 44:555–561

168. Seeman E, Szmukler GI, Formica C, Tsalamandris C, Mestrovic R (1992) Osteoporosis in anorexia nervosa: the influence of peak bone density, bone loss, oral contraceptive use, and exercise. J Bone Miner Res 7:1467–1474

169. Silverstein MN, Kelly PJ (1967) Osteoarticular manifestations of Gaucher's disease. Am J Med Sci 253:569–577

170. Singh M, Riggs BL, Beabout JW, Jowsey J (1972) Femoral trabecular-pattern index for evaluation of spinal osteoporosis. Ann Intern Med 77:63–67

171. Singh YM, Nagrath AR, Maini PS (1970) Changes in trabecular pattern of the upper end of the femur as an index of osteoporosis. J Bone Joint Surg Am 52:457–467

172. Smith R (1995) Idiopathic juvenile osteoporosis: experience of twenty-one patients. Br J Rheumatol 34:68–77

173. Smith R, Stevenson JC, Winearls CG, Woods CG, Wordsworth BP (1985) Osteoporosis of pregnancy. Lancet :1178–1180

174. Solomon BL, Wartofsky L, Burman KD (1993) Prevalence of fractures in postmenopausal women with thyroid disease. Thyroid 3:17–23

175. Squires JW, Pinch LW (1979) Heparin-induced spinal fractures. J Am Med Assoc 241:2417–2418

176. Steinbach HL, Gordan GS, Eisenberg E, Carne JT, Silverman S, Goldman L (1961) Primary hyperthyroidism: a correlation of roentgen, clinical, and pathologic features. Am J Roentgenol Radium Ther Nucl Med 86:239–243

177. Steinbach HL, Kolb FO, Gilfillan R (1954) A mechanism of the production of pseudofractures in osteomalacia (Milkman's syndrome). Radiology 62:388

178. Steinbach HL, Noetzli M (1964) Roentgen appearance of the skeleton in osteomalacia and rickets. Am J Radiol 91:955

179. Steinert H, Hahn K (1996) Wertigkeit der Drei Phasen Skelettszintigraphie zur Frühdiagnostik des Morbus Sudeck. Rofo Fortschr Geb Röntgenstr Neuen Bildgeb Verfahr 164:318–323

180. Sudeck P (1901) Über die akute (reflectorische) Knochenatrophie nach Entzündungen und Verletzungen an den Extremitäten und ihre klinischen Erscheinungen. Rofo 5:277
181. Sundaram M (1989) Renal osteodystrophy. Skeletal Radiol 18:415–426
182. Swezey RL (1970) Transient osteoporosis of the hip, foot and knee. Arthritis Rheum 94:858–868
183. Takada M, Steiner E, Genant HK (1994) Diagnostic imaging in chronic renal failure. J Jpn Soc Dial Ther 27:1281–1293
184. Thompson Jr RC (1973) Heparin osteoporosis. An experimental model using rats. J Bone Joint Surg Am SS:606
185. Todorovic Tirnanic M, Obradovic V, Han R, Goldner B, Stankovic D, Sekulic D, Lazic T, Djordjevic B (1995) Diagnostic approach to reflex sympathetic dystrophy after fracture: radiography or bone scintigraphy? Eur J Nucl Med 22:1187–1193
186. Toh SH, Claunch BC, Brown PH (1985) Effect of hyperthyroidism and its treatment on bone mineral content. Arch Intern Med 145:883–886
187. Trepman E, King TV (1992) Transient osteoporosis of the hip misdiagnosed as osteonecrosis on magnetic resonance imaging. Orthop Rev 21:1089–1091, 1094–1098
188. Urist MR (1960) Observations bearing on the problem of osteoporosis. In: Rodahl K, Nicholson JT, Brown EM Jr (eds) Bone as a tissue. McGraw-Hill, New York, pp 18–45
189. Vande Berg BE, Malghem JJ, Labaisse MA, Noel HM, Maldague BE (1993) MR imaging of avascular necrosis and transient marrow edema of the femoral head. Radiographics 13:501–520
190. Vetter U, Pontz B, Zauner E, Brenner RE, Spranger J (1992) Osteogenesis imperfecta: a clinical study of the first ten years of life. Calcif Tissue Int 50:36–41
191. Virtama P (1960) Uneven distribution of bone mineral and covering effect of non-mineralized tissue as reasons for impaired detectability of bone density from roentgenograms. Ann Med Int Fenn 49:57–65
192. Virtama P, Helela T (1969) Radiographic measurements of cortical bone. Acta Radiol (Stockh) [Suppl] 293
193. Wang YZ, Xing SZ, Hu JQ (1991) Reassessment on roentgenologic signs of early rickets. Roentgenopathologic correlations of 52 en block specimens. Chin Med J Engl 104:91–95
194. Wicks M, Garrett R, Vernon-Roberts B, Fazzalari N (1982) Absence of metabolic bone disease in the proximal femur in patients with fracture of the femoral neck. J Bone Joint Surg Br 64:319–323
195. Williamson MR, Boyd CM, Williamson SL (1990) Osteoporosis: diagnosis by plain chest film versus dual-photon bone densitometry. Skeletal Radiol 19:27–30
196. Wolbarst AB (1993) Dependence of attenuation on atomic number and photon energy. Physics of radiology. Appleton and Lange, Norwalk, pp 113–121

197. Zionts LE, Nash JP, Rude R, Ross T, Stott NS (1995) Bone mineral density in children with mild osteogenesis imperfecta. J Bone Joint Surg Br 77:143–147

12 Assessment of Vertebral Fracture

M. Jergas and D. Felsenberg

Introduction

In everyday clinical practice radiologists visually analyze radiographs of the thoracolumbar spine in the lateral projection to identify vertebral fractures in patients whose clinical indications suggest trauma, osteoporosis, malignancy, or acute back pain. While diagnosing the vertebral fracture in question, the interpreter also considers the potential differential diagnoses of this deformity. The radiologist's decision can be aided by additional radiographic projections such as anteroposterior or oblique views and by complementary examinations such as bone scintigraphy, computed tomography, and magnetic resonance imaging. Thus in a clinical environment the detection of vertebral fractures seldom poses great difficulties.

For epidemiological studies and clinical drug trials in osteoporosis research, requirements and expectations differ considerably from those in a clinical environment. For research purposes, the examinations are frequently performed without specific clinical indications and without therapeutic ramifications, while in clinical practice differential diagnosis and therapeutic decisions are of greatest interest.

The diagnostic procedures available for vertebral fracture assessment are usually restricted to lateral radiographs of the thoracolumbar spine. Furthermore, the number of subjects to be reviewed is often quite large, requiring an efficient assessment procedure. The qualitative assessment of vertebral fractures is affected by subjective factors because it depends heavily on the individual reader's training and experience, and the usual techniques of visual assessment may be insufficient in a research environment, where "objective" and reproducible tests are required. Since vertebral fractures represent a frequently used endpoint in clinical and epidemiological studies on osteoporosis, several methods have been proposed to meet the demands of research on the diagnosis of prevalent and incident vertebral fractures [11, 12, 29, 43, 44]. As with other fractures, vertebral fractures have characteristic features that allow a distinct description and classification, for example, gradations in severity, the permanent nature of the deformity and the possibility of a repeat fracture at the same site (Table 12-1).

Early reports on osteoporosis in the imaging literature gave descriptions primarily of the radiographic findings of osteopenia and the associated vertebral

Table 12-1 Comparison of features of vertebral fractures with other fractures (modified from Kleerekoper et al. [45])

Characteristic	Vertebral Fractures	Other Fractures
Severity	Graded	Mostly all or none
Impaction	invariable	Rare
Restoration of shape	Not possible	Common
Refracture at the same site	Common	Rare
Trauma	Mostly minimal, often not recalled	Common, usually severe
Absence of pain	Highly variable	Rare

deformities [2, 42, 61]. Common patterns of the disease, such as the "diminution of vertebrae in various forms" or the "crookedness and shortening of the spine" were observed, and several terms for the description of the associated vertebral deformities, for example, "fish vertebra," were introduced. Based on these findings, several standardized approaches have been developed to assess vertebral fractures. Wedging of vertebrae led Fletcher to propose an "index of wedging" to describe normal variations in anterior heights in comparison with posterior heights [21]. This was the first description of a quantitative method to assess vertebral deformities, and the author concluded from his results in young men that in deviations from the normal values "the cause cannot be determined with certainty." An often described feature of the osteoporotic spine, the biconcavity of vertebrae, was used in the biconcavity index proposed by Barnett and Nordin to diagnose osteoporosis [4, 5]. Hurxthal was the first to describe in detail the measurement of vertebral heights for the purpose of assessing anterior wedge fractures [34]. These studies have been the starting points for many studies and methods that rely solely on the quantitative, morphometric assessment of vertebral fractures.

At the same time new ways to visually diagnose vertebral fractures were being developed. These methods also rely on the basic features of vertebral deformities, especially their distinct gradations, their permanence, and their possible refracture. These diagnostic approaches, in which vertebral fractures are visually assessed by radiologists or experienced clinicians, are generally referred to as standardized visual (or semiquantitative) assessments of vertebral deformities. These two methods, the quantitative morphometric and the standardized visual (semiquantiative), are the subject of this chapter.

Standardized Visual Assessment of Vertebral Fractures

Standardized visual assessment is the assignment of numeric scores to vertebral deformities or fractures, or their assignment to distinct categories, according to their shape or type and their severity in a definable and reproducible manner without making measurements of vertebral dimensions. Several standardized approaches to describing vertebral fractures have been proposed. They may serve to facilitate the diagnosis of osteoporosis and to assess the severity or progression of the disease or of singular vertebral deformities.

The first standardized approach was proposed by Smith and colleagues [78]. They introduced the following classification of vertebral deformities as diagnosed from lateral radiographs of the thoracolumbar spine for the purpose of diagnosing the severity of osteoporosis:

- Indeterminate: borderline or equivocal findings, questionable loss of bone density and trabecular thinning, no vertebral body deformity
- Grade 1: overall density loss and trabecular markings, endplate deformities and biconcavities, definite wedging of one or more vertebral bodies
- Grade 2: further loss of density and of trabecular markings, endplate deformities and biconcavities, definite wedging of one or more vertebral bodies
- Grade 3: severe demineralization, extensive biconcavities, marked wedging or collapse of several vertebral bodies

As with the biconcavity index of Barnett and Nordin, the approach by Smith and colleagues grades only the vertebra with the most severe deformity on the radiograph. The patient is assigned a grade of normal, indeterminate, or osteoporotic (1–3, depending on the most severe deformity). This means that the spinal radiographs are evaluated on a per patient, not a per vertebra, basis. In the context of epidemiological studies or drug trials, this approach has some serious limitations. A follow-up of vertebral deformities is almost impossible because of the per patient evaluation, which does not take changes in individual vertebrae into account. Even for the assessment of the present status of a patient, this method provides only a relatively crude measure for the severity of osteoporosis. Smith's classification never gained widespread acceptance and was applied in only a few studies.

In contrast to the method of Smith and colleagues, Meunier proposed an approach in which each vertebra is graded according to its shape or deformity [58]. Grade 1 is assigned to a normal vertebra that has no deformity; grade 2 to a biconcave vertebra; and grade 4 to an endplate fracture or a wedged or crushed vertebra (Fig. 12-1). Vertebral bodies T3 (or T7) to L4 are evaluated [55,59]. A radiological vertebral index (RVI) can be calculated as the sum of the grades of all vertebrae, or as the quotient of this sum and the number of the vertebrae. The consideration of individual vertebral deformities makes the RVI suitable for assessing the extent of osteoporosis in a given individual and for follow-up examinations. A major limitation of this method is that it assesses only the type of the vertebral deformity, i.e., biconcavity versus fracture. The severity of the fracture is not assessed at all. In a baseline examination for prevalent fractures, each fracture, whether diminutive or severe, would have the same weight in the RVI. In follow-up examinations this means that refractures may not be detected at all. With its distinction between biconcavity and fracture, this approach introduced the concept of "vertebral deformity," as opposed to vertebral fracture. However, this method did not expressly attempt to distinguish nonfracture deformities, such

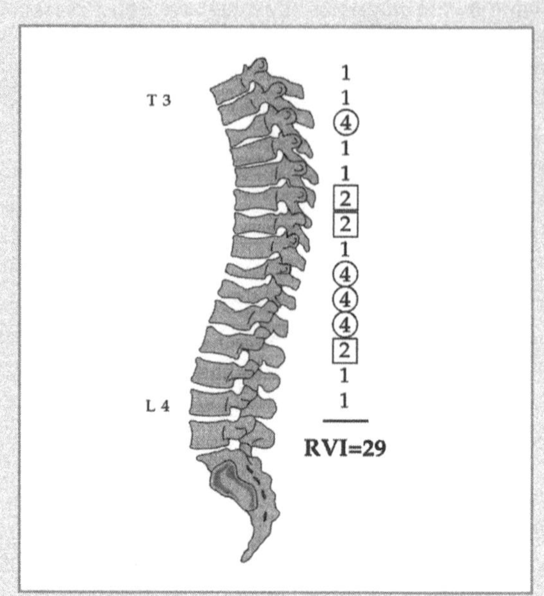

Fig. 12-1 Meunier's radiological vertebral index (RVI). Depending on the type of deformity a grade of 1 (normal vertebra), 2 (biconcavity), or 4 (endplate, wedge, or crush fracture) is assigned to a vertebra. The sum of the grades is the RVI

as degenerative remodeling, from actual fractures. The RVI has been applied in clinical drug trials that evaluated the fracture rate in patients with fluoride and calcitonin medication [59]. Overall, however, the RVI has never gained wide acceptance in epidemiological studies or clinical drug trials.

Kleerekoper and colleagues modified Meunier's radiological vertebral index and introduced the vertebral deformity score (VDS) [45]. In the VDS each vertebra from T4 to L5 is assigned an individual score from 0 to 3, depending on the type of deformity. This grading scheme is based on the reduction in the anterior, middle, and posterior vertebral heights (h_a, h_m, and h_p, respectively). A vertebral deformity (graded 1–3) is present when h_a, h_m, or h_p is reduced by at least 4 mm or 15% (Fig. 12-2). A VDS of 0 is assigned to a normal vertebra that has no reduction in any vertebral height. VDS of 1 corresponds to a vertebral endplate deformity, with h_a and% being normal. A wedge deformity with a reduction in h_a and, to a lesser extent, h_m is assigned a VDS of 2. A compression deformity, which is assigned a VDS of 3, is characterized by a reduction in all three vertebral heights. If one graded all vertebrae from T4 to L5 using this score, the minimum VDS possible for the whole spine would be 0 (all vertebrae intact), and the maximum score possible would be 42 (compression fractures of all vertebrae).

However, as with Meunier's RVI, the VDS still relies very much on the type of deformity, i.e., the vertebral shape, and there would have to be changes in verte-

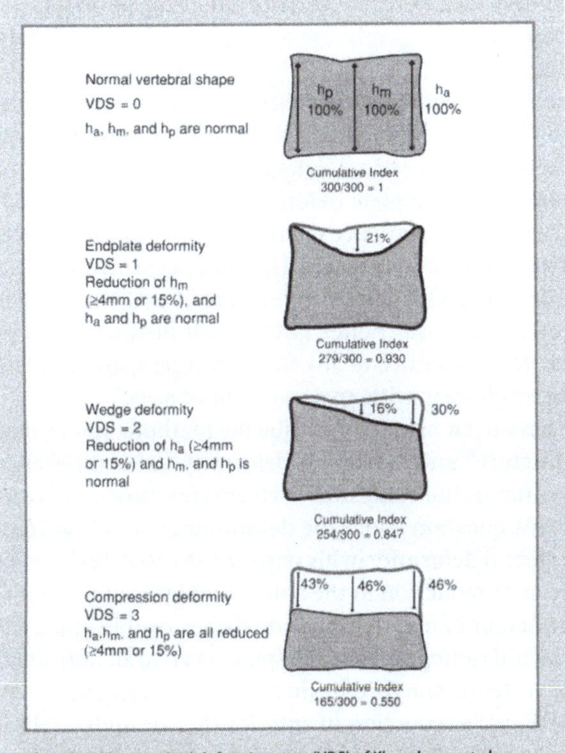

Fig. 12-2 The vertebral deformity score (VDS) of Kleerekoper et al. A grade of zero is assigned to a normal vertebra. A reduction in any vertebral height (h3, hm, tip) by at least 4 mm or 15% is assigned a grade of 1–3, depending on which height(s) is involved. A quantitative evaluation is also possible (cumulative index)

bral shape in order to account for incident vertebral fractures on follow-up radiographs. The grades do not necessarily reflect the progression of a vertebral fracture or its magnitude. Furthermore, most vertebral fractures appear to consist of a combination of wedge and endplate deformities, and less frequently posterior deformities. Therefore a reader's distinction among these deformities is often extremely arbitrary. Taking the possibly continuous character of vertebral deformities into consideration, the authors expanded their method by adding a quantitative component to it. Assigning a value of 100% to each of h_a, h_m, and h_p for each normal vertebra, reductions in these heights can be measured and expressed as percentage reduction from normal. A cumulative score can thus be calculated for each of the measured vertebrae (Fig. 12-2). This extension of the method is already beyond the scope of a standardized visual (semiquantitative) evaluation of vertebral fractures. A major limitation of this quantitative method, and one that applies in part also to its semiquantitative component (a height reduction of 4 mm or 15% for the diagnosis of vertebral deformity), is the accurate evaluation of the height reduction. Ideally, vertebral deformities can be diagnosed only when corresponding baseline radiographs are available, and one is certain about the normal vertebral height.

Nielsen and coworkers evaluated both interobserver agreement and intraobserver reproducibility of the VDS [65]. Between two observers the agreement on the presence of the different types of vertebral deformity ranged from 74% to 87%, with the poorest agreement for endplate deformities (VDS 1). The agreement between the two observers on the presence of any fracture was 87%. A better agreement between the two observers was reached for the absence of any fractures (fracture/nonfracture dichotomy), where an agreement of 94% was reported. The intraobserver reproducibility was better both for all distinct kinds of deformities and for the presence or absence of any fracture. Again, for endplate fractures the reproducibility was lowest, with an agreement of 88%.

The terminology that we have been using to describe the methods sometimes varies between "vertebral fracture" and "vertebral deformity." This difference represents a substantial question in the context of vertebral fracture diagnosis. Kleerekoper actually raises this question about the definition of vertebral fractures in comparison with vertebral deformity in his paper on the VDS [45]. There he defines vertebral fracture as "a reduction in the anterior height with or without a reduction in posterior height of a vertebral body that is readily apparent on naked eye inspection on lateral radiographs of the spine (even to an untrained observer)." In contrast to the vertebral fracture, he then defines a permanent vertebral deforming event (PVDE) as "a reduction in anterior (h_a), or midvertebral (h_m), or posterior (h_p) height beyond an arbitrarily set value and occurring between one lateral spine radiograph and a subsequent one obtained after a specified time interval." This definition narrows PVDEs to incident vertebral deformities or fractures. From the first definition of a vertebral fracture it is clear that PVDEs can become vertebral fractures (corresponding to a VDS 2 or 3) or vertebral deformities (VDS 1 or endplate deformity). Changes in the midvertebral height are not included in the definition of a vertebral fracture. This may be regarded as quite an arbitrary definition that is probably based on the understanding that biconcave vertebrae are not necessarily vertebral fractures. In fact, this distinction between endplate deformities and vertebral fractures may not be relevant in that end-plate deformities may be associated with osteoporosis and also may be predictors of future fractures.

A vertebral deformity is not always a vertebral fracture, but a vertebral fracture is always a vertebral deformity. From the perspective of the radiologist there is a long list of potential differential diagnoses for vertebral deformities, and the correct qualitative classification of vertebral deformities can be achieved only by visual inspection and expert interpretation of a radiograph. This perspective on vertebral fracture diagnosis is probably best reflected in the semiquantitative fracture assessment proposed by Genant [24, 27]. Here the severity of a fracture is assessed solely by visual determination of the extent of a vertebral height reduction and morphological change, and vertebral fractures are differentiated from other, nonfracture deformities. The approximate degree of height reduction determines the assignment of grades to a vertebra. This method is referred to as semiquantitative assessment of vertebral fractures. Unlike the other approaches, the type of the deformity (wedge, biconcavity, or compression) is no longer linked to the grading of a fracture in this approach. Thoracic and lumbar vertebrae from T4 to L4 are graded on visual inspection and without direct vertebral measurement as normal (grade 0), mildly deformed (grade 1: approximately a 20%–25% reduction in anterior, middle, and/or posterior height and a 10%–20% reduction in the projected vertebral area), moderately deformed (grade 2: approximately a 25%–40% reduction in anterior, middle, and/or posterior height and a 20%–40% reduction in the projected vertebral area), and severely deformed (grade 3: approximately a 40% or greater reduction in anterior, middle, and/or posterior height and the projected vertebral area). The authors gave a grade 0.5 to designate "borderline" vertebrae that show some deformation but cannot be clearly assigned to grade 1 fractures. In addition to height reductions, careful attention is given to alterations in the shape and configuration of the vertebrae relative to adjacent vertebrae and expected normal appearances. These features add a strong qualitative aspect to the interpretation and also render this method less readily definable as either qualitative or quantitative. Nevertheless, in experienced or highly trained hands, it makes the approach both relatively sensitive and specific. From this semiquantitative assessment a spinal fracture index (SFI) can be calculated as the sum of all grades assigned to the vertebrae divided by the number of the evaluated vertebrae. An illustration of the grading scheme is given in Fig. 12-3.

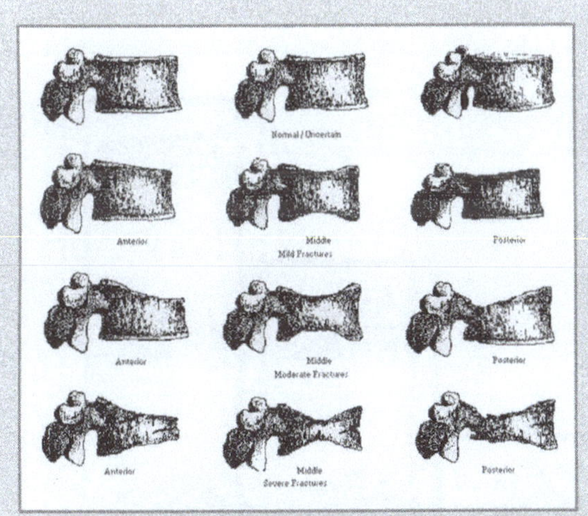

Fig. 12-3 Genant's grading scheme for a semiquantitative evaluation of vertebral fractures. The drawings illustrate normal vertebrae (top row) and mild to severe fractures (respectively, in the following rows). The size of the reduction in the anterior, middle, or posterior height is reflected in a corresponding fracture grade, from 1 (mild) to 3 (severe). (Drawing courtesy of Dr. C.Y. Wu)

Assessing the severity of the deformation as the reduction in vertebral height means (especially for the interpretation of incident fractures) that refractures of preexisting vertebral fractures may be assessed using this approach. This is an advantage of Genant's approach over the other standardized visual approaches; since it considers the continuous character of vertebral fractures, it makes possible a meaningful interpretation of follow-up radiographs (Fig. 12-4). Furthermore, this approach has no requirement for (inevitably arbitrary) decisions regarding wedge, endplate, or crush deformities, since most fractures contain combinations of these features and are influenced by the local biomechanics of the spinal level involved.

It has been argued that the diagnosis of mild vertebral fractures in particular, as used in Genant's semiquantitative grading scheme, may be quite subjective, and that these fractures may be unrelated to osteoporosis. However, mild fractures detected with this method are also associated with a lower bone density than normal, and they also predict future vertebral fractures, although to a lesser extent than moderate or severe fractures do [6]. For the diagnosis of incident fractures, other limitations may apply. Generally, incident fractures are more easily identified qualitatively on serial radiographs since a direct comparison with baseline radiographs is possible. Using Genant's semiquantitative grading scheme for the assessment of incident fractures, however, the reader may sometimes feel that even though a further height reduction is seen in a vertebra, it may not be justified to assign a higher grade to the incident fracture in comparison with the preexisting prevalent fracture since some degree of settling or remodeling generally occurs.

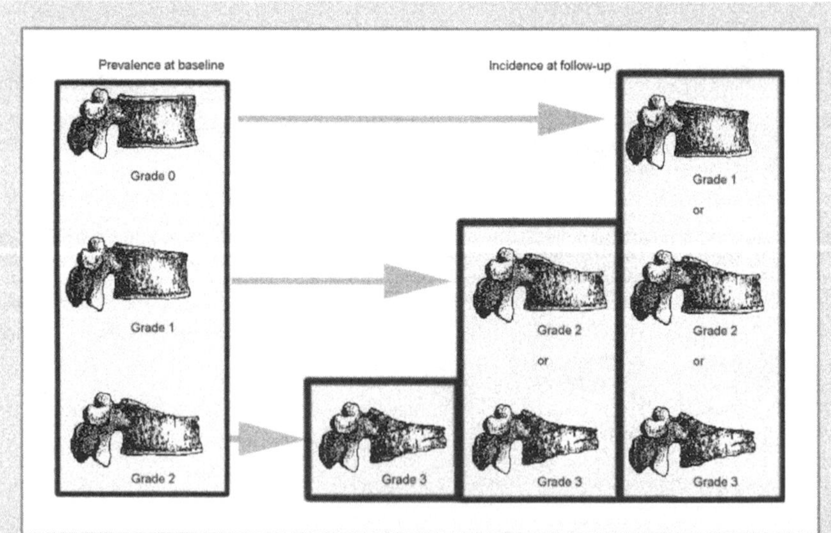

Fig. 12-4 Diagnosing incident vertebral fractures using Genant's semiquantitative grading scheme. Incident fracture may occur in nonfractured as well as in previously fractured vertebrae (Drawing courtesy of Dr. C.Y. Wu)

Both the intra- and the interobserver agreement for the diagnosis of prevalent and incident vertebral fractures were found to be excellent, indicating that Genant's semiquantitative grading scheme is highly reproducible among trained readers [27, 49, 88]. Even relatively inexperienced readers can assess vertebral fractures using this grading scheme with good results. Nevertheless, a clear limitation to the studies on intra- and interobserver agreement of Genant's method is that all readers, while initially trained at different institutions, underwent centralized and standardized specific training for semiquantitative fracture assessment. This implies that the agreement reached in this study may be higher than can be usually expected across different geographic centers. The semiquantitative grading scheme by Genant has been applied in a number of epidemiological studies and pharmaceutical trials through the 1980s until today [18, 33, 85–87].

Quantitative Morphometric Assessment of Vertebral Fractures

In quantitative morphometry the diagnosis of vertebral deformities relies on the measurement of distinct vertebral dimensions. Typically these are the anterior, the middle (or central), and the posterior heights: h_a, h_m, and h_p [7, 10, 17, 34, 53, 56, 57, 60, 74–76]. In some studies vertebral area and width are also assessed [19, 31, 62, 80]. Figure 12-5 shows normal values for the three vertebral heights for T4–L4 from a large epidemiological study [7]. This graph shows the typical pattern of the vertebral heights for the designated vertebral levels. Depending on the radiographic technique, the way in which the vertebral dimensions are obtained, and the population studied, the results from different studies may vary. Thus accurate assessment of vertebral dimensions within a population for the purpose of defining reliable normative data or to diagnose vertebral deformities depends on the quality and consistency of the techniques used. Banks et al. have proposed a protocol for obtaining radiographs of the lumbar and thoracic spine that is giv-

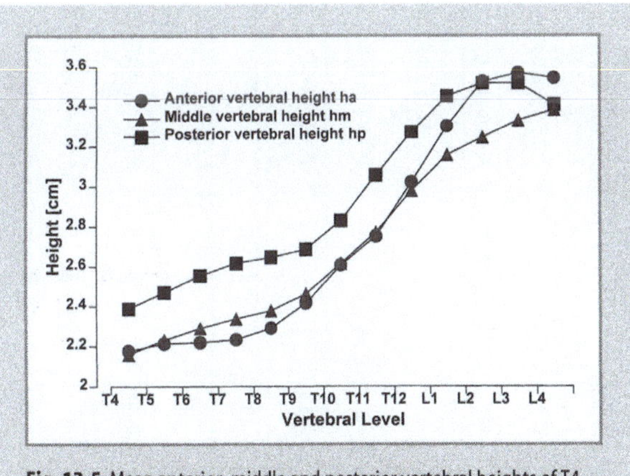

Fig. 12-5 Mean anterior, middle and posterior vertebral heights of T4 through L4 as derived from the Study of Osteoporotic Fractures [7]

Table 12-2 Radiographic techniques for anteroposterior and lateral radiographs of the lumbar and thoracic spine (adapted from [3])

Factor	Setting or instruction			
	AP thoracic spine	Lateral thoracic spine	AP lumbar spine	Lateral lumbar spine
Patient position	Supine on Bucky table	Lateral (ideally left) on Bucky table	Supine on Bucky table	Lateral on Bucky table
Focal spot size	<1.3 mm			
Total filtration	>3.0 mm Al			
Antiscatter grid radio	r=12:1; 40/cm			
Focal film distance	100–120 cm, standardized			
Voltage	60–70 kVp	60–85 kVp	70–80 kVp	80–100 kVp
Automatic exposure control	Central chamber	Chambers deselected	Central chamber	Chambers deselected
Exposure time	<0.5 s (manual)	<0.4 s, or 4 s and a high mA for breathing technique	<0.4 s	<1.0 s
Film screen combination	Speed class 400			
Film size	18x43 cm for normal spine; 35x43 cm for scoliotic spine	18x43 cm for normal spine; 35x43 cm for kyphotic spine	30x40 cm	18x43 cm for normal spine; 30x40 cm for severe lordotic spine
Centering point	Midline at T7 level	5 cm anterior to T7 spinous process	Midline at L3 level (usually lower costal margin)	10 cm anterior to L3 spinous process
Arms	By side	Raised at right angles to the body with the elbows flexed	By side	Raised at right angles to the body
Legs		Hips and knees flexed	Knees raised with feet on table	Hips and knees flexed
Lead rubber		On X-ray table, posterior to thoracic spine		On X-ray table, posterior to lumbar spine
Respiration	Arrested inspiration to lower diaphragm	Arrested expiration		
Radiation protection	Lead protective waist apron	Lead rubber gonad protection		

en in Table 12-2 [3]. A breathing technique for obtaining radiographs of the thoracic spine in the lateral projection cannot be recommended generally; even though it improves visualization of the lower thoracic vertebrae, the radiation dose is higher (approx. 0.65 mSv vs. 0.3 mSv), and for reasons of radiation protection, the application of this technique has been prohibited in some countries.

The requirements for a standardization of techniques also applies to the registration of vertebral dimensions. In the first studies published on quantitative morphometry, the investigators used translucent rulers or calipers [14,36,56,69]. The application of these instruments for the measurement of vertebral heights has some disadvantages, however. The measurements are relatively imprecise; often measurements are made only to the nearest millimeter. Furthermore, the results must be transcribed manually. This can result in an immense workload in large studies, and there is a risk of transcription errors. These shortcomings have led investigators to develop new procedures to simplify the registration of vertebral dimensions. The measurement of vertebral dimensions by so-called point-digitization, or simply "digitization," of radiographs facilitates the evaluation considerably [38,62,82]. In most studies, digitizing radiographs means entering specific coordinates into a computer for computation of vertebral dimensions. The coordinates are entered by marking certain points using a pointing device on a radiograph that has been placed on a digitizing tablet (Fig. 12-6). A digitizing tablet is a special data entry device that can transmit precise coordinates to a computer. For digitizing radiographs the tablet has a special translucent surface with background illumination, similar to a radiographic view box. A reader sets marks by means of a cursor-like input device that is equipped with fine crosshairs to allow an exact point placement. The marked points are transmitted and stored as local coordinates in the computer. Vertebral heights are then calculated from the stored coordinates.

There is no uniform approach for marking digitization points, and different institutions have applied point digitization differently [62, 82]. Six-point digitization is the most widely used technique [79, 82]. The four-corner points of the vertebral body are marked, as well as an additional point in the middle of the upper and lower endplates (Fig. 12-7). Other reported methods include eight- and ten-point digitization [57, 62]. One important difference between these techniques is the placement of points in the middle of the vertebral endplates. In case the outer contours of the endplates are not perfectly superimposed, a rather frequent finding, the middle points in six-point digitization are chosen in the center between the upper and the lower contours. With eight- and ten-point digitization two points are placed in the middle of the upper and lower contours, respectively. The middle height is then calculated as the average of the two resulting middle heights, or as one height of which the endpoints are the centers between the marked points on the vertebral contours. McCloskey also recorded an additional "minimum height" in cases of an obvious endplate fracture [53]. In ten-point digitization, further points are placed in the middle of the anterior and posterior contours of the vertebral body. These additional digitization points are used

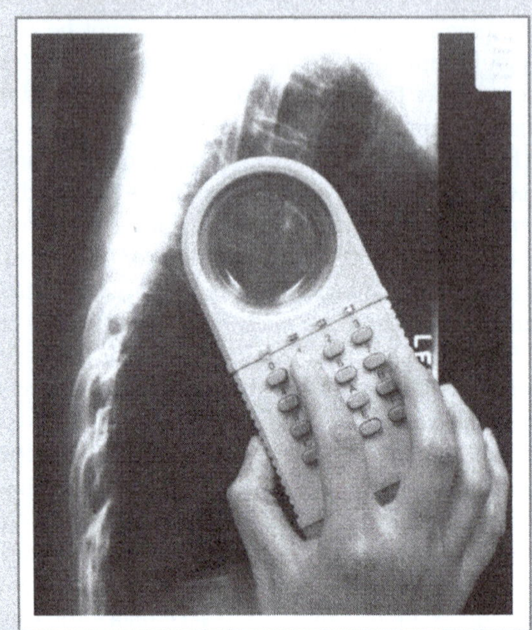

Fig. 12-6 Point digitization for the quantitative morphometric assessment of vertebral fractures. Points are placed at the endpoints of the anterior, middle, and posterior heights using a translucent cursor on a digitizing table

only for the calculation of vertebral area. A comparative study between six- and ten-point digitization shows 5% larger vertebral area for six-point digitization [62]. Point digitization techniques such as the ones described have been used in numerous studies, and the technical requirements are well established. These show reasonable precision errors of 1%–9% for vertebral heights and 3%–11% for the vertebral area on the same film [53, 62, 64, 79, 80, 82]. A good knowledge of the radiographic anatomy of the spine is required for the accurate and reproducible application of point digitization.

A very different approach was presented by Brinckmann et al., who published results for vertebral dimensions in a young normal population [9]. These authors used a digitization technique entering multiple digitization points only few millimeters apart to exactly describe the vertebral contours. Reference points, for example, the corner points, are determined in a second step. Using this technique, a precise definition of vertebral dimensions is feasible. Based on these reference points, a number of vertebral dimensions are calculated. However, the authors do not use absolute distances but rather quotients from heights or angles to account for differences in the projection between the radiographs, for example, magnification error. However, although the effect of differences in the projection may be reduced by this technique, it cannot be eliminated completely. The precision error

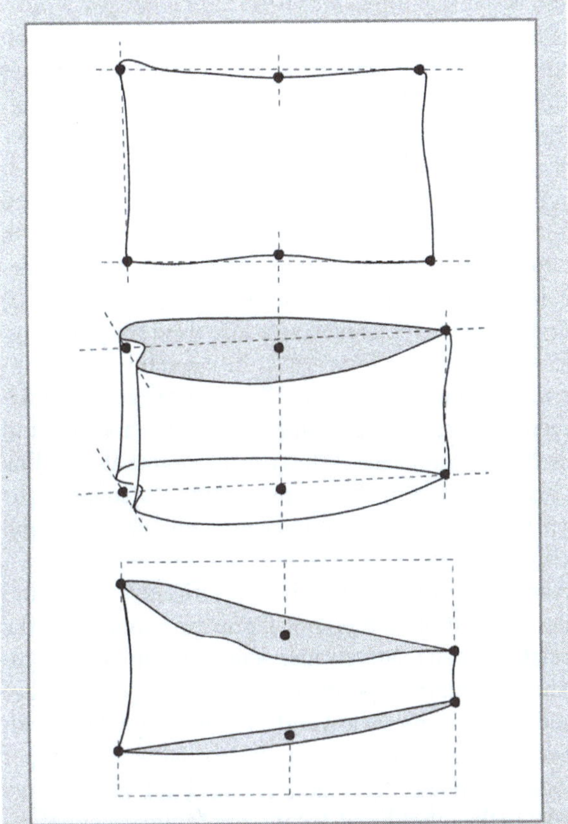

Fig. 12-7 In six-point-digitization the endpoints of the vertebral heights are marked directly on the vertebra. *Above*, point placement on a vertebra that is ideally projected with perfect superposition of the vertebral contours. *Below*, when the vertebra is rotated and oblique, point placement is more difficult

for this method is given as 1%–1.6% for the determination of typical quotients. Frobin et al. recently published normative data for vertebral heights, disk height and sagittal plane displacement for lumbar vertebrae using this technique [22]. As of yet there are no results existing for an application of this technique to identify vertebral deformities in osteoporosis.

Most investigators measure the vertebral heights directly on the radiographs. Another technique is to first trace the vertebral contours for the radiographs onto transparent paper and then measure the vertebral dimensions from the tracings [14,15,23,67]. This introduces another potential source of error that is determined by the accuracy of the tracing. Gallagher et al. found that the precision error roughly doubled when two sets of tracings from the same radiographs were used [23].

Some investigators assessed vertebral dimensions from digital images of radiographs [1, 19, 20, 41, 72, 73]. These digital images are generally obtained from an electronic capture of conventional radiographs using a video-camera or other scanning devices, such as flatbed scanners. This technique is also referred to as digitization. Depending on the method used, the image resolution can be on the order of 0.2 mm or better. The resulting files are relatively large. For example, a radiograph of the thoracic spine (35.6x43.2 cm) scanned at 0.2 mm spatial resolution and 3600 levels of gray (12-bit depth) may take up approximately 6–8 megabytes of disk space. High-resolution monitors may be required to visualize these images adequately. Adami et al. used a classic six-point digitization technique with digital images [1]. In the approach by Evans and colleagues, who also used six-point digitization on digital images of conventional radiographs, the operator must manually choose the four corner points of a vertebra [19]. The software automatically identifies midpoints between the corresponding upper and lower anterior and posterior corner points. Then the operator selects the true midpoints along a line joining these automatically placed midpoints best representing the edges of the vertebral body. Intraobserver variation for height measurements was 3.1% and interobserver variation was 5.3%.

Using digitized films for vertebral morphometry has specific advantages and disadvantages. The digitization process often does not capture the contrast of the original radiographs appropriately when relatively inexpensive commercial scanners are used. This may result in a substantially poorer quality of the digitized image in comparison with its original. For example, Evans and colleagues could not evaluate T4 in 24%, and T5 in 5% of all patients due to poor image quality in the upper thoracic region [19]. Of all other vertebrae less than 2% could not be evaluated because of poor image quality. On the other hand, techniques for image enhancement can be applied to digitally captured radiographs. Often structures that were partially hidden previously can thus the revealed. Several investigators have applied a number of different techniques for acquiring radiographic images in digitized form and for determining vertebral dimensions from digital images.

An interactive semiautomated method for vertebral height measurements was published by the Rédei and colleagues [70]. For this purpose the films are scanned using a high-resolution laser film digitizer. In the first step these authors use edge-enhancement filters to highlight vertebral edges. The operator then marks several control points along the anterior and posterior borders of the vertebrae. The computer connects the points with a smooth curve. Then the operator deposits endplate lines fitting the contours of the endplates, and following this the computer replaces the intersecting lines with boxes. The operator marks the lowest and highest points of the endplates, and the computer corrects the endplate contours accordingly for vertebral height determinations.

Felsenberg and Kalidis, in close cooperation with Kalender, proposed an automated technique for measuring vertebral dimensions from digitized radiographs [20, 41]. This method is based on contour finding algorithms as they are applied for an automated placement of slices in quantitative computed tomography (Fig. 12-8)

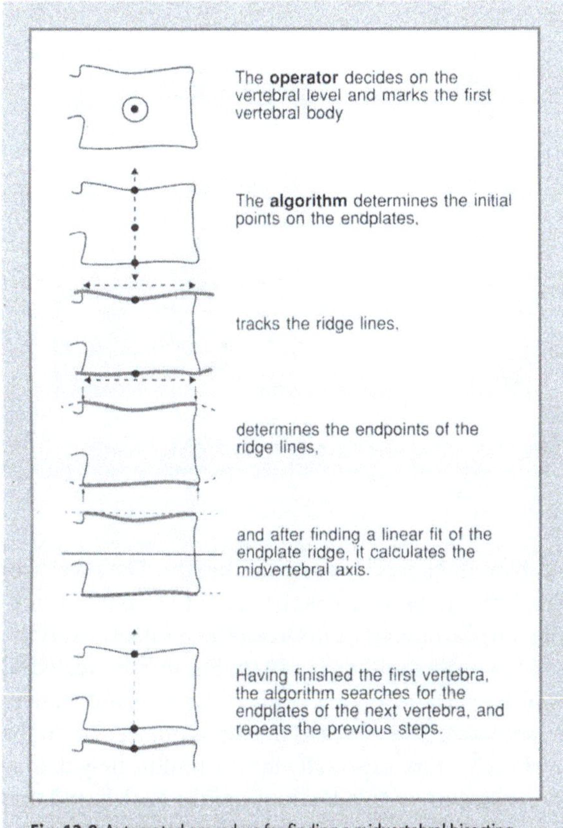

Fig. 12-8 Automated procedure for finding a midvertebral bisecting line by Kalender et al. This method is used to determine the midvertebral slice in computed tomography

[40]. As a first step the operator places a starting point in the center of the first vertebral body to be studied. The automated algorithm then starts searching for the vertebral endplates in both cranial and caudal directions. Finding points on the endplates as a local maximum the algorithm then defines the vertebral contours including ventral and dorsal boundaries. Having defined the first vertebra, the algorithm starts searching for the next endplate, and so on. This process continues until all vertebrae within a defined region of interest are found. The program allows for an interactive correction of the automatically defined vertebral contours through the operator. Following the determination of the vertebral contours a line is fitted parallel to the vertebral endplates, and the midvertebral plane is then defined as the bisector of the angle between these two fitting lines. The midvertebral plane is used for calculating the vertebral heights (Fig. 12-9): the vertebral body is subdivided into five equal vertical segments. In the first segment the algorithm automatically seeks the greatest perpendicular distance between both the upper and lower endplates and the angle bisector. The sum of

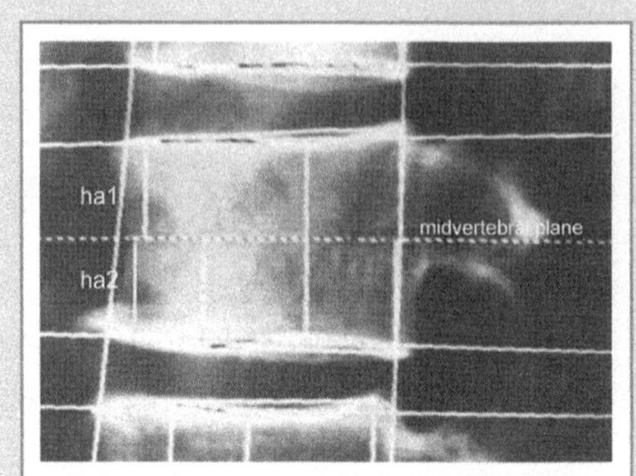

Fig. 12-9 Automated measurements of vertebral heights using the approach by Felsenberg and Kalender [20]. The anterior height is the sum of ha1 and ha2

these two distances corresponds to the anterior vertebral height. The measurement is limited to the anterior fifth of the vertebral body. In the middle three-fifths of the vertebral body the smallest distance between the endplates and the bisecting line is determined in the same manner to obtain the middle vertebral height. In the posterior fifth of the vertebral body, again, the greatest distances are determined. With such an automated determination slight differences in the manual determination of vertebral heights, especially for the middle height, may be observed. In a preliminary evaluation of this method Kalidis et al. found that approximately 60% of all radiographs could be analyzed using this automated method with only minimal interaction by the operator; 36% of all radiographs required in part extensive corrections by the operator, and 4% could not be analyzed at all [41]. The precision errors for vertebral height measurements using this approach were between 0.07 and 1.9%.

A special technique for obtaining images for quantitative morphometry is dual X-ray absorptiometry (DXA). For this a lateral image of the lumbar and thoracic spine is obtained using a DXA scanner. Following the acquisition of the image, a quantitative morphometric analysis of the vertebrae is performed. Since this method for acquiring spine images is performed with DXA scanners, it has been called morphometric X-ray absorptiometry (MXA) [37].

Both major manufacturers of DXA equipment, Hologic and Lunar, have implemented MXA in their latest models of DXA scanners. In all densitometers the MXA scan is performed as a lateral DXA study of the whole thoracolumbar spine with the patient in supine position. Once acquired, the scans are analyzed by a reader according to the rules of quantitative morphometric analysis outlined above. The point placement for vertebral height determination is semiautomated, and the two manufacturers follow somewhat different approaches with respect to scan acquisition and point placement. With Hologic, lateral morphometry scans cover T4–L4. The first vertebra to be evaluated is usually L4, and the operator determines its position from a "scout scan" of the spine in the posteroanterior (PA) projection. The PA scan is also called "centerline scan" because the information from the centerline of the spine is used to maintain a constant distance between the center of the spine and the X-ray tube at all visits. After determining the vertebral levels on the PA scan, the reader performs the lateral scan of the spine starting at mid-L5. Depending on the imaging mode, the scan time for the lateral scan takes between 6 and 25 min. The obtained images usually are dual-energy images. However, the software also allows for the depiction of a less noisy single-energy image. For better visualization the images may be magnified on the screen. Based on the reader's first point placements, the software computes an estimate of the vertebral dimensions that may be checked and adjusted by the reader.

As opposed to the Hologic scanners, the starting point of the lateral spine scan for the Lunar scanners is determined by positioning a laser spot 1 cm above the iliac crest. The scan length is determined by measuring the distance between the iliac crest and the armpit. While accurate in most patients, the starting point is not correct in some because of the normal anatomic variation of the position of the iliac crest in relation to the vertebral levels. The average lateral morphometry scan takes approximately 35 s at 1.2 cm/s scan speed. After the scan the program automatically identifies vertebral levels, proposes labeling, and indicates the assumed vertebral centers based on gray-scale histograms of the scanned regions. The operator may then change the settings if they appear incorrect (which happens especially in regions with great variation of contrast). After the center-points are determined, the program establishes a coordinate system, and six points defining the anterior, middle, and posterior heights are placed automatically on the vertebral endplates [51]. In addition to the automated algorithms the software provides tools for image enhancements to facilitate visual analysis of the images and the manual correction of digitization points. Examples of MXA scans obtained on densitometers from both manufactureres are shown in Figs. 12-10 and 12-11.

The principal error sources for MXA differ from those of conventional radiography to some extent. A comparative analysis of MXA and conventional radiography with respect to its application in quantitative morphometry is given in Table 12-3. The low radiation dose (approx. 15–50 µSv for MXA as compared to approx. 1500 µSv for a lateral thoracolumbar radiograph) and the reduction in projection errors make MXA a promising option for assessing vertebral dimensions in the context of clinical drug trials and epidemiological studies [8]. However, the radiation dose for MXA scans is certainly higher than it is for regular DXA scans. This has some significance for clinical practice because it is no longer the case that no special protection is necessary for the technician when performing MXA scans, or even DXA scans using devices employing the latest fan beam technology [68].

Clinical experience with MXA scanners is limited. Steiger et al. performed the first major study on MXA [83, 84]. Precision errors for anterior, middle, and posterior height measurements were 4.3%, 3.7%, and 4.5%, respectively. The preci-

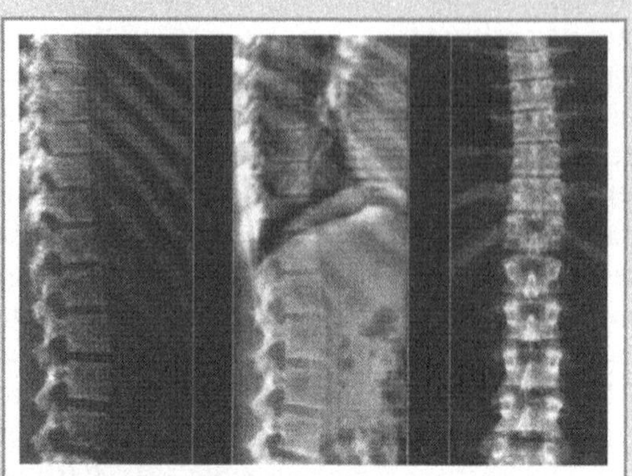

Fig. 12-10 Morphometric X-ray absorptiometry (MXA) scan using a Hologic QDR 4500 DXA scanner. Shown are dual- and single-energy images as well as the centerline scan. The centerline scan in the posteroanterior projection is obtained before the morphometry scan to control patient positioning and to determine the starting point of the morphometry data

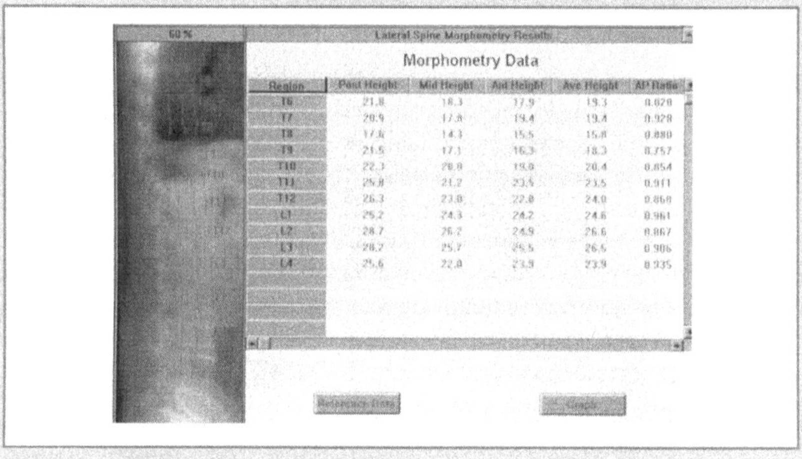

Fig. 12-11 Morphometric X-ray absorptiometry scan and morphometry data for the Lunar Expert scanner

sion error for all heights was worst in the upper thoracic spine due to the relatively poor visualization of the vertebrae in this region. This observation is confirmed by the data of Lang et al. who found that in only 10 of 16 patients could T4–L4 be identified, and in 15 of 16 patients T6–L4 [47]. There is a good correlation between vertebral dimensions as measured with MXA and quantitative morphometry on conventional radiographs. Gowin and colleagues presented results for accuracy and precision errors of MXA measurements in vitro. Using the European spine phantom as a standard, accuracy errors for two MXA devices for

Table 12-3 Positive ($\uparrow$) and negative ($\downarrow$) aspects of morphometric X-ray absorptiometry and conventional radiography for handling error sources in the assessment of vertebral fracture using quantitative morphometry

Error source	Morphometric X-ray absorptiometry	Conventional radiograph
Exposure parameters	$\uparrow$ Digital acquisition allows for image postprocessing $\downarrow$ Problems in adipose patients, exposure parameters relatively invariable	$\uparrow$ Exposure parameters may be altered easily, e.g., to adjust for increased soft tissue $\downarrow$ Faulty exposure relatively common, changes in serial radiographs possible
Focus-film distance	$\uparrow$ Fixed focus-film-distance	$\downarrow$ May be altered manually and may be prone to error if standardized protocol is not followed
Patient positioning	$\uparrow$ Highly standardized, no problems in normal patient anatomy $\downarrow$ Correct starting point for scan not always found, does not allow for compensation of scoliosis	$\uparrow$ Flexible positioning may allow for compensation of scoliosis $\downarrow$ Prone to differences in positioning, especially if performed by different technicians
Patient anatomy	$\downarrow$ Compensation for scoliosis not possible, anomalous segmentation may be missed	$\uparrow$ Allows for some correction of scoliosis, normal variants may be recognized more easily $\downarrow$ changes in positioning, e.g., to compensate for scoliosis may not be repeated in serial radiographs
Film processing	$\uparrow$ Complete digital acquisition allows for digital postprocessing	$\downarrow$ May have substantial impact on film quality
Point placement	$\uparrow$ Semiautomated procedure may allow for efficient point placement $\downarrow$ Relatively low resolution may make identification of vertebral contours and degenerative changes difficult; automated procedures may imply false accuracy, and points may be accepted too easily by operator	$\uparrow$ High-resolution usually allows for good identification of vertebral contours $\downarrow$ Point placement sometimes subjective; differentiation of degenerative changes and normal variants require expertise from the operator

vertebral height measurements were 2.3% and 4.9%, respectively, as compared to 2.0% for vertebral height measurements performed on a conventional radiograph. For measurements of fractured vertebrae using vertebral specimens, precision errors for MXA were between 5.1% and 6.0%, and 4.0% for the measurements performed using standard morphometry on conventional radiographs [28]. The authors also note that in its current application there is still room for improvement, especially in regard to the visibility of vertebral levels in regions with great soft tissue variability and in the overall resolution of the DXA image for a better definition of the vertebral contours. With respect to the image resolution the conventional radiograph is still far superior to the MXA image.

Defining Vertebral Deformity Using Quantitative Morphometry

An early contribution to the assessment of vertebral deformity was a study by Fletcher [21]. This author calculated an index of wedging, the quotient of anterior and posterior vertebral height, as a measure of vertebral deformity. Fletcher described the distribution of the index of wedging in 575 men aged 50 years or younger. In this study the author concluded that if the index of wedging falls below a given threshold, one cannot definitely determine the origin of the deformity. Fletcher uses the diminution of only the anterior height to define vertebral deformity. Thus only deformities involving the anterior vertebral height, i.e., compression fracture and anterior wedging, are identified using this method. Similarly, Jensen and Tougaard proposed a method for follow-up measurements of osteoporosis [36]. Measuring only the anterior height, these authors report a good reproducibility of 1.4–3.2 for single vertebrae and 0.9% for a combination of vertebrae using their method. Again, only the anterior heights are measured, and thus, this method may be useful just for serial assessment of osteoporotic compression fractures or anterior wedge fractures. A significant aspect of this study is the technique that was applied to measure the anterior height (Fig. 12-12). The method proposed by Barnett and Nordin to assess biconcave deformity was used as a diagnostic tool for the assessment of osteoporosis [4, 5]. The authors calculated a lumbar spine score from the middle and anterior heights of one lumbar vertebra that was centered best. An osteoporosis is diagnosed if the quotient from middle and anterior height is less than 80%. The Barnett-Nordin index of the spine is poorly correlated with bone density, and it is rarely used in today's diagnosis of osteoporosis [39].

In 1968 Hurxthal assessed vertebral deformities quantitatively using a technique which already includes basic elements of today's techniques for measuring vertebral dimensions [34]. The author extensively describes the measurement of anterior, middle, and posterior heights as well as that of the intervertebral disk space. Since the influence of projection on vertebral dimensions is considered extensively in this study, this article became a classic reference of quantitative morphometry. Hurxthal proposed only one fracture definition in his article: the anterior compression fracture was defined as a 4 mm reduction in the anterior

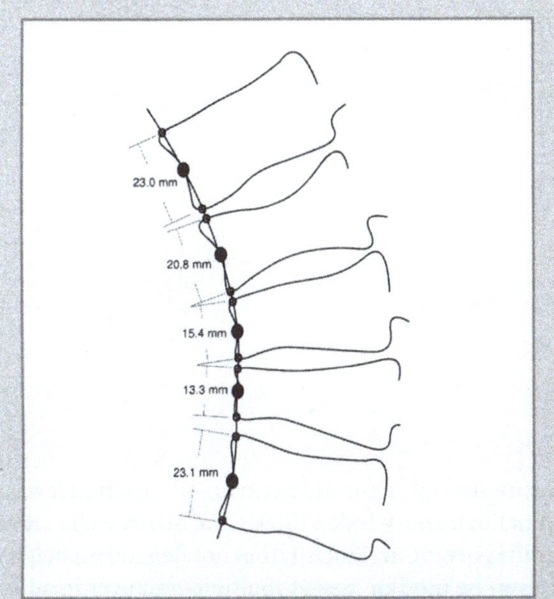

Fig. 12-12 For the determination of anterior vertebral height, Jensen and Tougaard proposed drawing a line along the waist of the vertebrae that follows the curvature of the spine. The endpoints for anterior height measurements are placed at the intersections of this line with the vertebral endplates

height in comparison to the posterior height. Hedlund and coworkers measured the anterior and posterior vertebral heights and vertebral body depth, and they then calculated various parameters such as vertebral wedging, vertebral area, and the difference between the anterior heights of adjacent vertebral bodies [31]. As a threshold for diagnosing vertebral fracture the authors used a reduction of 2 SD from normative values. Sensitivity and specificity of the used parameters ranged from 24.2% and 96.2% (for vertebral area) to 85.5% and 100% (for differences in anterior vertebral heights of adjacent vertebral bodies). Using identical thresholds for the reduction in anterior and posterior heights the authors found most vertebral fractures in the middle and lower thoracic spine. The parameters described in this section and given in Table 12-4 are still used in various clinical and epidemiological studies for diagnosing vertebral deformities.

Minne and coworkers presented a model for diagnosing vertebral fractures comparing the anterior, middle, and posterior vertebral heights to the respective heights of the fourth thoracic vertebra [60]. The expected vertebral heights are expressed as a third order function: $f(x)=ax^3+bx^2+cx+1$, with $f(x)$ being the relative vertebral heights and x representing the vertebral level between Th4 and L5. Based on normative data the authors proposed an equation system that defines the normal range of vertebral heights. The differences between the lower thresh-

Table 12-4 Dimensions and parameters in quantitative morphometry

Parameters measured	
Anterior vertebral height	H_a
Middle (or central) vertebral height	H_m
Posterior vertebral height	H_p
Upper vertebral width	W_u
Lower vertebral width	W_l
Parameters calculated	
Wedging	H_a/H_p $(H_a-H_p)/H_p$
Biconcavity	H_m/H_p
Compression	H_p/H_p+1, H_p/H_p-1 $(H_p-H_p+1)/H_p$

old value and the actually measured heights are added up for all vertebral levels, and the result is called the spinal deformity index (SDI). The SDI is well suited for following vertebral deformities over time. Since it does not depend on neighboring vertebral level, it may even be used in case of multiple fractures in adjacent vertebrae. There are limitations to this approach. The fourth thoracic vertebra, being the standard for the calculation of normal ranges, often is not depicted in an ideal fashion on radiographs of the thoracic spine. Often there are overlying structures that make the correct assessments of vertebral dimensions at this level impossible. In this case, and if the vertebra is fractured, another vertebra must replace the fourth thoracic vertebra as the standard. Furthermore, since the correlation between vertebral dimensions is getting worse the further apart the vertebrae are, describing vertebral heights based on normalization for T4 may not account sufficiently for natural variability in the lumbar spine. Raymakers and colleagues also presented a model of vertebral dimensions for the whole spine based on mathematical equations [69]. Using the individual vertebral dimensions, and excluding abnormally low values, the parameters for the equation are adapted from the measured heights. Vertebral deformities, called vertebral deforming events (VDE) by the authors are defined by a reduction in a vertebral height of 15% or more below the estimated value. Smith-Bindman and colleagues also used a mathematical transformation to describe the radiographic area of the vertebral body [80]. The authors calculated an index of radiographic area (IRA) based on normal vertebrae using a fourth order mathematical function. The IRA is calculated as the sum of the absolute or relative deviation of the vertebral area from the respective expected values. A good correlation exists between the IRA and Genant's visual SFI as well as between IRA and bone density.

Several methods have been proposed for the diagnosis of prevalent vertebral deformities. For example, one can use an absolute reduction in vertebral height, [34]. The use of a percentage reduction from normal values is another possibility (Fig. 12-13) [20]. Using a constant threshold of 0.75 for H_a/H_p and H_m/H_p for

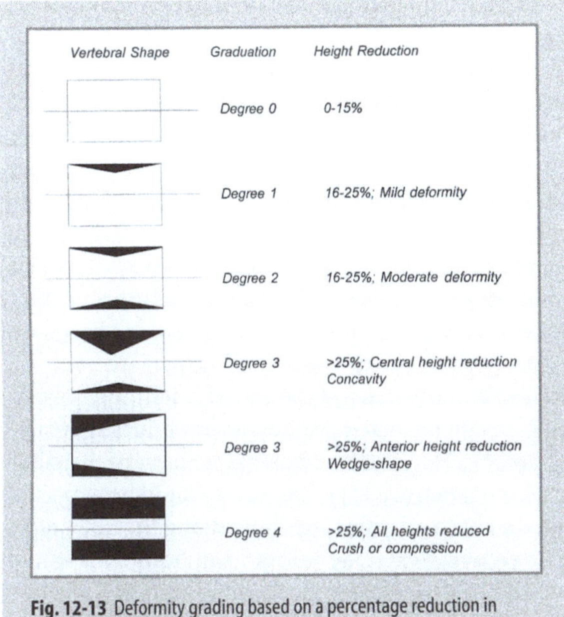

Fig. 12-13 Deformity grading based on a percentage reduction in vertebral height [20]

defining vertebral fracture, Harrison and coworkers found that singular vertebral deformities in the midthoracic spine were not associated with a low bone mineral density [30]. The authors concluded that such deformities may be degenerative changes that are not related to osteoporosis. Both absolute and proportional reductions (that are not based on normative data) may not be the adequate means for diagnosing vertebral deformity. Physiological changes in the vertebral shape with age require a comparative analysis with age-adjusted normative data for a reliable diagnosis of vertebral deformity. McCloskey and colleagues found that using a fracture threshold of 3 SD, depending on the vertebral level, the proportional reduction in the quotient H_a/H_p was between 14.4% and 26.7% [53]. Other parameters revealed a similar behavior. Melton and coworkers used normative values from healthy persons to define adjusted height quotients for each vertebral level [56]. Using a threshold of 0.85 for the adjusted quotients for H_a/H_p, H_m/H_p, H_p/H_p+1, or H_p/H_p-1 showed a significant effect on fracture prevalence when compared to unadjusted values. Davies and colleagues revised their criteria with the help of a radiologist's readings [15]. Using a low prevalence cohort, the threshold values were adjusted for the radiologist's call. The thresholds were 4.05 and 2.5 SD for a compression fracture and a wedge fracture, respectively. Using these thresholds in a different study cohort with higher fracture prevalence, sensitivity and specificity were 73.9% and 99.3, respectively. The National Osteoporosis Foundation working group on vertebral fractures recommended that in studies involving community populations, prevalent fractures be defined on the basis of a reduction of 3 SD or more from normal mean ratios of dimensions for the particular vertebral level [13, 17].

Defining normative data is probably one of the greatest problems in quantitative morphometry. There are some differences between normative data from different study cohorts as presented in the literature, and although there are some common tendencies in the distribution of normative values along the spine, differences in the normal values are sometimes quite substantial (Fig. 12-14). Thus, it is not possible to simply transfer normative data between different studies, or between different populations [48, 66, 75]. Differences in the exposure settings, digitizing technique, and statistical analysis of normative data are further sources of differences. Moreover, in some studies normative data are based on pre- or perimenopausal women, in others postmenopausal women are used [14, 23, 32, 56, 60]. Black et al. proposed a mathematical method for defining normative values based on the assumption that normative values of vertebral height quotients (H_a/H_p, H_m/H_p, H_p/H_{p-1} and H_p/H_{p+1}) show a normal (gaussian) distribution, and that most vertebrae are not fractured [7]. Fractures would be expected to be on both ends of the gaussian curve significantly influencing the normative values. Trimming the curve by removing extreme values from both ends would result in a curve better reflecting the distribution of vertebral dimensions in a normal population. Black and colleagues calculated the mean and the standard deviation for the normal population based on a truncated gaussian distribution. The standard deviations calculated using this method differed by 5%–20% from those based on uncorrected data. It is of advantage that using this method, normative data can be calculated from a study sample of fractured and nonfractured

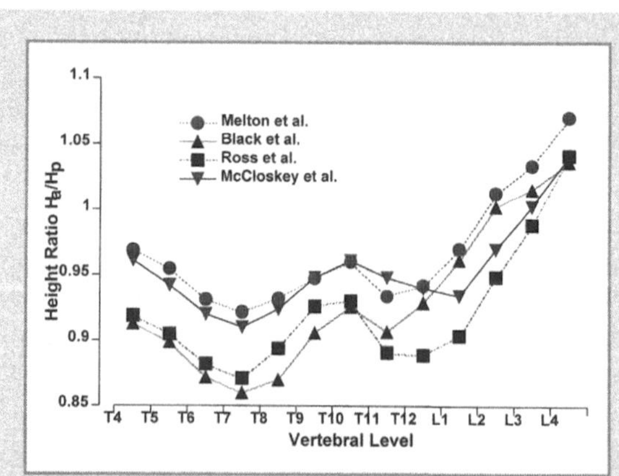

Fig. 12-14 Normative data for the quotient from anterior to posterior height from various studies using quantitative morphometry to assess vertebral fracture show consistently smaller quotients in the middle thoracic spine and the thoracolumbar junction [7, 53, 56, 74]. The differences in the normal values may be due to differences in the populations or differences in the exposure settings, digitizing technique, and statistical analysis of normative data

persons without requiring a previous qualitative reading to exclude fractured persons. On the other hand, using this approach some normal vertebrae, especially in the upper range of the gaussian distribution, may be misclassified and also some vertebrae that are fractured or otherwise deformed may be falsely classified as being normal. In populations where a high fracture prevalence may be expected, this approach may be unreliable. Melton and coworkers used a different approach to trim extreme values from the frequency distributions [57]. An iterative algorithm calculating threshold values was applied to the data until there were no data left that would meet the exclusion criteria. Mean and standard deviation were then calculated from the remaining data.

Ross and colleagues emphasize that applying normative data for diagnosing vertebral fractures may result in a relatively large number of nonidentified fractures [74]. For example, using a 3SD threshold for diagnosing fractures, only 76% of wedge fractures, and 86% of the compression fractures would be detected, with the specificity being 99.9%. Lowering the fracture threshold to 2 SD would increase the sensitivity to 90% and 92%, respectively but at the cost of a reduced specificity of 97.7%. Since, in comparison to nonfractured vertebrae, fractured vertebrae are relatively rare, the specificity of a method is a very sensitive issue. Especially in clinical drug trials an increased number of false positives may impair the statistical power (Table 12-5). For prevalent fractures Ross and colleagues therefore proposed a model in which normative values are adjusted based upon the average vertebral heights of the individual patient measured [76]. Applying this method to identify incident vertebral fractures the authors found that this approach detected a greater number of true-positive fractures and produced a smaller number of false-positive results.

Vertebral fractures are often identified when one parameter falls below a threshold value. McCloskey and colleagues proposed a model where two conditions had to be met for vertebral fracture diagnosis [54]. The authors introduced a predicted posterior height which is calculated as the average of the four neighboring heights [52]. This predicted posterior height allows a more accurate assessment of the posterior height, especially when deformities are present in adjacent segments. The criteria for vertebral fracture detection are given in Table 12-6. Using these criteria in a group of patients with metastasizing breast cancer the authors esti-

Table 12-5 Definition of prevalent vertebral fractures by McCloskey et al. [53]. H_{pp} is the expected posterior height which is calculated from the 4 adjacent vertebral heights

Type of deformity	Criteria
Endplate fracture	H_m/H_p and $H_m/H_{pp} < (\text{mean } H_m/H_p - 3\text{ SD})$
Anterior wedging	H_a/H_p and $H_a/H_{pp} < (\text{mean } H_a/H_p - 3\text{ SD})$
Posterior wedging	$H_p/H_{pp} < (\text{mean } H_p/H_{pp} - 3\text{ SD})$ and $H_a/H_p > (\text{mean } H_a/H_p + 3\text{ SD})$
Compression	$H_p/H_{pp} < (\text{mean } H_p/H_{pp} - 3\text{ SD})$ and $H_a/H_{pp} > (\text{mean } H_a/H_p - 3\text{ SD})$

Table 12-6 Interrelationship between fracture threshold and fracture prevalence in 2992 women from the Study of Osteoporotic Fracture. The absolute number and the percentage of women having one or more vertebral fractures according to the respective definition are given [7]

Fracture definition	Prevalence	
	n	Percent
Mean–2 SD	1891	63.2
Mean–2.5 SD	1160	38.8
Mean–3 SD	735	24.6
Mean–15%	844	28.2
Mean–20%	374	12.5

mated that only 8% of the newly diagnosed fractures were false positives. Since no gold standard exists, no estimates can be made about the sensitivity of this approach. With the use of such strict criteria, however, the number of fractures may be underestimated. Table 12-5 summarizes several approaches for vertebral fracture definition.

There are few references in regard to the diagnosis of incident vertebral fractures. In drug trials new fractures are usually assessed in comparison to baseline radiographs (Table 12-7). Riggs and colleagues defined incident vertebral fracture as a 15% or greater reduction in the quotients H_a/H_p or H_m/H_p or in any vertebral height [71]. Relatively small changes in point placement and projection may result in false-positive incident fractures especially for small vertebrae if a percentage reduction in a vertebral height or a height quotient are applied for fracture diagnosis. Applying an additional condition that must be met, an absolute threshold, may somewhat improve the accuracy of this approach [88]. An absolute reduction in height or height quotient may also be applied as the sole criterion for diagnosis of incident fracture [45]. McCloskey and colleagues proposed a point-prevalence approach for diagnosing incident vertebral fractures [53]. Using criteria for prevalent fractures for both baseline and follow-up radiographs, the difference in fractures between the two radiographs corresponds to the number of new vertebral fractures. Using criteria for prevalent fractures for incident fracture diagnosis avoids a number of problems arising from the direct comparison of two radiographs, such as different projection of vertebrae, magnification effects, etc. However, in this case the limitations that apply for the diagnosis of prevalent fractures also apply here, and the criteria for fracture definition must be chosen carefully since they have a significant impact on sensitivity and specificity.

Table 12-7 Quantitative assessment of vertebral fracture: alphabetical listing including year of publication

Reference	Parameters measured	Parameters calculated	Normative data	Fracture definition	Comment
Barnett and Nordin [4]	H_a, H_m	H_m/H_a	None	<0.8	Diagnosis of osteoporosis, based on evaluation of 1 vertebra
Black et al. [7]	H_a, H_m, H_p	H_a/H_m, H_m/H_p, H_p/H_p-1, H_p/H_p+1	Study cohort, trimming fixed percentage from tails and calculate mean and SD from truncated Gaussian (normal) distribution	Several, based on SD reduction and relative (%) height reduction.	
Davies et al. [14]	H_a, H_p	$(H_a-H_p)/H_p$, $(H_p-H_p-1)/H_p$-1	Healthy pre- and perimen opausal women, adjusted for extreme values	Value below adjusted minimum	
Davies et al. [15]	H_a, H_p	$(H_a-H_p)/H_p$, H_p-H_p+1)/ H_p+1	Healthy pre- and perimenopausal women	Wedge fracture ≤ -2.5 SD, compression fracture ≤ -4.05 SD	Threshold based on visual evaluation
Eastell et al. [17]	H_a, H_m, H_p	$(H_p-H_a)/H_p$, $(H_p-H_m)/H_p$, $(H_p+1-H_p)H_p$+1	Healthy postmenopausal women	More than 3 SD from mean	Fracture grading: grade 1 (3–4 SD) and grade 2 (>4 SD)
Evans et al. [19]	H_a, H_m, H_p, WI	$(H_p-H_a)/H_p$, $(H_p-H_m)/H_p$, $(H_p-H_p+1)H_p$, $(WI-H_p)/WI$	Study cohort	3 SD below mean	
Fletcher [21]	H_a, H_p	Index of wedging=H_p/H_a	Study cohort	1 SD below mean	
Hedlund and Gallagher [31]	H_a, H_p, W	$(H_p-H_a)/H_p$, $(H_a-H_a+1)/H_a$, $2*sin-1((H_p-H_a)/W)$	Healthy pre-, peri- and postmenopausal women	More than 2 SD from mean	
Hurxthal [34]	H_a, H_m, H_p	None	None	$H_p-H_a \geq 4$ mm	
Jensen and Tougaard [36]	H_a	None	None	None	Follow-up of osteoporosis

H_a, Anterior vertebral height; H_m, middle vertebral height; H_p, posterior vertebral height; WI, lower vertebral width; W, vertebral width; SD, standard deviation.

Table 12-7 Continue: Quantitative assessment of vertebral fracture: alphabetical listing including year of publication

Reference	Parameters measured	Parameters calculated	Normative data	Fracture definition	Comment
McCloskey et al. [53]	H_a, H_m, H_p	H_m/H_p, H_m/H_{pp}, H_a/H_p, H_a/H_{pp}, H_p/H_{pp}	Healthy women aged 45–50	Two criteria must be met, e.g. wedge fracture: H_a/H_p and $H_a/H_{pp} <$(mean Ha/H_p−3 SD)	Similar definition for other types of deformity, point-prevalence for incident fractures
Melton et al. [56]	H_a, H_m, H_p	H_a/H_p, H_m/H_p, H_p/H_p+1, H_p/H_p-1	Study cohort, adjusted normative data from subgroup	15% r eduction in any quotient	
Melton et al. [57]	H_a, H_m, H_p	H_a/H_p, H_m/H_p, H_p/H_p+1, H_p/H_p-1	Study cohort, trimming of the frequency distribution	3 SD below mean	
Minne et al. [60]	H_a, H_m, H_p	Spinal deformity index (SDI)	Healthy men and women	Falling short of reference range	Polynomial function of normative data; vertebral dimensions adjusted to T4
Raymakers et al. [69]	H_a, H_m, H_p	Spine fracture index (SFI)	Pre- and perimenopausal women, individually adjusted	Deviation of ≥15% from expected value	Calculation of expected vertebral heights using mathematical function
Riggs et al. [71]	H_a, H_m, H_p	H_a/H_p, H_m/H_p, H_p/H_p+1, H_p/H_p-1	None	More than 15% deviation from adjacent vertebral bodies (prevalent) or from baseline adiographs (incident)	
Ross et al. [76]	H_a, H_m, H_p		Study cohort, trimming of the frequency distribution and calculation of individual normative values	3 SD from individual Z score	
Smith-Bindman et al. [80]	H_a, H_m, H_p, projected area	Index of radiographic area (IRA)	Premenopausal women	Adjusted height or area below 1st percentile of normative values	Calculation of expected areas using mathematical function; vertebral areas adjusted to T4

H_a, Anterior vertebral height; H_m, middle vertebral height; H_p, posterior vertebral height; WI, lower vertebral width; W, vertebral width; SD, standard deviation.

Applying Standardized Visual and Quantitative Morphometric Diagnosis of Vertebral Fracture

Standardized visual assessment and quantitative morphometry are two completely different approaches for assessing vertebral deformities which are often regarded to be competitive. Evaluating the accuracy of the right approach to define vertebral fracture is difficult since a gold standard that is required for such a test must be a product of a different approach, and thus should itself be subject to testing. There are substantial differences between both approaches in their description of vertebral deformities. The most substantial difference is that through the reading in standardized visual assessments of vertebral deformities, a qualitative component is added to the evaluation that allows the distinction of fracture from nonfracture deformities. Quantitative morphometry lacks this "feature." However, it is because of this qualitative element that quantitative morphometry was introduced. Radiologists may not always agree on the nature of a deformity, and they may read the same deformities with different results on another day, introducing some subjectivity through the visual assessment [16, 35]. A joint reading session may improve the diagnostic accuracy, and marking vertebral levels on baseline films may also be helpful for a consistent identification of vertebral levels to avoid misclassifications when evaluating serial radiographs. The latter point also applies to quantitative morphometry. There also should be a clear standardization for fracture definition and a thorough training of the readers to ensure good agreement between readers. If these necessary preconditions are met, standardized visual assessment of vertebral fracture is a reliable approach to diagnose vertebral fractures [27, 65].

There are few studies comparing standardized visual assessment and quantitative morphometry. Melton and colleagues found that when applying their methodology for vertebral fracture diagnosis, fracture rates were comparable to visual reading [56]. However, complete agreement on the basis of individual vertebrae was only 75%. Hansen et al. also applied both methods for vertebral fracture detection. Depending on the approach the prevalence in 70-year- old women was between 33% and 85% (Fig. 12-15) [29]. Li and coworkers found a moderate agreement between quantitative morphometry and a consensus reading using Genant's standardized visual approach. The results from quantitative morphometry using a 2.5 SD of vertebral height ratios as fracture threshold yielded the best agreement with the consensus reading. Depending on the cutoff value, fracture prevalence on a per vertebra basis ranged from 7.48% at 4.0 SD to 20.6% at 2.0 SD [49]. Applying a number of different methods for diagnosing vertebral fracture using quantitative morphometry Smith-Bindman and colleagues found that there was no acceptable agreement between these methods and standardized visual reading [79]. Similarly, Genant et al. found that there still was substantial disagreement between standardized visual assessment of vertebral fracture and quantitative morphometry for both prevalent and incident vertebral fractures [25]. Black et al. compared four quantitative morphometric approaches for frac-

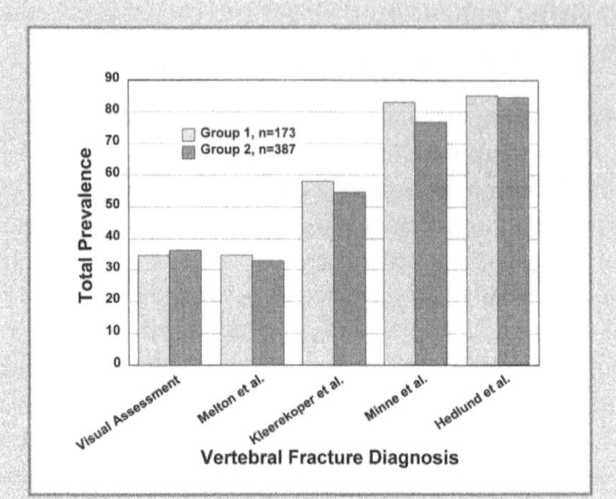

Fig. 12-15 Deformity grading based on a percentage reduction in vertebral height [20]. The two groups consisted of 70-year-old women, recruited at an interval of 10 years.

ture definition and Genant's semiquantitative approach and assessed their relationship to clinical criteria including bone density, height loss since age 25 years, back pain, and incidence of subsequent deformity in 503 thoracolumbar radiographs. The authors found that three of the four quantitative methods as well as the standardized visual approach provided similar relationships to clinical criteria [6].

Adami and coworkers compared several methods for the diagnosis of incident vertebral fractures and found quite substantial differences in sensitivity and specificity between the various methods [1]. However, the gold standard used in this study, a 1-mm reduction in vertebral height, is certainly questionable. McCloskey et al. compared their approach for vertebral fracture definition with those of Eastell et al. and Melton et al. in two cohorts with low and high fracture prevalence (Fig. 12-16) [54]. There was poor agreement between the three methods in the low prevalence cohort and a good agreement in women with high fracture prevalence. There was a greater difference in bone density between the fractured and nonfractured women in the low prevalence group when applying McCloskey's approach as compared to the others. There was also a stronger association between vertebral fractures and backaches for McCloskey's fracture definition. One must keep in mind, however, that this result may have been influenced by the stricter criteria of McCloskey's approach, and while probably being more specific, its sensitivity is not known since no gold standard exists. The results presented by McCloskey and colleagues are confirmatory of other studies [53, 54, 81]. Comparing the methods of Hedlund and Gallagher, Melton et al., Davies et al. and Minne et al., Sauer and coworkers found a moderate agreement between the these methods [77]. Using comparisons between baseline and follow-up radiographs the

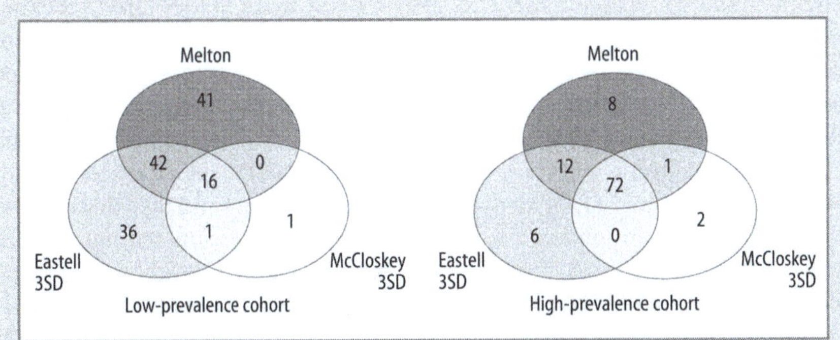

Fig. 12-16 Agreement among three quantitative morphometric approaches to define vertebral deformities in a low- and high-prevalence group. The proportion of patients identified by all three methods was 11.6% in the low-prevalence group and 72% in the high-prevalence group

authors also compared how many vertebrae were diagnosed normal on follow-up radiographs that were diagnosed fractured at baseline. With Minne's approach only 0.7% of the previously "fractured" vertebrae were diagnosed normal on the follow-up radiographs while with the other methods 8.5%–10.9% of the previously diagnosed fractures "vanished."

Being independent of subjective, qualitative criteria may be regarded both as a strength and as a weakness of quantitative morphometry. Since with this method only vertebral dimensions are assessed, all deformations that fulfill certain criteria are regarded as fractured or deformed. Quantitative morphometry cannot determine the nature of a deformity, and thus misdiagnoses of nonfracture deformities are possible. The number of misdiagnosed fractures depends heavily on the method used, and since there is no gold standard, there is no way in which to determine the genuine proportion of misdiagnosed fractures. Mann et al. studied the misclassification of vertebral deformities in 144 men and found that 36 vertebral bodies in 14 men showed deformities from Scheuermann's disease, and of these 39% showed a greater than 15% reduction in the anterior height [50]. Using a threshold of 2 SD below the mean for a H_a/H_p quotient, only one deformity would have been diagnosed as fractured.

The phenomenon of "vanishing" fractures in quantitative morphometry has been widely discussed [63, 77]. Having excluded incident vertebral fractures from their analysis, Genant et al. found that on follow-up radiographs the classification of vertebrae according to standard deviation categories changed by at least 1 SD in a large number of vertebrae compared to the baseline classification [25]. The most probable explanations for this phenomenon are differences in projection between baseline and follow-up radiographs or misregistration of digitization points. Using strict criteria for incident fracture may reduce the risk of "vanishing" fractures but at the cost of sensitivity. Gallagher et al. found that increasing the focus-film distance by 10 cm was associated with a 6.4% reduction in the posterior height, a 5.5% reduction in the anterior height, and a 3.5% reduction in vertebral area [23]. Brinckmann et al. also showed that the measured vertebral dimensions depended strongly on the centering of the X-ray beam and on patient positioning [9]. Correcting vertebral dimensions for baseline measurements based on some reference points, for example, nonfractured vertebrae, seems to be too difficult and time consuming to perform [46]. In this case the trained reader certainly has a great advantage over quantitative morphometry. The experienced radiologist or clinician may easily identify different projections and take these differences between radiographs into account when evaluating spine radiographs for incident vertebral fractures. Therefore, in general, serial radiographs of a patient should be viewed together so that incident fractures can be readily identified.

There are some limitations other than the inherent subjectivity of the reader to standardized visual approaches as well. For example, from morphometric data on normal subjects we know that vertebrae in the midthoracic spine and in the thoracolumbar junction are slightly more wedged than in other regions of the spine (Figs. 12-5, 12-14). As a result normal variations may be misinterpreted as mild vertebral deformities, and this may falsely increase prevalence values for vertebral fractures from visual readings in the specific regions. The same applies to a lesser extent to the lumbar spine, where some degree of biconcavity is frequently seen. Accurate diagnosis of prevalent fractures, which requires distinguishing between normal variations and the degenerative changes from true fractures, still depends on the experience of the observer.

The National Osteoporosis Foundation's Working Group on Vertebral Fractures recently put together some procedural requirements for the assessment of vertebral fractures [13]. This report found that both standardized visual approaches and quantitative morphometry may be used in clinical trials for assessing prevalent as well as incident vertebral deformities recognizing the strengths and the weaknesses of the two methods. The recommendations of this group for applying qualitative reading for vertebral fracture diagnosis are:
- Assessments should be performed by a radiologist or trained clinician who has specific expertise in the radiology of osteoporosis.
- Qualitative and semiquantitative assessments should be performed according to a written protocol of fracture definitions, which are sufficiently detailed that the readings can be reproduced by other experts. Reference to an atlas of standard films or illustrations may be helpful. It is recommended that a standardized protocol be developed by a consensus of expert radiologists.
- The definition of fracture should include deformities of the endplates and anterior borders of vertebral bodies, as well as generalized collapse of a vertebral body.
- Grading of the extent of each fracture should employ discrete, mutually exclusive categories. An atlas of standard films and illustrations may again help to assure consistency.

In clinical trials the National Osteoporosis Foundation Working Group suggests to also include changes in bone mass, height loss, pain and disability, and quality of life as outcome variables. It is expected that these outcome variables should be associated with the presence of vertebral fractures. To reduce the workload associated with quantitative morphometry, Black et al. tested a visual triage system in which only those films with evidence of deformity were assessed with quantitative morphometry [6]. The triage rarely missed deformities, and, of utmost importance for its application in clinical studies, it did not affect the performance of quantitative or semiquantitative methods for vertebral fracture assessment.

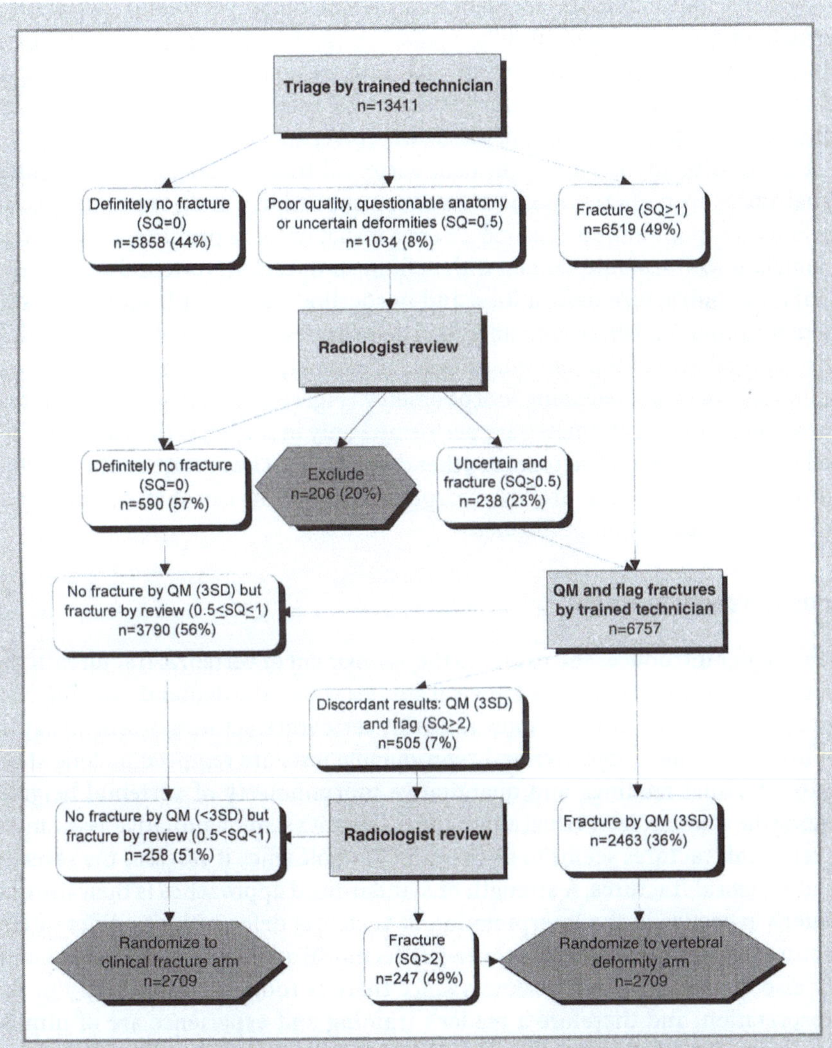

Fig. 12-17 Flowchart for assessment of prevalent fractures in a clinical drug trial [26]. Fracture assessment comprises a visual triage by a trained technician, standardized visual (semiquantitative) assessment by an experienced radiologist, and quantitative morphometric analysis. *SQ*, Semiquantitative evaluation using Genant's grading scheme; *QM*, quantitative morphometry; *SD*, standard deviation

Similar results are reported by Genant et al. who found that visual triage identified all films on which at least one moderate vertebral fracture was present [25]. Thus visual triage may be regarded a time-saving as well as cost-effective procedure in the context of large clinical trials or epidemiological studies.

Serial radiographs of a patient should always be viewed together in order to accomplish a thorough and reliable analysis of all new deformities. The blinding of readers to the temporal sequence of radiographs should be avoided. Most experts believe that knowing the temporal order of serial radiographs enhances the reader's ability to assess incident fractures. Because a vertebral fracture is a permanent event that is unlikely to vanish on follow-up radiographs, temporal blinding does not appear to be of any use: most readers easily identify a temporal sequence of films by new deformities as well as by progressive disc degeneration and osteophyte formation, which are universal among the elderly.

A composite approach to prevalent vertebral fracture diagnosis combining visual and morphometric methods has been applied in a multicenter drug trial, the Fracture Intervention Trial [26]. Here a visual triage is performed by trained technicians who separate women with definite or uncertain vertebral deformities (artifacts, nonfracture deformities, and borderline fractures) from those without deformities. Vertebrae with uncertain deformities are then judged by a radiologist (second arm of the semiquantitative triage) and finally the triaged "abnormal" cases are evaluated using morphometry (Fig. 12-17). Thus semiquantitative assessment and morphometry are performed only in study participants who are likely to have vertebral fractures or other deformities. The semiquantitative evaluation by the radiologist and the morphometric results can then be compared and a final adjudication performed.

Summary and Conclusion

This chapter introduces the reader to the assessment of vertebral fractures in the context of clinical and epidemiological studies where the demands are different from a clinical environment. Approaches for vertebral fracture assessment in this environment where objective and reproducible tests are required include standardized visual readings and quantitative morphometry of vertebral heights. Among the standardized visual approaches, Genant's semiquantitative assessment of vertebral fractures seems to be the most suitable since it assesses the severity of all vertebral fractures. A strength of standardized approaches is their use of a reader's expertise in the interpretation of vertebral deformities to differentiate fracture from nonfracture deformities or technical artifacts. On the other hand, this also constitutes their weakness since there is room for subjectivity in the interpretation, and therefore a reader's training and experience are of utmost importance for a valid use of standardized visual techniques.

Quantitative morphometry was introduced to reduce the subjectivity that is inherent to standardized visual approaches. In quantitative morphometry vertebral heights and/or vertebral area are measured, and several other measures, such as height quotients, are derived from these basic measurements. The technique for data acquisition in quantitative morphometry usually is point digitization on conventional radiographs, and recently more sophisticated techniques, such as semiautomated and automated height measurements on digitized radiographs and MXA have been employed. The latter technique significantly reduces radiation exposure of the patient, and if image quality can be improved, it may be the method of choice for vertebral fracture assessment in clinical drug trials and epidemiological studies.

The diagnosis of vertebral deformities in quantitative morphometry is based on comparisons with normative data. The choice of threshold values determines sensitivity and specificity of a method. Quantitative morphometry may be influenced adversely by differences in the radiographic technique and by differences in the digitization technique. Since there is no qualitative evaluation in quantitative morphometry, it cannot readily distinguish fracture deformities from nonfracture deformities. Both standardized visual reading and quantitative morphometry have become accepted methods for evaluation of vertebral deformities in clinical drug studies and in epidemiological research. The combination of a standardized visual technique and quantitative morphometry system enhances the overall accuracy for diagnosing vertebral fractures. A visual triage performed by trained technicians to select only those films of persons with evidence of vertebral deformities for quantitative morphometry is both a time-saving and cost-effective procedure in the context of large clinical trials or epidemiological studies.

References

1. Adami S, Gatti D, Rossini M, Adamoli A, James G, Girardello S, Zamberlan N (1992) The radiological assessment of vertebral osteoporosis. Bone 13 [Suppl]:S33-S36
2. Albright F, Smith PH, Richardson AM (1941) Postmenopausal osteoporosis. Its clinical features. JAMA 116:2465–2474
3. Banks LM, van Kuijk C, Genant HK (1995) Radiographic technique for assessing osteoporotic vertebral deformity. In: Genant HK, Jergas M, van Kuijk C, (eds) Vertebral fracture in osteoporosis. Radiology Research and Education Foundation, San Francisco, pp 131–147
4. Barnett E, Nordin BEC (1960) The radiological diagnosis of osteoporosis: a new approach. Clin Radiol 11:166–174
5. Barnett E, Nordin BEC (1961) Radiological assessment of bone density. I. The clinical and radiological problem of thin bones. Br J Radiol 34:683–692
6. Black D, Palermo L, Nevitt MC, Genant HK, Epstein R, San Valentin R, Cummings SR, the Study of Osteoporotic Fractures Research Group (1995) Comparison of methods for defining prevalent vertebral deformities: the study of osteoporotic fractures. J Bone Miner Res 10:890–902
7. Black DM, Cummings SR, Stone K, Hudes E, Palermo L, Steiger P (1991) A new

approach to defining normal vertebral dimensions. J Bone Miner Res 6:883–892

8. Blake G, Lewis M, Steiger P, Fogelman I (1994) Patient dosimetry for morphometric X-ray absorptiometry. J Bone Miner Res 9 [Suppl 1]:S406

9. Brinckmann P, Frobin W, Biggemann P, Hilweg D, Seidel S, Burton K, Tillotson M, Sandover J, Atha J, Quinell R (1994) Quantification of overload injuries of thoracolumbar vertebrae in persons exposed to heavy physical exertions or vibration at the work-place. I. the shape of vertebrae and intervertebral disks – study of a young, healthy population and a middle-aged control group. Clin Biomechan 9:S1–S83

10. Burger H, van Daele PLA, Grashuis K, Hofman A, Grobbee DE, Schütte HE, Birkenhäger JC, Pols HAP (1997) Vertebral deformities and functional impairment in men and women. J Bone Miner Res 12:152–157

11. Cooper C, Atkinson EJ, Kotowicz M, O'Fallon WM, Melton III LJ (1992) Secular trends in the incidence of postmenopausal vertebral fractures. Calcif Tissue Int 51:100–104

12. Cooper C, O'Neill T, Silman A (1993) The epidemiology of vertebral fractures. Bone 14:S89–S97

13. Cummings SR, Melton LJ III, Felsenberg D, National Osteoporosis Foundation Working Group on Vertebral Fracture (1995) Report: assessing vertebral fractures. J Bone Miner Res 10:518–523

14. Davies KM, Recker RR, Heaney RP (1989) Normal vertebral dimensions and normal variation in serial measurements of vertebrae. J Bone Miner Res 4:341–349

15. Davies KM, Recker RR, Heaney RP (1993) Revisable criteria for vertebral deformity. Osteoporosis Int 3:265–270

16. Deyo RA, McNiesh LM, Cone III RO (1985) Observer variability in the interpretation of lumbar spine radiographs. Arthritis Rheum 28:1066–1070

17. Eastell R, Cedel SL, Wahner HW, Riggs BL, Melton III LJ (1991) Classification of vertebral fractures. J Bone Miner Res 6:207–215

18. Ettinger B, Block JE, Smith R, Cummings SR, Harris ST, Genant HK (1988) An examination of the association between vertebral deformities, physical disabilities and psycho-social problems. Maturitas 10:283–296

19. Evans SF, Nicholson PHF, Haddaway MJ, Davie MWJ (1993) Vertebral morphometry in women aged 50–81 years. Bone Miner 21:29–40

20. Felsenberg DF, Kalender WA (1995) Computer-assisted morphometry of vertebral fractures. In: Genant HK, Jergas M, van Kuijk C (eds) Vertebral fracture in osteoporosis. Radiology Research and Education Foundation, San Francisco, pp 309–317

21. Fletcher H (1947) Anterior vertebral wedging – frequency and significance. Am J Roentgenol 57:232–238

22. Frobin W, Brinckmann P, Biggemann M, Tillotson M, Burton K (1997) Precision measurement of disc height, vertebral height and sagittal plane displacement from lateral radiographic views of the lumbar spine. Clin Biomech 12:S1–S64

23. Gallagher JC, Hedlund LR, Stoner S, Meeger C (1988) Vertebral morphometry: normative data. Bone Miner 4:189–196

24. Genant HK (1990) Radiographic assessment of the effects of intermittent cyclical treatment with etidronate. In: Christiansen C, Overgaard K (eds) 3rd international conference on osteoporosis 3. Osteopress, Copenhagen, pp 2047–2054

25. Genant HK, Jergas M, Palermo L, Nevitt M, San Valentin R, Black D, Cummings SR (1996) Comparison of semiquantitative visual and quantitative morphometric assessment of prevalent and incident vertebral fractures in osteoporosis. J Bone Miner Res 11:984–996

26. Genant HK, Nevitt MC, Black D, Palermo L, Jergas M, Cummings SR (1993) Assessment of prevalent vertebral fractures combining visual, semiquantitative and morphometric analyses. J Bone Miner Res 8 [Suppl 1]:S338

27. Genant HK, Wu CY, van Kuijk C, Nevitt M (1993) Vertebral fracture assessment using a semi-quantitative technique. J Bone Miner Res 8:1137–1148

28. Gowin W, Dießel E, Mews J, Hoja T, Felsenberg D (1997) Wirbelkörpermorphometrie mit DXA/MXA-Geräten – ein Gerätevergleich. Fortschr Rontgenstr 166:140–145

29. Hansen M, Overgaard K, Nielsen V, Jensen G, Gotfredsen A, Christiansen C (1992) No secular increase in the prevalence of vertebral fractures due to postmenopausal osteoporosis. Osteoporosis Int 2:241–246

30. Harrison JE, Patt N, Müller C, Bailey TA, Budden FH, Josse RG, Murray TM, Sturtridge WC, Strauss A, Goodwin S (1990) Bone mineral mass associated with postmenopausal vertebral deformities. Bone Miner 10:243–251

31. Hedlund LR, Gallagher JC (1988) Vertebral morphometry in diagnosis of spinal fractures. Bone Miner 5:59–67

32. Hedlund LR, Gallagher JC, Meeger C, Stoner S (1989) Change in vertebral shape in spinal osteoporosis. Calcif Tissue Int 44:168–172

33. Heuck A, Block J, Glüer CC, Steiger P, Genant HK (1989) Mild versus definite osteoporosis: comparison of bone densitometry techniques using different statistical models. J Bone Miner Res 4(6):891–900

34. Hurxthal L (1968) Measurement of anterior vertebral compressions and biconcave vertebrae. Am J Roentgenol 103:635–644

35. Jensen GF, McNair P, Boesen J, Hegedüs V (1984) Validity in diagnosing osteoporosis. Eur J Radiol 4:1–3

36. Jensen KK, Tougaard L (1981) A simple X-ray method for monitoring progress of osteoporosis. Lancet 2:19–20

37. Jergas M, Lang TF, Fuerst T (1995) Morphometric X-ray absorptiometry. In: Genant HK, Jergas M, van Kuijk C (eds) Vertebral fracture in osteoporosis. Radiology Research and Education Foundation, San Francisco, pp 331–348

38. Jergas M, San Valentin R (1995) Techniques for the assessment of vertebral dimensions in quantitative morphometry. In: Genant HK, Jergas M, van Kuijk C (eds) Vertebral fracture in osteoporosis. Radiology Research and Education Foundation, San Francisco, pp 163–188

39. Jergas M, Uffmann M, Escher H, Schaffstein J, Nitzschke E, Köster O (1994)

Visuelle Beurteilung konventioneller Röntgenaufnahmen und duale Röntgenabsorptiometrie in der Diagnostik der Osteoporose. Z Orthop Grenzgeb 132:91–98

40. Kalender WA, Brestowsky H, Felsenberg D (1988) Bone mineral measurements: automated determination of the midvertebral CT section. Radiology 168:219–221

41. Kalidis L, Felsenberg D, Kalender W, Eidloth H, Wieland E (1992) Morphometric analysis of digitized radiographs: description of automatic evaluation. In: Ring EFG (ed) Current research in osteoporosis and bone mineral measurement II: British Institute of Radiology, London, pp 14–16

42. Kienböck R (1931) Die Krankheiten der Wirbelsäule im Röntgenbild. Wien Klin Wochenschr 44:232–234

43. Kleerekoper M, Nelson DA (1992) Vertebral fracture or vertebral deformity? Calcif Tissue Int 50:5–6

44. Kleerekoper M, Nelson DA, Peterson EL, Tilley BC (1992) Outcome variables in osteoporosis trials. Bone 13:S29–S34

45. Kleerekoper M, Parfitt AM, Ellis BI (1984) Measurement of vertebral fracture rates in osteoporosis. In: Christiansen C, Arnaud CD, Nordin BEC, Parfitt AM, Peck WA, Riggs BL (eds) Copenhagen international symposium on osteoporosis, 3–8 June 1984. 1. Glostrup Hospital, Department of Clinical Chemistry, Copenhagen, pp 103–108

46. Kuiper JW, van Kuijk C, van Bogedom J (1993) Vertebral deformity indices: influence of X-ray technique and patient width (abstract). Calcif Tissue Int 52:173

47. Lang T, Takada M, Gee R, Wu C, Li J, Hayashi-Clark C, Schoen S, March V, Genant HK (1997) A preliminary evaluation of the Lunar Expert-XL for bone densitometry and vertebral morphometry. J Bone Miner Res 12:136–143

48. Lau EMC, Chan HHL, Woo J, Lin F, Black D, Nevitt M, Leung PC (1996) Normal ranges for vertebral height ratios and prevalence of vertebral fracture in Hong Kong Chinese: a comparison with American Caucasians. J Bone Miner Res 11:1364–1368

49. Li J, Wu CY, Jergas M, Genant HK (1995) Diagnosing prevalent vertebral fracture: a comparison between quantitative morphometry and a standardized visual (semiquantitative) approach. In: Genant HK, Jergas M, van Kuijk C (eds) Vertebral fracture in osteoporosis. Radiology Research and Education Foundation, San Francisco, pp 271–279

50. Mann T, Oviatt SK, Wilson D, Nelson D, Orwoll ES (1992) Vertebral deformity in men. J Bone Miner Res 7:1259–1265

51. Mazess RB (1993) Morphometric X-ray absorptiometry. United States, Lunar Corporation, Madison

52. McCloskey EV, Kanis JA (1994) Assessing vertebral deformities (letter). Osteoporosis Int 4:117–119

53. McCloskey EV, Spector TD, Eyres KS, Fern ED, O'Rourke N, Vasikaran S, Kanis JA (1993) The assessment of vertebral deformity: a method for use in population studies and clinical trials. Osteoporosis Int 3:138–147

54. McCloskey EV, Spector TD, Khan S, Sirtori P, Nagatsuka K, Kanis JA (1993) Prevalence of vertebral deformity and concordance between definitions of fracture. In: Christiansen C, Riis B (eds) Fourth international symposium on osteoporosis and consensus development conference. Osteopress, Hong Kong, pp 62–64

55. Megard M, Pitiot-Rousset M, Boissel JP, Andre-Fouet X, Meunier P (1976) Comparaison de l'indice des travees femorales et de l'indice radiologique vertebral. Lyon Med 235:85–93

56. Melton LJ III, Kan SH, Frye MA, Wahner HW, O'Fallon WM, Riggs BL (1989) Epidemiology of vertebral fractures in women. Am J Epidemiol 129:1000–1011

57. Melton LJ III, Lane AW, Cooper C, Eastell R, O'Fallon WM, Riggs BL (1993) Prevalence and incidence of vertebral deformities. Osteoporosis Int 3:113–119

58. Meunier P (1968) La dynamique du remaniement osseux humain, étudiée par lecture quantitative de la biopsie osseuse, Lyon

59. Meunier PJ, Bressot C, Vignon E, Edouard C, Alexandre C, Courpron P, Laurent J (1978) Radiological and histological evolution of post-menopausal osteoporosis treated with sodium fluoride-vitamin D-calcium. Preliminary results. In: Courvoisier B, Donath A, Baud CA (eds) Fluoride and bone. Huber, Bern, pp 263–276

60. Minne HW, Leidig G, Wüster C, Siromachkostov L, Baldauf G, Bickel R, Sauer P, Lojen M, Ziegler R (1988) A newly developed spine deformity index (SDI) to quantitate vertebral crush fractures in patients with osteoporosis. Bone Miner 3:335–349

61. Nathanson L, Lewitan A (1941) Deformities and fractures of the vertebrae as a result of senile and presenile osteoporosis. Am J Roentgenol 46:197–202

62. Nelson D, Peterson E, Tilley B, O'Fallon W, Chao E, Riggs BL, Kleerekoper M (1990) Measurement of vertebral area on spine X-rays in osteoporosis: reliability of digitizing techniques. J Bone Miner Res 5:707–716

63. Nelson DA, Kleerekoper M, Peterson EL (1994) Reversal of vertebral deformities in osteoporosis: measurement error or "rebound"? J Bone Miner Res 9:977–982

64. Nicholson PHF, Haddaway MJ, Davie MWJ, Evans SF (1993) Vertebral deformity, bone mineral density, back pain and height loss in unscreened women over 50 years. Osteo Int 3:300–307

65. Nielsen VAH, Pødenphant J, Martens S, Gotfredsen A, Riis BJ (1991) Precision in assessment of osteoporosis from spine radiographs. Eur J Radiol 13:11–14

66. O'Neill TW, Varlow J, Felsenberg D, Johnell O, Weber K, Marchant F, Delmas PD, Cooper C, Kanis J, Silman AJ (1994) Variation in vertebral height ratios in population studies. J Bone Miner Res 9:1895–1907

67. Osman AA-H, Bassiouni H, Koutri R, Nijs J, Geusens P, Dequeker J (1994) Aging of the thoracic spine: distinction between wedging in osteoarthritis and fracture in osteoporosis – a cross-sectional and longitudinal study. Bone 15:437–442

68. Patel R, Blake GM, Batchelor S, Fogelman I (1996) Occupational dose to the radi-

ographer in dual X-ray absorptiometry: a comparison of pencil-beam and fan-beam systems. Br J Radiol 69:539–543

69. Raymakers JA, Kapelle JW, van Berensteijn ECH, Duursma SA (1990) Assessment of osteoporotic spine deformity: a new method. Skeletal Radiol 19:91–97

70. Rédei J, Ouyang X, Engelke K, Song SM, Genant HK (1995) Technical considerations for digital image processing. In: Genant HK, Jergas M, van Kuijk C (eds) Vertebral fracture in osteoporosis. Radiology Research and Education Foundation, San Francisco, pp 293–308

71. Riggs BL, Seeman E, Hodgson SF, Taves PR, O'Fallon WM (1982) Effect of the fluoride/calcium regimen on vertebral fracture occurrence in postmenopausal osteoporosis. N Engl J Med 306:446–450

72. Rosenthal DI, Cohen GL, Rosol MS (1995) Digital morphometry in a large-scale international osteoporosis clinical trial. In: Genant HK, Jergas M, van Kuijk C (eds) Vertebral fracture in osteoporosis. Radiology Research and Education Foundation, San Francisco, pp 319–330

73. Rosol M, Moore R, Chew F, Dupuy D, Palmer W, Rosenthal D (1993) A digital method of vertebral morphometry. J Bone Miner Res 9 [Suppl 1]:S278

74. Ross PD, Davis JW, Epstein RS, Wasnich RD (1992) Ability of vertebral dimensions from a single radiograph to identify fractures. Calcif Tissue Int 51:95–99

75. Ross PD, Wasnich RD, Davis JW, Vogel JM (1991) Vertebral dimension differences between Caucasian populations, and between Caucasians and Japanese. Bone 12:107–112

76. Ross PD, Yhee YK, He Y-F, Davis JW, Kamimoto C, Epstein RS, Wasnich RD (1993) A new method for vertebral fracture diagnosis. J Bone Miner Res 8:167–174

77. Sauer P, Leidig G, Minne HW, Dudeck G, Schwarz W, Siromachkostov L, Ziegler R (1991) Spine deformity index (SDI) versus other objective procedures of vertebral fracture identification in patients with osteoporosis. J Bone Miner Res 6:227–238

78. Smith RW, Eyler WR, Mellinger RC (1960) On the incidence of senile osteoporosis. Ann Intern Med 52:773–781

79. Smith-Bindman R, Cummings SR, Steiger P, Genant HK (1991) A comparison of morphometric definitions of vertebral fracture. J Bone Miner Res 6:25–34

80. Smith-Bindman R, Cummings SR, Steiger P, Genant HK (1991) The index of radiographic area (IRA): a new approach to grading the severity of vertebral fractures. Bone Miner 15:137–150

81. Spector TD, McCLoskey EV, Doyle DV, Kanis JA (1993) Prevalence of vertebral fracture in women and the relationship with bone density and symptoms: the Chingford study. J Bone Miner Res 8:817–822

82. Spencer NE, Steiger P, Cummings SR, Genant HK (1990) Placement for points for digitizing spine films. J Bone Miner Res 5:S247

83. Steiger P, Cummings SR, Genant HK, Weiss H (1994) Morphometric X-ray absorptiometry of the spine: correlation in vivo with morphometric radiography. Osteoporosis Int 4:238–244

84. Steiger P, Weiss H, Stein JA (1993) Morphometric X-ray absorptiometry of the spine: a new method to assess vertebral osteoporosis. In: Christiansen C, Riis B (eds) 1993 Proceedings of the 4th International Symposium on Osteoporosis and Consensus Development Conference. 4th International Symposium on Osteoporosis, Hong Kong, p 292

85. Storm T, Thamsborg G, Sørensen HA, Kollerup G, Genant HK, Sørensen OH (1992) Long-term treatment with intermittent cyclical etidronate: effect on bone mass and fracture rate. J Bone Miner Res 7 [Suppl 1]:S117

86. Storm T, Thamsborg G, Steiniche T, Genant HK, Sørenson OH (1990) Effect of intermittent cyclical etidronate therapy on bone mass and fracture rate in women with postmenopausal osteoporosis. N Engl J Med 322:1265–1271

87. Watts NB, Harris ST, Genant HK, Wasnich RD, Miller PD, Jackson RD, Licata AA, Ross P, Woodson GCI, Yanover MJ, Mysiw J, Kohse L, Rao MB, Steiger P, Richmond B, Chesnut CHI (1990) Intermittent cyclical etidronate treatment of postmenopausal osteoporosis. N Engl J Med 323:73–79

88. Wu CY, Li J, Jergas M, Genant HK (1995) Diagnosing incident vertebral fracture: a comparison between quantitative morphometry and a standardized visual (semiquantitative) approach. In: Genant HK, Jergas M, van Kuijk C (eds) Vertebral fracture in osteoporosis. Radiology Research and Education Foundation, San Francisco, pp 281–291

13 Basic Considerations and Definitions in Bone Densitometry

M. Jergas and M. Uffmann

Bone densitometry has become an established tool for diagnosing and following up patients with disorders affecting the bone mineralization. The development of bone densitometry has certainly been driven by the need to overcome the inherent shortcomings of plain radiography for assessing bone density [17, 79]. Several studies show that the agreement between radiologists for the assessment of the bone mineral status based on radiographs of the spine is only moderate [30, 66]. This may be even more a problem when one tries to assess changes in bone density based on conventional radiography. Semiquantitative methods such as Saville's, Singh's, or Jhamaria's osteoporosis indices are of limited value, and some quantitative scores such as the Barnett-Nordin index at the spine do not really demonstrate a good correlation with bone density [6, 67, 68, 112, 114]. Therefore a number of methods for quantitatively assessing a person's bone status to overcome the imperfections of plain radiography have been developed. With these methods a completely new terminology has evolved including various acronyms and definitions that are in part specific to some methods, or that are used for diagnostic purposes.

Acronyms in Bone Densitometry

When acronyms are used for a method it is usually evidence of its general widespread acceptance. However, acronyms in the medical field are used excessively, and some may even have several meanings depending on the context they are used in. The field of bone densitometry has definitely become a playground for acronyms. We therefore begin with a short overview of acronyms commonly used in bone densitometry:

- Bone densitometry
    - Single-photon absorptiometry: SPA
    - Dual-photon absorptiometry: DPA
    - Single X-ray absorptiometry: SXA (also SEXA)
    - Dual X-ray absorptiometry: DXA (also DEXA, rarely DER, DEPR, QDR, DPX)
    - Quantitative computed tomography: QCT
    - Peripheral quantitative computed tomography: pQCT
- Quantitative ultrasound: QUS
    - Speed of sound: SOS

- Amplitude-dependent speed of sound: ad-SOS
- Ultrasound transmission velocity (synonymous with speed of sound) UTV
- Broadband ultrasound attenuation: BUA

Most acronyms are made up from the initial letters of a name, such as QCT for quantitative computed tomography. Except for dual X-ray absorptiometry there has never been any controversy about the acronyms for densitometric methods. The introduction of dual X-ray absorptiometry in 1987 was closely linked to marketing by the major manufacturers of the densitometers [119]. Therefore a multitude of synonyms exist for dual X-ray absorptiometry, such as DEXA (dual-energy X-ray absorptiometry), DER (dual-energy radiography), DEPR (dual-energy projection radiography), QDR (quantitative digital radiography), and DPX (dual-photon X-ray absorptiometry). Some of these acronyms are linked to tradenames of manufacturers, and since the method is derived from dual-photon absorptiometry (DPA), and to avoid favoring a particular manufacturer, DXA has been proposed as the acronym for dual X-ray absorptiometry [34, 131]. In the recent years quantitative ultrasound (QUS) measures have been added to the diagnostic toolbox of osteoporosis, and with the introduction of this new technique, the list of acronyms has continued to grow. The commonly used acronyms for these methods are also listed above.

Bone Mineral Density Is Not Bone Mineral Density Is Not Bone Mineral Density

A person's bone status may be assessed in a number of ways (Table 13-1). Most established methods still rely on the attenuation of an X-ray beam by the bone, and it is a common feature of these methods that the results are expressed in the form of bone mineral density (BMD). However, the first thing that the reader must learn here is that bone density as measured by one method does not necessarily corre-

Table 13-1 Terminology and units used in radiogrammetry, bone densitometry and quantitative ultrasound

Terminology	Acronym	Unit	Method
Radiogrammetry			
Combined cortical thickness	CCT	cm	Conventional radiography
Cortical area		cm^2	
Bone Densitometry			
Bone mineral content	BMC	g	SPA, SXA, DPA, DXA
Bone mineral density (linear)	BMD	g/cm	SPA, SXA
Bone mineral density (area)	BMD	g/cm^2	SPA, SXA, DPA, DXA
„Standardized" bone mineral density	sBMD	mg/cm^2	DXA
Bone mineral density (volumetric)	BMD	g/cm^3	QCT, pQCT, (DXA)
Bone mineral apparent density	BMAD	g/cm^3	DXA
Quantitative ultrasound			
Speed of sound	SOS, UTV	m/s	QUS
Broadband ultrasound attenuation	BUA	dB/MHz	QUS

spond to bone density as measured by another method. The *American Heritage Dictionary* defines density as "a. the amount of something per unit measure, esp. per unit length, area, or volume. b. the mass per unit volume of a substance under specified or standard conditions of pressure and temperature" [3]. The latter definition is well known to anyone who has ever attended physics class at school, and this meaning of density usually applies when one talks about density. However, it is the first definition that corresponds more closely to the meaning of density as the term is used in bone densitometry. To understand why this is so, one must take a close look at the techniques applied to measure bone density.

The first technique applied to quantitatively measure bone density was photodensitometry, or radiographic absorptiometry [54, 88, 118]. In radiographic absorptiometry a radiograph of the peripheral skeleton with an aluminum or hydroxyapatite reference wedge included is taken. After film processing bone and reference wedge are evaluated; a small spot on the bone of interest and the reference wedge are measured using a photodensitometer. The density of a defined region of interest is then compared to that of the aluminum wedge. The result for bone density is usually given in millimeters of aluminum equivalent if the reference step consists of aluminum, or in millilmeters of hydroxyapatite equivalent. Thus bone density as measured by photodensitometry is not a true bone mass per volume but rather the attenuation over a selected small area adjusted for a given reference standard. The three dimensions of the body part are reduced to two dimensions due to the nature of the technique that is applied.

One would expect that such a measure depends on skeletal size since it is affected by the thickness of the bone of interest. As with photodensitometry, there are a number of methods based on projection techniques that measure bone mass over an area rather than a volume. Today's most popular methods that employ a projection technique for assessing bone density are SXA and DXA [64]. Most of these techniques therefore give bone density in grams per square centimeter, as an area density. With some early SPA devices, the predecessor of SXA, bone density is sometimes even given as linear density of grams per centimeter when only one line is acquired. The only densitometric method that measures true volumetric bone density is QCT. This generates a slice of a distinct thickness, and bone density is measured from a region of interest placed in the vertebral body or any other bone. The slice thickness usually applied in spinal QCT is 1 cm, and depending on the method the region of interest may consist of purely trabecular bone or a combination of cortical and trabecular bone [11, 24, 33, 74]. There are models for projection techniques, especially for DXA, that allow for an adjustment for the bone volume and give some estimate for a true volumetric bone density [12, 15, 62, 105]. However, these models are approximations that may not always meet reality.

Some researchers and clinicians do not use a correction for bone dimensions at all, and simply express the results from densitometry as the measured bone mass of an object, or bone mineral content (BMC), given in grams. Since the BMC of a bone partly depends on its size, BMC usually displays a strong correlation with bone dimensions and other anthropometric parameters such as height and weight [62]. The latter correlation is reduced when BMC is corrected for bone dimensions such as area, and there is no association between body height or weight and true volumetric bone density as measured with QCT [62].

To make things more complicated, bone density as measured on the device from one manufacturer cannot necessarily be compared with density from that of another. Thus, although excellent correlations exist between the measurements of the same sites performed on densitometers of the different manufacturers, the application of different standards to determine the BMC of a given object and different algorithms for edge detection and thresholding make comparisons difficult [83, 106, 121]. These technical variations result in considerable differences in the absolute BMD values for the individual patient that depend on which machine is used. In an effort to standardize BMD measurements, representatives of the major DXA manufacturers agreed to standardize their BMD results on the bases of in vivo and in vitro measurements [35, 100].

The European spine phantom was engineered with the intention of intercomparing bone density results independently of the device being used [73]. Based on the results from cross-calibration between scanners the standardization committee proposed a new standardized BMD for the spine with the main advantage that distinct reference populations that exist for one scanner may be transferred to another [35]. Although for individual patients scanners from different manufacturers may yield similar results when expressed as standardized bone density, owing to unique software specifications it still may not be advisable to employ more than one type of scanner for serial assessment of bone density. The standardization of bone density measurements for the hip is more difficult than that for the spine, and efforts are also being made to standardize bone density measurements of the hip.

For QCT the problem is somewhat different. Several researchers have looked at differences resulting from the use of solid and liquid calibration phantoms [21, 44]. For clinical practice it is important to notice that QCT measurements with solid-state phantoms typically yield 10%–15% higher results than with liquid phantoms. This must be considered when comparing the results in an individual patient to normative data, and when assessing longitudinal changes in BMD in cases in which the calibration standard has changed [40]. Slight differences have also been observed for QCT measurements on different CT scanners [4]. Thorough cross-calibration may adjust for most of these differences provided a consistent technique including the choice of the region of interest is applied.

Quantity Versus Quality: Diagnosing Osteoporosis with Quantitative Ultrasound Techniques

Ultrasound techniques used to assess material properties are established methods in industrial material testing. In contrast to measurements of BMD, they seem to measure different properties of bone [48, 65, 77, 84]. While the concept of bone density measurements is quite intuitive, ultrasound measurements are not that easy to understand. When applying ultrasound measurements for the diagnosis of osteoporosis, the results are usually not images but rather pure numbers. Thus, these ultrasound techniques are also called quantitative ultrasound (QUS). Two measurement techniques have been applied, one of which is the speed of sound (SOS) passing through the bone, sometimes also referred to as ultrasound transmission velocity, and the other is the attenuation of the ultrasound beam passing through the bone [53, 55, 81]. The SOS is calculated from the transit time of an ultrasound wave through bone and the width or diameter of this bone, expressed in meters per second. Scattering and absorption are the main mechanisms that contribute to the attenuation of the ultrasound wave penetrating a material. Ultrasound attenuation strongly depends on the frequency of the ultrasound wave employed. With the use of a low-frequency range (approx. 200–600 kHz) the attenuation is an almost linear function of frequency. In QUS the attenuation of the ultrasound wave is measured over a low-frequency range, and the slope of the regression line is the "broadband ultrasound attenuation" value (BUA), given in decibels per megahertz (dB/MHz). Both SOS and BUA are related to bone density, trabecular orientation, proportion of trabecular and cortical bone, composition of organic and inorganic components, and fatigue damage to the bone. Thus QUS of the bone depends on a variety of factors, and their respective contributions to the ultrasound parameters are hard to grasp.

There are some variations to the basic measures of QUS, for example, the amplitude-dependent SOS, the SOS along the cortical shell of a bone, and the ultrasound reflection velocity [2, 5, 26, 45, 103]. Except for the ultrasound reflection velocity, the other ultrasound measurements have already been commercially introduced. With the amplitude-dependent speed of sound (ad-SOS) the user may not always measure a velocity that is based on the first signal of the ultrasound wave that passed through the bone but rather on a later signal depending on the magnitude of the signal received. Thus, the ad-SOS does depend not only on the true SOS but also on the attenuation of the ultrasound beam that tends to be greater in osteoporotic patients. This approach tends artificially to increase the difference between osteoporotic and nonosteoporotic persons, offering a potential benefit over the regular velocity measurements for diagnostic purposes. One manufacturer of QUS devices has also introduced another combined measure called "stiffness." This parameter is calculated from both SOS and BUA values, and although this approach may simplify the interpretation of both values it is not yet clear whether it truly offers additional useful information.

Commercial QUS systems exist for measurements at various sites such as the calcaneus, tibia, patella, and the phalanges. The results acquired with devices from various manufacturers can seldom be easily compared, even when the same site is measured. There is even less standardization in this field than in that of bone densitometry, and considering the rapid new developments including ultrasound imaging for better positioning and the competition among the manufacturers in this emerging market one may not expect any standardization soon.

Being in Conformity to Fact: Accuracy

Again using a definition of the *American Heritage Dictionary*, being accurate means to be "in exact conformity to fact" [3]. How does this translate to bone densitometry and QUS. In fact, it is quite simple to determine the accuracy of a radiographic method to measure bone density. The measured BMC may generally be compared directly to the ash weight of the measured bone. For most methods of bone densitometry an excellent correlation exists between the measured BMC and the ash weight. Depending on the method, however, there may be some discrepancy between the ash weight and the absolute BMC. For example, single-energy QCT measurements are strongly dependent on the fat content of the bone marrow. Thus in single-energy QCT the presence of marrow fat, especially in the elderly, may result in underestimating the true bone density by up to 30% [42, 85]. Dual-energy QCT corrects for this error at the cost of increased radiation dose and potentially poorer reproducibility [32, 43, 70, 109]. In general the magnitude of the offset between the measured and the actual bone mass is not a problem as long as a good correlation between these two measures exists. Table 13-2 includes some numbers of the accuracy for some densitometric techniques.

Table 13-2 Precision, accuracy error, and radiation dose of currently used techniques for the assessment of bone density

Technique	Accuracy (%)	Precision (%)	Radiation exposure (mSv)[a]
Conventional radiography			
Lateral thoracic spine			500–1100
Lateral lumbar spine			1300–2700
Photodensitometry (hand)	5	1–2	<5
SPA/SXA	1–2	4–6	1
DPA			
Lumbar spine	2–11	2–3	5
Proximal femur		2–5	3
DXA			
Lumbar spine PA pencil beam	1–10	1	1–2.5
Lumbar spine PA fan beam	1-100	1	10–60
Lumbar spine lateral	8–10	1–6	3
Proximal femur	6	1–2	1–6
Radius	5	1	1
Whole body	3	1	3
QCT			
Single-energy QCT	5–15	1.5–4	50–300
Dual-energy QCT	3–6	4–6	150–1000
pQCT			
Radius trabecular	2–8	1–2	1
Radius total	2–8	1–2	1
Quantitative ultrasound			
SOS calcaneus		.3–1.2	
BUA calcaneus		1.3–3.8	

[a] Radiation exposure is given as effective dose equivalent [56, 57, 61, 70]. For comparison: the annual exposure from natural background irradiation is approximately 2400 μSv.

There is currently no way to judge the accuracy of QUS measurements. The reason for this is that there is no known correlate for that which one measures quantitatively by the QUS parameters. Both measures appear to be affected by a number of quantitative and qualitative factors, and no single correlate for any QUS measure exists.

Being Within Specified Limits: Precision and Its Impact on Serial Bone Mass Measurements

The *American Heritage Dictionary* definition of being precise is "capable of, resulting from, or designating an action, performance, or process executed or successively repeated within close specified limits" [3]. In bone densitometry, precision is about the ability of a method reproducibly to measure bone density with the intent to reliably monitor changes in bone density or QUS parameters over time.

Bone density measurements have long suffered from inadequate performance in precisely assessing changes in bone density over time. A number of improvements have been implemented to make bone densitometry more precise. For example, rectilinear scanning has improved the precision of SPA [124]; better image quality and visualization of the scanned region resulting in a more accurate definition of the bone edges are important factors for the improved precision of DXA over that of DPA [90,125]. Automated algorithms for defining the midvertebral slice and the regions of interest have improved the precision of single- and dual-energy QCT [72,117]. Precision errors for a number of techniques are given in Table 13-2.

One sees in Table 13-2 that some methods have very small precision errors, such as ultrasound velocity measurements, and others relatively large precision errors, such as QCT. One should therefore expect methods with small precision errors to be better suited for assessing serial changes in bone density or even for stratifying patients as healthy or osteoporotic. However, there is an important flaw in such a simplistic view of the precision error. For example, a precision error (coefficient of variation) of 1% is given for DXA of the spine in a number of publications. The precision error of ultrasound transmission velocity is reported to be as low as 0.2%. From this one would clearly favor ultrasound velocity over DXA. However, looking at the difference between old and young normals, this difference is only 5% for the ultrasound velocity, and it is approximately 30% for DXA. Thus, for stratification of patients the precision error must be compared to the population standard deviation, the difference between young and old persons, and most importantly to the difference between healthy and osteoporotic patients. For most methods the precision error is too small to be of clinical significance in this respect.

Another important issue is the serial assessment of bone density in patients. To detect serial changes in a patient the precision error should be smaller than the expected changes. Therefore a standardized precision has been proposed that relates the precision error to the average annual change in an individual patient [38, 95, 96]. Standardized precision may be defined as the ratio of the precision error to the average annual rate of change for that parameter in a reference population. Given a precision error of 0.01 g/cm² for DXA, and an annual rate of loss of 0.01 g/cm², the standardized precision would be 1. Comparing this result to an ultrasound velocity measurement one finds that at a precision error of 1.5 m/s and an annual rate of loss of 0.4 m/s the standardized precision is approximately 4, although the coefficient of variation in a young normal population is 0.1%.

The coefficient of variation nevertheless plays a role in considering the magnitude of changes required to detect bone density with high confidence. For example, Cummings and colleagues estimated that based on two-point measurements and a 2% precision error bone density changes in individual patients must be greater than 5.5% to be detected with 95% confidence using a two-tailed estimation for confidence intervals [13]. Genant and colleagues proposed a one-tailed approach over the two-tailed approach, which would reduce the required changes in bone density to greater than 3.6% [31]. Both the changes to accurately predict the bone density change and the standardized precision are important in determining when bone density measurements are be repeated, and what measures can be taken to improve precision for serial bone density measurements. It has been found that bone loss rates have a smaller variability over long follow-up time than a short follow-up time [50]. Changes in fracture risk as indicated by BMD measurements are unlikely to occur in periods shorter than 3–5 years [51]. Verheij et al. proposed that duplicate measurements should be performed to pinpoint the results in the method's precision, and they recommended that follow-up periods be at least 1 year [122].

Using the coefficient of variation as a measure for the reproducibility of a method may actually underestimate the true reproducibility by about 30%. Glüer and coworkers recently published a study on the assessment of reproducibility using a root mean square of the standard deviation which more accurately reflects the precision error [37]. Similar statistical approaches have been applied previously by other authors [82, 105, 115]. However, in the majority of studies the coefficient of variation is still used when reproducibility is calculated. These two measures for precision cannot be compared directly, and there is certainly a need for standardizing the way of calculating the precision error.

Which Site To Measure?

Some of the methods in bone densitometry may only be applied to measuring peripheral sites such as the radius and the calcaneus. The methods that are restricted to these sites are single-energy methods that cannot correct for greater soft tissue inhomogeneities and QUS techniques that can be applied only in very close contact to the bone. Other methods such as DPA and SXA/DXA are not restricted to the peripheral skeleton, and sites such as the spine or the hip may be measured. For QCT no restrictions apply other than those due to the lack of specific software for various measurement sites or by the design of the scanner, for example, specific peripheral QCT scanners.

The measurement site has become an important issue in bone densitometry since trabecular bone is regarded as metabolically more active than cortical bone [25]. Because of this higher bone turnover it is desirable to measure bone density at a site with a relatively large amount of trabecular bone. Furthermore, one may wish to measure bone density at a site where osteoporotic fractures frequently occur [133, 134]. In conclusion, preferred sites for measuring bone density are the ultradistal radius, lumbar spine, proximal femur, and calcaneus. Table 13-3 gives the relative amount of mineral content from trabecular and cortical bone at these measurement sites. Using projection techniques such as SPA/SXA or DPA/DXA one always measures a combination of cortical and trabecular bone since these two compartments are projected on top of each other and cannot be separated. QCT is the only method that allows separate assessment of these two bone compartments.

It has been documented that weight-bearing activity has an effect both on BMD and on QUS [69, 130]. The effect of physical activity on site-specific bone density and on bone size may be quite substantial in professional athletes [19, 46]. However, in normal controls these differences are usually much smaller. It has been shown that the association between bone density measured at weight-bearing sites, such as the calcaneus, and future fractures is comparable to that of bone density measured at other sites [9].

Currently there are only limited data on whether a combination of multiple sites improves the diagnostic capability or fracture prediction over that of measuring BMD at only one site. Results from several studies are controversial, with some authors favoring the measurement of a second site, for example, femur in addition to the lumbar spine, for identifying patients at risk for osteoporosis [80, 129]. Using thresholds for diagnosing osteoporosis from bone density measurements, it has been shown that simply adjusting the threshold for a single site measurement identifies as many women at risk for fracture as do multiple site measurements [8, 36, 63]. However, it is of concern that different women may be identified at risk [108]. Therefore, although there may not be a compelling reason routinely to perform bone densitometry of both spine and hip in one patient, if there is evidence of artifacts that make BMD results of one site unreliable, for example,

Table 13-3 Trabecular and cortical bone mineral content at various measurement sites (adapted from Vogel [123])

Measurement site	Bone mineral content from trabecular bone	Weight bearing
Calcaneus	95%	Yes
Lumbar vertebra	50%–70%	Yes
Distal radius	30%–40%	No
Proximal radius	4%	No
Proximal femur	Highly variable depending on region of interest	Yes

anatomic variations, severe degenerative changes or fractures, measuring a second site may be useful for the assessment of a person's bone mineral status. For general clinical practice the interpretation and value of multiple site measurements are still uncertain.

Interpretation of Bone Densitometry for Diagnosing Osteoporosis and Predicting Future Fractures

The definition of osteoporosis is a much debated issue among researchers, health officials, and clinicians. Often the clinical diagnosis of osteoporosis is associated with the presence of characteristic fractures. However, these fractures should be regarded as the sequelae of a qualitative and quantitative deterioration of bone tissue leading to increased fragility of the bones. Thus osteoporosis may rather be defined by means of bone quantity and bone quality. Albright defined osteoporosis as "that category of decreased bone mass where the disturbance is a failure of the osteoblasts to lay down bone matrix" [1]. Bone densitometry is a technique for assessing bone mass noninvasively, and recently a definition of osteoporosis based on results from bone densitometry has been published by a World Health Organization study group [132]. In women osteoporosis can be diagnosed if the BMD or BMC value is 2.5 SD below the mean of a young reference population. Kanis and coworkers commented on this definition and gave diagnostic categories that may be applied to white women [75, 76]:
- Normal: a BMD or BMC value not less than 1 SD below the young adult mean value
- Low bone mass (or osteopenia): a BMD or BMC value between 1 and 2.5 SD below the young adult mean value
- Osteoporosis: a BMD or BMC value more than 2.5 SD below the young adult mean value
- Severe osteoporosis (or established osteoporosis): a BMD or BMC value more than 2.5 SD below the young adult mean value in the presence of one or more fragility fractures

This definition uses the T score as a diagnostic measure as it has already long been used in bone densitometry. Bone density results are typically compared to those of age-, sex-, and race-matched controls. T and Z scores have been introduced for the interpretation of results from bone densitometry. The Z score gives the patient's results as the deviation from the mean of age-matched controls divided by the standard deviation, which is an indicator of biological variability. The T score is usually referenced to the peak bone mass of young normal adults and is calculated similarly to the Z score.

The use of a threshold for diagnosing osteoporosis as proposed by the WHO working group is derived from the concept of a so-called "fracture threshold." Epidemiological studies show that the rate of prevalent fractures increases substantially below a certain value. For clinical use the "fracture threshold" is generally set relatively arbitrarily at 2 SD below the mean of a young normal population or a suitable reference population [91,101,102]. From a clinical perspective this concept offers significant guidance for therapeutic and diagnostic procedures. On the other hand, the term "fracture threshold" in its literal sense may be misleading because of the substantial overlap between fracture and nonfracture patients. Speaking in terms of bone mass, an absolute discrimination between these groups is not possible. Furthermore, this discrimination is not the goal of bone mass measurements. Rather they should be used to assess the risk of future fractures, and must be understood as the probability of an adverse event (the fracture), not as absolute prediction. Osteoporosis should be understood as the lower part of a continuum of bone density, with the greatest risk among those subjects with lowest absolute BMD values ("gradient of risk") [127].

Apart from these very basic limitations of a fracture threshold there are some quite practical considerations that make the use of a fracture threshold based on a T score very controversial [10]. Probably the most important issue is the use of an appropriate reference database. Recent studies have shown that there may be limited agreement between a manufacturer's reference database and data derived from a study population [86,87]. The T score cutoff points between different sites of BMD measurement, even within the same region, for example, total hip, femoral neck, trochanter, identify different proportions of patients and create different risk groups [10, 93]. This is even more a problem in regard to multiple anatomic sites, such as spine and hip: densitometric results from different sites disagree in a large number of patients.

Using a fracture threshold based on a comparison to young normals to define osteoporosis is a concept that does not do justice to the complexity of the disease even though bone density must currently be regarded as the most important contributor to osteoporotic fractures. Bone density has been found to be significantly associated with the risk of future fracture in many prospective studies [9, 14, 27–29, 58–60, 92, 98, 113, 120]. This association is partly independent of age and other significant predictors of fracture such as falls, cognizance, and mobility [16]. The differences between the various densitometric techniques in predicting future osteoporotic fracture of any type is marginal [9]. However, it seems that bone density measurements at the site of fracture perform better than measurements at other sites [89]. Retrospective, or cross-sectional, and prospective study designs generally deliver comparable results [116]. There is currently no evidence that measuring a second site improves the diagnostic capability of bone densitometry. However, as noted above, measuring a second site may identify a number of different patients at risk for osteoporosis. From long-term prospective studies it can be concluded that peak bone density and bone loss are important predictors of subsequent fracture, and that fracture can be predicted over a longer period of time [29, 49, 116]. Bone density predicts fracture even in very elderly persons [29, 60, 97]. However, some fractures, such as the femoral neck fracture, may be more strongly influenced by other risk fractures at a higher age.

QUS has a predictive capability similar to bone densitometry without showing a close correlation to the quantitative measures of bone density [7, 23, 39]. Considering the results from the first prospective studies QUS may soon be an alternative to bone density measurements in clinical practice [47, 52, 107]. From the perspective that bone densitometry and QUS independently predict fractures, these measures actually seem complementary rather than competitive.

Simple geometric measures of the bones such as hip axis length and vertebral depth may also be derived from images of bone densitometry scans and are also predictive of hip fracture or vertebral fracture independent of bone density [20, 111]. In addition, prevalent fractures are strong predictors of future fracture and must be considered when therapeutic intervention is planned [78, 110, 128]. Overall, there are various risk factors that contribute to the fragility of bone and to osteoporotic fracture.

Radiation Exposure in Bone Densitometry

Ever since the days of DXA, radiation exposure has almost become a nonissue in discussions of bone densitometry. With the early pencil-beam DXA scanners it was possible to perform a scan with a very low dose, on the order of 1 μSv [57, 70]. The radiation dose to the operator was also extremely low, and there was therefore no need for a special radiation protection, and the operator's desk could be placed next to the densitometer. This has changed somewhat with the latest models of bone densitometers, using a fan beam design rather than a pencil-beam design, and with increased efforts to improve image quality, especially for the purpose of creating a diagnostic image for the assessment of vertebral fracture. With these scanners the radiation dose to both the patient and the radiographer is considerably higher than with scanners using a pencil-beam mode [18, 99]. Patel and colleagues have estimated that the ambient dose equivalent rate is similar to that of a radionuclide bone scan [104]. Therefore the authors propose stricter precautions for the radiographers involved in DXA scanning such as increasing the distance between the operator and the densitometer or using scan modes with short scanning times. An overview of the radiation exposure to the patient using various methods for bone densitometry is given in Table 13-2. Considering the annual dose equivalent from natural background radiation, the radiation exposure from bone densitometry is quite small. Furthermore, due to the age distribution of the patients usually studied with bone densitometry, the risk of radiation-induced damage is outweighed by a potentially greater benefit from bone mineral measurements.

Quality Control in Bone Densitometry

Bone density is an endpoint in numerous clinical drug trials and epidemiological studies that often involve multiple densitometers and serial assessment of bone density in individual patients. It is of importance that bone densitometry results be comparable between different sites, and for serial measurements the densitometer must provide a consistent performance over the course of the study [22, 41, 94, 126]. Consistent measurements over time are not only of concern in clinical drug trials but are essential in everyday clinical practice. To control for a consistent performance, a quality control scan of a known standard is performed every day, and the results from this quality control scan are then compared to other scan data in a quality control database. The standard used for these daily quality control scans differs with the manufacturer and may consist of anthropomorphic phantoms or geometric objects of known density. For cross-calibration purposes and for longitudinal quality control Kalender and colleagues have manufactured a special semianthropomorphic phantom, the European spine phantom, that may be applied across densitometers from different manufacturers and for both QCT and DXA [71, 73].

Summary and Conclusion

Bone densitometry and QUS have become important tools for the quantitative assessment of osteoporosis. The widespread introduction and acceptance of these methods has been accompanied by a new terminology and new concepts for making the results of bone densitometry applicable in clinical practice. The methods differ with respect to precision (deviation based on multiple measurements), accuracy (reliability that the measured value reflects true BMC), and sensitivity (capability to readily separate an abnormal state from the normal or to readily detect changes over time in a patient or a population). Furthermore, the densities measured do not always correspond to each other. Projection techniques such as DXA allow assessment only of an area density while QCT allows true volumetric bone density to be assessed. Depending on the site of measurement, projection techniques always assess combinations of trabecular and cortical bone to various amounts. With QCT it is possible to assess either component separately. QUS techniques have recently been added as a diagnostic tool assessing "bone quality" rather than bone quantity.

T scores and Z scores are diagnostic concepts in osteoporosis relying on comparisons with young normals and age-matched controls. A recent definition of osteoporosis issued by the WHO relies on the definition of osteoporosis based on a fixed threshold (T score ≤ 2.5 SD). However, since no absolute discrimination is possible between fractured and nonfractured patients, bone mass measurements should rather be used as an estimate of the probability of an adverse event (the fracture), not as absolute prediction.

References

1. Albright F (1947) Osteoporosis. Ann Intern Med 27:861–882
2. Alenfeld F, Wüster C, Goetz M, Beck C, Ziegler R (1995) Diagnostic value of

ultrasound measurements of bone mineral density on the metacarpals in healthy and osteoporotic subjects. Bone 16:147S

3. American Heritage Dictionary (1985) Houghton Mifflin, Boston

4. Andresen R, Radmer S, Banzer D, Felsenberg D, Wolf KJ (1994) Quantitative Knochenmineralgehaltsbestimmung (QCT). Systemvergleich baugleicher Computertomographen. Rofo Fortschr Geb Röntgenstr Neuen Bildgeb Verfahr 160:260–265

5. Antich PP, Pak CYC, Gonzales J, Anderson J, Sakhaee K, Rubin C (1993) Measurement of intrinsic bone quality in vivo by reflection ultrasound: correction of impaired quality with slow-release sodium fluoride and calcium citrate. J Bone Miner Res 8:301–311

6. Barnett E, Nordin BEC (1960) The radiological diagnosis of osteoporosis: a new approach. Clin Radiol 11:166–174

7. Bauer DC, Glüer CC, Genant HK, Stone K (1995) Quantitative ultrasound and vertebral fracture in post menopausal women. J Bone Miner Res 10:353–358

8. Black D, Bauer DC, Lu Y, Tabor H, Genant HK, Cummings SR (1995) Should BMD be measured at multiple sites to predict fracture risk in elderly women? J Bone Miner Res 10 [Suppl 1]:S140

9. Black D, Cummings SR, Genant HK, Nevitt MC, Palermo L, Browner W (1992) Axial and appendicular bone density predict fractures in older women. J Bone Miner Res 7:633–638

10. Black DM, Palermo L, Genant HK, Cummings SR (1996) Four reasons to avoid the use of BMD T-scores in treatment decisions for osteoporosis. J Bone Miner Res 11:S118

11. Boonen S, Cheng XG, Nijs J, Nicholson PHF, Verbeke G, Lesaffre E, Aerssens J, Dequeker J (1997) Factors associated with cortical and trabecular bone loss as quantified by peripheral conputed tomography (pQCT) at the ultradistal radius in aging women. Calcif Tissue Int 60:164–170

12. Carter DR, Bouxsein ML, Marcus R (1992) New approaches for interpreting projected bone densitometry data. J Bone Miner Res 7:137–145

13. Cummings SR, Black D (1986) Should perimenopausal women be screened for osteoporosis? Ann Intern Med 104:817–823

14. Cummings SR, Black DM, Nevitt MC, Browner W, Cauley J, Ensrud K, Genant HK, Palermo L, Scott J, Vogt TM (1993) Bone density at various sites for prediction of hip fractures. Lancet 341:72–75

15. Cummings SR, Marcus R, Palermo L, Ensrud KE, Genant HK (1994) Does estimating volumetric bone density of the femoral neck improve the prediction of hip fracture? A prospective study. J Bone Miner Res 9:1429–1432

16. Cummings SR, Nevitt MC, Browner WS, Stone K, Fox K, Ensrud K, Cauley J, Black D, Vogt T (1995) Risk factors for hip fractures in white women. N Engl J Med 332:767–773

17. Doyle FH, Gutteridge DH, Joplin GF, Fraser R (1967) An assessment of radiological criteria used in the study of spinal osteoporosis. Br J Radiol 40:241–250

18. Eiken P, Kolthoff N, Bärenholdt O, Hermansen F, Nielsen SP (1994) Switching from DXA pencil-beam to fan-beam. II: Studies in vivo. Bone 15:671–676

19. Etherington J, Harris PA, Nandra D, Hart DJ, Wolman RL, Doyle DV, Spector TD (1996) The effect of weight bearing exercise on bone mineral density: a study of female ex-elite athletes and the general population. J Bone Miner Res 11:1333–1338

20. Faulkner KG, Cummings SR, Glüer CC, Palermo L, Black D, Genant HK (1993) Simple measurement of femoral geometry predicts hip fracture: the study of osteopotic fractures. J Bone Miner Res 8:1211–1217

21. Faulkner KG, Glüer CC, Grampp S, Genant HK (1993) Cross calibration of liquid and solid QCT calibration standards: corrections to the UCSF normative data. Osteoporosis Int 3:36–42

22. Faulkner KG, McClung MR (1995) Quality control of DXA instruments in multicenter trials. Osteoporos Int 5:218–27

23. Faulkner KG, McClung MR, Coleman LJ, Kingston-Sandahl E (1994) Quantitative ultrasound of the heel: correlation with densitometric measurements at different skeletal sites. Osteoporosis Int 4:42–47

24. Felsenberg D, Kalender WA, Banzer D, Schmilinsky G, Heyse M, Fischer E, Schneider U (1988) Quantitative computertomographische Knochenmineralgehaltbestimmung. Fortschr Rontgenstr 148:85–89

25. Frost HM (1964) Dynamics of bone remodelling. In: Frost HM (ed) Bone biodynamics. Little Brown, Boston, pp 315–334

26. Funck C, Wüster C, Alenfeld FE, Pereira-Lima JFS, Fritz T, Meeder PJ, Götz M, Ziegler R (1996) Ultrasound velocity of the tibia in normal German women and hip fracture patients. Calcif Tissue Int 58:390–394

27. Gärdsell P, Johnell O, Nilsson BE (1990) The predictive value of forearm bone mineral content measurements in men. Bone 11:229–232

28. Gärdsell P, Johnell O, Nilsson BE (1991) The predictive value of bone loss for fragility fractures in women: a longitudinal study over 15 years. Calcif Tissue Int 49:90–94

29. Gärdsell P, Johnell O, Nilsson BE, Gullberg B (1993) Predicting various fragility fractures in women by forearm bone densitometry: a follow-up study. Calcif Tissue Int 52:348–353

30. Garton MJ, Robertson EM, Gilbert FJ, Gomersall L, Reid DM (1994) Can radiologists detect osteopenia on plain radiographs? Clin Radiol 49:118–122

31. Genant HK, Block JE, Steiger P, Glüer CC, Ettinger B, Harris ST (1989) Appropriate use of bone densitometry. Radiology 170:817–822

32. Genant HK, Boyd DP (1977) Quantitative bone mineral analysis using dual energy computed tomography. Invest Radiol 12:545–551

33. Genant HK, Cann CE, Ettinger B, Gordan GS (1982) Quantitative computed tomography of vertebral spongiosa: a sensitive method for detecting early bone loss after oophorectomy. Ann Intern Med 97:699–705

34. Genant HK, Glüer CC, Faulkner KG, Majumdar S, Harris ST, Engelke K, van KC (1992) Acronyms in bone densitometry. Radiology 184:878

35. Genant HK, Grampp S, Glüer CC, Faulkner KG, Jergas M, Engelke K, Hagiwara S, van Kuijk C (1994) Universal standardization for dual X-ray absorptiometry: patient and phantom cross-calibration results. J Bone Miner Res 9:1503–1514

36. Genant HK, Lu Y, Mathur AK, Fuerst TP, Cummings SR (1996) Classification based on DXA measurements for assessing the risk of hip fractures. J Bone Miner Res 11:S120

37. Glüer CC, Blake G, Lu Y, Blunt BA, Jergas M, Genant HK (1995) Accurate assessment of precision errors: how to measure the reproducibility of bone densitometry techniques. Osteoporos Int 5:262–270

38. Glüer CC, Blunt B, Engelke K, Jergas M, Grampp S, Genant HK (1994) "Characteristic follow-up time" – a new concept for standardized characterization of a technique's ability to monitor longitudinal changes. Bone Miner 25 [Suppl 2]:S40

39. Glüer CC, Cummings SR, Bauer DC, Stone K, Pressman A, Mathur A, Genant HK (1996) Osteoporosis: association of recent fractures with quantitative ultrasound findings. Radiology 199:725–732

40. Glüer CC, Engelke K, Jergas M, Hagiwara S, Grampp S, Genant HK (1993) Changes in calibration standards for quantitative computed tomography: recommendations for clinical practice. Osteoporosis Int 3:286–287

41. Glüer CC, Faulkner KG, Estilo MJ, Engelke K, Rosin J, Genant HK (1993) Quality assurance for bone densitometry research studies: concept and impact. Osteoporosis Int 3:227–235

42. Glüer CC, Genant HK (1989) Impact of marrow fat on accuracy of quantitative CT. J Comput Assist Tomogr 13:1023–1035

43. Glüer CC, Reiser UJ, Davis CA, Rutt BK, Genant HK (1988) Vertebral mineral determination by quantitative computed tomography (QCT): accuracy of single and dual energy measurements. J Comput Assist Tomogr 12:242–258

44. Goodsitt MM (1992) Conversion relations for quantitative CT bone mineral density measured with solid and liquid calibration standards. Bone Miner 19:145–158

45. Guglielmi G, Giannantempo GM, Scillitani A, Chiodini I, Liuzzi A, Cammisa M (1996) Phalangeal QUS, QCT and DXA in healthy, postmenopausal and osteoporotic women. Osteoporosis Int 6:S207

46. Haapasalo H, Sievanen H, Kannus P, Heinonen A, Oja P, Vuori I (1996) Dimensions and estimated mechanical characteristics of the humerus after long-term tennis loading. J Bone Miner Res 11:864–872

47. Hans D, Dargent-Molina P, Schott AM, Seber JL, Cormier C, Kotzli PO, Delmas PD, Pouilles JM (1996) Ultrasonographic heel measurements to predict hip fracture in the elderly. Lancet 348:511–514

48. Hans D, Fuerst T, Duboeuf F (1997) Quantitative ultrasound bone measurement. Eur Radiol 7:S43–S50

49. Hansen MA, Overgaard K, Riis BJ, Christiansen C (1991) Role of peak bone

mass and bone loss in postmenopausal osteoporosis: 12 year study. BMJ 303:961–964

50. He Y-F, Davis JW, Ross PD, Wasnich RD (1993) Declining bone loss rate variability with increasing follow-up time. Bone Miner 21:119–128

51. He Y-F, Ross PD, Davis JW, Epstein RS, Vogel JM, Wasnich RD (1994) When should bone density measurements be repeated? Calcif Tissue Int 55:243–248

52. Heaney RP, Avioli LV, Chesnut III CH, Lappe J, Recker RR, Brandenburger GH (1995) Ultrasound velocity through bone predicts incident vertebral deformity. J Bone Miner Res 10:341–345

53. Heaney RP, Avioli LV, Chestnut CH, Lappe J, Recker RR, Brandburger GH (1989) Osteoporotic bone fragility: detection by ultrasound transmission velocity. JAMA 261:2986–2990

54. Heuck F, Schmidt E (1960) Die quantitative Bestimmung des Mineralgehaltes des Knochens aus dem Röntgenbild. Fortschr Rontgenstr 93:523–554

55. Hosie CJ, Smith DA, Deacon AD, Langton CM (1987) Comparison of broadband ultrasonic attenuation of the os calcis and quantitative computed tomography of the distal radius. Clin Phys Physiol Meas 8:303–308

56. Huda W, Bissessur K (1990) Effective dose equivalents, HE, in diagnostic radiology. Med Phys 17:998–1003

57. Huda W, Morin RL (1996) Patient doses in bone mineral densitometry. Br J Radiol 69:422–425

58. Hui SL, Slemenda CW, Carey MA, Johnston CC Jr (1995) Choosing between predictors of fractures. J Bone Miner Res 10:1816–1822

59. Hui SL, Slemenda CW, Johnston CC (1988) Age and bone mass as predictors of fracture in a prospective study. J Clin Invest 81:1804–1809

60. Hui SL, Slemenda CW, Johnston CC (1989) Baseline measurement of bone mass predicts fracture in white women. Ann Intern Med 111:355–361

61. ICRP (1977) Recommendations of the International Commission on Radiation Protection (ICRP). ICRP publication 26. Pergamon, Oxford

62. Jergas M, Breitenseher M, Gluer CC, Yu W, Genant HK (1995) Estimates of volumetric bone density from projectional measurements improve the discriminatory capability of dual X-ray absorptiometry. J Bone Miner Res 10:1101–1110

63. Jergas M, Fuerst T, Grampp S, Uffmann M, Glüer CC, Genant HK (1995) Assessment of spinal osteoporosis with dual X-ray absorptiometry of the spine and femur. Radiology 197 (P):362

64. Jergas M, Grampp S, Hagiwara S, Lang P, Bendavid EJ, Genant HK (1993) Perspectives on bone densitometry: past /present/future. J Bone Miner Metab 11 [Suppl 1]:S7–S16

65. Jergas M, Köster O (1993) Ultraschallverfahren in der Diagnostik der Osteoporose. Ultraschall Med 14:136–143

66. Jergas M, Uffmann M, Escher H, Glüer CC, Young KC, Grampp S, Köster O, Genant HK (1994) Interobserver variation in the detection of osteopenia by

radiography and comparison with dual X-ray absorptiometry (DXA) of the lumbar spine. Skeletal Radiol 23:195–199

67. Jergas M, Uffmann M, Escher H, Schaffstein J, Nitzschke E, Köster O (1994) Visuelle Beurteilung konventioneller Röntgenaufnahmen und duale Röntgenabsorptiometrie in der Diagnostik der Osteoporose. Z Orthop Grenzgeb 132:91–98

68. Jhamaria NL, Lal KB, Udawat M, Banerji P, Kabra SG (1983) The trabecular pattern of the calcaneum as an index of osteoporosis. J Bone Joint Surg Br 65:195–198

69. Jones PRM, Hardmann AE, Hudson A, Norgan NG (1991) Influence of brisk walking on the ultrasonic attenuation of the calcaneus in previously sedentary women aged 30–61 years. Calcif Tissue Int 49:112–115

70. Kalender WA (1992) Effective dose values in bone mineral measurements by photon absorptiometry and computed tomography. Osteoporosis Int 2:82–87

71. Kalender WA (1992) A phantom for standardization and quality control in spinal bone mineral measurements by QCT and DXA: design considerations and specifications. Med Phys 19:583–586

72. Kalender WA, Brestowsky H, Felsenberg D (1988) Bone mineral measurements: Automated determination of the midvertebral CT section. Radiology 168:219–221

73. Kalender WA, Felsenberg D, Genant HK, Fischer M, Dequeker J, Reeve J (1995) The European Spine Phantom – a tool for standardization and quality control in spinal bone mineral measurements by DXA and QCT. Eur J Radiol 20:83–92

74. Kalender WA, Felsenberg D, Louis O, Lopez P, Klotz E, Osteaux M, Fraga J (1989) Reference values for trabecular and cortical vertebral bone density in single and dual-energy quantitative computed tomography. Eur J Radiol 9:75–80

75. Kanis JA, Melton III LJ, Christiansen C, Johnston CC, Khaltaev N (1994) The diagnosis of osteoporosis. J Bone Miner Res 9:1137–1141

76. Kanis JA, WHO Study Group (1994) Assessment of fracture risk and its application to screening for postmenopausal osteoporosis: synopsis of a WHO report. Osteoporosis Int 4:368–381

77. Kaufman JJ, Einhorn TA (1993) Perspectives: ultrasound assessment of bone. Osteoporosis Int 8:517–525

78. Kotowicz MA, Melton LJ III, Cooper C, Atkinson EJ, O'Fallon WM, Riggs LB (1994) Risk of hip fracture in women with vertebral fracture. J Bone Miner Res 9:599–605

79. Lachmann E, Whelan M (1936) The roentgen diagnosis of osteoporosis and its limitations. Radiology 26:165–177

80. Lai K, Rencken M, Drinkwater BL, Chesnut CH III (1993) Site of bone density measurement may affect therapy decision. Calcif Tissue Int 53:225–228

81. Langton CM, Palmer SB, Porter RW (1984) The measurement of broadband ultrasound attenuation in cancellous bone. Eng Med 13:89–91

82. Larnach TA, Boyd SJ, Smart RC, Butler SP, Rohl PG, Diamond TH (1992) Reproducibility of lateral spine scans using dual energy X-ray absorptiometry. Calcif Tissue Int 51:255–258

83. Laskey MA, Flaxman ME, Barber RW, Trafford S, Hayball MP, Lyttle KD, Crisp AJ, Compston JE (1991) Comparative performance in vitro and in vivo of Lunar DPX and Hologic QDR-1000 dual energy X-ray absorptiometers. Br J Radiol 64:1023–1029

84. Laugier P, Giat P, Berger G (1994) New ultrasonic methods of quantitative assessment of bone status. Eur J Ultrasound 1:23–38

85. Laval-Jeantet AM, Roger B, Bouysse S, Bergot C, Mazess RB (1986) Influence of vertebral fat content on quantitative CT density. Radiology 159:463–466

86. Lehmann R, Wapniarz M, Randerath O, Kvasnicka HM, John W, Reincke M, Kutnar S, Klein K, Allolio B (1995) Dual-energy X-ray absorptiometry at the lumbar spine in German men and women: a cross-sectional study. Calcif Tissue Int 56:350–354

87. Looker AC, Wahner HW, Dunn WL, Calvo MS, Harris TB, Heyse SP, Johnston CC, Lindsay RL (1995) Proximal femur bone mineral levels of US adults. Osteoporosis Int 5:389–409

88. Mack PB, O'Brian AT, Smith JM, Bauman AW (1939) A method for estimating degree of mineralization of bones from tracings of roentgenograms. Science 89:467

89. Marshall D, Johnell O, Wedel H (1996) Meta-analysis of how well measures of bone mineral density predict occurrence of osteoporotic fractures. BMJ 312:1254–1259

90. Mazess R, Chesnut III CH, McClung M, Genant HK (1992) Enhanced precision with dual-energy X-ray absorptiometry. Calcif Tissue Int 51:14–17

91. Mazess RB (1987) Bone density in the diagnosis of osteoporosis: thresholds and breakpoints. Calcif Tissue Int 41:117–118

92. Melton LJ III, Atkinson EJ, O'Fallon WM, Wahner HW, Riggs BL (1993) Long-term fracture prediction by bone mineral assessed at different skeletal sites. J Bone Miner Res 8:1227–1233

93. Melton LJ III, Chrischilles EA, Cooper C, Lane AW, Riggs BL (1992) How many women have osteoporosis? J Bone Miner Res 7:1005–1010

94. Miller CG (1993) Bone density measurements in clinical trials: the challenge of insuring optimal data. Br J Clin Res 4:113–120

95. Miller CG, Herd RJM, Ramalingam T, Fogelman I, Blake GM (1993) Ultrasonic velocity measurements through the calcaneus: which velocity should be measured? Osteoporosis Int 3:31–35

96. Moris M, Peretz A, Tjeka R, Negaban N, Wouters M, Bergmann P (1995) Quantitative ultrasound bone measurements: normal values and comparison with bone mineral density by dual X-ray absorptiometry. Calcif Tissue Int 57:6–10

97. Nevitt M, Johnell O, Black DM, Ensrud K, Genant HK, Cummings SR (1994) Bone mineral density predicts non-spine fractures in very elderly women. Osteoporosis Int 4:325–331

98. Nguyen T, Sambrook P, Kelly P, Jones G, Lord S, Freund J, Eisman J (1993) Prediction of osteoporotic fractures by postural instability and bone density. BMJ 307:1111–1115

99. Njeh CF, Apple K, Temperton DH, Boivin CM (1996) Radiological assessment of a new bone densitometer – the Lunar EXPERT. Br J Radiol 69:335–340

100. Nord RH (1992) Work in progress: a cross-correlation study on four DXA instruments designed to culminate in inter-manufacturer standardization. Osteoporosis Int 2:210–211

101. Nordin BEC (1987) The definition and diagnosis of osteoporosis. Calcif Tissue Int 40:57–58

102. Odvina CV, Wergedal JE, Libanati CR, Schulz EE, Baylink DJ (1988) Relationship between trabecular vertebral body density and fractures: a quantitative definition of spinal osteoporosis. Metabolism 37:221–228

103. Orgee JM, Foster H, McCloskey EV, Khan S, Coombes G, Kanis JA (1996) A precise method for the assessment of tibial ultrasound velocity. Osteoporosis Int 6:1–7

104. Patel R, Blake GM, Batchelor S, Fogelman I (1996) Occupational dose to the radiographer in dual X-ray absorptiometry: a comparison of pencil-beam and fan-beam systems. Br J Radiol 69:539–543

105. Peel NFA, Eastell R (1994) Diagnostic value of estimated volumetric bone mineral density of the lumbar spine in osteoporosis. J Bone Miner Res 9:317–320

106. Pocock NA, Sambrook PN, Nguyen T, Kelly P, Freund J, Eisman JA (1992) Assessment of spinal and femoral bone density by dual X-ray absorptiometry: comparison of Lunar and Hologic instruments. J Bone Miner Res 7:1081–1084

107. Porter R, Miller C, Grainger D, Palmer S (1990) Prediction of hip fracture in elderly women: a prospective study. BMJ 301:638–641

108. Pouilles JM, Tremollieres F, Ribot C (1993) Spine and femur densitometry at the menopause: are both sites necessary in the assessment of the risk of osteoporosis? Calcif Tissue Int 52:344–347

109. Reinbold WD, Adler CP, Kalender WA, Lente R (1991) Accuracy of vertebral mineral determination by dual-energy quantitative computed tomography. Skeletal Radiol 20:25–29

110. Ross PD, Genant HK, Davis JW, Miller PD, and Wasnich RD (1993) Predicting vertebral fracture incidence from prevalent fractures and bone density among non-black, osteoporotic women. Osteoporosis Int 3:120–126

111. Ross PD, Huang C, Davis JW, Wasnich RD (1995) Vertebral dimension measurements improve prediction of vertebral fracture incidence. Bone 16:257S–262S

112. Saville PD (1967) A quantitative approach to simple radiographic diagnosis of osteoporosis: its application to the osteoporosis of rheumatoid arthritis. Arthritis Rheum 10:416–422

113. Seeley DG, Kelsey J, Jergas M, Nevitt MC (1996) Predictors of ankle and foot fractures in older women. J Bone Miner Res 11:1347–1355

114. Singh YM, Nagrath AR, Maini PS (1970) Changes in trabecular pattern of the upper end of the femur as an index of osteoporosis. J Bone Joint Surg Am 52:457–467
115. Slosman DO, Rissoli R, Donath A, Bonjour J-P (1990) Vertebral bone mineral density measured laterally by dual-energy X-ray absorptiometry. Osteoporosis Int 1:23–29
116. Stegman MR, Recker RR, Davies KM, Ryan RA, Heaney RP (1992) Fracture risk as determined by prospective and retrospective study designs. Osteoporos Int 2:290–297
117. Steiger P, Block JE, Steiger S, Heuck A, Friedlander A, Ettinger B, Harris ST, Glüer CC, Genant HK (1990) Spinal bone mineral density measured with quantitative CT: effect of region of interest, vertebral level, and technique. Radiology 175:537–543
118. Stein I (1937) The evaluation of bone density in the roentgenogram by the use of an ivory wedge. Am J Roentgenol 37:678–682
119. Stein JA, Lazewatsky JL, Hochberg AM (1987) Dual energy X-ray bone densitometer incorporating an internal reference system. Radiology 165(P):313
120. Torgerson DJ, Campbell MK, Thomas RE, Reid DM (1996) Prediction of perimenopausal fracture by bone density and other risk factors. J Bone Miner Res 11:293–297
121. Tothill P, Fenner JAK, Reid DM (1995) Comparisons between three dual-energy X-ray absorptiometers used for measuring spine and femur. Br J Radiol 68:621–629
122. Verheij LF, Blokland AK, Papapoulos SE, Zwinderman AH, Pauwels EKJ (1992) Optimization of follow-up measurements of bone mass. J Nucl Med 33:1406–1410
123. Vogel JM (1987) Application principles and technical considerations in SPA. In: Genant HK (ed) Osteoporosis update 1987. Radiology Research and Education Foundation, San Francisco, pp 219–231
124. Vogel JM, Anderson JT (1972) Rectilinear transmission scanning of irregular bones for quantification of mineral content. J Nucl Med 13:13–18
125. Wahner HW, Dunn WL, Brown ML, Morin RL, Riggs BL (1988) Comparison of dual-energy X-ray absorptiometry and dual photon absorptiometry for bone mineral measurements of the lumbar spine. Mayo Clin Proc 63:1075–1084
126. Wahner HW, Looker A, Dunn WL, Walters LC, Hauser MF, Novak C (1994) Quality control of bone densitometry in a national health survey (NHANES III) using three mobile examination centers. J Bone Miner Res 9:951–60
127. Wasnich R (1987) Fracture prediction with bone mass measurements. In: Genant HK (ed) Osteoporosis update 1987. Radiology Research and Education Foundation, San Francisco, pp 95–101
128. Wasnich RD, Davis JW, Ross PD (1994) Spine fracture risk is predicted by non-spine fractures. Osteoporosis Int 4:1–5
129. Wasnich RD, Ross PD, Davis JW, Vogel JM (1989) A comparison of single and

multi-site BMC measurements for assessment of spine fracture probability. J Nucl Med 30:1166–1171
130. Williams JA, Wagner J, Wasnich R, Heilbrun L (1984) The effect of long-distance running upon appendicular bone mineral content. Med Sci Sports Exercise 16:223–227
131. Wilson CR, Collier BD, Carrera GF, Jacobson DR (1990) Acronym for dual-energy X-ray absorptiometry. Radiology 176:875
132. World Health Organization (1994) Assessment of fracture risk and its application to screening for postmenopausal osteoporosis. WHO, Geneva
133. Jones CD, Laval-Jeantet AM, Laval-Jeantet MH, and Genant HK (1987) Importance of measurement of spongious vertebral bone mineral density in the assessment of osteoporosis. Bone 8:201–206
134. Melton III LJ, Thamer M, Ray NF, Chan JK, Chesnut III CH, Einhorn TA, Johnston CC, Raisz LG, Silverman SL, and Siris ED (1997) Fractures attributable to osteoporosis: report from the National Osteoporosis Foundation. J Bone Miner Res 12:16–23

14 Radiogrammetry and Radiographic Absorptiometry

C. van Kuijk and H. K. Genant

Introduction

This chapter addresses the methods of radiogrammetry (translated freely as "measuring dimensions on radiographs") and radiographic absorptiometry ("measuring the X-ray absorption on radiographs"). Both techniques have been used widely in the past, and especially the latter continues to be used in the present as a straightforward, relatively simple and inexpensive technique for the assessment of skeletal status. Its use is primarily in osteoporosis, which is defined as loss of bone leading to fractures. Radiographic absorptiometry also has strong roots and applications in dental research, as is discussed below.

This chapter presents an overview of the history of these techniques and current applications. These techniques have been riding the waves of scientific interest and neglect over the past 60 years, and the history of these techniques is a subject of its own. While the current applications are in fact new versions of older ones, with advancing technologies especially in computer sciences and computerized image processing and image-acquisition, interesting and exciting issues are still emerging.

History

Radiogrammetry

Bone dimensions have long been measured, in fact, since it became apparent that the skeleton could be imaged with X-ray techniques. One of the first descriptions of these measurements assessing aging bone was the paper by Barnett and Nordin published in 1960 [1]. They introduced a femoral score (measured at the femoral shaft), a hand score (measured at the shaft of the second metacarpal), and a spine score (measurement of the midvertebral height and the anterior vertebral height). The femoral and hand scores are both measurements of cortical thickness at the respective sites. Since then a large number of papers have been published on the use of bone dimension measurements in the assessment of osteoporosis. Several dimensions can be measured, such as total bone width, cortical thickness, the ratio of cortical width to total bone width, and the cortical area. These measurements are usually performed on radiographs depicting tubular bones [2–4]. More recently Meema et al. have published several papers discussing radiogrammetry of the radius and the second metacarpal, maintaining that radiogrammetry is suitable for screening in osteoporosis [5–8]. Rico and coworkers have also published several papers using radiogrammetry in a variety of studies including those on the treatment of osteoporosis [9–13]. The number of recent papers on radiogrammetry of the metacarpal, phalangeal, and forearm bones, however, is limited, and these publications come primarily from a few dedicated research groups.

A recent promising addition to this field is the measurement of the hip axis length both on standard X-rays of the hip and on images acquired by bone densitometers. This approach was first published by Faulkner et al. in 1993 [14].

While measurements were formerly carried out manually using standard rulers, with today's computer science and image processing tools the more recent techniques are applied on digitized images and provide for semiautomated measurements of bone dimensions.

Radiographic Absorptiometry

When did radiographic absorptiometry emerge? This is not easy to answer. In searching for the first reference to this technique in the literature, one gains the impression that in the first decades of this century considerable scientific knowledge was distributed among individual researchers by means of personal communications ("scientific letters"), usually within the confines of their specific scientific societies. Specifying the first publication would be very difficult, and those interested in medical history are encouraged to take on the challenge. One of the first papers is in a series of superb scientific works presented by Hodge et al., who published ten papers titled "Factors Influencing the Quantitative Measurement of the Roentgen-Ray Absorption in Tooth Slabs," with a variety of subtitles [15–24]. This series was based on earlier work by Warren et al. published in the *American Journal of Roentgenology and Radium Therapy*, April 1934 [25]. This paper introduced an aluminum wedge to compare the radiographic optical density of the tooth with a "known" standard. The idea of using a "known" standard as reference material was attributed to Wilsey at the Eastman Kodak Company according to this paper. We are not in fact certain that this was really the first description of the aluminum-wedge design for its use in radiographic absorptiometry. However, it is certain that the whole concept of radiographic absorptiometry in the dental field is at least 60 years old, which makes it by far the oldest method of the densitometry tools discussed in this volume.

One of the first applications in bone research was that of Stein from the University of Pennsylvania [26], who described the design of an ivory step wedge to quantify bone density in radiographs. According to this paper the first reference to an ivory wedge (in fact ivory disks of known size) was by Endtz [27] from the University of Leiden, the Netherlands (1934). Also from the University of Pennsylvania came a paper by Mack et al. in 1939 [28]. They described the design of an apparatus for radiographic absorptiometry based on earlier work by Sanders from Pennsylvania State College in 1937. In a 1949 paper Mack et al. [29] described various upgradings and refinements of their apparatus. Radiographic absorptiometry gained substantially in interest during the 1960s as it was used to assess bone loss in astronauts [30].

Techniques for image analysis were facilitated by the advent of computers. The first use of a digital computer in radiographic absorptiometry was described by the same group of researchers in 1969 [31].

In dental research the technique also enjoyed renewed interest, and several papers appeared in the 1970s discussing the dental applications of radiographic absorptiometry [32–34].

Attention in bone research was then attracted by single-photon absorptiometry (SPA) and later by dual-photon absorptiometry (DPA), quantitative computed tomography (QCT), dual X-ray absorptiometry (DXA) and quantitative ultrasound (QUS) emenged. However, radiographic absorptiometry continued to be carried out, and recently this conventional technique has gained renewed interest because it is simple and inexpensive, both of which features are important in times of economic constraints.

Outline of Present Techniques

Radiogrammetry

Radiogrammetry in osteoporosis now has two major applications in osteoporosis research. The first is in measurement of the phalangeal and metacarpal indices. This is based on the fact that when osteopenia develops, the cortical thickness of these small tubular bones decreases while the medullary cavity enlarges due to endosteal resorption of bone. The second application is in measurement of geometric dimensions of the hip (especially the hip axis length) which a large epidemiological study has shown to be a strong predictor of hip fractures [14].

The oldest application is the measurement of dimensions on images of tubular bones, the basic idea of which is simple: One measures the outside diameter of the tubular bone (D) and its inside diameter (d) (Fig. 14-1). The ratio (D–d)/D is called the cortical index, D–d being the combined cortical thickness. When endosteal resorption occurs, the cortical shell becomes thinner while the medullary cavity enlarges; in this case the cortical index and the combined cortical thickness decrease.

These measurements are usually performed on the metacarpal bones and, rarely, the radius. The precision errors with these techniques are generally in the order of 3%. One of the major deficiencies of the technique is that it does not measure intracortical porosity or the resorption of trabecular structures, both well-known features of bone loss.

The measurement of geometric dimensions in the hip has no direct relationship to osteopenia. It is speculated that the hip axis length has some correlation

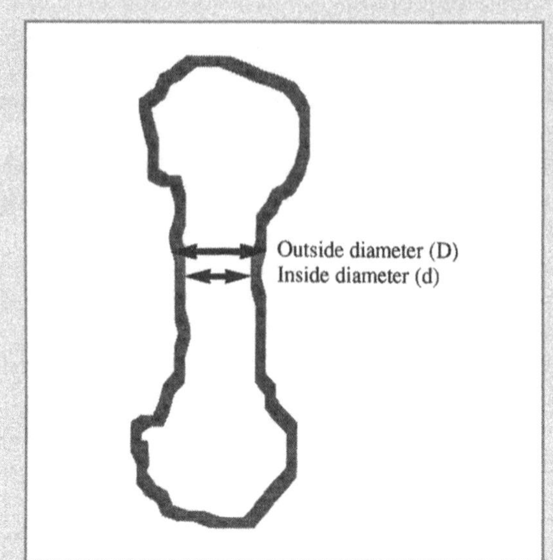

Fig. 14-1 Drawing of radiogrammetric measurement in a tubular bone. The inner (medullary cavity: d) and outer diameter (total bone width: D) of the bone is measured. Several indices can be calculated from these simple measurements

with the biomechanical stress forces within the femur and as such could be an indirect measure of bone strength. Although the hip axis length is related to hip fracture risk, the actual explanation for this relationship is not known. The hip axis length can be measured both on standard radiographs of the hip(s) [35] and on images acquired with some of the devices also used for bone densitometry, such as DXA [14, 36, 37], and on femoral scout views or three-dimensional reconstructions of the femur from computed tomography. In addition to hip axis length, several other geometric dimensions within the femur have been measured, such as the femoral head width, shaft width, and neck-shaft angle. The resolution of DXA images does not allow an accurate measurement of the actual hip axis length, and a surrogate measurement is performed from below the lateral aspect of the greater trochanter to the inner pelvic rim [14]. The precision error of these semiautomated measurements is approximately 1%–2%.

Radiographic Absorptiometry

Several methods are currently in use. One of these is the method developed by CompuMed (Osteogram; California, USA). This technique makes two posteroanterior radiographs of the hand, one at 50 kVp and the other at 60 kVp using nonscreen film. An aluminum reference wedge is placed parallel to the middle phalanx of the index finger (Fig. 14-2). The radiographs are analyzed at a central laboratory. Bone

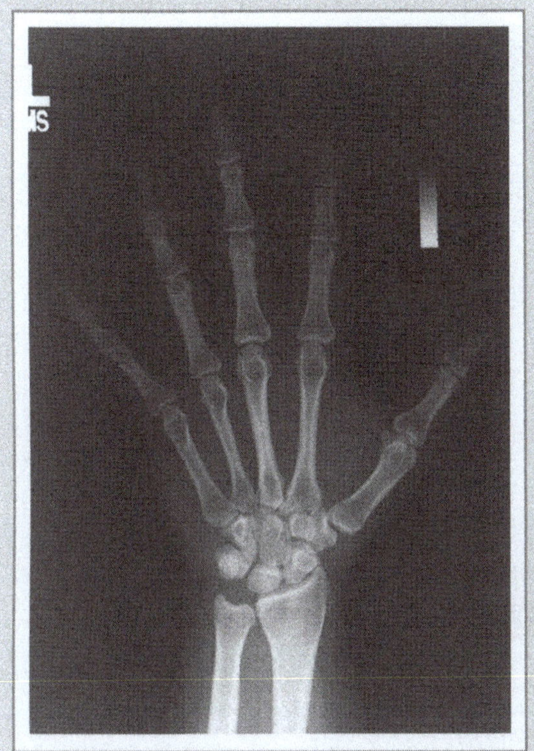

Fig. 14-2 Radiograph of a hand made for the CompuMed radiographic absorptiometry technique. A wedge is placed alongside the second finger for calibration purposes. Results are given in arbitrary units

mineral "density" is calculated in arbitrary units using the aluminum reference wedge as a calibration material. The software also encompasses a soft-tissue correction. Results from the two views are compared, and if found to be in agreement (less than 3% difference), the results are averaged. If the difference between the measurements is more than 3%, the films are rejected, and repeats are requested by the central laboratory. The short-term precision error is reported to be 1.5% (coefficient of variation) in vivo [38] and about 1% in vitro [39].

Other systems are those provided by NIM, (Osteoradiometer; Verona, Italy) for metacarpal bone and radius measurements [40, 41]; by Teijin (Bonalyzer; Tokyo, Japan) for radius measurements [42]; and by Chugai (Tokyo, Japan) for metacarpal measurements [43]. All systems are based on the same principles and have reported precision errors of about 2% [44].

A slightly different technique was developed by Trouerbach et al. [45, 46] at Erasmus University, Rotterdam, the Netherlands. In addition to the anteroposterior view of the hand, a lateral view of the index finger is made on the same screen using a dedicated cassette. A linear aluminum wedge is used as reference (Fig.

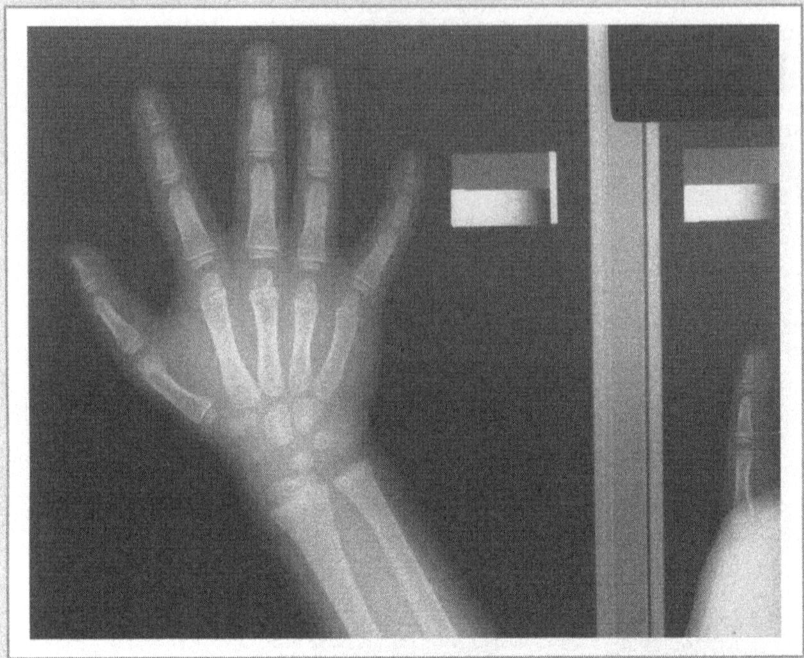

Fig. 14-3 Radiograph of a pediatric hand made according to the method developed by Trouerbach et al. An additional lateral view of the index finger is made on the same film together with a linear aluminum wedge. Optical densities are measured on the exact same anatomical location on both views of the index finger. Results can then be calculated in real density values. (Copyright: Department of Experimental Radiology, Erasmus University, Rotterdam, the Netherlands; courtesy of A.W. Zwamborn)

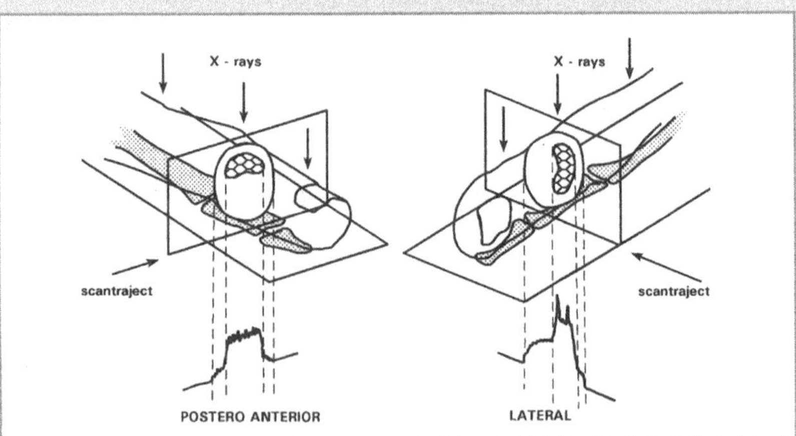

Fig. 14-4 Outline of measurement technique used for the radiographic absorptiometry method of Trouerbach et al. Optical densities are measured on the exact same anatomical location on both views of the index finger. Results can then be calculated in real density values. (Copyright: Department of Experimental Radiology, Erasmus University, Rotterdam, the Netherlands; courtesy of A.W. Zwamborn)

14-3). By combining measurements at the same anatomical level in the middle phalanx using both views a real density value can be calculated, and in addition a sophisticated soft-tissue correction is provided (Fig. 14-4).

Applications

Radiogrammetry is primarily used in research, while radiographic absorptiometry methods are used in research and clinical practice, the latter especially in Japan.

Radiogrammetry

Radiogrammetry has been used in a variety of studies. Van Hemert et al. [47] showed in a large epidemiological study that the relative cortical area (defined as $100x(D^2-d^2)/D^2$, in mm^2%) decreases an average of 1% in women aged 45–64 years. In another study the same authors [48] reported that the metacarpal cortical area (D^2-d^2) when used as a risk factor for osteoporotic fractures shows a clear trend towards more fractures when the cortical area is decreased. However, the sensitivity and specificity were relatively poor when it (in conjunction with other risk factors) was used as a screening test for fracture prediction.

Comparing a group of healthy peri- and postmenopausal women with a group of women with osteoporotic vertebral deformities, Meema et al. [6] showed that the measurement of combined cortical thickness (D–d) at the metacarpal bones can be useful in identifying osteoporotic women when a "fracture threshold" was used, defined as 2 SD below the mean of healthy young subjects. In subsequent studies these authors refined their technique by incorporating a measurement of the radius shaft [7, 8]. By combining both measurements to a summed combined cortical thickness parameter they claimed that their measurement had better discriminative power than DPA for the detection of osteoporotic vertebral deformities. Rico et al. [11] used radiogrammetry in a prospective study evaluating the effect of salmon calcitonin on bone mass. Total and regional bone mass measurements with DXA showed a 16% increase in axial bone mass and a 6% increase in the forearm bone mass in the treated group, while the untreated group lost bone mass significantly in most areas except the arm. The combined cortical thickness increased significantly (+12%) in the treated group. Another study comparing dual X-ray absorptiometry with quantitative ultrasound and radiogrammetry showed that all measurements were correlated significantly [13]. Weight was related to bone measurements with DXA results but not to bone measurements with QUS or radiogrammetry.

Wishart and coworkers compared metacarpal radiogrammetry with SPA and spinal QCT and concluded that radiogrammetry yields cross-sectional information about bone density and fracture risk comparable to that obtained by the other methods [49]. Derisqueburg and coworkers [50] used digitized images and home-made software to measure the appropriate dimensions on standardized hand X-rays (precision of 1%) and found that radiogrammetry can be of value in mass screening for osteoporosis, although they also stated that radiogrammetry would not replace DXA and QCT as the preferred methods for bone densitometry. Adami et al. recently showed that the metacarpal index [(D–d)/D] is very moderately correlated with spinal, femoral, and forearm measurements with DXA. In addition, they showed a considerable precision error with their technique, ranging between 1.5%–5% [41].

The hip axis length has been shown to be a predictor of hip fracture independently of femoral bone density. Faulkner et al. [14] showed that a longer hip axis length as measured by DXA is associated with femoral neck fractures (odds ratio= 1.9 per SD). Glüer et al. [35] showed that several measurements on standardized pelvic films can predict femoral fractures. Measurements of the femoral shaft cortical thickness resulted in an odds ratio of 1.7, and those of the femoral neck cortical thickness resulted in an odds ratio of 1.4.

Radiographic Absorptiometry

Radiographic absorptiometry with the CompuMed method has been shown to have predictive power for vertebral deformities [44, 51]. The reported odds ratio is 1.7 per SD change, which is comparable to the predictive power determined for SXA and ultrasound measurements. Several studies have shown that the correlation of radiographic absorptiometry with SPA, DPA, SXA, DXA, and QCT at several skeletal sites (calcaneus, radius, spine, and hip) is typically between 0.4 and 0.8 [38, 51–53]. In a comparison of radiographic absorptiometry with DXA and QCT, Kleerekoper et al. reported that the average difference from peak adult bone mass was greatest for radiographic absorptiometry [52].

Grampp et al. [53] compared spinal QCT, pQCT, spinal DXA, femoral DXA, forearm DXA, QUS, and radiographic absorptiometry in an extensive multimodality study using various devices. The odds ratios for the distinction between healthy postmenopausal and osteoporotic postmenopausal women were 4.3 for spinal QCT, 2.4 for spinal DXA, 1.5–2.2 for femoral DXA, 1.9–2.2 for forearm DXA, 1.2–1.7 for pQCT, 1.0–2.1 for QUS, and 1.7–2.0 for radiographic absorptiometry (CompuMed and Chugai methods). However, the differences among sites and techniques were statistically nonsignificant using age-adjusted ROC analysis. This study and the comprehensive statistical analysis of the data suggests that radiographic absorptiometry is at least as good as the other bone densitometry techniques in discriminative power, with the possible exception of spinal QCT, which showed superior performance over the other techniques.

The annual age-related decline in bone equivalent values has been reported as 0.92% by the CompuMed method and 1.21% by the Bonalyzer method as assessed in a cross-sectional study [51]. The method developed by Trouerbach et al. [54] showed a decline of approximately 1% per year in the age range of 43–49 and 58–73 years in women and accelerated bone loss of approximately 2.5% per year in the age range 50–57 as assessed in a cross-sectional study. In men they found small decline of bone loss of 0.5% per year in the age range of 54–67 years but an accelerated bone loss of approximately 3% per year in the age range of 68–75 years [54]. In a longitudinal study the same authors reported somewhat less decline in bone equivalent values in women, although the number of patients in the latter study was smaller, and a potential selection bias at the follow-up phase and other cohort-effects were well possible [55]. The same method was also used to study the bone density in children [56, 57]. In a postmenopausal osteoporosis prevention study this method showed a treatment effect of two doses of tibolone after 2 years of treatment. However, in the same study QCT proved more powerful in detecting changes in bone density. The changes seen with QCT were larger and significantly different from those in the placebo group at a much earlier stage. This could be due both to differences between the two methods of measurement and to differences between the site of measurement (phalanx versus spine) [58].

Preliminary data from a study evaluating the accuracy and precision of the method provided by Chugai show an excellent correlation between the measurements and the ash weight of the metacarpal bones and an odds ratio comparable to that of forearm DXA comparing osteoporotic and nonosteoporotic women. However, the reproducibility of the measurement (3.5%) was somewhat disappointing [59, 60].

Future Developments

What is ahead for these techniques? New image acquisition techniques without the use of X-ray film will be used to acquire digital images of any part of the skeleton of interest. Connected workstations with image analysis tools will provide the user (semi-)automated analysis of radiogrammetry and radiographic absorptiometry. The level of precision, now already reaching 1% in specific research settings, will become available for routine clinical practice. The technique itself will not be the limiting factor. The limiting factor will be the clinical applicability. Monitoring drug efficiency for the prevention or treatment of low bone mass is one of the clinical applications. Radiogrammetry is not suitable for this as the expected change in cortical thickness or area is too small to be detected. Radiographic absorptiometry, however, can be and has been used for this purpose, but the results show that both DXA and QCT are more useful as they can measure bone density at sites with a higher turnover, such as the highly trabecular vertebral bodies in the spine. Another clinical application is that for detecting low bone mass to identify those at risk for osteoporosis. It is for this application that both radiogrammetry and radiographic absorptiometry play a potential role. The methods are inexpensive, relatively easy to perform, and readily accessible to most health care professionals throughout the world. The recently demonstrated capability of radiographic absorptiometry to predict fractures could make this method attractive as a first-line screening tool for identifying those at risk for osteoporosis.

Radiographic absorptiometry could also play an important role in pediatric densitometry. As radiographs of the hand are made routinely in pediatric subjects for the purpose of determining skeletal age and advancement, the addition of a calibration wedge on the film cassette is a minor effort which then facilitates radiographic absorptiometry.

In conclusion, there is still a potential role for these techniques. The use of radiographic absorptiometry for first-line screening of those at risk for osteoporosis and in pediatric densitometry seems to be especially promising.

References

1. Barnett E, Nordin BEC (1960) The radiological diagnosis of osteoporosis: a new approach. Clin Radiol 11:166–174
2. Horsman A, Simpson M (1973) The measurement of sequential changes in cortical bone geometry. Br J Radiol 48:471–476
3. Bloom RA, Pogrund H, Libson E (1983) Radiogrammetry of the metacarpal: a critical reappraisal. Skeletal Radiol 10:5–9
4. Kalla AA, Meyers OL, Parkyn ND, Kotze TJvW (1989) Osteoporosis screening – radiogrammetry revisited. Br J Rheumatol 28:511–517
5. Meema HE, Meema S (1969) Cortical bone mineral density versus cortical thickness in the diagnosis of osteoporosis: a roentgenologic-densitometric study. J Am Geriatric Soc 17:120–141
6. Meema HE, Meema S (1987) Postmenopausal osteoporosis: simple screening method for diagnosis before structural failure. Radiology 164:405–410
7. Meema HE (1991) Improved fracture threshold in postmenopausal osteoporosis by radiogrametric measurements: its usefulness in selection for preventive therapy. J Bone Miner Res 6:9–14
8. Meema HE, Meindok H (1992) Advantages of peripheral radiogrametry over dual-photon absorptiometry of the spine in the assessment of prevalence of osteoporotic vertebral fractures in women. J Bone Miner Res 7:897–903
9. Rico H, Revilla M, Cardenas JL, Villa LF, Fraile E, Martin FJ, Arribas I (1994) Influence of weight and seasonal changes on radiogrammetry and bone densitometry. Calcif Tissue Int 54:385–388
10. Rico H, Aguada F, Revilla M, Villa LF, Martin J (1994) Ultrasound bone velocity and metacarpal radiogrametry in hemodialyzed patients. Miner Electrolyte Metab 20:103–106
11. Rico H, Revilla M, Hernandez ER, Villa LF, Alvarez de Buergo M (1995) Total and regional bone mineral content and fracture rate in postmenopausal osteoporosis treated with salmon calcitonin: a prospective study. Calcif Tissue Int 56:181–185
12. Revilla M, de la Sierra G, Aguado F, Varela L, Jimenez-Jimenez FJ, Rico H (1996) Bone mass in Parkinson's disease: a study with three methods. Calcif Tissue Int 58:311–315

13. Aguado F, Revilla M, Hernandez ER, Villa LF, Rico H (1996) Behavior of bone mass measurements. Dual-energy X-ray absorptiometry total body bone mineral content, ultrasound bone velocity, and computed metacarpal radiogrammetry, with age, gonadal status, and weight in healthy women. Invest Radiol 31:218–222

14. Faulkner KG, Cummings SR, Black D, Palermo L, Glüer CC, Genant HK (1993) Simple measurement of femoral geometry predicts hip fracture: the study of osteoporotic fractures. J Bone Miner Res 8:1211–1217

15. Hodge HC, Van Huysen G, Warren SL (1935) Factors influencing the quantitative measurement of the roentgen-ray absorption of tooth slabs. I. Radiation factors. Am J Roentgenol Radiat Ther 34:523–528

16. Hodge HC, Van Huysen G, Warren SL (1935) Factors influencing the quantitative measurement of the roentgen-ray absorption of tooth slabs. II. Filter factors. Am J Roentgenol Radiat Ther 34:529–538

17. Hodge HC, Van Huysen G, Warren SL (1935) Factors influencing the quantitative measurement of the roentgen-ray absorption of tooth slabs. III. Mechanical factors of tube and machine. Am J Roentgenol Radiat Ther 34:678–691

18. Hodge HC, Bale WF, Warren SL, Van Huysen G (1935) Factors influencing the quantitative measurement of the roentgen-ray absorption of tooth slabs. IV. Absorption coefficient factors. Am J Roentgenol Radiat Ther 34:817–838

19. Hodge HC, Warren SL (1936) Factors influencing the quantitative measurement of the roentgen-ray absorption of tooth slabs. V. Theory of the step tablet. Am J Roentgenol Radiat Ther 36:391–407

20. Hodge HC, Van Huysen G, Wilsey RB, Warren S (1936) Factors influencing the quantitative measurement of the roentgen-ray absorption of tooth slabs. VI. Miscellaneous film factors. Am J Roentgenol Radiat Ther 36:531–549

21. Hodge HC, Wilsey RB, Van Huysen G, Warren SL (1937) Factors influencing the quantitative measurement of the roentgen-ray absorption of tooth slabs. VII. Sensitometric factors. Am J Roentgenol Radiat Ther 37:385–403

22. Hodge HC, Van Huysen G, Warren SL (1937) Factors influencing the quantitative measurement of the roentgen-ray absorption of tooth slabs. VIII. Emulsion factors. Am J Roentgenol Radiat Ther 37:529–542

23. Hodge HC, Van Huysen G, Warren SL (1938) Factors influencing the quantitative measurement of the roentgen-ray absorption of tooth slabs. IX. Tube-machine combination factors. Am J Roentgenol Radiat Ther 40:109–125

24. Hodge HC, Van Huysen G, Warren SL (1938) Factors influencing the quantitative measurement of the roentgen-ray absorption of tooth slabs. X. Tissue factors. Am J Roentgenol Radiat Ther 40:269–282

25. Warren SL, Bishop FW, Hodge HC, Van Huysen G (1934) A quantitative method for studying the roentgen-ray absorption of tooth slabs. Am J Roentgenol Radiat Ther 31:663–672

26. Stein I (1937) The evaluation of bone density in the roentgenogram by the use of ivory wedges. Am J Roentgenol Radiat Ther 37:678–682

27. Endtz AW (1934) Een methode om in vivo het kalkgehalte van het beenstelsel

te bepalen. Thesis, University of Leiden, the Netherlands. Boek-en Steen-drukkery, IJdo

28. Mack PB, O'Brien AT, Smith JM, Bauman AW (1939) A method for estimating the degree of mineralization of bones from tracings of roentgenograms. Science 89:46

29. Mack PB, Brown WN Jr, Trapp HD (1949) The quantitative evaluation of bone density. Am J Roentgenol Radiat Ther 61:807–825

30. Mack PB, LaChange PA, Vose GP, Vogt FB (1967) Bone demineralization of foot and hand of Gemini-Titan IV, V and VII astronauts during orbital flight. Am J Roentgenol Radiat Ther Nucl Med 100:503–511

31. Vogt FB, Meharg LS, Mack PB (1969) Use of a digital computer in the measurement of roentgenographic bone density. Am J Roentgenol Rad Ther Nucl Med 105:870–876

32. Plotnick IJ, Beresin VE, Simkins AB (1970) Study of in vivo radiographic densitometry. J Dent Res 49:1034–1041

33. Hedin M, Lundberg M, Wing K (1974) Measurement of fine structures in roentgenograms. I. A microdensitometric method. Acta Odont Scand 32:357–364

34. Matsue I, Collings CK, Zimmerman ER, Vail WC (1970) Microdensitometric analysis of human autogenous alveolar bone implants. J Periodont 41:489–495

35. Glüer CC, Cummings SR, Pressman A, Li J, GlŸer K, Faulkner KG, Grampp S, Genant HK and the study of osteoporotic fractures research group (1994) Prediction of hip fractures from pelvic radiographs: the study of osteoporotic fractures. J Bone Miner Res 9:671–677

36. Faulkner KG, McClung M, Cummings SR (1994) Automated evaluation of hip axis length for predicting hip fracture. J Bone Miner Res 9:1065–1070

37. Faulkner KG (1995) Letter to the editor: hip axis length and osteoporotic fractures. J Bone Miner Res 10:506–508

38. Ravn P, Overgaard K, Huang C, Ross PD, Green D, McClung M, for the EPIC study group (1996) Comparison of bone densitometry of the phalanges, distal forearm and axial skeleton in early postmenopausal women participating in the EPIC study. Osteoporosis Int 6:308–313

39. Yang SO, Hagiwara S, Engelke K, Dhillon MS, Guglielmi G, Bendavid EJ, Soejima O, Nelson DL, Genant HK (1994) Radiographic absorptiometry for bone mineral measurement of the phalanges: precision and accuracy study. Radiology 192:857–859

40. Maggio D, Pacifici R, Cherubini A, Aisa MC, Santucci C, Cucinotta, Senin U (1995) Appendicular cortical bone loss after the age 65: sex-dependent event? Calcif Tissue Int 56:410–414

41. Adami S, Zamberlan N, Gatti D, Zanfisi C, Braga V, Broggini M, Rossini M (1996) Computed radiographic absorptiometry and morphometry in the assessment of postmenopausal bone loss. Osteoporosis Int 6:8–13

42. Seo GS, Shraki M, Aoki C, Chen J-T, Aoki J, Imose K, Togawa Y, Inoue T (1994) Assessment of bone density in the distal radius with computer assisted X-ray densitometry (CXD). Bone Miner 27:173–182

43. Hayashi Y, Yamamoto K, Fukunage M, Ishibashi T, Takahashi T, Nishii Y (1990) Assessment of bone mass by image analysis of metacarpal bone roentgenograms: a quantitative digital image processing (DIP) method. Radiat Med 8:173–178

44. Yates AJ, Ross PD, Lydick E, Epstein RS (1995) Radiographic absorptiometry in the diagnosis of osteoporosis. Am J Med 98(2A):41S–47S

45. Trouerbach WT (1982) Radiographic aluminum equivalent value of bone: the development of a registration method and some clinical applications. Thesis, Erasmus University Rotterdam, the Netherlands

46. Trouerbach WT, Hoornstra K, Birkenhäger JC, Zwamborn AW (1985) Roentgendensitometric study of the phalanx. Diagn Imag 54:64–77

47. Van Hemert AM, Vandenbroucke JP, Hofman A, Valkenburg HA (1990) Metacarpal bone loss in middle-aged women: "horse racing" in a 9-year population based follow-up study. J Clin Epidemiol 43:579–588

48. Van Hemert AM, Vandenbroucke JP, Birkenhäger JC, Valkenburg HA (1990) Prediction of osteoporotic fractures in the general population by a fracture risk score. Am J Epidemiol 132:123–135

49. Wishart JM, Horowitz M, Bochner M, Need AG, Nordin BEC (1993) Relationships between metacarpal morphometry, fore-arm and vertebral bone density and fractures in postmenopausal women. Br J Radiol 66:435–440

50. Derisquebourg T, Dubois P, Devogelaer JP, Meys E, Duquesnoy B, Nagant de Deuxchaisnes C, Delcambre B, Marchandise X (1994) Automated computerized radiogrammetry of the second metacarpal and its correlation with absorptiometry of the forearm and spine Calcif Tissue Int 54:461–465

51. Ross PD, Huang C, Davis J, Imose K, Yates J, Vogel J, Wasnich R (1995) Predicting vertebral deformity using bone densitometry at various skeletal sites and calcaneus ultrasound. Bone 16:325–332

52. Kleerekoper M, Nelson DA, Flynn MJ, Pawluszka AS, Jacobsen G, Peterson EL (1994) Comparison of radiographic absorptiometry with dual-energy X-ray absorptiometry and quantitative computed tomography in normal older white and black women. J Bone Miner Res 9:1745–1749

53. Grampp S, Genant HK, Mathur A, Lang P, Jergas M, Takada M, Glüer CC, Lu Y, Chavez M (1997) Comparisons of non-invasive bone mineral measurements in assessing age-related loss, fracture discrimination, and diagnostic classification. J Bone Miner Res 12:697–711

54. Trouerbach WT, Birkenhäger JC, Schmitz PIM, Van Hemert AM, Van Saase JLCM, Colette HJA, Zwamborn AW (1988) A cross-sectional study of age-related loss of mineral content of phalangeal bone in men and women. Skeletal Radiol 17:338–343

55. Trouerbach WT, Vecht-Hart CM, Colettte HJA, Slooter GD, Zwamborn AW, Schmitz PIM (1993) Cross-sectional and longitudinal study of age-related bone loss in adult females. J Bone Miner Res 8:685–691

56. Trouerbach WT, de Man SA, Gommers D, Zwamborn AW, Grobbee DE (1991) Determinants of bone mineral content in children. Bone Miner 13:55–67

57. Van Teunenbroek A, Mulder P, De Muinck Keizer-Schrama, Van Kuijk C, Grashuis J, Van Bodegom JW, Drop S (1995) Radiographic absorptiometry of the phalanges in healthy children and in girls with Turner Syndrome. Bone 17:71–78

58. Berning B, Van Kuijk C, Kuiper JW, Coelingh Bennink HJT, Kicovic PM, Fauser BCJM (1996) Effects of two doses of tibolone on trabecular and cortical bone loss in early postmenopausal women: a two-year randomized, placebo-controlled study. Bone 19:395–399

59. Hagiwara S, Yang S-O, Dhillon MS, Engelke K, Guglielmi G, Young K, Nelson DL, Genant HK (1993) Precision and accuracy of photodensitometry of metacarpal bone (digital image processing). J Bone Miner Res 8(S1):S346

60. Hagiwara S, Engelke K, Takada M, Yang S-O, Guglielmi G, Jergas M, Glüer CC, Dhillon MS, Nelson DL, Genant HK (1997) Accuracy and diagnostic sensitivity of radiographic absorptiometry of the second metacarpal (submitted)

15 Single- and Dual-Energy: X-Ray Absorptiometry

J. E. Adams

Introduction

Osteoporosis is the most common of the metabolic disorders of bone. The condition is characterised by reduced bone mass and easy (fragility) fracture. Such fractures can occur in any site but are most frequent in the wrist, spine (vertebral body) and hip – areas of the skeleton rich in trabecular bone. Such fractures, and particularly those in the hip, result in considerable morbidity (pain, deformity, loss of height with vertebral fractures) and even mortality, with enormous socio-economic consequences. Treatment of established osteoporosis is difficult and often unsatisfactory, although in recent years diphosphonates (etidronate, alendronate) have been introduced which show encouraging results in increasing bone mass and reducing fracture incidence [1, 2]. Previously treatment strategies favoured prevention of osteoporosis by maximising peak bone mass, minimising age related and postmenopausal bone loss (hormone replacement therapy), avoiding risk factors, and ensuring adequate dietary intake of calcium and appropriate exercise. There is a growing demand from patients, general medical practitioners and specialists (obstetricians, orthopaedic surgeons, rheumatologists and endocrinologists) for clinical services that provide for the detection, assessment and management of osteoporosis [3, 4]. Whether a fracture is sustained depends on a variety of factors including the propensity to fall and the response to falling [5, 6]. However, bone mineral density (BMD) is the single most important determinant as to whether or not a fracture occurs [7, 8] (Fig. 15-1). Reduced bone mass is therefore a useful predictor of increased fracture risk [9–11].

Methods of measuring BMD are pertinent to the detection of osteopenia and identification of those individuals at risk of easy fracture so that appropriate interventions may be made, and to the assessment of the efficacy of either prevention or treatment of osteoporosis. Estimation of spinal bone mineral content (BMC) from bone density on conventional radiographs is insensitive and inaccurate if vertebral fractures are not present, since the subjective assessment is influenced by radiographic exposure factors, patient size and film processing techniques [12, 13]. Additionally the presence of clinical risk factors (life-style, diet and family history of osteoporosis) are relatively insensitive in predicting the presence of osteopenia [14]. These factors have fuelled the need for objective, non-invasive methods of bone densitometry which ideally should be accurate, precise (repro-

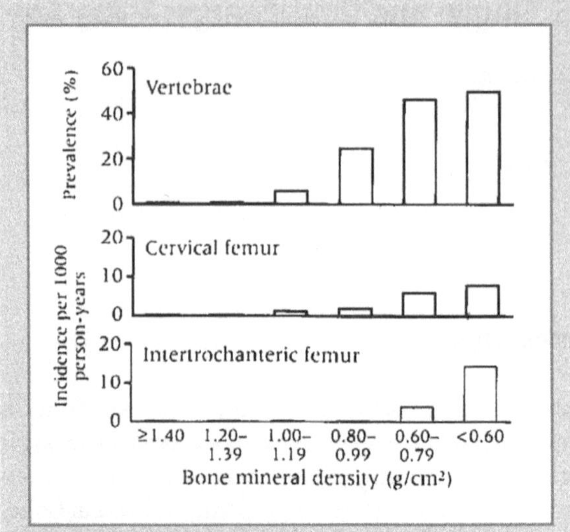

Fig. 15-1 Estimated prevalence of vertebral fractures by lumbar spine BMD and estimated incidence of cervical and intertrochanteric hip fractures by cervical and intertrochanteric BMD, respectively, among women 35 years of age in Rochester, Minn. There is an increase in fractures as BMD falls. (From [8], with permission)

ducible), sensitive, inexpensive and involve a minimal exposure to ionising radiation. Several of the photon absorptiometric techniques now available for bone densitometry come close to these ideal requirements [3, 4, 15]. Single-photon absorptiometry (SPA) was first introduced in 1963 for application to measurements in the appendicular skeleton. Subsequently dual-photon absorptiometry (DPA) was developed for application to sites in the axial skeleton. These techniques have now been superseded by single-energy X-ray absorptiometry (SXA) and dual-energy X-ray absorptiometry (DXA). DXA is now the most widely applied method of bone densitometry, but there are other established (quantitative computed tomography, QCT), promising (broadband ultrasound attenuation, BUA) and research (quantitative magnetic resonance, QMR; high-resolution and micro-computed tomography, finite element analysis, compton scattering and neutron activation analysis) techniques also available [16–18].

Past Radionuclide Methods

Single-Photon Absorptiometry

SPA was introduced by Cameron and Sorenson in 1963 [19]. The method overcame the problems for radiographic photodensitometric techniques caused by polychromatic X-rays and non-uniformity of film sensitivity and development by using a single-energy γ-ray source (^{125}I, photon energy 27.3 keV or americium

241, photon energy 59.4 keV) and a scintillation detector to measure transmitted photons. The radionuclide source and detector were coupled and scanned in a rectilinear fashion across the area of interest. To correct for overlying soft tissue the anatomical site in which BMD was being measured must be surrounded either by water, water bags or water equivalent mouldable material, with an addition correction for adipose tissue being made [20] (Fig. 15-2). The technique was generally applicable only to peripheral skeletal sites, including the os calcis [21], but measurements were most often performed in the non-dominant forearm [22–24]. Early equipment used an horizontal scan with the hand in a pronated position. Subsequently, vertical scans with the hand gripping a rod in a water bath provided improved precision (Fig. 15-2). Bone density measurements were provided as BMC in grams per centimetre of bone length or as BMD in grams per square centimetre. This is an areal rather than a true volumetric density and is calculated from BMC divided by bone width, the margins of the bone being detected automatically from the scan data. BMD is a less precise measure than is BMC but partially compensates for the effect of patient size on bone density and is a better indicator of fracture risk. SPA measured integral (cortical and trabecular) bone and was applied to different sites along the shaft of the radius, which contain differing proportions of cortical and trabecular bone [16, 20] (Fig. 15-3). The midshaft consists entirely of cortical bone, in the distal metaphysis there is a cortical/trabecular ratio of 6:1, and in the ultradistal site trabecular bone (up to 95%) predominates [25]. The os calcis has a cortical/trabecular ratio of 5/95 [16].

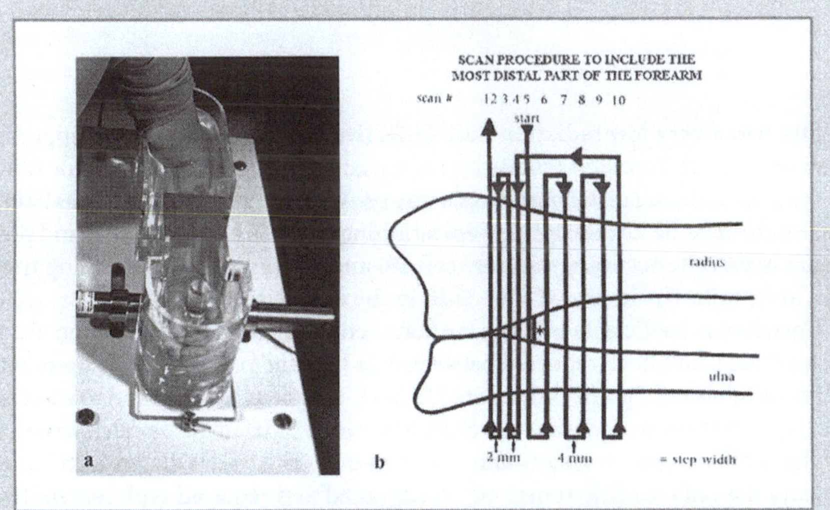

Fig. 15-2 a Single-photon absorptiometer (Nuclear Data SPA scanner). The nondominant arm is placed in a water bath with the hand gripping a rod to avoid rotation of the wrist. **b** The radionuclide source (125ᵢ) and coupled detector scan in a rectilinear fashion in two sites (proximal and ultradistal) of the forearm, after determination of the 8-mm gap* between radius and ulna

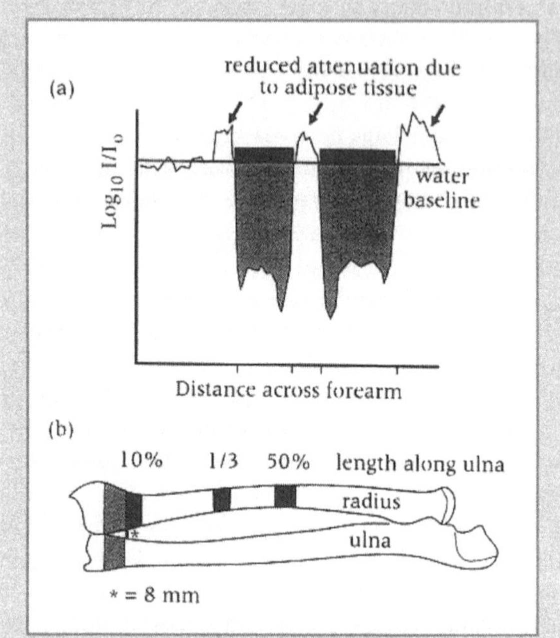

Fig. 15-3 a Graph of SPA log10 transmitted photon intensity against distance across the forearm. **b** Typical sites for single-photon absorptiometry forearm densitometry. The sites have different percentages of cortical and trabecular bone; the midshaft is entirely cortical bone; in the distal metaphysis the cortical/trabecular ratio is 6:1; in the ultradistal site trabecular bone (75%–95%) predominates. These latter sites for scanning are located by the scanning equipment automatically finding the 8-mm gap between the distal radius and ulna (From [20], with permission)

SPA had a very low radiation dose (effective dose equivalent, EDE, approximately 0.6μ Sv). Precision (coefficient of variation, CV) in the forearm for BMC in the mid-shaft and distal metaphysis was 1%. With the shape of the bones being less uniform in the ultradistal site repositioning errors are more critical, and precision is 2%–3%. Accuracy was between 4% and 6% [25, 26]. The scanning time was 10–15 min. The in vivo CV for BMC in the os calcis was 1.2% [27].

Correlation coefficients between the bone density in the lumbar spine and ultradistal radius have been reported between 0.52 [28] and 0.64 [29]. Measurements in the os calcis are significantly related to body weight and height and to exercise [30, 31], and there is moderate correlation between BMD in the os calcis and that in the lumbar spine (r=0.77) and distal radius (r=0.71). With an half-life of 60 days the radionuclide source of ^{125}I degraded and required replacement two or three times a year. SPA was a widely used and established bone density technique, the results of which were predictive of fracture risk in the appendicular skeleton, hip and spine [32, 33]. SPA has now been superseded by SXA in which the radionuclide source has been replaced by a low-dose X-ray source.

Dual-Photon Absorptiometry

The limitation of SPA was that it could be applied only to peripheral skeletal sites. DPA was introduced in the 1960s to enable bone density measurements to be made in more clinically relevant sites such as the spine, hip and whole body [34–37]. The simultaneous measurement of radiation of two different energies allows for the correction of soft tissue and fat of the torso without the need for a water bath. The most widely used radionuclide was ^{153}Gd that produces photons at energies of 44 and 100 keV. The transmitted photons of the two energies were counted separately by scintillation detectors. The low- (44 keV) and high-energy (100 keV) photons were attenuated differently in bone and soft tissue. The difference in relative attenuations allowed the mass of bone mineral in the beam to be calculated and expressed as BMC in grams or as an areal bone density BMD in grams per square centimetre. From scanning of the whole body could be derived total body mineral, lean (muscle) and fat contents [36]. The equipment scanned in a rectilinear fashion and because of the low photon flux, images were of low spatial resolution (3 mm) and took a considerable scanning time (lumbar spine 30 min, whole body 40–60 min), which limited precision (2%–4%) due to patient movement during scanning. In DPA an assumption was made that soft tissue is of uniform composition but of unknown thickness, but this is not so in practice and non-uniform thickness of adipose tissue contributes to accuracy errors of up to 9%. Due to decay the radionuclide source had to be replaced annually. DPA has now been replaced by DXA.

Present Photon Absorptiometric Methods

Although SPA and DPA were widely used and provided many valuable clinical and research data, they had limitations. These resulted from the photon source being provided by a radionuclide. This decayed and needed to be replaced regularly and had a low photon flux which caused scanning times to be long and spatial resolution to be poor. These limitations have been overcome in SXA and DXA by photons being produced from a low-dose X-ray source instead of from a radionuclide source. With the higher photon flux (50–1000 times greater) scanning speeds are increased (to less than 5 min per site) and spatial resolution improved with consequent enhancement of precision (better than 1% for lumbar spine) [38–40].

Single-Energy X-Ray Absorptiometry

The physical principles of SXA are the same as SPA except that the photon source is an X-ray system (55 kV, 300 A with K-edge filtration and solid state detectors; Osteometer MediTech, Roedovre, Denmark). If a single-energy X-ray beam is used then the arm is placed in a water bath to allow correction for soft tissue overlying bone. If a dual-energy X-ray beam is used the water bath is not necessary. The equipment is relatively compact and mobile (Fig. 15-4); scanning takes about

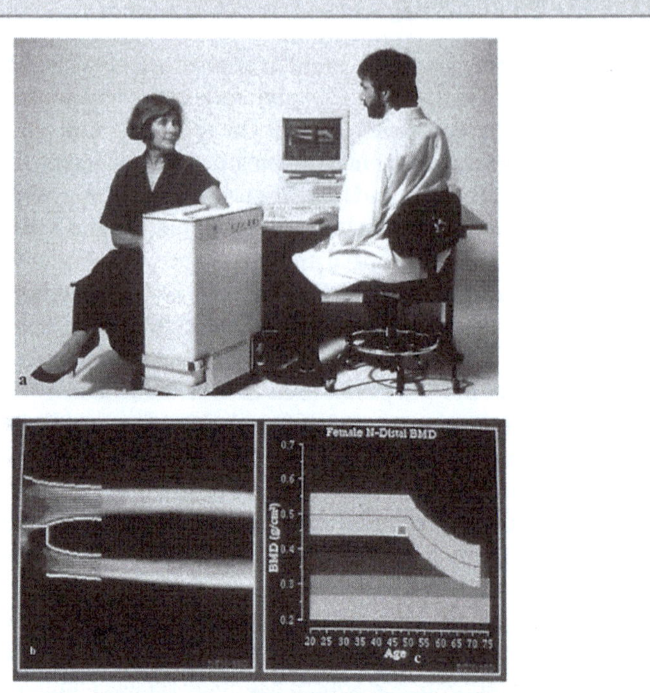

Fig. 15-4 SXA for measuring BMD in the forearm. **a** Scanning equipment and patient in position for scan. **b,c** Scan of distal radius with areas of analysis outlined (distal and ultradistal sites) BMD result plotted inrelation to appropriate reference range. (Courtesy of Osteometer, Meditech, Roedovre, Denmark, with permission)

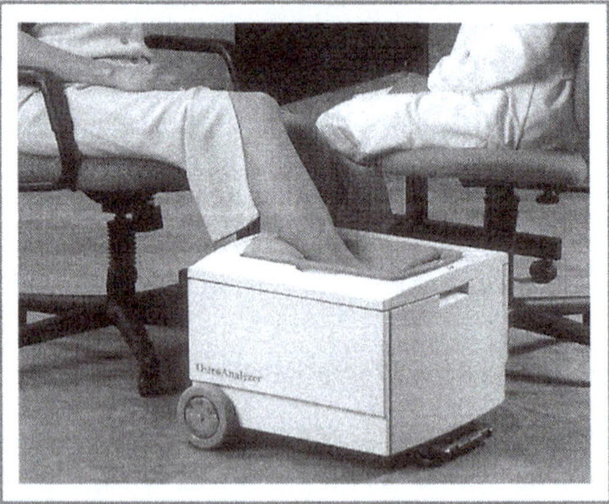

Fig. 15-5 SXA 3000 Osteo Analyzer. For measuring BMD in the os calcis. Scanning equipment and patient in position for scan. (Courtesy of Dove Medical Systems; Norland Medical Systems, Newbury Park, California, USA, with permission)

5 min. The position of the forearm is standardised by the patient gripping a vertical rod. The scans are performed in a rectilinear fashion in a distal (87% cortical bone) and ultradistal (predominantly [65%] trabecular bone) site. Results are expressed as BMC (in g) or BMD (in g/cm²). Accuracy is 3%, precision is better than 1% and radiation dose EDE is 0.1µ Sv.

There is also an SXA scanner specific to measurement of BMD in the os calcis (Osteo Analyzer SXA 3000 manufactured by Dove Medical Systems, a subsidiary of Norland Medical Systems, Newbury Park, California, USA; Fig. 15-5). Scanning is performed in 2 min; precision is better than 1%.

Dual-Energy X-Ray Absorptiometry

The physical principles of DXA are similar to those of DPA except that a low-dose X-ray tube replaces the gadolinium as a source of photons [41–43]. The first commercially available DXA scanner was introduced in 1987. X-ray beams of two peak energies are produced by a variety of techniques by different manufacturers. The energies used are selected to optimise separation of the mineralised and soft tissue

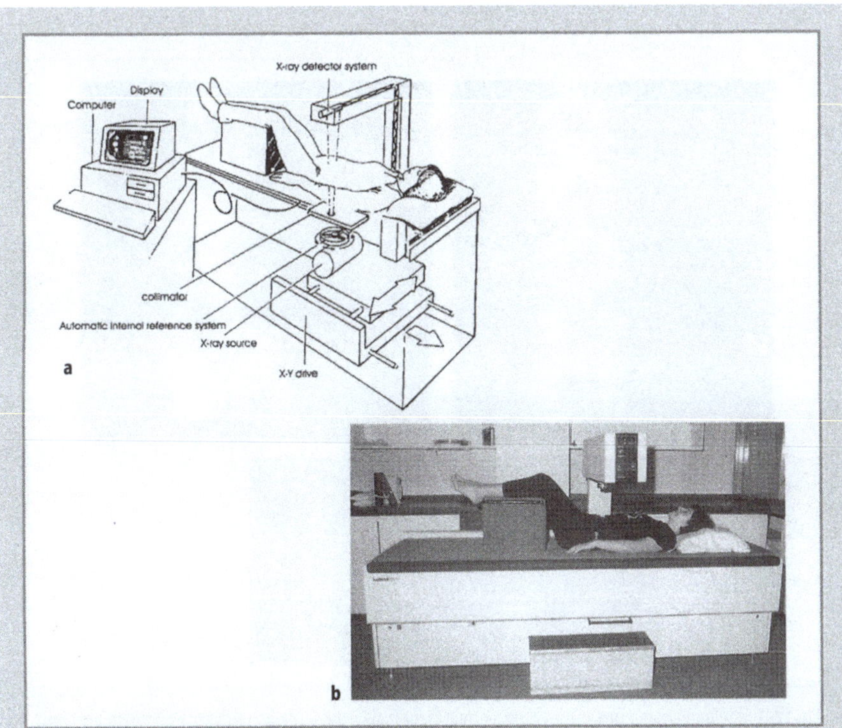

Fig. 15-6 DXA. **a** Schematic diagram showing principles of DXA with the X-rays from the source passing through the rotating calibration disc and the patient. (From Hologic, with permission) **b** Patient positioned on DXA scanner (Lunar DPX-L) for scanning of the lumbar spine

components of the area analysed. Scanners manufactured by Hologic (Waltham, Massachusetts, USA) use an energy switching system in which the X-ray tube potential is switched rapidly from 70–140 kVp alternating at 60/s. The problems of beam hardening and background radiation usually associated with polychromatic beams produced by X-ray tubes in quantitative applications are overcome by appropriate corrections and simultaneous calibration by continuously interposing known amounts of bone and soft tissue equivalent material in the beam. This reference calibration material is mounted on a disc which rotates synchronously with the X-ray pulses (Fig. 15-6).

The scanners manufactured by the Lunar Corporation (Madison, Wisconsin, USA), Norland Medical Systems (Fort Atkinson, Wisconsin, USA) and Sopha (Buc Cedex, France) use a constant potential X-ray source combined with a rare earth filter with energy-specific absorption characteristics due to K-edges of the atomic structure of the element (K-edge filtration). The K-edge filter separates the X-ray distribution into two separate components of 'high' and 'low' energy photons (70 keV and 40 keV using cerium; 45 keV and 80 keV using a samarium filter) [40, 44, 45]. The technique is most commonly applied to scanning of the lumbar spine (L1–L4; Fig. 15-7), femoral neck (regions of analysis include neck, trochanter,

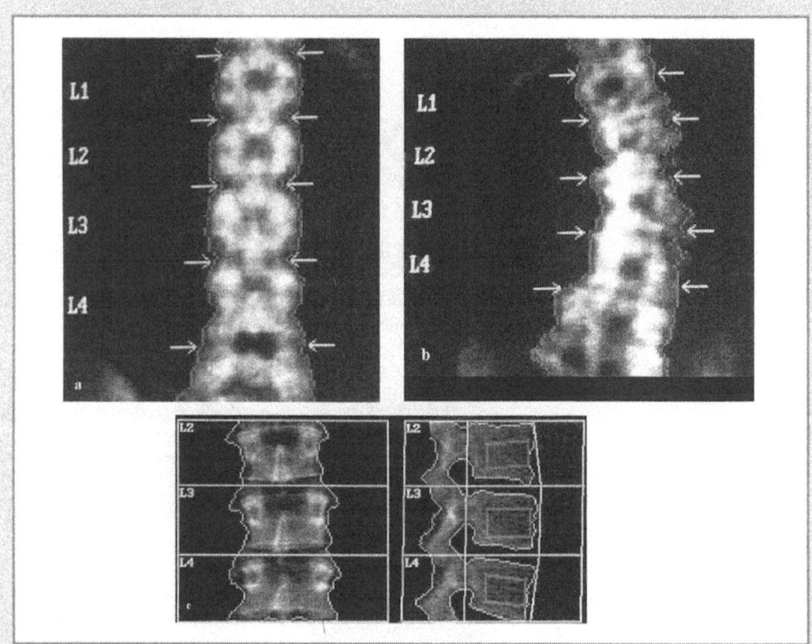

Fig. 15-7 DXA lumbar spine. **a** PA scan of the normal lumbar spine. **b** PA DXA of the lumbar spine with scoliosis and associated hyperostotic changes with osteophytes at L2/3 and L3/4. The scoliosis makes scanning difficult and the osteophytes cause over-estimation of BMD. **c** PA (left) and lateral (right) DXA scans. From such scans estimates of 'volumetric' bone density can be calculated; the lateral DXA scan has a higher proportion of trabecular bone than PA DXA, and can exclude hyperostotic changes which cause inaccuracies in PA DXA

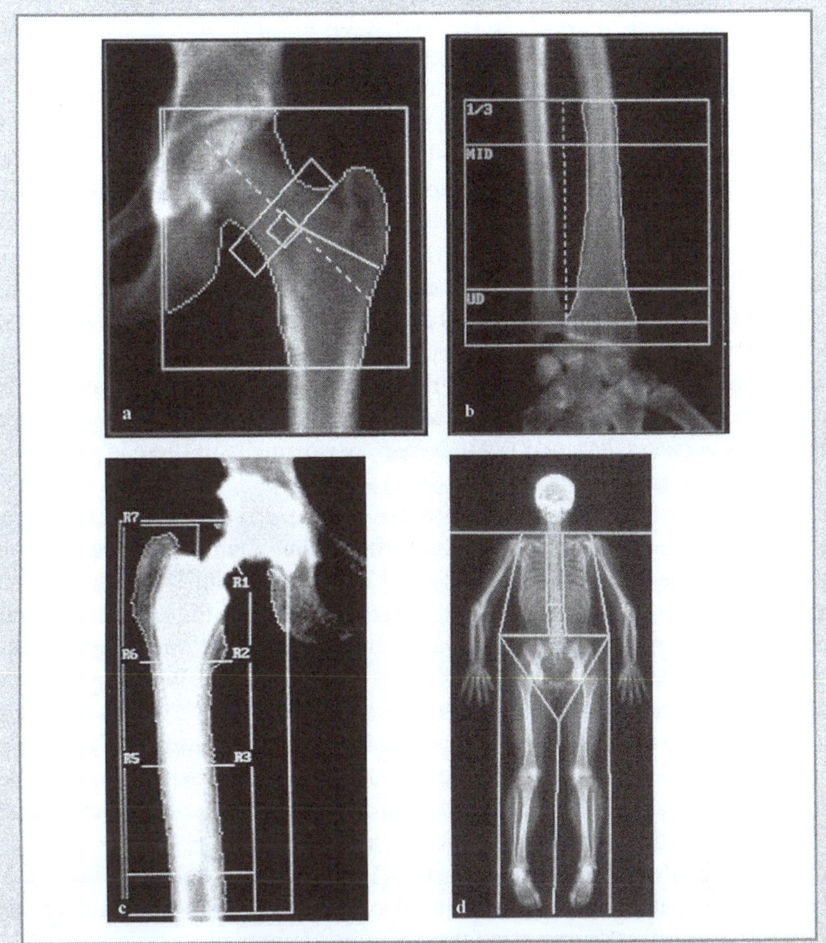

Fig. 15-8 DXA. **a** Hip showing ROIs analysed: femoral neck (oblong box), Ward's area (box) and trochanter. **b** Forearm showing ROIs analysed ultradistal (UD), distal shaft (MID) and shaft (1/3). **c** Hip following arthroplasty with ROIs of analysis around prosthesis. **d** Whole body with regional areas of analysis (head, chest, pelvis, arms and legs). With appropriate software programmes information on whole and regional body composition (muscle and fat mass) can be obtained. (From Hologic, with permission)

Ward's area and total hip) and whole body (Fig. 15-8). DXA measures integral bone density with cortical/trabecular ratios of 50/50 in the lumbar spine (PA), 10/90 in lateral projection lumbar spine, 60/40 in the proximal femur and 80/20 in the whole body [16].

Positioning for Scanning. The patient is positioned supine on the scanning table. When the lumbar spine is being examined, the hips and knees are flexed over a support so as to eliminate the lumbar lordosis and flatten the spine to the table top (Fig. 15-6). For scanning of the femoral neck the leg is slightly abducted and internally rotated by use of a positioning device to bring the femoral neck parallel to the scan table to avoid foreshortening of the femoral neck which would cause the BMD to be increased (same BMC in smaller area of bone). Different leg positions can cause significant errors in BMD measured by DXA in the proximal femur (0.9% to 4.5% in the neck; 1.0% to 6.7% at Ward's area and 0.4% to 3.1% in trochanter) [46] and can be reduced by use of a positioning jig rather than the manufacturers' foot block [47]. For whole body scanning it is imperative that all parts of the body (including arms) are included in the scan field for precise results.

Technical Aspects and Applications. The original DXA scanners have a collimated pencil beam (1.5 mm as compared to 5–8 mm in DPA) of X-rays aligned and mechanically connected to a scintillation detector. Scanning is performed in a rectilinear fashion. Scan times for such first generation scanners is 15 min per site examined, and up to 30–40 min for whole body scans in large individuals. Cross-calibration between DPA and DXA has been performed and there is good correlation between the techniques ($r>0.94$) [39, 48–51].

The accuracy of DXA is similar to that of DPA at 3%–8% [52–54]. Much has been published on the precision of DXA in the various anatomical sites to which it is applied to measure bone density [55–62]. The precision for PA measurements of the spine is 0.5%–2%, but usually better than 1%; for the proximal femur between 1% and 5%, depending on the anatomic site analysed, being better in the neck and trochanter (1%–2%) than in Ward's area (2.5%–5%). Positioning of the femoral neck is critical to maintaining good precision [46, 47]. Ward's area may be more sensitive to changes in BMD since it contains a relatively higher proportion of trabecular bone than other sites measured in the proximal femur. However, the small area sampled and repositioning errors in this projected area result in inferior precision, so limiting its use in clinical practice.

Precision achievable in all sites measured is better in normal individuals than in osteoporotic patients. Precise measures require dedicated, skilled and highly motivated technical staff operating the scanning equipment.

DXA body scanners are being used increasingly to measure BMD in the forearm [63, 64]. Scanning is performed with the patient sitting on a chair next to the scanner table with the forearm resting on the table top, the hand pronated and, on some scanners, secured on a positioning board and restraining strap. BMD measurements are made in the ultradistal (predominantly trabecular bone), distal (designated MID radius) and shaft (designated 1/3 radius, predominantly cortical bone) regions of the forearm (Fig. 15-8).

There is also now available a desktop DXA scanner specific to scanning the forearm (pDEXA Norland Medical Systems, Fort Atkinson, Wisconsin, USA; Fig. 15-9). Scanning takes about 5 min to perform, and measurements are made in the distal radius and ulna (predominantly trabecular bone) and in the shaft of the radius and ulna (cortical bone).

In research studies whole body scans provide measures of total body and regional bone density (Fig. 15-8). With appropriate software information on body

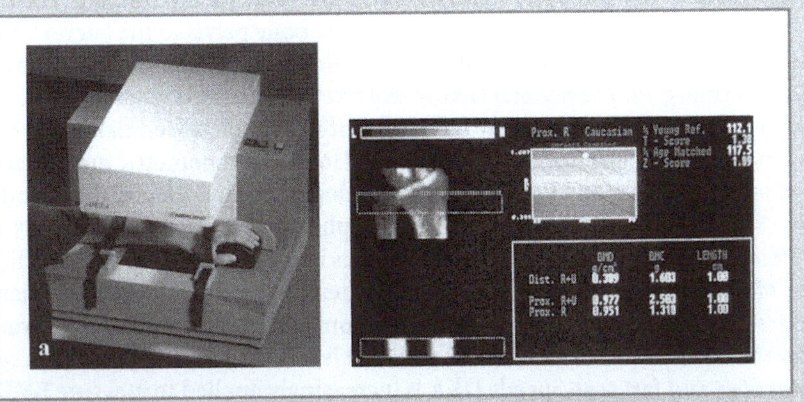

Abb. 15-9 a Desktop DXA scanner (pDEXA) for measuring bone density in two sites in the forearm with patient positioned for scanning. **b** Monitor display of sites scanned in the forearm with bone density results displayed. (From Norland Medical Systems, with permission)

composition (lean muscle and fat mass) can be obtained from whole body scans. Measurement of body composition is an area of considerable expansion and importance in the research application of DXA since the results are well correlated with other indirect measures of body mass [65–70]. Body composition assessment by DXA has been applied to children and young adults (4–26 years old) [71]. However, some investigators have reported significant differences in DXA body composition measurements between DXA scanners and compared with other reference methods [72–74]. Because of these discrepancies there is a need for an internationally agreed standard soft tissue phantom against which all DXA scanners used in body composition research can be calibrated [75]. Short term precision for total body and forearm BMD lies between 0.8% and 1.3% [76].

DXA has been used to study regional bone density around prostheses following hip arthroplasty, for which specific software analysis programmes are available [77] (Fig. 15-8). There is a growing demand for appropriate analysis programmes to perform DXA bone density in bone specimens and small experimental animals in which scanning is now feasible [78, 79]. Application of DXA scanning to other established and novel anatomical sites (calcaneum, mandible, hand) has been described [80, 81]. Although no specific software analysis programmes may be available commercially for scanning these sites, software for scanning conventional sites (e.g. forearm) can be used and analysis be performed by manual placements of regions of interest (ROIs).

Bone density measurement in the os calcis, either on conventional DXA scanners with special software analysis programmes or using specific equipment (Osteo Analyzer) is becoming increasingly important [82–84].

DXA scans have also been used for anatomical morphometric measurements. In 1994 Faulkner et al. [85] reported the automation of measurement of hip axis length (HAL) from DXA scans and its predictive value for hip fracture. The HAL is the distance between the inner margin of the bony pelvis to the lateral border of the femur along a line drawn through the midline of the femoral neck and parallel to its margins. The normal HAL in women was 10.5±0.62 cm; HAL of 11.0 cm increased risk of hip fracture twofold; HAL of 11.5 cm increased risk of hip fracture by a factor of four. DXA has been applied to the morphometric measurement of other long bones [86]. With technical developments in DXA and the introduction of fan beam X-ray sources vertebral morphometry is feasible [87] (Fig. 15-10).

Precision of DXA is not affected by changes in the anteroposterior (AP) diameter of patients over a wide range, except when they are very obese (AP diameter greater than 28 cm) or in children, in whom additional soft tissue equivalent material needs to be added if the AP diameter is less than 10 cm. With its low radiation dose and fast scan speeds DXA is increasingly applied to measure BMD in neonates, infants and children, enabling the study of skeletal development [88–94]. Precision levels of 2.8% are reported for DXA bone density in infants [95], and of 1.95% for BMC and 5.35% for fat for body composition in piglets and neonates [96]. Specific scanning software is required to achieve good precision and optimise accuracy when scanning small objects (neonates, children, bone specimens and small animals), using smaller pixel areas for analysis than in scanning of adults. There are some problems in using DXA for clinical diagnosis in children. There are as yet limited reference data [97] available compared to those which are available for the adult population. Additionally, DXA measurements are greatly influenced by patient size, which other techniques (QCT) are not, and skeletal status in children is not only related to sex and chronological age but also to puber-

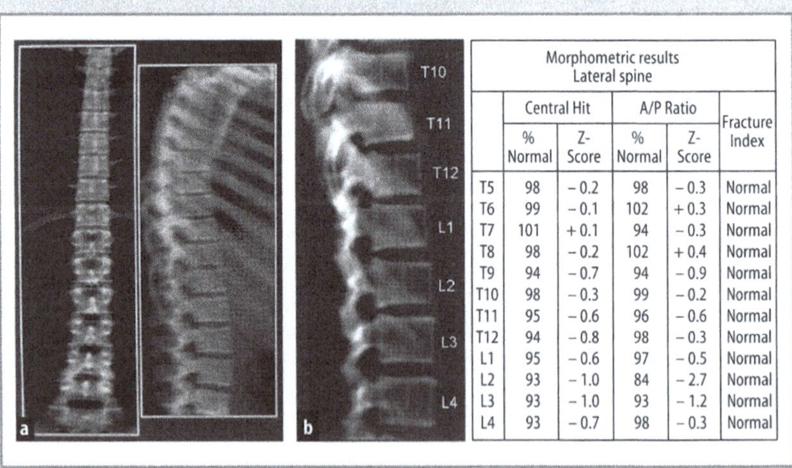

	Morphometric results Lateral spine				
	Central Hit		A/P Ratio		Fracture Index
	% Normal	Z-Score	% Normal	Z-Score	
T5	98	− 0.2	98	− 0.3	Normal
T6	99	− 0.1	102	+ 0.3	Normal
T7	101	+ 0.1	94	− 0.3	Normal
T8	98	− 0.2	102	+ 0.4	Normal
T9	94	− 0.7	94	− 0.9	Normal
T10	98	− 0.3	99	− 0.2	Normal
T11	95	− 0.6	96	− 0.6	Normal
T12	94	− 0.8	98	− 0.3	Normal
L1	95	− 0.6	97	− 0.5	Normal
L2	93	− 1.0	84	− 2.7	Normal
L3	93	− 1.0	93	− 1.2	Normal
L4	93	− 0.7	98	− 0.3	Normal

Fig. 15-10 a Postero-anterior (left) and lateral (right) DXA scan of the thoracic and lumbar spine for vertebral morphometry. (From Hologic, with permission). **b** Lateral thoracolumbar DXA scan showing morphometric measurements and results. (From Lunar Corporation, with permission)

tal stage, on which there are limited published data in relation to bone densitometry.

Sources of Error and Technical Developments. In posteroanterior (PA) DXA of the spine the BMD is an areal density of integral bone which includes both the vertebral body and neural arch (cortical/trabecular bone ratio 50:50). All the mineral within the path of the photon beam contributes to the BMD. Extraneous calcification, such as in the walls of the aorta, and more particularly degenerative disc and apophyseal joint disease with consequent hyperostosis, causes inaccuracies and over-estimation of BMD [98–101] (Fig. 15-7). This limits the usefulness and sensitivity of PA spinal DXA in the elderly population in whom such degenerative changes are commonly present (>60%) at age 70 years or more. This has led to the development of lateral DXA scanning of the lumbar spine [102–105] (Fig. 15-7). On some of the early-generation scanners this required the patient to be repositioned for scanning in the lateral decubitus position. This limited precision and was difficult and impractical with some patients, particularly those with osteoporosis. On scanners with mobile "C" arms lateral scanning can be performed with the patient remaining in the supine position, which has practical advantages and better precision than scanning in the decubitus position [106]. Precision for lateral DXA scanning in the decubitus position is 2.8%–5.9% [102, 103] but is improved with the patient remaining in the supine position; being 1.6% in normal individuals and 2% in osteoporotic patients [107]. Ideally one would like to be able to make BMD measurements in all four lumbar vertebrae (L1 and L4) on lateral DXA, but L1 and L2 may have ribs superimposed and, more significantly, L4 is frequently overlapped by the ilium [108, 109]. In some patients therefore only the analysis from L3 is available.

Lateral DXA permits exclusion of degenerative changes from BMD results and an ROI positioned in the centre of the vertebral body contains a higher proportion of trabecular bone (cortical/trabecular ratio 10:90). This makes lateral DXA more sensitive to change in BMD than PA DXA, but the poorer precision of lateral DXA limits its usefulness in longitudinal studies. Lateral DXA discriminates better than PA DXA between healthy subjects and those with spinal osteoporosis (vertebral fracture) [110] and glucocorticoid-induced bone loss [111]. Estimates of "volumetric" bone density calculated from projectional PA and lateral DXA measurements enhance this discriminatory capability between vertebral fracture and non-fracture groups [112] (Fig. 15-7).

Falsely high spinal BMD on PA DXA may be caused by other aetiologies including a vertebral wedge or crush fracture, Paget's disease of bone, sclerotic metastases and vertebral haemangioma. Large differences in BMD of lumbar vertebrae in an individual should alert the interpreter to such artifacts. Vertebral fractures may be suspected by reduced vertical height of the vertebra involved. Previous spinal surgery with metallic pinning or plating may render results of spinal DXA meaningless. Other artifacts (calcified lymph nodes, residual Myodil) overlying the lumbar spine may also adversely influence results. Non-uniformity of the soft-tissue baseline adjacent to the spine (i.e. ribs at L1) cause elevation of the density of this soft tissue and as a consequence an underestimation of BMD in the bone [40]. Although the image quality of DXA has improved greatly over the past decade (Fig. 15-10) with spatial resolution for DPA being 3 mm to that for third-generation DXA scanners being 0.5–0.7 mm (compared with 0.1 mm of radiographs) [40] there are not yet the scientific data to prove that DXA images can be used for interpretation of pathology. Appropriate radiographs may therefore be required to define the aetiology of discrepant BMD in a vertebra or other anatomical site scanned. It is therefore imperative that all DXA scans be scrutinised by the individual reporting the BMD results.

Spinal scoliosis, severe kyphosis and anomalous vertebral segmentation [113] (Fig. 15-7) may make DXA scanning technically difficult and limit its clinical usefulness and precision. With regard to DXA scanning in paediatric studies Koo et al. [114] reported that covering the step phantom with a cotton blanket, small non-metallic objects and tissue freezing had no significant effect but movement artifact, radiographic contrast media and non-metallic orthopaedic casts significantly interfered with BMC and BMD, as did operator selection of ROI on whole body scans.

The introduction of a fan beam source of X-rays, a strip of detectors and mobile "C" arm units (Lunar Expert; Hologic 4500 Acclaim) during the past 2–3 years has resulted in faster scan times (5 min or less per site scanned) and improved spatial resolution of images (Fig. 15-11). The higher photon flux enables lateral imaging of the entire spine (single or dual energy) from which morphometric X-ray absorptiometry analyses of vertebral fractures can be made (Fig. 15-10). Such sophisticated scanners may be more expensive than the first generation scanners by a factor of two.

Such technical developments, which are inevitable, and differences between scanners cause difficulties in longitudinal studies and clinical practice, since results may not be comparable. A system upgrade can affect the scanner performance and as a consequence patient results [115, 116]. Due to different calibration criteria and edge detection algorithms used by the various DXA manufacturers BMD results are not interchangeable, and there may be differences of up to 12% between scanners (Lunar>Hologic) [72, 117–121]. Changing from the pencil-beam to fan-beam geometry has been shown to result in differences in BMD [122, 123], morphometric measurements (HAL 7.5% greater on fan beam scanner) [124] and longitudinal rates of bone loss [125].

It is possible to correct for most of these differences and inconsistencies by rigid quality assurance programmes [126–129], and cross-calibration procedures are essential in all departments performing bone densitometry and in pharmaceutical trials [130–132]. There is, through the International DXA Standardisation Committee, agreement between manufacturers of DXA equipment to attempt to standardise BMD results from different scanners through appropriate cross-calibration in patients and a universal phantom (European Spine Phantom) [133,134]. Such standardised BMD results may well be available within the next 12 months

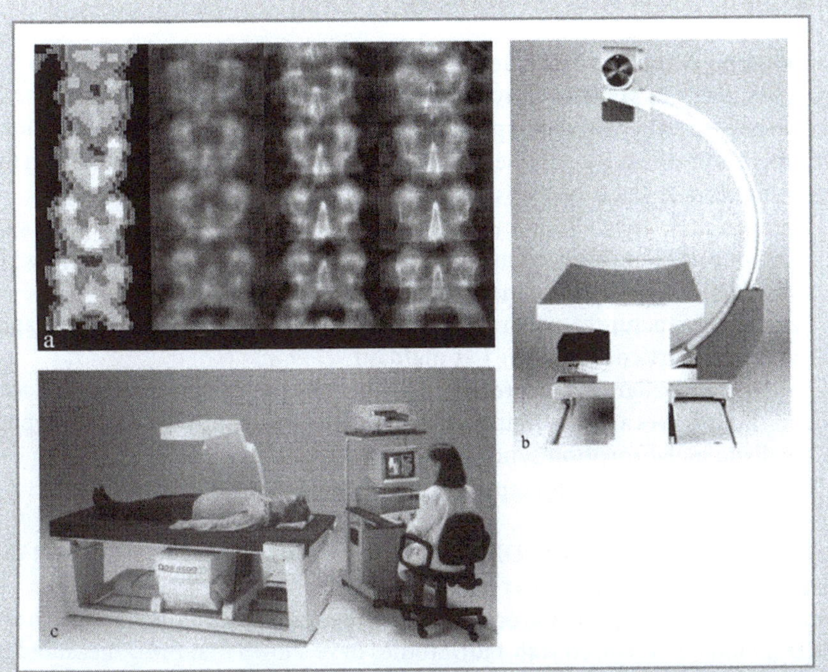

Fig. 15-11 a PA spine images of the same subject acquired (left to right) on DP3 (DPA), DPX (pencil-beam DXA), DPX-IQ and EXPERT XL (fan-beam DXA) showing marked improvement in spatial resolution and image quality. (From Lunar Corporation, with permission). **b** Most recent third-generation of DXA scanner (Lunar Expert) which has a fan beam source of X-rays and a strip of detectors providing rapid scanning (<5 min per site scanned), improved image quality, lateral spine scanning in the supine position and which has spine morphometry capabilities. **c** Third-generation DXA fan beam scanner manufactured by Hologic, Acclaim 4500

and would contribute significantly to consolidating DXA's role as the "gold standard" in clinical bone densitometry.

Radiation Dose. Radiation doses in the photon absorptiometric techniques of bone densitometry are extremely low. For SXA the EDE is less than 1μ Sv; for pencil-beam DXA 1μ Sv per site scanned (up to 6μ Sv in scans of the hip in women). This is little more than background radiation (2400μ Sv per annum) and compares very favourably with conventional radiographic examinations (60μ Sv for PA chest radiograph; 700–2000μ Sv for lateral spinal radiograph) [135, 136]. The radiation dose from fan-beam exposures is higher by a factor of about 10, but may be up to 62μ Sv [137]. As scattered radiation is higher from the fan beam X-ray source it is recommended that the operator be positioned at least 2 m from the scanning table when the scanner is in use [138, 139].

Indications for DXA Bone Densitometry

There has been much debate concerning the appropriate use of bone densitometry, particularly in population screening in women at the menopause [140, 141]. The cost-effectiveness of such a programme has not been established [142]. However, there is consensus that bone densitometry is appropriate for diagnosis in the following clinical situations [143–148]:
- Estrogen deficiency – in women with early (before age 45 years) natural, surgical- or radiation-induced menopause; or in selected cases at menopause to assist in decision on hormone replacement therapy
- Low trauma fractures, vertebral deformity or osteopenia noted on radiographs
- Long-term corticosteroid use (>5 mg/day)
- Causes of secondary osteoporosis (i.e. primary hyperparathyroidism – reduced bone mass serves as a determinant for surgical treatment; thyrotoxicosis; hypogonadism; malabsorption syndrome; postgastrectomy)
- Monitoring efficacy of therapy for osteoporosis

It is important that adequate DXA scanning facilities are available to meet this diagnostic requirement, conservatively estimated to be at least 600 scans per annum in a population of 300 000 [147]. There is much discussion on which site BMD should be measured [149, 150]. Studies have shown that BMD measured by different techniques in the same individual are variously correlated ($r=0.2–0.9$). Such variable correlations are to be expected since the techniques measure different types of bone (cortical, trabecular, integral) in various skeletal sites. However, because of the dispersion around the regression line of correlations between techniques BMD results obtained by one method cannot be used to predict the result which would be obtained by using another method in the same, or a different, anatomical site (Fig. 15-12) [3, 4]. In research studies the different techniques

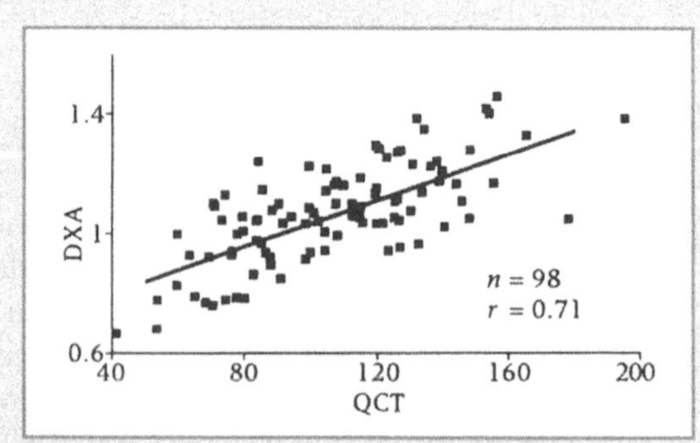

Fig. 15-12 Comparison of bone density measurements made in the same anatomical site (spine) but by different techniques, QCT (mg/cm²) and DXA (g/cm²), in the same individual, showing correlation but the results from one technique cannot be used to predict those which would be obtained by an alternative technique in the same anatomical site

provide complementary information. BMD measurements can be used to predict fracture risk. Any of the measurements can make general predictions of the risk of fracture, but for specific site fracture risk then BMD is best made in that particular anatomical site [151–155]. In a meta-analysis study [156] to determine relative risk of fracture for a decrease in BMD of 1 SD below age adjusted mean all measurement sites had similar predictive abilities (relative risk 1.5; confidence interval 1.4–1.6) except for measurement at the spine for predicting vertebral fractures (relative risk 2.3; confidence interval 1.9–2.8) and measurements at the hip for hip fractures (relative risk 2.6; confidence interval 2.0–3.5). Predictive ability for fracture of decrease in bone mass is similar to (or for hip and spine measurements, better than) that of a 1-SD increase in blood pressure for stroke and better than a 1-SD increase in serum cholesterol concentration for cardiovascular disease. BMD can therefore predict fracture risk but cannot identify individuals who will fracture. For sensitivity to change measurement in metabolically active trabecular bone (QCT) is preferred, so long as precision of the technique is good [157].

DXA is now the most widely available technique for bone densitometry studies and is the accepted "gold standard" in pharmaceutical trials assessing the efficacy of therapeutic interventions in osteoporosis. DXA is generally applied to the lumbar spine and hip, anatomic sites important for osteoporotic fracture. These measures suffice in clinical diagnosis, although the results in the spine in the elderly population may be invalidated because of the presence of hyperostotic and degenerative changes. Whether cheaper and more portable methods (SXA, pDEXA, BUA) of bone densitometry can substitute for the more expensive and generally "fixed" DXA units has still to be substantiated scientifically. Mobile DXA units in customised cabins may be the most appropriate cost-effective solution to provide the diagnostic bone density needs of a community.

Interpretation of DXA Bone Densitometry and Reference Ranges

In order to interpret BMD results in an individual patient it is essential to have appropriate race- and sex-matched BMD reference ranges, since there are ethnic differences in BMD and fracture prevalence [158–160]. The patient's result can then be expressed as a standard deviation (SD; Z score), percentage of expected or percentile of mean for age and sex, or as a SD (T score), percentage of expected or percentile of young normals (peak bone mass). The presently favoured method is Z and T scores [161]. The World Health Organisation [162] has defined "osteopenia" as T score between –1 and –2.5 and "osteoporosis" as T score of below –2.5 and severe osteoporosis as T score below –2.5 together with fragility fractures. There is not yet, however, consensus on how these diagnostic definitions of bone density might most appropriately be related to therapeutic intervention. BMD reference ranges are generally provided by the manufacturers of DXA scanners or can be drawn from published studies. There is no universally accepted study design for the collection of reference data, and the mean and SD of BMD are therefore influenced by inclusion/exclusion criteria, data analysis and geographic and epidemiological differences between populations. Some differences (up to 0.5 SD) have been observed between reference data drawn from the American white population provided by the equipment manufacturers and studies of different nationalities [163, 164] with variations within national reference data utilised [165]. This was the stimulus to a multicentre study within Europe (European Community Concerted Action Group) to develop appropriate BMD reference phantoms and gather European BMD reference data [166–168]. It is essential that appropriate BMD references ranges are available in order to correctly categorise patients for clinical diagnosis and management. There may be less variation in DXA reference data for total hip BMD than that for femoral neck; cross-manufacturer standardisation on total hip BMD is therefore proposed for the future (P. Steiger, personal communication).

In longitudinal studies of large cohorts of patients BMD measurements are performed at 6-month intervals. However, in individual patients a minimum period of 1 year, and preferably 2 years, should elapse between measures to ensure change in BMD is significant (change must be approximately x3 precision error to be significant), unless large changes in bone density are expected [169, 170]. The ideal interval of time between BMD measurements in an individual patient would be related to the technique used and its precision, the site of measurement (axial or appendicular skeleton), the type of bone measured (cortical, trabecular or integral) and the expected rate of change in bone density.

Conclusions

DXA (and SXA) are important non-invasive methods of bone densitometry that provide precise and acceptably accurate measures of BMD in the clinically relevant sites of osteoporotic fractures of spine, hip and wrist, and additionally in the os calcis, with extremely low radiation doses to patients. From the results obtained those individuals with osteoporosis or at risk of fracture can be identified and appropriate therapeutic or other interventions made (life-style factors, diet, exercise, etc.). Scanners vary in cost from approximately U.K. £20 000 for SXA, £40 000–50 000 for first-generation pencil-beam DXA scanners to around £100 000 for the latest generation of fan-beam scanners with spinal morphometry capabilities. DXA scanners are becoming more widely available, particularly in the developed countries of the world, and they play an increasingly important role in clinical practice and therapeutic trials assessing the efficacy of new therapies for osteoporosis [1, 2]. Some inaccuracies occur in BMD measured in the spine by DXA through degenerative and hyperostotic changes and vertebral fracture which limits the technique's usefulness in the elderly population and those with severe spinal osteoporosis. DXA measurements in other sites (proximal femur, forearm, os calcis) may be more appropriate in the elderly. Technical developments and variations between scanners produced by different manufacturers can result in significant differences in BMD and reference ranges. Such differences can largely be compensated for by appropriate cross-calibration and rigid quality assurance programmes in therapeutic trials and in all departments performing bone densitometry. Departments should check their own precision, ideally calculated by the root mean square average of the standard deviation of three or four repeat measurements in 14 individuals [171], and not rely on precisions provided by the manufacturer, which are generally related to repeat scanning of phantoms or normal individuals rather than patients. Optimum precision is achieved if a few, permanent, highly motivated, skilled and experienced operators are performing bone densitometry, rather than having a large number of rotating technical staff operating the scanners.

There have been several different terms and acronyms used for dual-energy X-ray absorptiometry including dual-energy radiography (DER), dual-energy X-ray absorptiometry (DXA or DEXA), dual-energy radiographic absorptiometry (DRA) and quantitative digital radiography (QDR). This leads to some confusion and standardisation of terminology, in addition to calibration and measurement units, is desirable. DXA is the preferred abbreviation for dual-energy X-ray absorptiometry [172, 173].

References

1. Chestnut CH, McClung MR, Ensrud KE, Bell NH, Genant HK, Harris ST, Singer FR, Stock JL, Yood RA, Delmas PD, Kher U, Pryor-Tillotson S, Santora AC (1995) Alendronate treatment of postmenopausal osteoporotic woman: effect of multiple dosages on bone mass and remodeling. Am J Med 99:144–151
2. Liberman UA, Weiss SR, Bröll J, Minne HW, Quan H, Bell NH, Rodriguez-Portales J, Downs Jr RW, Dequeker J, Favus M, Seeman E, Recker RR, Capizzi T, Santora II AC, Lombardi A, Shah RV, Hirsch LJ, Karpf DB (1995) Effect of oral alendronate on bone mineral density and the incidence of fractures in postmenopausal osteoporosis. N Engl J Med 333:1437–1443
3. Adams JE (1995) Quantitative measurements in osteoporosis. In: Tovey FI, Stamp TCB (eds) Measurement in metabolic bone disease. Parthenon, London, pp 107–142
4. Jergas M, Genant HK (1995) Quantitative bone mineral analysis. In: Resnick D (ed) Diagnosis of bone and joint disease. Saunders, Philadelphia, pp 1854–1884
5. Prudham G, Evans JG (1981) Factors associated with falls in the elderly: a community study. Age Ageing 10:141–146
6. Kelsey JL, Hoffmann S (1987) Risk factors for hip fractures. N Engl J Med 316:404–406
7. Melton LJ (1988) Epidemiology of fractures. In: Riggs BL, Melton LJ (eds) Osteoporosis: aetiology, diagnosis and management. Raven, New York, pp 111–131
8. Riggs BL, Melton JJ (1986) Medical progress: involutional osteoporosis. N Engl J Med 314:1676–1684

9.   Hui SL, Slemenda W, Johnston CC (1989) Baseline measurement of bone mass predicts fracture in white women. Ann Intern Med 111:355–361

10. Ross PD, Davis JW, Vogel JM, Wasnich RD (1990) A critical review of bone mass and the risk of fractures in osteoporosis. Calcif Tissue Int 46:149–161

11. Wasnich RD, Ross PD, Heilbrun LK, Vogel JM (1985) Prediction of post-menopausal fracture risk with use of bone mineral measurements. Am J Obstet Gynecol 153:745–751

12. Doyle FH, Gutteridge DH, Joplin GF, Fraser R (1967) An assessment of radio-logical criteria used in the study of spinal osteoporosis. Br J Radiol 40:241–250

13. Masud T, Mootoosamy I, McCloskey EV, O'Sullivan MP, Whitby EP, King D, Matson MB, Doyle DV, Spector TD (1996) Assessment of osteopenia from spine radiographs using two different methods – the Chingford Study. Br J Radiol 69:451–456

14. Cooper C, Shah S, Hand DJ, Adams JE, Compston J, Davie M Woolf A (1991) Screening for vertebral osteoporosis using individual risk factors. Osteoporos Int 2:48–53

15. Adams JE (1992) Osteoporosis and bone mineral densitometry. Curr Opin Radiol 4:11–19

16. Faulkner KG, Gluer CC, Majumdar S, Lang P, Engelke K, Genant HK (1991) Non invasive measurements of bone mass, structure and strength: current methods and experimental techniques. Am J Radiol 157:1229–1237

17. Guglielmi G, Gluer CC, Majumdar S, Blunt B, Genant HK (1995) Current methods and advances in bone densitometry. Eur Radiol 5:129–139

18. Grampp S, Jergas M, Lang P, Genant HK, Gluer CC (1996) Quantitative assessment of osteoporosis: current and future trends. In: Sartoris DJ (ed) osteoporosis: diagnosis and treatment. Dekker, New York, pp 232–265

19. Cameron JR, Sorenson J (1963) Measurement of bone mineral in vivo: an improved method. Science 142:230–232

20. Whitehouse RW (1991) Methods for measuring bone mass. Curr Imaging 3:213–220

21. Vogel JM, Wasnich RD, Rodd PD (1988) The clinical relevance of calcaneus bone mineral measurements: a review. Bone Miner 5:35–58

22. Cameron JR, Mazess RB, Sorenson JA (1968) Precision and accuracy of bone mineral determination by direct photon absorptiometry. Invest Radiol 3:141–150

23. Tothill P (1988) Photon Absorptiometry. In: Galasko CBS, Isherwood I (eds) Imaging techniques in orthopaedics. Springer, Berlin Heidelberg New York, pp 251–257

24. Mazess RB, Wahner HM (1988) Nuclear medicine and densitometry. In: Riggs BL, Melton LJ (eds) Osteoporosis: etiology, diagnosis and management. Raven, New York, pp 251–295

25. Price RI, Barnes MP, Gutteridge DH, Baron-Hay M (1989) Ultradistal and cortical forearm bone density in assessment of postmenopausal bone loss and non-axial fracture risk. J Bone Miner Res 4:149–154

26. Nilas L, Borg J, Gotfredsen A, Christiansen C (1985) Comparison of single and dual-photon absorptiometry in post menopausal bone mineral loss. J Nucl Med 26:1257–1262

27. Wasnich RD, Rodd PD, Heilbrun LK, Vogel JM (1987) Selection of the optimal site for fracture risk prediction. Clin Orthop 216:262–269

28. Nilas L, Borg J, Gotfredsen A, Christiansen C (1985) Comparison of single- and dual-photon absorptiometry in postmenopausal bone mineral loss. J Nucl Med 26:1257–1262

29. Nilas L, Gotriedsen A, Hadberg A, Christiansen C (1988) Age-related bone loss in women evaluated by the single and dual photon technique. Bone Miner 4:95–103

30. Vogel JM (1987) Application principles and technical considerations in SPA. In: Genant HK (ed) Osteoporosis update. Radiology Research and Education Foundation, San Francisco, pp 219–231

31. Williams JA, Wagner J, Wasnich R, Heilbrun L (1984) The effect of long-distance running upon appendicular bone mineral content. Med Sci Sports Exerc 16:223–227

32. Cummings SR, Black DM, Nevitt MC (1990) Appendicular bone density and age predict hip fracture in women. J Am Med Assoc 263:665–668

33. Black DM, Cummings SR, Genant HK, Nevitt MC, Palermo L, Browner W (1992) Axial and appendicular bone density predict fractures in older women. J Bone Miner Res 7:633–638

34. Dunn WL, Wahner HW, Riggs BL (1980) Measurement of bone mineral content in human vertebrae and hip by dual photon absorptiometry. Radiology 136:485–487

35. Krolner B, Neilson SP (1980) Measurement of bone mineral content (BMC) of the lumbar spine. Theory and application of a new two-dimensional dual photon attenuation method. Scand J Clin Lab Invest 40:653–663

36. Peppler WW, Mazess RB (1981) Total body bone mineral and lean body mass by dual-photon absorptiometry. Calcif Tissue Int 33:353–359

37. Wahner HW, Dunn WL, Mazess (1985) Dual photon (Gd-153) absorptiometry of bone. Radiology 156:203–206

38. Sartoris DJ, Resnick D (1989) Dual-energy radiographic absorptiometry for bone densitometry. Am J Radiol 152:241–246

39. Gluer CC, Steiger P, Selvidge R, Elliensen-Kliefoth K, Hayashi C, Genant HK (1990) Comparative assessment of dual-photon absorptiometry and dual-energy radiography. Radiology 174:223–228

40. Mazess RB (1995) Dual-energy X-ray absorptiometry for the management of bone disease. Phys Med Rehabil Clin North Am 6:507–537

41. Nelson DA, Bown EB, Flynn MJ, Cody DD, Shaffer S (1991) Comparison of dual photon and dual-energy X-ray bone densitometers in a clinic setting. Skeletal Radiol 20:591–595

42. Kelly TL, Slovik DM, Schoenfeld DA, Neer RM (1988) Quantitative digital radiography versus dual photon absorptiometry of the lumbar spine. J Clin Endocrinol Metab 67:839–844

43. Cullum ID, Ell PJ, Ryder JP (1989) X-ray dual-photon absorptiometry: a new method for measurement of bone density. Br J Radiol 62:587–592

44. Kellie SE (1992) Measurement of bone density with dual-energy X-ray absorptiometry (DEXA). J Am Med Assoc 267:286–294

45. Wahner HW, Fogelman I (1994) The evaluation of osteoporosis: dual energy X-ray absorptiometry in clinical practice. Dunitz, London

46. Wilson CR, Fogelman I, Blake GM, Rodin A (1991) The effect of positioning on dual-energy X-ray absorptiometry of the proximal femur. Bone Miner 13:69–76

47. Goh JC, Low SL, Bose K (1995) Effect of femoral rotation on bone mineral density measurements with dual energy X-ray absorptiometry. Calcif Tissue Int 57:340–343

48. Mazess RB, Barden HS (1988) Measurement of bone by dual-photon absorptiometry (DPA) and dual-energy X-ray absorptiometry (DEXA) Ann Chir Gynaecol 77:197–203

49. Slosman DO, Rizzoli R, Buchs B, Piana F, Donath A, Bonjour JP (1990) Comparative study of the performance of X-ray and gadolinium 153 bone densitometers at the level of the spine, femoral neck and femoral shaft. Eur J Nucl Med 17:3–9

50. Adachi JD, Webber CE (1991) The interchangeability of radioisotope and X-ray based measurements of bone density. Br J Radiol 64:217–220

51. Lees B, Stevenson JC (1992) An evaluation of dual-energy X-ray absorptiometry and comparison with dual-photon absorptiometry. Osteoporos Int 2:146–152

52. Ho CP, Kim RW, Schaffler MB, Sartoris DJ (1990) Accuracy of dual-energy radiographic absorptiometry of the lumbar spine: cadaver study 176:171–173

53. Edmondston SJ, Singer KP, Price RL, Breidahl PD (1993) Accuracy of dual-energy X-ray absorptiometry for the determination of bone mineral content in the thoracic and lumbar spine: an in-vitro study. Br J Radiol 66:309–313

54. Hagiwara S, Lane N, Engelke K, Sebastian A, Kimmel DB, Genant HK (1993) Precision and accuracy of rat whole body and femur bone mineral determination with dual X-ray absorptiometry. Bone Miner 22:57–68

55. Lilley J, Walters BC, Heath DA, Droc Z (1991) In vivo and in vitro precision of bone density measured by dual energy X-ray absorptiometry. Osteoporos Int 1:141–146

56. Orwell ES, Eviatt SK (1991) Longitudinal precision of dual-energy X-ray absorptiometry in a multicentre study. J Bone Miner Res 6:191–197

57. Pouilles JM, Tremollieres F, Todorovsky N, Ribot C (1991) Precision and sensitivity of dual-energy X-ray absorptiometry in spinal osteoporosis. J Bone Miner Res 6:997–1002

58. Mazess R, Chestnut CH, McClung M, Genant HK (1992) Enhanced precision with dual-energy X-ray absorptiometry. Calcif Tissue Int 51:14–17

59. Sievänen H, Oja P, Vuori I (1992) Precision of dual-energy X-ray absorptiometry in determining bone mineral density and content of various skeletal sites. J Nucl Med 33:1137–1142

60. Sievänen H, Kannus P, Oja P, Vuori I (1993) Precision of dual-energy X-ray absorptiometry in the upper extremities. Bone Miner Res 20:235–243

61. Fuleihan GE, Testa MA, Angell JE, Porrino N, Leboff MS (1995) Reproducibility of DXA absorptiometry: a model for bone loss estimates. J Bone Miner Res 10:1004–1014

62. Reginster JY, Deroisy R, Zegels B, Jupsin I, Albert A, Franchimont P (1995) Long-term performance in vitro and in vivo of dual-energy X-ray absorptiometry. Clin Rheumatol 14:180–186

63. Larcos G, Wahner HW (1991) An evaluation of forearm bone mineral measurement with dual-energy X-ray absorptiometry. J Nucl Med 32:2101–2106

64. Ryan PJ, Blake GM, Fogelman I (1992) Measurement of forearm BMD in normal women by dual-energy X-ray absorptiometry. Br J Radiol 65:127–131

65. Haarbo J, Gotfredsen A, Hassager C, Christiansen C (1991) Validation of body composition by dual-energy X-ray absorptiometry (DEXA). Clin Physiol 11:331–341

66. Compston JE, Bhambhara M, Lasky MA, Murphy S, Khaw KT (1992) Body composition and bone mass in postmenopausal women. Clin Endocrinol 37:426–431

67. Fuller NJ, Laskey MA, Elia M (1992) Assessment of the composition of major body regions by dual energy X-ray absorptiometry (DEXA) with special reference to limb muscle mass. Clin Physiol 12:253–266

68. Svendsen OL, Haarbo J, Hassager C, Christiansen C (1988) Accuracy of measurement of body composition by dual-energy X-ray absorptiometry in vivo. Am J Clin Nutr 57:605–608

69. Herd RJM, Blake GM, Parker JC, Ryan PJ, Fogelman I (1993) Total body studies in normal British women using dual-energy X-ray absorptiometry. Br J Radiol 66:303–308

70. Kohrt WM (1995) Body composition by DXA: tried and true? Med Sci Sports Exerc 27:1349–1354

71. Ogle GD, Allen JR, Humphries IR, Lu PW, Briody JN, Morley K, Howman-Giles R, Cowell CT (1995) Body composition assessment by dual-energy X-ray absorptiometry in subjects aged 4–26 y. Am J Clin Nutr 61:746–753

72. Tothill P, Avenelli A, Love J, Reid DM (1994) Comparisons between Hologic, Lunar and Norland dual-energy X-ray absorptiometers and other techniques for whole body soft-tissue measurements. Eur J Clin Nutr 48:781–794

73. Johansson AG, Forslund A, Sjodin A, Mallmin H, Hambraeus L, Ljunghall S (1993) Determination of body composition – a comparison of dual-energy X-ray absorptiometry and hydrodensitometry. Am J Nutr 57:323–326

74. Ellis JK, Shypailo RJ, Pratt JA, Pond WG (1994) Accuracy of dual-energy X-ray absorptiometry for body composition measurements in children. Am J Clin Nutr 60:660–665

75. Paton NIJ, Macallan DC, Jebb SA, Pazianas M, Griffin GE (1995) Dual-energy X-ray absorptiometry results differ between machines (letter). Lancet 346 (I):899–900

76. Nuti R, Martini G, Righe G, Frediani B, Turchetti V (1991) Comparison of total body measurements by dual-energy X-ray absorptiometry and dual-photon absorptiometry. J Bone Miner Res 6:681–687

77. McCarthy CK, Steinberg CG, Agren M, Leahy D, Wyman E, Baran DT (1991) Quantifying bone loss from the proximal femur after total hip arthroplasty. J Bone Joint Surg Br 73:774–778

78. Griffin MC, Kimble R, Hopfer W, Pacifici R (1993) Dual-energy X-ray absorptiometry of the rat: accuracy, precision and measurement of bone loss. J Bone Miner Res 8:795–800

79. Pastoureau P, Chomel A, Bonnet J (1995) Specific evaluation of localized bone mass and bone loss in the rat using dual-energy X-ray absorptiometry subregional analysis. Osteoporos Int 5:143–149

80. Laval-Jeantet AM, Bergot C, Williams M, Davidson K, Laval-Jeantet M (1995) Dual-energy X-ray absorptiometry of the calcaneus: comparison with vertebral X-ray absorptiometry and quantitative computed tomography. Calcif Tissue Int 56:14–18

81. Horner K, Devlin H, Alsop CW, Hodgkinson IM, Adams JE (1996) Mandibular bone mineral density as a predictor of skeletal osteoporosis. Br J Radiol 69:1019–1025

82. Szücs J, Johnson R, Granhed H, Hansson T (1992) Accuracy, precision and homogeneity effects in the determination of the bone mineral content with dual photon absorptiometry in the heel bone. Bone 13:179–183

83. Yamada M, Ito M, Hayashi K, Nakamura T (1993) Calcaneus as a site for assessment of bone mineral density: evaluation in cadavers and healthy volunteers. AJR 161:621–627

84. Kotzki PO, Buyck D, Leroux JL, Thomas E, Rossi M, Blotman F (1993) Measurement of the bone mineral density of the os calcis as an indication of vertebral fracture in women with lumbar osteoarthritis. Br J Radiol 66:55–60

85. Faulkner KT, McClung M, Cummings SE (1994) Automated evaluation of hip axis length for predicting hip fracture. J Bone Miner Res 9:1065–1070

86. Sieranen H, Kannus P, Oja P, Vuori I (1994) Dual-energy X-ray absorptiometry is also an accurate and precise method to measure the dimensions of human long bones. Calcif Tissue Int 54:101–105

87. Felsenberg D, Gowin W, Diessel E, Armburst S, Mews J (1995) Recent developments in DXA quality of new DXA/MXA devices for densitometry and morphometry. Eur J Radiol 20:179–184

88. Glastre C, Braillon P, David L, Cochat P, Meunier PJ, Delmas PD (1990) Measurement of bone mineral content of the lumbar spine by dual-energy X-ray absorptiometry in normal children: correlations with growth parameters. J Clin Endocrinal Metab 70:1330–1333

89. De Schepper J, Derde MP, Van den Broeck M, Piepsz A, Jonckheer MH (1991) Normative data for lumbar spine bone mineral content in children: influence of age, height, weight and pubertal state. J Nucl Med 32:216–220

90. Ott SM (1991) Bone density in adolescents. N Engl J Med 23:1646–1647

91. Southard RN, Morris JD, Mahan JD, Hayes JR, Torch MA, Sommer A, Zipf WB (1991) Bone mass in healthy children: measurement with quantitative DXA. Radiology 179:735–738

92. Braillon PM, Salle BL, Brunet J (1992) Dual-energy X-ray absorptiometry measurement of bone mineral content in newborns: validation of the technique. Paediatr Res 32:77–80

93. Salle BL, Braillon P, Glorieux FH (1992) Lumbar bone mineral content measured by dual-energy X-ray absorptiometry in newborns and infants. Acta Paediatr 81:953–958

94. Hori C, Tsukahara H, Fujui Y, Kawamitsu T, Konishi Y, Yamamoto K, Ishii Y, Sudo M (1995) Bone mineral status in preterm-born children: assessment by dual-energy X-ray absorptiometry. Biol Neonate 68:254–258

95. Koo WW, Massom LR, Walters J (1995) Validation of accuracy and precision of dual-energy X-ray absorptiometry for infants. J Bone Miner Res 10:1111–1115

96. Picaud JC, Rigo J, Nyamugato K, Milet J, Senterre J (1996) Evaluation of dual-energy X-ray absorptiometry for body composition assessment in piglets and term human neonates. Am J Clin Nutr 63:157–163

97. Lu PW, Briody JN, Ogle GD, Morley K, Humphries IR, Allen J, Howman-Giles R, Sillence D, Cowell CT (1994) Bone mineral density of total body, spine and femoral neck in children and young adults: a cross-sectional and longitudinal study. J Bone Miner Res 9:1451–1458

98. Orwoll ES, Oviatt SK, Mann T (1990) The impact of osteophytic and vascular calcifications on vertebral mineral density measurement in men. J Clin Endocrinol Metab 70:1202–1207

99. Laskey MA, Crisp AJ, Compston JE, Khaw KT (1993) Heterogeneity of spine bone density. Br J Radiol 66:480–483

100. Frohn J, Wilken T, Falk S, Stutte HJ, Kollath J, Hor G (1991) Effect of aortic sclerosis on bone mineral measurements by dual-photon absorptiometry. J Nucl Med 32:259–262

101. Franck H, Munz M, Scherrer M (1995) Evaluation of dual-energy X-ray absorptiometry bone mineral measurement – comparison of a single-beam and fan-beam design: the effect of osteophytic calcification on spine bone mineral density. Calcif Tissue Int 56:192–195

102. Rupich R, Pacifici R, Griffin M, Vered I, Susman N, Avioli LV (1990) Lateral dual-energy radiography: a new method for measuring vertebral bone density: a preliminary study. J Clin Endocrinol Metab 70:1768–1770

103. Slosman DO, Rizzoli R, Donath A, Bonjour J-P (1990) Vertebral bone mineral density measured laterally by dual-energy X-ray absorptiometry. Osteoporos Int 1:23–29

104. Uebelhart D, Duboeuf F, Meunier PJ, Delmas PD (1990) Lateral dual-photon absorptiometry: a new technique to measure bone mineral density at the lumbar spine. J Bone Miner Res 5:525–531

105. Mazess BR, Gifford CA, Bisek JP, Barden HS, Hansen JA (1991) DEXA measurement of spine density in the lateral projection I. Methodology. Calcif Tissue Int 49:235–239

106. Blake GM, Jagathesan T, Herd RJ, Fogelman I (1994) Dual-energy X-ray absorptiometry of the lumbar spine: the precision of paired anterioposterior/lateral studies. Br J Radiol 67:624–630

107. Del Rio L, Pons F, Huguet M, Setoain FJ, Setoain J (1995) Anterioposterior versus lateral bone mineral density of spine assessed by dual X-ray absorptiometry. Eur J Nucl Med 22:407–412

108. Jergas M, Breitenseher M, Gluer CC, Black D, Lang P, Grampp S, Engelke K, Genant HK (1995) Which vertebrae should be assessed using lateral dual-energy X-ray absorptiometry of the lumbar spine. Osteoporos Int 5:196–204

109. Rupich RC, Griffin MG, Pacifici R, Alvioli LV, Susman N (1992) Lateral dual-energy radiography: artifact error from rib and pelvic bone. J Bone Miner Res 7:97–101

110. Guglielmi G, Grimston SK, Fischer KC, Pacifici R (1994) Osteoporosis: diagnosis with lateral and posteroanterior dual X-ray absorptiometry compared with quantitative CT. Radiology 192:845–850

111. Reid IR, Evans MC, Stapleton J (1992) Lateral spine densitometry is a more sensitive indicator of glucocorticoid-induced bone loss. J Bone Miner Res 7:1221–1225

112. Jergas M, Breitenseheer M, Gluer CC, Yu W, Genant HK (1995) Estimates of volumetric bone density from projectional measurements improve the discriminatory capability of dual X-ray absorptiometry. J Bone Miner Res 10:1101–1110

113. Peel NFA, Johnson A, Barrington NA, Smith TWD, Eastell R (1993) Impact of anomalous vertebral segmentation on measurements of bone mineral density. J Bone Miner Res 8:719–723

114. Koo WW, Walters J, Bush AJ (1995) Technical considerations of dual-energy X-ray absorptiometry-based bone mineral measurements for paediatric studies. J Bone Miner Res 10:1998–2004

115. Simmons A, Barrington SF, Archbold LJ, O'Doherty MJ, Coakley AJ (1995) Assessment of changes in dual-energy X-ray absorptiometry performance following a system upgrade. Nucl Med Commun 17:331–341

116. Spector E, Le Blanc A, Shackelford L (1995) Hologic QDR 2000 whole-body scans: a comparison of three combinations of scan modes and analysis software. Osteoporos Int 5:440–445

117. Tothill P, Avenell A, Reid DM (1994) Precision and accuracy of measurements of whole-bone mineral: comparisons between Hologic, Lunar and Norland dual-energy X-ray absorptiometers. Br J Radiol 67:1210–1217

118. Tothill P, Fenner JA, Reid DM (1995) Comparisons between three dual-energy X-ray absorptiometers used for measuring spine and femur. Br J Radiol 68:621–629

119. Blake GM, Tong CM, Fogelman I (1991) Intersite comparison of the Hologic QDR-1000 dual energy X-ray bone densitometer. Br J Radiol 64:440–446

120. Laskey MA, Flaxman ME, Barber W, Trafford S, Hayball MP, Lyttle KD, Crisp AJ, Compston JE (1991) Comparative performance in vitro and in vivo of

Lunar DPX and Hologic QDR-1000 dual energy X-ray absorptiometers. Br J Radiol 64:1023–1029

121. Nelson D, Feingold M, Mascha E, Kleerkoper M (1992) Comparison of single photon and dual-energy X-ray absorptiometry of the radius. Bone Miner 18:77–83

122. Eiken P, Barenholdt O, Bjorn Jensen L, Gram J, Pors Nielsen S (1994) Switching from DXA pencil-beam to fan beam. I Studies in vitro at four centres. Bone 15:667–670

123. Bouyoucef SE, Cullen ID, Ell PJ (1996) Cross-calibration of a fan-beam X-ray densitometry with a pencil-beam system. Br J Radiol 69:522–531

124. Faulkner KG, Genant HK, McClung M (1995) Bilateral comparison of femoral bone density and hip axis length from single and fan beam DXA scans. Calcif Tissue Int 56:26–31

125. Peel NF, Eastell R (1995) Comparison of rates of bone loss from the spine measured using two manufacturers' densitometers. J Bone Miner Res 10:1796–1801

126. Gluer CC, Faulkner KG, Estilo MJ, Engelke K, Rosin J, Genant HK (1993) Quality assurance for bone densitometry research studies: concept and impact. Osteoporos Int 3:227–235

127. Miller CG (1993) Bone density measurements in clinical trials: the challenge of ensuring optimal data. Br J Clin Res 4:113–120

128. Wahner HW, Looker A, Dunn WL, Walters LC, Hauser MF, Novak C (1994) Quality control of bone densitometry in a National Health Survey (NHANES III) using three mobile examination centres. J Bone Miner Res 9:951–960

129. Faulkner KG, McClung MR (1995) Quality control of DXA instruments in multicenter trials. Osteoporos Int 5:218–227

130. Nord RH (1992) Work in progress: a cross-calibration study of four DXA instruments designed to culminate in inter-manufacturer standardization. Osteopor Int 2:210–211

131. Finkelstein JS, Butler JP, Cleary RL, Neer RM (1994) Comparison of four methods for cross-calibrating dual-energy X-ray absorptiometers to eliminate systematic errors when upgrading equipment. J Bone Miner Res 9:1945–1952

132. Abrahamsen B, Gram J, Hansen TB, Beck-Nielsen H (1995) Cross-calibration of QDR-2000 and QDR-1000 dual-energy X-ray densitometers for bone mineral and soft tissue measurements. Bone 16:385–390

133. Genant HK, Grampp S, Gluer CC, Faulkner KG, Jergas M, Engelke K, Hagiwara S, Van Kuijk C (1994) Universal standardisation for dual X-ray absorptiometry: patient and phantom cross-calibration results. J Bone Miner Res 9:1503–1514

134. Kalender WA, Felsenberg D, Genant HK, Dequeker J, Reeve J (1995) The European Spine Phantom: a tool for standardisation and quality control in spinal bone mineral measurement by DXA and QCT. Eur J Radiol 20:83–92

135. Kalender WA (1992) Effective dose values in bone mineral measurements by photon absorptiometry and computed tomography. Osteoporos Int 2:82–87

136. Huda W, Morin RL (1996) Patient doses in bone mineral densitometry. Br J Radiol 69:422–425

137. Eiken P, Kolthoff N, Barenholdt O, Hermansen F, Pors Nielsen S (1994) Switching from DXA pencil-beam to fan-beam. II studies in vivo. Bone 15:671–676

138. Njeh CF, Apple K, Temperton DH, Boivin CM (1996) Radiological assessment of a new bone densitometer: the Lunar Expert. Br J Radiol 69:335–340

139. Patel R, Blake GM, Batchelor S, Fogelman I (1996) Occupational dose to the radiographer in dual X-ray absorptiometry: a comparison of pencil-beam and fan-beam systems. Br J Radiol 69:539–543

140. Cummings SR, Black D (1986) Should peri-menopausal women be screened for osteoporosis? Ann Int Med 104:817–823

141. Melton LJ, Eddy DM, Johnston CC (1990) Screening for osteoporosis. Ann Intern Med 112:516–528

142. Tostestan ANA, Rosenthal DI, Melton LJ, Weinstein MC (1990) Cost effectiveness of screening perimenopausal white women for osteoporosis: bone densitometry and hormone replacement therapy. Ann Intern Med 113:594–603

143. Cummings SR (1987) Bone mineral densitometry. Ann Intern Med 107:932–936

144. Genant HK, Block TE, Steiger P, Gluer CC, Ettinger B, Harris ST (1989) Appropriate use of bone densitometry. Radiology 170:817–822

145. Johnson CC, Melton LJ, Lindsay R, Eddy DM (1989) Clinical indications for bone mass measurement. A report from the Scientific Advisory Board of the National Osteoporosis Foundation. J Bone Miner Res 4 [Suppl 2]:1–28

146. Johnson CC, Slemender CW, Melton LJ (1991) Clinical use of bone densitometry. N Engl J Med 324:1105–1109

147. Advisory Group on Osteoporosis, Barlow DH (Chairman) (1994) Report for the Department of Health, UK, pp 61–62

148. Compston JE, Cooper C, Kanis JA (1995) Bone densitometry in clinical practice. BMJ 310:1507–1510

149. Slemenda CW, Johnson CC (1988) Bone mass measurement: which site to measure. Am J Med 84:643–645

150. Need AG, Nordin BEC (1990) Which bone to measure. Osteoporos Int 1:3–6

151. Ross PD, Wasnich RD, Heilbrun LK, Vogel JM (1987) Definition of spine fracture threshold based upon prospective fracture risk. Bone 8:271–278

152. Cummings SR, Black DM, Nevitt MC, Browner WS, Cauley JA, Genant HK, Mascioli SR, Scott JC, Seeley DG, Steiger P, Vogt TM, Study of Osteoporotic Fractures Research Group (1990) Appendicular bone density and age predict hip fracture in women. J Am Med Assoc 263:665–668

153. Black DM, Cummings SR, Genant HK (1992) Axial and appendicular bone density predict fractures in older women. J Bone Miner Res 6:633–638

154. Cummings SR, Black DM, Nevitt MC, Browner W, Cauley J, Ensrund K, Genant HK, Palermo L, Scott J, Vogt TM, Osteoporotic Fractures Research Group (1993) Bone density at various sites for prediction of hip fractures. Lancet 341:72–75

155. Gardsell P, Johnell O, Nilsson BE, Gullberg B (1993) Predicting various fragility fractures in women by forearm densitometry: a follow-up study. Calcif Tissue Int 52:348–353

156. Marshall D, Johnell O, Wedel H (1996) Meta-analysis of how well measures of bone mineral density predict occurrence of osteoporotic fracture. BMJ 312:1254–1259

157. Reinbold WD, Genant HK, Reiser UJ, Harris ST, Ettinger B (1986) Bone mineral content in early postmenopausal and postmenopausal osteoporotic women: comparison of measurement methods. Radiology 160:469–478

158. Patel DN, Pettifor JM, Becker PJ (1993) The effect of ethnicity on appendicular bone mass in white, coloured and Indian school children. S Afr Med J 83:847–853

159. Anderson JJ, Pollitzer WS (1994) Ethnic and genetic differences in susceptibility to osteoporotic fracture. Adv Nutr Res 9:129–149

160. Tobias JH, Cook DG, Chambers TJ, Dalzell N (1994) A comparison of bone mineral density between Caucasian, Asian and Afro-Caribbean women. Clin Sci 87:587–591

161. Parfitt AM (1990) Interpretation of bone densitometry measurements; disadvantages of a percentage scale and a discussion of some alternatives. J Bone Min Res 5:537–540

162. World Health Organisation (1994) Assessment of fracture risk and its application to screening for postmenopausal osteoporosis. Technical report series 843. WHO, Geneva

163. Kroger H, Heikkinen J, Laitinen K, Kotaniemi A (1992) Dual energy X-ray absorptiometry in normal women: a cross-sectional study of 717 Finnish volunteers. Osteoporos Int 2:135–140

164. Looker AC, Wahner HW, Dunn WL, Calvo MS, Harris TB, Heyse SP, Johnston CC, Lindsay RL (1995) Proximal femur bone mineral levels of US adults. Osteoporos Int 5:389–409

165. Simmons A, O'Doherty MJ, Barrington SF, Coakley AJ (1995) A survey of dual-energy X-ray absorptiometry (DEXA) normal reference ranges used within the UK and their effect on classification. Nucl Med Commun 16:1041–1053

166. Dequeker J, Pearson J, Reeve J, Henley M, Bright J, Felsenberg D, Kalender W, Laval-Jeantet AM, Ruegsegger P, Adams J, Diaz Curiel M, Fischer M, Galan F, Geusens P, Hyldstrup L, Jaeger P, Kotzki P, Kröger H, Lips P, Mitchell A, Louis O, Perez Cano R, Pols H, Reid DM, Ribot C, Schneider P, Lunt M (1995) Dual-energy X-ray absorptiometry – cross-calibration and normative reference ranges for the spine; results of a European Community Concerted Action. Bone 17:247–254

167. Pearson J, Dequeker J, Reeve J, Felsenberg D, Henley M, Bright J, Lunt M, Adams J, Diaz Curiel M, Galan F et al (1995) Dual energy X-ray absorptiometry of the proximal femur: normal European values standardised with the European Spine Phantom. J Bone Miner Res 10:315–324

168. Pearson J, Ruegsegger P, Dequeker J, Henley M, Bright J, Reeve J, Kalender W, Felsenberg D, Laval-Jeantet AM, Adams JE et al (1995) European semi-anthropomorphic phantom for the cross-calibration of bone densitometers: assessment of precision, accuracy and stability. Bone Miner 27:109–120

169. Ross PD, Davis JW, Wasnick RD, Vogel JM (1991) The clinical application of serial bone mass measurements. Bone Miner 12:189–199

170. Verheij LF, Blokland JA, Papapoulos SE, Zwinderman AH. Pauwels EK (1992) Optimization of follow-up measurements of bone mass. J Nucl Med 33:1406–1410

171. Gluer CC, Blake G, Lu Y, Blunt BA, Jergas M, Genant HK (1995) Accurate assessment of precision errors: how to measure the reproducibility of bone densitometry techniques. Osteoporos Int 5:262–280

172. Wilson CR, Collier D, Carrera GF, Jacobson DR (1990) Acronym for dual-energy X-ray absorptiometry. Radiology 176:875

173. Genant HK, Gluer CC, Faulkner KG, Majumdar S, Harris ST, Engelke K, van Kuijk C (1992) Acronyms in bone densitometry (letter). Radiology 184:878

16 Quantitative Computed Tomography at the Axial Skeleton

G. Guglielmi, T. F. Lang, M. Cammisa, and H. K. Genant

Introduction

Quantitative computed tomography (QCT) is an established technique for measuring bone mineral density (BMD) in the axial spine and appendicular skeleton [1–3]. Because it provides cross-sectional images, QCT is uniquely able to provide separate measurements of trabecular and cortical bone BMD as well as a true volumetric mineral density in grams per cubic centimeter. In this application QCT has been used for assessment of vertebral fracture risk [4, 5], measurement of age-related bone loss [6–8], and follow-up of osteoporosis and other metabolic bone diseases [9]. This chapter assesses the current capabilities of QCT at different skeletal sites, and reviews recent technical developments such as fast three-dimensional data acquisition and high-resolution image acquisition and processing techniques, in which novel information about bone strength may be obtained through analysis of trabecular microarchitecture.

Spinal QCT

The fundamental advantage of spinal QCT for noninvasive bone mineral measurement lies in the high responsiveness and biomechanical importance of vertebral trabecular bone. The method is usually applied to the spine to measure trabecular bone in consecutive vertebrae (usually two to four vertebrae of T12–L4) using commercial CT scanners and a bone mineral reference standard to calibrate each scan. Based on a lateral localizer image, or scoutview (Fig. 16-1), single 8- to 10-mm-thick sections are obtained through the midplane of each of these vertebrae using a low-dose technique (Fig. 16-2; 50 µSv for four axial slices and 30 µSv for the localizer image), with the gantry angled parallel to the vertebral endplates. A region of interest (ROI) is manually positioned in the anterior portion of trabecular bone of the vertebral body for analysis [4, 10–12]. In some approaches this region of interest may be positioned automatically [13, 14]. For optimal reproducibility the selection of scan plane and ROIs may be performed using computer-assisted localization to provide separate BMD measurements of trabecular bone, cortical rim of the vertebral body, and integral bone [13,14]. Care must be taken to exclude the basivertebral vein and sclerotic foci. The CT density of the selected area of interest within a slice through a vertebral body is mea-

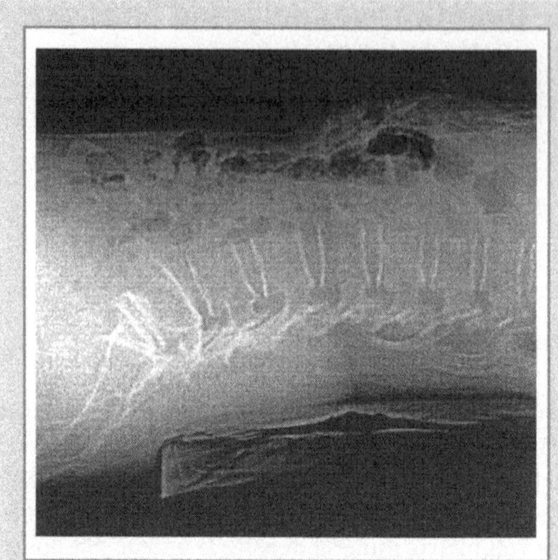

Fig. 16-1 Localizer image used to determine midvertebral positions for CT slices

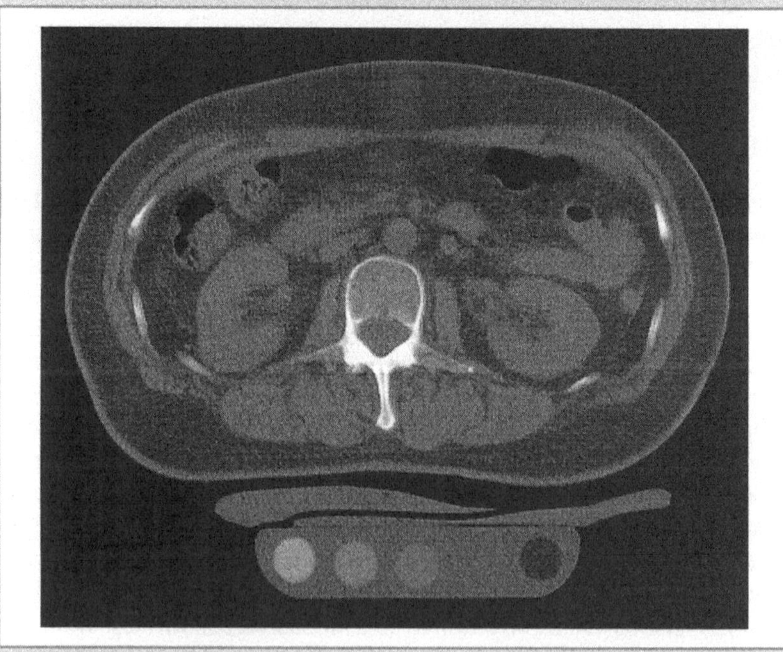

Fig. 16-2 A 10-mm-thick CT slice through the middle of L2. QCT calibration phantom is positioned under the patient

sured in Hounsfield units (HU; also known as CT number) where water=o HU and air =–1000 HU. Conversion to grams per cubic centimeter is carried out by using linear regression to relate the CT number of the trabecular bone to that of the compartments of the calibration standard. The calculated densities for the vertebrae are averaged and compared to those of a normative population [7, 10, 15].

Several bone mineral calibration techniques are currently available. Liquid calibration reference phantoms (e. g., the Cann-Genant standard) containing varying concentrations of dipotassium hydrogen phosphate (K_2HPO_4) [4] have seen considerable initial use. The utility of this type of phantom may be constrained by the limited long-term stability of the calibration solutions. Therefore solid hydroxyapatite calibration phantoms have also come into widespread use. Simultaneous calibration techniques such as those described above correct to some extent for scanner instabilities and for variable beam hardening, which depends on patient size and shape. Nonsimultaneous calibration, in which an anthropomorphic tissue equivalent phantom is scanned after the patient, has also been investigated [16]. Recently some studies have reported promising results on a new QCT technique in which paraspinal muscle and subcutaneous fat served for internal calibration [17,18]; however, only limited studies have been carried out to date.

It should be noted that the various calibration standards show systematic differences, and it is important that serial evaluations employ the same reference phantom [19]. If this is not possible, duplicate measurement on the old and new standard need to be carried out on the same day to determine the offset. It is possible to employ a reference database acquired on one calibration standard to patients scanned on another only if the normative data are adjusted by a cross-calibration analysis [20–22].

QCT can be performed in single-energy (SEQCT) or dual-energy (DEQCT) modes, which differ in accuracy, precision, and radiation [23, 24]. The presence of marrow fat within trabecular bone may cause the standard SEQCT technique to underestimate BMD by 10%–15% [25]. Provided that QCT scans are acquired at low effective energies (i. e., 80–90 kVp) the clinical relevance of the fat error is usually small, however, given the use of age-matched databases [26]. DEQCT techniques have been devised using either pre- or postprocessing methods [27, 28]. Such techniques may improve accuracy, but at the price of increased precision errors [29, 30]. The in vivo precision and accuracy errors of QCT are approximately 2%–4% and 4%–15%, respectively [9, 24] and are generally higher than those observed for posteroanterior dual-X-ray absorptiometry (DXA) of the spine and comparable with those of lateral DXA.

The diagnostic efficacy of QCT for vertebral fracture and bone loss is based on the ability to assess vertebral trabecular bone separately. Several recent studies have compared QCT and DXA measurements in this regard [31-38]. In a retrospective study Yu et al. [39] found that spinal trabecular BMD assessed by QCT shows a larger decrement between age-matched vertebrally fractured and non-fractured populations than DXA in either the posteroanterior or lateral projections and also found that low spinal trabecular BMD confers higher relative risk for vertebral fracture (odds ratio 3.67) than did lateral or posteroanterior DXA (odds ratio 2.00 and 1.54 respectively). Other studies have demonstrated similar results showing larger decrements between vertebrally fractured and nonfractured groups for QCT than for posteroanterior or lateral DXA. Jergas et al. demonstrated that volumetric BMD estimates based on paired anteroposterior and lateral DXA scans had greater discriminatory capability (odds ratio 2.87) than anteroposterior (1.47) or lateral DXA (1.88) alone, but spinal trabecular BMD showed the best discriminatory power (3.17) [41]. In addition to its biomechanical importance, spinal trabecular bone has high metabolic activity, and this is manifested in relative of bone loss rates between DXA and QCT. In a cross-sectional study of 108 postmenopausal women Guglielmi et al. measured overall bone loss rates of 1.96% per year with QCT compared with 0.97% and 0.45%, respectively, with lateral and posteroanterior DXA [6].

Measurement of BMD Using Volumetric CT Images of the Spine and Hip

Spinal QCT is based on two-dimensional analysis of the trabecular bone compartment in 5- or 10-mm-thick axial slices through the lumbar midvertebral bodies. Although the single-slice approach is useful for spinal BMD quantification, three-dimensional approaches are optimal for analysis of highly complex structures, such as the proximal femur. These volumetric techniques encompass the entire object of interest either with stacked-slice or spiral CT scans and can employ anatomic landmarks to automatically define coordinate systems for reformatting of the CT data into anatomically relevant projections.

Current quantitative analysis of the proximal femur is based on DXA technology, which provides an integral bone mass measurement which is normalized by the projected area, resulting in a size-dependent areal BMD [40, 41]. Extension of QCT to the proximal femur is desireable for both diagnostic and serial studies in that this technique can sample the highly responsive trabecular bone compartment and provide a true volumetric density measurement.

Development of hip QCT techniques have been hindered by the the acquisition time required to encompass the hip with a large number of slices and by the need for specialized workstations capable of handling the large volume of image data. However, with the advent of helical CT systems equipped with inexpensive and powerful workstations, these obstacles have been greatly reduced, and femoral volumetric QCT should be clinically feasible, given the existence of appropriate image processing techniques to reproducibly delineate volumes of interest in the proximal femur. Several researchers have examined automated algorithms to accomplish this. Heitz et al. [42] have developed a femoral neck fixed coordinate system operated in conjunction with a second-derivative based edge detection technique to determine volumes of interest (VOIs), while Sartoris et al. [43] and Bhasin et al. [44] have employed threshold-driven edge detection methods to isolate the entire compartment of trabecular bone in the proximal femur. Recently

Lang et al. [45] have presented an approach to semiautomatically define integral and trabecular VOIs in the femoral neck and intertrochanteric subregions (Fig. 16-3) and to measure geometric quantities such as the femoral neck cross-sectional area and cross-sectional moment of inertia. For trabecular BMD measurements the in vivo precision of this method was found to range from 0.6% to 1.1% depending on the VOI assessed.

While there have been relatively few efforts to develop proximal femur QCT for clinical use, a larger number of investigators have focused on establishing the relationship between QCT measurements and biomechanical strength assessed in vitro. Several investigators have examined the relationship between QCT density measures and femoral strength assessed in a loading configuration simulating a single-legged stance and producing mostly fractures of the femoral neck [46–48]. In general, significant but relatively modest relationships (R^2=0.4–0.7) between BMD and femoral strength have been found [46–48]. Reasoning that most fractures are due to falls, Lotz and Hayes [49] developed a loading configuration which simulated a fall to the side, with impact on the posterolateral aspect of the greater trochanter. In this mode, which produced mostly intertrochanteric fractures, they measured a very high correlation of trabecular trochanteric BMD

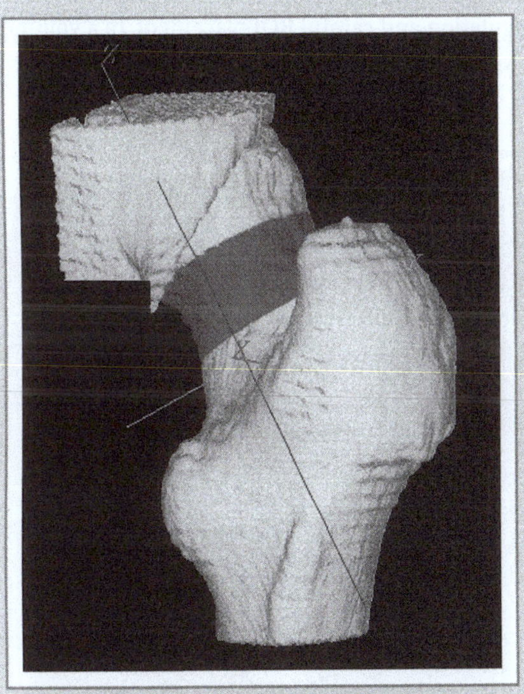

Fig. 16-3 Isosurface reconstruction of proximal femur imaged in vivo with QCT. Integral femoral neck VOI is overlaid on CT data. Axes of femoral neck based coordinate system are overlaid on image

(R^2=0.87) with femoral strength. Lang et al. applied their analysis technique to scans of proximal femurs which were later fractured in both single-legged stance and fall-to-the-side modes [45]. These results confirmed those of Lotz and Hayes for trabecular BMD in the fall mode and found moderate correlations between BMD and single-legged stance fracture load, as did previous observers. However, when the stance-mode strength data were corrected for femoral neck cross-sectional area and axis length, the BMD measurements (integral or trabecular) explained approx. 90% of the residual variance in the data.

Thus, based on good precision and strong correspondence of the BMD and geometry measurements to biomechanical strength measures, hip QCT shows the potential for both diagnostic and serial assessments. The advent of helical CT systems and powerful but inexpensive computer workstations, in conjunction with the increased availability of CT scan time, should make this approach increasingly clinically attractive.

In the spine the use of volumetric QCT measurements should affect precision more than discriminatory capability. Their potential to improve the precision of spinal measurements is related to the use of three-dimensional anatomic landmarks to guide the placement of volumes of interest and to the use of image alignment techniques to ensure that the VOIs are accurately repositioned in serial scans. Currently, single-slice QCT techniques are highly operator dependent, requiring careful slice positioning and angulation and careful ROI placement. In a volumetric approach, on the other hand, an image of the entire vertebral body is acquired,

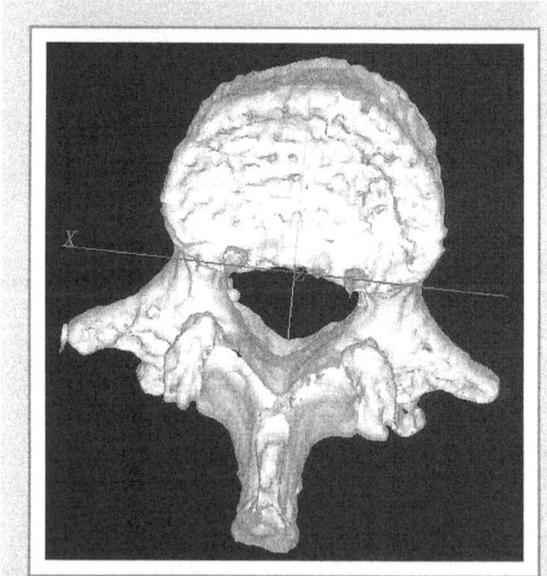

Fig. 16-4 Isosurface reconstruction of L2 vertebral body from volumetric QCT data. Axes of vertebral coordinate system are overlaid on image

and the VOIs may be determined and repositioned in software. With a volumetric acquisition it is possible to employ landmarks such as the vertebral endplates to determine the three-dimensional orientation of the vertebral body (Fig. 16-4), thus removing the need for careful slice positioning by the operator and improving the accuracy of the measurement in cases of pronounced lordotic or scoliotic curvature. It is also possible to define new trabecular and integral VOIs which contain most of the bone in the vertebral centrum. Although measuring a larger volume of tissue may enhance precision, these new regions are highly correlated with the midvertebral subregions assessed with standard QCT techniques [50] and may not contain significant new information about vertebral strength. Consequently, volumetric studies of regional BMD, which examine specific subregions of the centrum [51] that may vary in their contribution to vertebral strength, and studies of the cortical shell [52], the condition of which may be important for vertebral strength in osteoporotic individuals, are of interest for future investigation.

High-Resolution Imaging of Trabecular Microarchitecture Using CT

The goal of high-resolution CT techniques is to assess the arrangement of the trabeculae rather than the bone mass or density. Although the mean BMD assessed in a volume of interest is an important determinant of bone strength, there is evidence that the architecture of the trabeculae and the thickness of the cortical shell are determinants as well. Research approaches to assess the trabecular network involve both adaptation of existing clinical CT systems (spatial resolution approx. 500–700 μm) to this task as well as development of ultrahigh-resolution μCT systems (20–200 μm) for scanning of bone specimens or of the peripheral skeleton, particularly at the distal radius and phalanges. This section focuses on the adaptation of existing body CT scanners for high-resolution measurements.

Several investigators have hypothesized that the status of the vertebral microarchitecture should be reflected in measurements of regional BMD. Sandor et al. [53, 54] presented a technique in which the trabecular bone in the midvertebral centrum was subdivided into small regions arranged in a radial pattern similar to a spider's web. BMD showed a characteristic regional distribution with maxima situated at the lateral and anterior portions of the vertebral body. These maxima showed the highest age-related BMD loss. Cody and Flynn developed a technique which assessed regional BMD [51, 55] in volumetric images of the vertebral body by distributing 18 cylindrical regions of interest through the vertebral centrum. These subvolumes had high intercorrelations, and there was no specific region which was more sensitive than the others in vertebral fracture prediction. However, in a later analysis Flynn found that pattern classification methods [56] identified vertebral architectural density patterns that potentially provide enhanced fracture discrimination.

Reasoning that a wide variation in the gray-scale values inside the QCT ROI was indicative of a robust trabecular architecture, Braillon et al. [57] suggested using the standard deviation of the BMD values as a parameter reflective of the trabecular structure in the lumbar vertebral bodies. Engelke et al. [58] applied this approach to 218 women, including both normal and vertebrally fractured subjects. However, the results did not support the contention that the standard deviation could be used to improve vertebral fracture assessment over BMD alone. However, if higher radiation doses and higher magnifications are employed to improve depiction of the trabecular structure, then this technique may show more promise.

High-resolution thin-slice tomography performed with standard body CT scanners may be employed to better resolve the trabecular network. Such images typically have pixel sizes of 0.18–0.3 mm and slice thicknesses of 1–1.5 mm (Fig. 16-5). The depiction of the trabeculae is limited by the spatial resolution of these systems, typically around 600 μm and the low radiation doses involved. While this imaging approach does not accurately represent the trabecular structure (trabecular thickness approx. 100–150 μm and spacing approx. 500–700 μm), it may be possible to extract some measures of trabecular texture. However, the results may vary substantially according to which image processing technique is used. Some investigational work using thin-slice tomography has been published recently by Chevalier et al. [59]. They measured a feature termed the trabecular fragmentation index (length of the trabecular network divided by the number of discontinuities) to separate osteoporotic subjects from normal subjects. However, this index did not readily separate postmenopausal osteoporotic women with vertebral fractures from normal or osteopenic subjects. A similar trabecu-

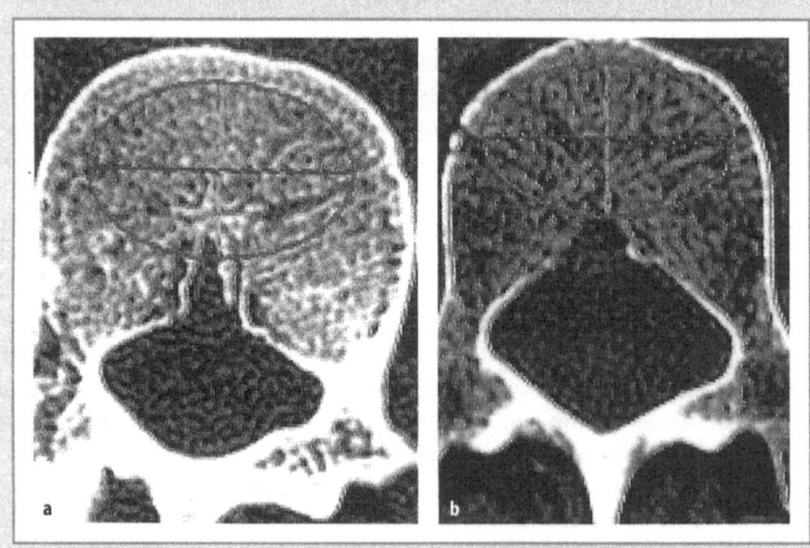

Fig. 16-5 High-resolution spinal CT acquisitions through the middle of L1 (identically thresholded and windowed). **a** A 35-year old man. **b** A 60-year old woman; note the dimunition of the trabecular network

lar texture analysis approach was also reported by Ito et al. [60]. Wang et al. [61] applied a textural analysis (BV/TV, I.Th, N.Br) to a group of osteopenic women ($T_{\text{DXA spine or hip}} \leq 2.5$), containing a subset of vertebrally fractured subjects. They found that these textural measures were moderately correlated to trabecular BMD ($R^2 = 0.55$–0.75) and also discriminated fractured and nonfractured subjects ($p < 0.03$), as did BMD. However, when the textural measures were adjusted for BMD, the difference was no longer statistically significant.

In summary, while the measures of trabecular structure described above may discriminate between fractured and nonfractured subjects, there is currently no evidence that these measures improve assessment of vertebral strength compared to BMD alone. This situation may change depending on technical improvements. In addition to diagnostic measurements, it is also of interest to explore the performance of these measures for longitudinal studies. It is possible that the representation of trabecular structure afforded by standard CT systems will prove useful for clarifying the action of drug therapies.

Conclusion

QCT is a widely available method for diagnostic and serial assessment of vertebral fracture risk and metabolic bone disease. There are over 40 000 CT scanners worldwide and these may be adapted to densitometric measurements with a relatively modest investment in a calibration standard and software incorporating a normative database and simple image analysis tools. QCT measurements of spinal trabecular BMD are strongly associated with vertebral fracture and demonstrate significant changes with age, disease, and the progress of therapy. The ability to selectively assess vertebral trabecular bone provides superior discriminatory capability for vertebral fracture than either anteroposterior or lateral DXA and QCT measurements demonstrate a larger rate of bone loss.

While QCT has important advantages with respect to DXA, it also has some limitations, such as the high degree of operator dependence, limited access to CT scanners, and absence of a technique to assess the proximal femur, which have constrained its clinical acceptance. It is hoped that new developments in volumetric QCT will address some of these limitations by providing rapid and highly precise volumetric measurements at the spine and proximal femur. It is also possible that use of high-resolution vertebral CT images will provide new information about trabecular architecture which improves both vertebral fracture risk assessment and serial assessment of therapy compared to BMD alone.

References

1. Genant HK, Cann CE, Ettinger B, Gordan GS (1982) Quantitative computed tomography of vertebral spongiosa: a sensitive method for detecting early bone loss after oophorectomy. Ann Intern Med 97:699–705

2. Guglielmi G, Glüer CC, Majumdar S, Blunt BA, Genant HK (1995) Current methods and advances in bone densitometry. Eur Radiol 5:129–139

3. Rüegsegger P, Elsasser U, Anliker M, Gnehm H, Kind H, Prader A (1976) Quantification of bone mineralization using computed tomography. Radiology 121:93–97

4. Cann CE, Genant HK (1980) Precise measurement of vertebral mineral content using computed tomography. J Comput Assist Tomogr 4:493–500

5. Pacifici R, Rupich R, Griffin M, Chines A, Susman N, Avioli LV (1990) Dual energy radiography versus quantitative computed tomography for the diagnosis of osteoporosis. J Clin Endocrinol Metab 70:705–710

6. Guglielmi G, Grimston SK, Fisher KC, Pacifici R (1994) Osteoporosis: diagnosis with lateral and posteroanterior dual X-ray absorptiometry compared with quantitative CT. Radiology 192:845–850

7. Block JE, Smith R, Glüer CC, Steiger P, Ettinger B, Genant HK (1989) Models of spinal trabecular bone loss as determined by quantitative computed tomograhy. J Bone Miner Res 4:249–257

8. Kalender WA, Klotz E, Süss C (1987) Vertebral bone mineral analysis: an integrated approach. Radiology 164:419–423

9. Genant HK, Steiger P, Block JE, Glüer CC (1987) Quantitative computed tomography: update 1987. Calcif Tissue Int 41:179–186

10. Genant HK, Block JE, Steiger P, Glüer CC (1987) Quantitative computed tomography in the assessment of osteoporosis. In: Genant HK (ed) Osteoporosis update 1987. University of California Press, Berkeley, pp 49–71

11. Firooznia H, Golimbu C, Rafii M, Schwartz MS, Alterman ER (1984) Quantitative computed tomography assessment of spinal trabecular bone: II. In osteoporotic women with and without vertebral fractures. J Comput Tomogr 8:99–103

12. Genant HK, Glüer CC, Steiger P, Faulkner KG (1992) Quantitative computed tomography for the assessment of osteoporosis. In: Moss AA, Gamsu G, Genant HK (eds) Computed tomography of the body. Saunders, Philadelphia, pp 523–549

13. Kalender WA, Brestowsky H, Felsenberg D (1988) Bone mineral measurements: automated determination of the midvertebral CT section. Radiology 168:219–221

14. Steiger P, Block JE, Steiger S, Heuck A, Friedlander A, Ettinger B, Harris ST, Glüer CC, Genant HK (1990) Spinal bone mineral density by quantitative computed tomography: effect of region of interest, vertebral level, and technique. Radiology 175:537–543

15. Guglielmi G, Giannatempo GM, Blunt BA, Grampp S, Glüer CC, Cammisa M, Genant HK (1995) Spinal bone mineral density by quantitative computed tomography in a normal Italian population. Eur Radiol 5:269–275

16. Cann CE (1987) QCT applications: comparison of current scanners. Radiology 162:257–261

17. Boden SD, Goodenough DJ, Stockham CD, Jacobs E, Dina T, Allman RM (1989)

Precise measurement of vertebral bone density using computed tomography without the use of an external reference phantom. J Digit Imag 2:31–38

18. Gudmundsdottir H, Jonsdottir B, Kristinsson S, Johanesson A, Goodenough DJ, Sigurdsson G (1993) Vertebral bone density in Icelandic women using quantitative computed tomography without an external reference phantom. Osteoporos Int 3:84–89

19. Suzuki S, Yamamuro T, Okumura H, Yamamoto I (1991) Quantitative computed tomography: comparative study using different scanners with two calibration phantoms. Br J Radiol 64:1001–1006

20. Goodsitt MM (1992) Conversion relations for quantitative CT bone mineral density measured with solid and liquid calibration standards. Bone Miner 19:145–148

21. Faulkner KG, Glüer CC, Grampp S, Genant HK (1993) Cross calibration of liquid and solid QCT calibration standards: corrections to UCSF normative data. Osteoporos Int 3:36–43

22. Glüer CC, Engelke K, Jergas M, Hagiwara S, Grampp S, Genant HK (1993) Changes in calibration standards for quantitative computed tomography: recommendations for clinical practice. Osteoporos Int 3:286–287

23. Genant HK, Boyd DP (1977) Quantitative bone mineral analysis using dual energy computed tomography. Invest Radiol 12:545–551

24. Cann CE, Genant HK (1983) Single versus dual-energy CT for vertebral mineral quantification. J Comput Assist Tomogr 7:551–552

25. Laval-Jeantet AM, Roger B, Bouysse S, Bergot C, Mazess RB (1986) Influence of vertebral fat content on quantitative CT density. Radiology 159:463–466

26. Glüer CC, Genant HK (1989) Impact of marrow fat on accuracy of quantitative CT. J Comput Assist Tomogr 13:1023–1035

27. Reinbold WD, Genant HK, Reiser UJ, Harris ST, Ettinger B (1986) Bone mineral content in early-postmenopausal osteoporotic women and postmenopausal women: comparison of measurements methods. Radiology 160:469–478

28. Glüer CC, Reiser UJ, Davis CA, Rutt BK, Genant HK (1988) Vertebral mineral determination by quantitative computed tomography (QCT): accuracy of single and dual energy measurements. J Comput Assist Tomogr 12:242–258

29. Pacifici R, Susman N, Carr PL, Birge SJ, Avioli LV (1987) Single and dual energy tomography analysis of spinal trabecular bone: a comparative study in normal and osteoporotic women. J Clin Endocrinol Metab 64:209–214

30. Reinbold WD, Adler CP, Kalender WA, Lente R (1991) Accuracy of vertebral mineral determination by dual-energy quantitative computed tomography. Skel Radiol 20:25–29

31. Cann CE, Genant HK, Kolb FO, Ettinger B (1985) Quantitative computed tomography for prediction of vertebral fracture risk. Bone 6:1–7

32. Heuck A, Block J, Glüer CC, Steiger P, Genant HK (1989) Mild versus definitive osteoporosis: comparison of bone densitometry techniques using different statistical models. J Bone Miner Res 4:891–899

33. Sambrook P, Barlett C, Evans R, Hesp R, Katz D, Reeve J (1985) Measurements

of lumbar spine bone mineral: a comparison of dual photon absorptiometry and computed tomography. Br J Radiol 58:621–624

34. Ross PD, Genant HK, Davis JW, Wasnich RD (1993) Predicting vertebral fracture incidence from prevalent fractures and bone density among non-black, osteoporotic women. Osteoporos Int 3:120–126

35. Larnach TA, Boyd SJ, Smart RC, Butler SP, Rohl PG, Diamond TH (1992) Reproducibility of lateral spine scans using dual energy X-ray absorptiometry. Calcif Tissue Int 51:255–258

36. Rupich R, Pacifici R, Griffin MG, Vered I, Susman N, Avioli LV (1990) Lateral dual energy radiography: a new method for measuring vertebral bone density: a preliminary study. J Clin Endocrinol Metab 70:1768–1770

37. Slosman DO, Rizzoli R, Donath A, Bonjour JP (1990) Vertebral bone mineral density measured laterally by dual-energy X-ray absorptiometry. Osteoporos Int 1:23–29

38. Reid IR, Evans MC, Stapleton J (1992) Lateral spine densitometry is a more sensitive indicator of glucocorticoid-induced bone loss. J Bone Miner Res 7:1221–1225

39. Yu W, Glüer CC, Grampp S, Jergas M, Fuerst T, Wu CY, Lu Y, Fan B, Genant HK (1995) Spinal bone mineral assessment in postmenopausal women: a comparison between dual X-ray absorptiometry and quantitative computed tomography. Osteoporos Int 5:433–439

40. Cummings S, Marcus R, Palermo L, Ensrud K, Genant HK (1994) Does estimating volumetric bone density of the femoral neck improve the prediction of hip fracture? J Bone Miner Res 9:1429–1432

41. Jergas M, Breitenseher M, Glüer CC, Yu W, Genant HK (1995) Estimates of volumetric bone density from projectional measurements improve the discriminatory capability of dual X-ray absorptiometry. J Bone Miner Res 10:1101–1110

42. Heitz M, Kalender W (1994) Evaluation of femoral density and strength using volumetric CT and anatomical coordinate systems. Bone 25:S11

43. Sartoris DJ, Andre M, Resnick C, Resnick D (1986) Trabecular bone density in the proximal femur: quantitative CT assessment. Radiology 160:707–712

44. Bhasin S, Sartoris DJ, Fellingham L, Zlatkin MB, Andre M, Resnick D (1988) Three-dimensional quantitative CT of the proximal femur: relationship to vertebral trabecular bone density in postmenopausal women. Radiology 167:145–149

45. Lang T, Heitz M, Keyak J, Genant HK (1996) A 3D anatomic coordinate system for hip QCT. Osteoporos Int 6:S203

46. Esses SI, Lotz JC, Hayes WC (1989) Biomechanical properties of the proximal femur determined in vitro by single-energy quantitative computed tomography. J Bone Miner Res 4:715–722

47. Alho A, Høiseth A, Torstein H (1989) Bone-mass distribution in the femur. Acta Orthop Scand 60:101–104

48. Smith M, Cody DD, Goldstein S, Cooperman A, Matthews L, Flynn M (1992) Proximal femoral density and its correlation to fracture load and hip-screw penetration load. Clin Orthop 283:244–251

49. Lotz JC, Hayes WC (1990) Estimates of hip fracture risk from falls using quantitative computed tomography. J Bone Joint Surg Am 72:689–700
50. Lang T, Augat P, Heitz M, Genant HK (1996) Volumetric QCT of the spine: comparison to single-slice QCT and DXA. J Bone Miner Res 11:479
51. Cody DD (1991) Correlations between vertebral regional bone mineral density (rBMD) and whole bone fracture load. Spine 16:146–154
52. Hangartner TN, Gilsanz V (1993) Measurement of cortical bone by computed tomography. Calcif Tissue Int 52:160
53. Sandor T, Felsenberg D, Kalender W, Brown E (1991) Global and regional variations in the spinal trabecular bone: single and dual energy examinations. J Clin Endocrinol Metab 72:1157–1168
54. Sandor T, Felsenberg D, Kalender W, Clain A, Brown E (1992) Compact and trabecular components of the spine using quantitative computed tomography. Calcif Tissue Int 50:502–506
55. Cody DD, Flynn MJ, Vickers DS (1989) A technique for measuring regional bone mineral density in human lumbar vertebral bodies. Med Phys 16:766–772
56. Flynn MJ, Cody DD (1993) The assessment of vertebral bone macroarchitecture with X-ray computed tomography. Calcif Tissue Int 53:S170-175
57. Braillon PM, Bochu M, Meunier PJ (1993) Quantitative computed tomography (QCT): a new analysis of bone quality in osteoporosis and osteomalacia. Calcif Tissue Int 52:166
58. Engelke K, Grampp S, Glüer CC, Jergas M, Yang SO, Genant HK (1995) Significance of QCT bone mineral density and its standard deviation as parameters to evaluate osteoporosis. J Comput Assist Tomogr 19:111–116
59. Chevalier F, Laval-Jeantet AM, Laval-Jeantet M, Bergot C (1992) CT image analysis of the vertebral trabecular network in vivo. Calcif Tissue Int 51:8–13
60. Ito M, Ohki M, Hayashi K, Yamada M, Uetani M, Nakamura T (1995) Trabecular texture analysis of CT images in the relationship with spinal fracture. Radiology 194:55–59
61. Wang X, Lang T, Heitz M, Ouyang X, Engelke K, Genant HK (1996) Comparison of spinal trabecular structure analysis and QCT spinal BMD: an in vivo, low-dose pilot study. J Bone Miner Res 11:S474

17 Peripheral Quantitative Computed Tomography

P. Schneider and C. Reiners

Development of the pQCT Technology

Access to measurement of bone density by absorptiometry has been limited to planar information due to its ability to deliver only projections of the bones that are investigated. Some researchers realized this lack of capability of the available techniques and tried to develop systems offering three-dimensional information. The aim was to provide a view inside the bone into the spongiosa compartment, which is known to have a high turnover. It was expected to see changes in bone mass occurring earlier in this compartment than in compact bone or in a projected mixture of trabecular and compact bone.

The first attempt at developing a method capable of three-dimensional evaluation of bones was done at the University of Würzburg in 1969 [1]. It was a simple profile scanner, taking perpendicular profiles of the midphalanx and assuming an elliptical shape based on the main ellipsoid axes. The scanner used an ^{125}I photon source. A further and more sophisticated attempt was published in the Proceedings of the International Conference on Bone Mineral Measurement 1973 in Chicago [2], when Rüegsegger and coworkers described an iterative method which came very close to computed tomography as proposed by Hounsfield [3]. A few years later the group had developed a ^{125}I based system offering true computed tomographic images at a higher resolution than the conventional systems available [4]. This has led to much interest and to several derivatives for research purposes [5–9]. In the early 1980s a simple device was developed in Würzburg following the profile finger-scanner method. The system was able to perform translate-rotate scans at very variable parameter settings. An approach similar to Rüegsegger's first method produced a least-squares algorithm for the contour detection of long bones [10].

We have favored the use of small computer units in order to make such systems affordable for a large community of scientists and physicians. Due to the constantly increasing power of personal computers we were soon able to handle the large amount of operations required for the calculation of backprojected computer tomographic images. With a system similar to Rüegsegger's ^{125}I based scanner we achieved first clinical results in comparison to the conventional techniques of single-photon (SPA) and dual-photon absorptiometry (DPA) [11]. Sensitivity and specificity of the prototype system for peripheral quantitative computed tomography (pQCT) was acceptable but not superior to those of the other techniques. The reason for this was probably the biased selection of osteoporosis cases by using a threshold decision with DPA as the gold standard. Other clinical groups later presented promising results concerning sensitivity and specificity of the method [12]. Clinical results were also published in the pediatric field [13].

The prototype system developed at Würzburg still had some disadvantages, such as the lack of ability to perform a scout scan. Although reproducibility in the hand of a trained technician was acceptable, it had to be improved considerably to be of commercial interest. A German company (Stratec Electronic) was contracted to design a completely new ^{125}I based system for quantitative computed tomography of the radius in cooperation with the University of Würzburg. This first commercially successful SCT900 scanner used five CdTl semiconductor crystals as radiation detectors [14]. Approximately 40 of these scanners were built and distributed in Europe. A γ-ray based pQCT scanner system termed Oscar, pioneered by a group in the United Kingdom, was reported to be ready for commercialization, but it didn't appear on the market for some unknown reasons [15].

In the meantime Rüegsegger and coworkers had made substantial improvements in their pQCT technology [16] and had attempted to commercialize it for performing a multislice technique at both the forearm and the lower limbs with remarkably high resolution. Their system incorporated two advantages: an X-ray source with much higher photon flux at a higher energy than ^{125}I and a more powerful computer technology. The multislice technique could thus be performed at reasonable speed and high resolution [17], allowing the analysis of structural features of the bones. The drawback, however, was the price three times as expensive as the Stratec system, which limited its distribution. Some 20 units of this Densiscan system were produced by the Swiss company ScancoMedical.

The increasing demand for affordable pQCT scanners and the requirements concerning scanning speed and resolution led to further design changes in the Stratec pQCT scanner. An X-ray tube with appropriate filtering techniques was developed and accompanied by a better collimating system, resulting in higher image resolution and shorter scanning time. To date the XCT900 unit and its derivatives XCT960 and XCT960A have been delivered to over 800 sites worldwide for clinical and research purposes by Norland/Stratec.

Technical Aspects of pQCT

The two commercially distributed pQCT scanner types are second-generation systems using the translate-rotate technique with a multidetector head for different acquisition angles. Only one (noncommercial) pQCT scanner prototype is known to use the fan-beam rotation technique [5]. pQCT scanners are generally limited to the translate-rotate scanning technique due to the preferred type of X-ray tubes. The tubes are operated in constant current mode without extensive cooling other than by an oil reservoir. The limited gantry space therefore also limits the size of the tubes. The entire instrument must also meet stringent criteria concerning the cost of the components.

^{125}I based systems became practically unimportant because of their limitation to objects of small diameters. Energy selection of the X-ray spectrum must be adapted to the special requirements of quantitative bone scanning. Ideally in single energy mode it is below 60 keV [18] for best discrimination between fat/water and bone mineral. It must be somewhat above 30 keV because of the high absorption in thick tissue layers. Different filtering techniques are applied to achieve a small half-band width of the spectrum (Fig. 17-1), such as a combination of Al, Cu, and Ce. Dual-energy techniques in pQCT have not been introduced into routine.

Finite band width of the spectra requires a correction for energy dispersion. This phenomenon, known as "beam hardening effect," may be corrected by pre- or by postprocessing. The Stratec system uses a preprocessing correction, based on aluminum step phantoms [14]. The residual error is fairly small. A comparative test suggested that the early version of the ^{125}I based SCT900 scanner had an incorrect correction algorithm [19]. However, the observed error was due to an inadequate collimation system. Fortunately, only a few of these collimators have been installed in earlier SCT900 units.

For image reconstruction a backprojection algorithm published by Shepp and Logan [20] is commonly used. This allows a linear programming code which can be used on personal computers (PCs). Higher level computers, such as array processors, require a different type of reconstruction code [21]. The filtered back projection code was especially adapted for runtime-efficient use on PCs [11] and installed in Stratec devices. On the IBM AT the code for the calculation of one slice of 72 angle steps in a 128^2 matrix took 12 min, whereas on Pentium processors it now takes less than 1 s. Image resolution depends on the collimating system and

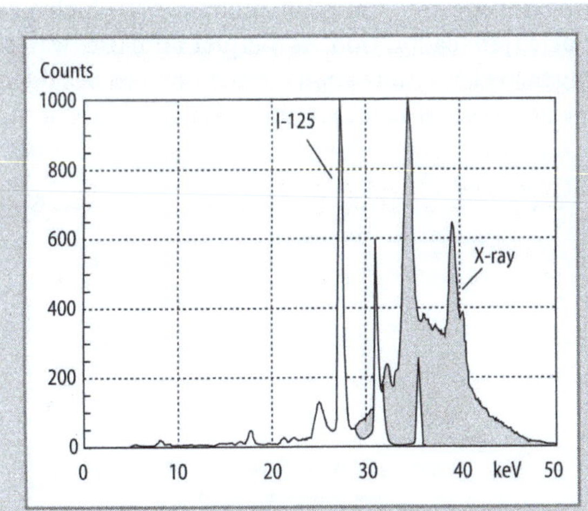

Fig. 17-1 Spectra of I-125 photon source and the X-ray source of the XCT900, filtered with Al, Cu, and Ce. The mean energy optimally discriminates bone mineral and fat/water equivalent tissue

the scanning mode. For the regular Stratec systems the pixel resolution is 1/128 of the variable scanning diameter. At a scanning diameter of 72–80 mm this results in a pixel resolution of 0.59–0.63 mm. Scanners especially designed for small animals use the same pixel matrix, but both the scanning diameter and the collimators are much smaller, resulting in a pixel resolution of 0.05–0.1 mm. The true image resolution of the human system is 0.8 mm as determined by a modulation transfer function. The more sophisticated Densiscan offers an image resolution of 0.2 mm in a high-resolution mode [21], whereas the fan-beam prototype has a spatial resolution of 0.6 mm [5]. The new series of Norland/Stratec XCT2000 and XCT3000 scanners offers a variable image resolution ranging from 0.02 to 0.5 mm using variable matrix sizes of up to 400×400.

The pQCT systems are calibrated arbitrarily. Several aspects may be considered. Bone consists of a certain amount of water- and fat-equivalent tissue and mineral components. One may choose an appropriate ratio of fat/water to simulate the relationships in bone marrow. This usually leads to the use of some type of resin as calibration material. Various concentrations of hydroxyapatite are added (Fig. 17-2) to simulate bone. The resin may also be selected to simulate the density of water. In this case trabecular bone may present with negative mineral content if bone marrow contains material (mostly fat) that is less dense than water and of very low mineral content. The calibration may also be based on dry bone [21]. However, this results in high values for bone mineral content in vivo, which do not reflect the true volumetric mineral content as measured by Archimedes' principle. In addition, omitting a soft tissue component in the calibration leads to high values for the mineral content, with the appreciable side effect of better precision figures [22]. These conditons are realized in the Densiscan device.

The Stratec machine uses the European forearm phantom (EFP) which was developed for a multicenter trial [23] for calibration. As this phantom uses water-equivalent soft tissue simulating material, a calibration correction must be added for the amount of fat found in vivo. A recent accuracy and precision study of the

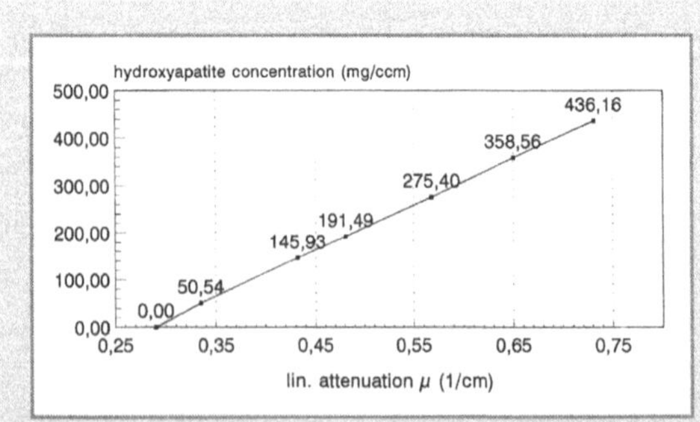

Fig. 17-2 Linearity of the XCT900 pQCT system, calibrated with hydroxyapatite/resin phantoms

Stratec scanner reported an accuracy error of 14% in comparing ashed bone versus the calibrated in vivo result [24]. Several factors may explain the finding in this experimental setting, but not all of these were discussed or presented in this study. The bone specimen may have been preserved with liquid different from the material used for calibration. Ashing of bone also may have changed its crystalline status by releasing crystal lattice water from bone minerals and collagen structure. This also does not comply with the situation in vivo or with the assumptions made for the calibration.

Hangartner has claimed that accuracy does not play an important role in pQCT technology [8]. However, for comparability between systems they should all be calibrated in the same way; otherwise the exact correction factor must be known. Different from planar absorptiometry systems, pQCT exhibits very high linearity within the range covered by the EFP and highly linear correction equations between the two pQCT systems of different manufacturers in the test [22]. It should be noted that the difference between the XCT900 device distributed in Europe and the XCT960 system for international distribution is a 40 mg/cm^3 calibration difference. The XCT960 is the only pQCT scanner approved by the United States Food and Drug Administration. An increasingly important factor is the radiation exposure. pQCT has the lowest effective dose equivalent of all densitometric techniques (except SPA), exposing the forearm to <0.1 µSv compared to 25 µSv of the abdomen scanned with axial QCT [18].

Precision

The precision of pQCT scanners depends on its intended use. When time-consuming multislice examinations are being performed, a series of consecutive, spaced CT slices allows precise recovery of the bone volume scanned at a previous session, provided that no modeling drift has changed the bone volume. This technique is based on comparison of the cross-sectional area, which is assumed to remain the same at the same cross-section in relation to the bone axis. An interpolation algorithm allows fine adjusting of the density result and changes in it. This technique is used in the Densiscan machine and in some research prototypes [5, 8, 21]. The Stratec machines provide software to perform multislice analysis with interpolative calculation of the results, based on the same method. This technique is used mainly in animal studies and in research studies in humans. Mostly single slice evaluation is used in regular clinical applications due to the shorter scanning time.

Despite justified criticism about inadequate use of the single-slice mode which may result in reduced precision, comprehensive means have been provided to control the precise location of a single CT slice in repeat measurements. This process has recently been fully automated and is operator independent. The precision that can be achieved manually by trained operators is sufficient to allow follow-up measurements in normal clinical use and is comparable with all other densitometry techniques (Table 17-1). In rapidly progressing diseases modeling

Table 17-1 reported in vivo and in vitro precision of pQCT devices for trabecular bone density in human bones (measured in mg/cm^3)

Reference	Precision (CV%)	Device	Method
Schneider et al. [11]	1.7	SCT900	In vivo
Reiners et al. [64]	0.8–1.5	SCT900	In vivo
Zander [65]	1.56	SCT900	In vivo
Hosie et al. [12]	1.26	SCT900	In vivo
Grampp et al. [68]	0.9–2.1	XCT960	In vivo
McClean et al. [5]	0.57	Prototype	In vivo
Hosie [19]	0.5	Oscar	In vivo
Stebler, Rüegsegger [21]	0.22	Densiscan	In vivo
Takada et al. [24]	1.85	XCT960	In vitro
Wapniarz et al. [66]	0.9	XCT900	In vitro
Zander [65]	0.22	XCT900	In vitro
Lehmann et al. [67]	0.18	XCT900	In vitro
Guglielmi et al. [69]	0.23	XCT900/XCT960	In vitro
McClean et al. [5]	0.12	Prototype	In vitro

drift is likely to change the investigated bone volume considerably over time. Then more or less sophisticated approaches may fail to relocate the measurement site. Whereas the Densiscan machine provided the best published in vivo precision figures in the hand of few experts, it has not been confirmed whether these can be achieved under the conditions of widespread use, comparable to that of the Stratec scanner systems. A new development that is currently under clinical evaluation, the Norland/Stratec XCT3000 system, offers several improvements over its predecessors XCT900 and XCT960, eliminating substantial differences to the Densiscan.

Clinical Evaluation of the pQCT Technology

In 1974 first clinical results have been reported by Rüegseggers group in a small number of patients [4]. The instrumentation allowed monitoring of very small changes in density of the appendicular trabecular bone. Subsequent work confirmed the value of the method to monitor very small changes of bone mineral mass in short periods of time either pharmacologcally induced [25–27] or due to disease [28–31]. Some investigations have documented the value of pQCT in comparison to other densitometric methods [11, 12, 32]. It should also be noted that the hypothesis of a bimodal frequency of bone loss measured in a relatively small number of women with the Densiscan in early menopause has not been confirmed [29]. One would expect here a normal distribution based on a larger number of cases.

To study the epidemiology of osteoporosis, densitometric methods should be simple and standardized. The results obtained with pQCT devices from different manufacturers should be comparable. This had been well noticed by the end of the 1980s, when other densitometry techniques appeared to be barely comparable between different manufacturers. Even at the same bone, the distal radius, the measurement sites of pQCT were not exactly comparable because of the wide variation of the radius along the axis and the slightly different sites which the investigators had chosen to measure the CT slices [7,14,28,33]. Therefore in the context of a large European multicenter trial (COMAC-BME) the standardization committee first had to agree on a standardized measurement site before the study could be attempted [34]. The COMAC-BME study included seven Stratec XCT900 scanners, one Stratec SCT900 scanner, and two Densiscan units.

Achieving intercomparability among the various scanners required in addition that a phantom was designed [23]. The EFP spanned most of the bone density values occurring in the radii of human subjects, including those suffering from osteoporosis. The outcome of the study showed several important aspects for peripheral densitometers. The older SPA technology performed less well than pQCT with regard to linearity and stability [22]. By means of the EFP, multicenter data could be jointly calibrated to achieve a larger normal data base for healthy individuals, resulting in the first multicenter data base for pQCT [35]. Along with German multicenter data of normals [36], reliable data bases became available for clinical use and for comparing regional differences in bone mineral content. The COMAC-BME study analysed sensitivity and specificity using the normal data and selected groups of osteoporotic patients. The nonsignificant differences among ROC curves showed that pQCT performed equally well in discriminating fracture cases (hip and spine) as did all other densitometric techniques. pQCT was therefore suggested as the method of choice when evaluating generalized bone loss [37]. The ROC curves for pQCT were very similar (Fig. 17-3) to those published earlier [32, 38] and to the recent results of Fuji et al. [39]. pQCT has also had an impact in the pediatric field and opened up new clinical perspectives in

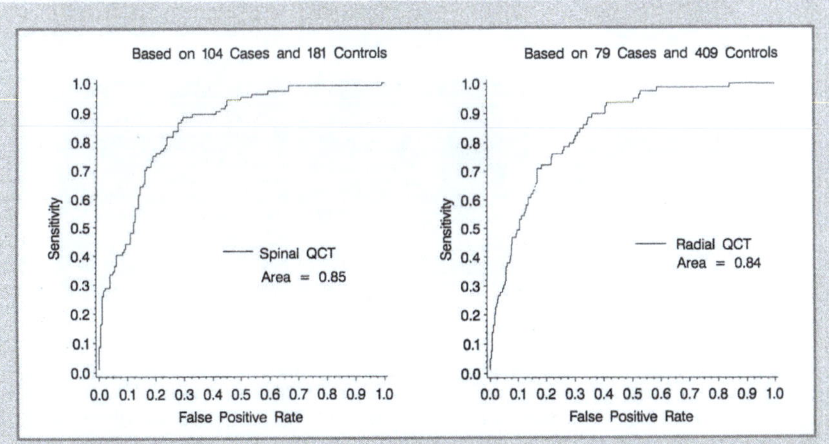

Fig. 17-3 ROC-curves of the axial QCT and the peripheral QCT of patients with spinal osteoporosis as the result of the COMAC-BME study

assessing bone mass and its development in children with various diseases [40–45]. New developments, such as the XCT3000, allow investigation of further aspects of bone mineral and architectural changes in humans at a number of sites (Fig. 17-4).

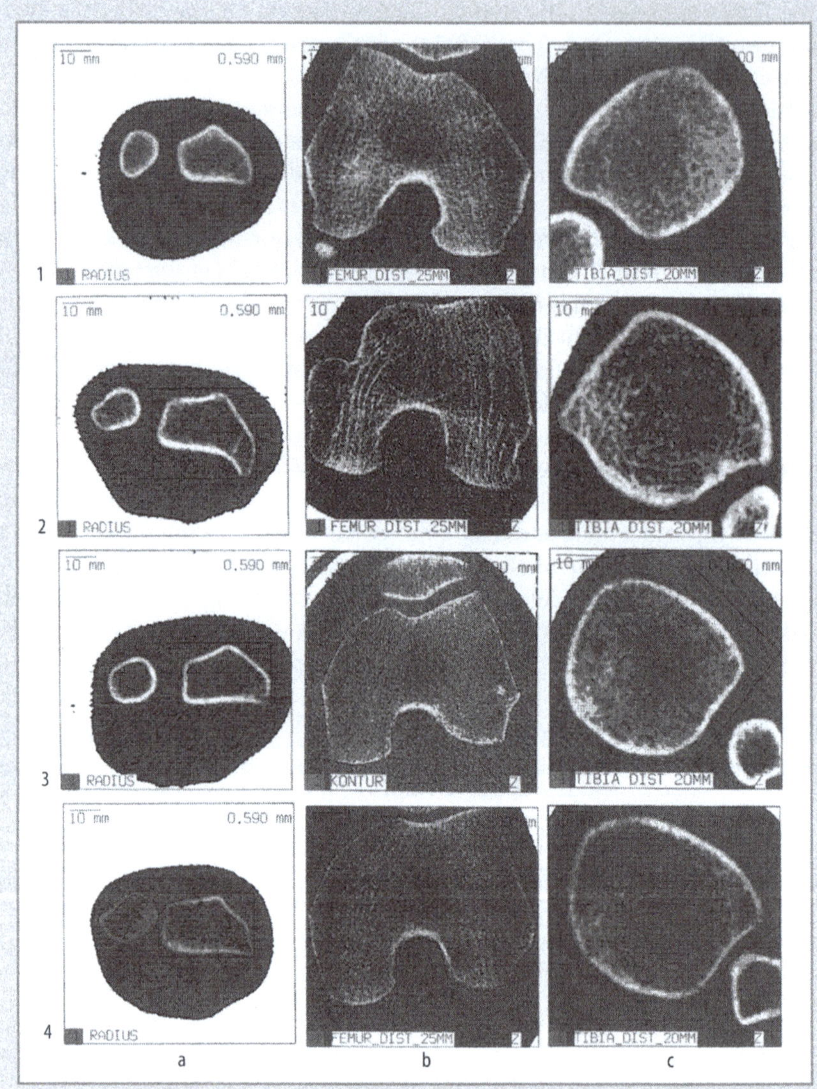

Fig. 17-4 Clinical examples of pQCT findings at standardized measurement sites. **a**, Distal forearm; **b**, distal femur; **c**, distal tibia; **1**, a normal healthy woman (24 years); **2**, a man with idiopathic osteoporosis (50 years), vertebral fractures; **3**, a woman with osteoporosis (70 years), vertebral fractures; **4**, a woman with osteomalacia due to primary hypoparathyroidism (72 years), vertebral and other fractures. The examples clearly show modeling drift and structural disintegrity in osteoporotic cases and undermineralized bone in osteomalacia compared to the normal case

Animal Models Assessed by pQCT

The specially built versions of the Norland/Stratec pQCT scanners had a substantial impact on drug studies in animals. Predominantly, pharmaceutical companies appreciated the advantages of the method [46–50]. It was recognized that pQCT in small animals is important to analyze the results of drug treatment. Some researchers found it to be more sensitive than dual-energy X-ray absorptiometry (DXA), allowing shorter duration of experiments [51]. pQCT can reliably measure changes in cancellous and cortical bone mass in small animals over time. It should be viewed as a technique complementary to static and dynamic histomorphometry, which does not replace either of these methods. A study by Sato [52] showed the change in mineral density in a rat tibia to be ten times greater than the precision of pQCT, whereas DXA failed due to edge detection problems. In the rat vertebra on the other hand, pQCT was unable to achieve acceptable precision in vivo due to positioning problems. A study by Jerome et al. [53] also reported that pQCT was potentially more sensitive than DXA because it could separate cancellous bone from cortical bone. These results suggest that pQCT may allow a reduction in the number of animals investigated and/or killed.

Noninvasive Estimation of Bone Stability

In contrast to all other methods, pQCT is a method capable of three-dimensional imaging which can therefore provide information related to the architecture of bone. In addition, it allows determination of the material property by examining the bone mass per volume unit. It may therefore be applied to noninvasive estimation of bone mechanical properties of the bone, exceeding the possibilities of standard densitometry [54]. Moreover, some sophisticated research machines even allow structural estimation at an almost microscopic level [55], simulating a noninvasive bone biopsy by µCT. Again, the widespread use of the Stratec pQCT system has opened part of these capabilities to a larger community of researchers. Excellent results have been obtained regarding correlations between pQCT-assessed mechanical parameters, such as the second moment of inertia and its derivatives, with ultimate failure load in animal bones [56] and most recently in human bones [57]. Interesting in vivo correlations of noninvasively measured bone strength to clinically relevant fractures are expected [58, 59]. The most exciting advances have been shown in pharmaceutical trials, demonstrating in vitro assessed changes of bone bending strength by pQCT due to pharmacological interactions [60–63]. This approach is considered the most relevant with regard to the desired improvement in bone stability in vivo, as the benefit of a drug application. In fact it would be consistent to use only a method providing this information.

Future Prospects

New developments are expanding the scope of pQCT from microscopic resolution for animal research to high resolution for research and clinical work in humans. After setting new standards in densitometry to overcome the limited information provided by conventional techniques, it is expected that the next generation of pQCT systems will open access to structural information for researchers and clinicians. Based on the positive results and more differentiated information in pharmaceutical research provided by pQCT, a similar impact is expected in larger clincal trials and in fields where DXA remains dominant.

Due to its high spatial resolution pQCT is more sensitive to immobilization and repositioning artifacts of the scanned regions. By taking into account this difficulty a cross-sectional view of separate bone compartments is provided, offering more detailed variables than any other densitometric method, down to a microscopic level. Structural analysis depends on these capabilities of pQCT. Animal models have shown that the assessment of metabolically more active bone compartments provides earlier information about the onset of disease or the effects therapy.

References

1. Börner W, Grehn S, Moll E (1969) Messung der Absorption des Fingerknochens mit einem I-125-Profilscanner. Quantitative Methode zur Erkennung der Osteoporose. Fortschr Röntgenstr 110:378–387
2. Rüegsegger P, Niederer P, Anliker M (1973) A method for the determination of the compacta area and the mean absorption density of human bones. In: Mazess RB (ed) Proceedings of the International Conference on Bone Mineral Measurements, Chicago, Illinois. DHEW publicaton no (NIH) 75-683, 30–38
3. Hounsfield GN (1973) Computerized transverse axial scanning (tomography). I. Description of system. Br J Radiol 46:1016–1022
4. Rüegsegger P, Elsasser U, Anliker M, Gnehm H, Kind H, Prader A (1976) Quantfication of bone mineralization using computed tomography. Radiology 121:93–97
5. McClean BA, Overton TR, Hangartner TN, Rathee S (1990) A special purpose X-ray fan beam CT scanner for trabecular bone density measurement in the appendicular skeleton. Phys Med Biol 35:11–19
6. Hosie CJ, Richardson NW, Gregoryn L (1985) A gamma-ray computed tomography scanner for the quantitative measurement of bone density. J Biomed Eng 7:30–34
7. Hesp R, Doré C, Page L, Summers R (1985) Normal values for trabecular and cortical bone in the radius measured by computed tomography. Clin Phys Physiol Meas 4:303–310

8. Hangartner TN, Overton TR (1982) Quantiative measurement of bone density using gamma-ray computed tomography. J Comput Assist Tomogr 6:1156 –62

9. Schulz E, Flowers C, Sauser DD, Brin BN, Wergedal JE, Baylink DJ (1990) The causes of bone scintigram hot spots in fluoride-treated osteoporotic patients. J Bone Miner Res 5:S201–204

10. Schneider P, Berger P, Moll E, Reiners C, Börner W (1985) Getrennte Messung von Kompakta- und Spongiosadichte mit einem Transversal-Rotations-Scanner: Bestimmung des Mineralgehalts am Radius mit einem Least-Square-Algorithmus. Fortschr Röntgenstr 143:178–182

11. Schneider P, Börner W, Mazess RB, Barden H (1988) The relationship of peripheral to axial bone density. Bone Miner 4:279–287

12. Hosie C J, Hart DM, Smith DAS, Al-Azzawi IF (1989) Differential effect of long-term oestrogen therapy on trabecular and cortical bone. Maturitas 11:137–145

13. Kruse K, Süss A, Büsse M, Schneider P (1987) Monomeric serum calcitonin and bone turnover during anticonvulsant treatment and in congenital hypothyroidism. J Pediatr 111:57–63

14. Schneider P, Börner W (1991) Periphere quantitative Computertomographie zu Knochenmineralmessung mit einem neuen speziellen QCT-Scanner. Fortschr Röntgenstr 154:229–348

15. Hosie CJ, Smith DAS (1986) Precision measurement of bone density with a special purpose computed tomography scanner. Br J Radiol 59:345–350

16. Rüegsegger P, Durand E, Dambacher MA (1991) Differential effects of ageing and disease on trabecular and compact bone density of the radius. Bone 12:99–105

17. Rüegsegger P, Durand E, Dambacher MA (1991) Localization of regional forearm bone loss from high resolution computed tomographic images. Osteoporosis Int 1:76–80

18. Lassmann M, Börner W (1993) Die Strahlenexposition bei Knochendichtemessungen. In: Holeczke F, Reiners C, Messerschmidt O (eds) Strahlenexposition bei neuen diagnostischen Verfahren. Fischer, Stuttgart, pp 51–63

19. Hosie CJ (1993) Measurement of trabecular bone density in the distal radius by two gamma ray computed tomography scanners. Physiol Meas 14:269–276

20. Shepp LA, Logan BF (1974) The Fourier reconstruction of a head section. IEEE Trans Nucl Sci NS-21:21–43

21. Stebler B, Rüegsegger P (1983) Kleincomputertomograph für quantitative Knochenuntersuchungen in den Extremitäten des Menschen. Biomed Tech 28:196–205

22. Pearson J, Rüegsegger P, Dequeker J, Henley M, Bright J, Reeve J, Kalender W, Felsenberg D, Laval-Jeantet AM, Adams J, Birkenhäger JC, Fischer M, Geusens P, Hesch RD, Hyldstrup L, Jaeger P, Johnson R, Kröger H, Van Lingen A, Mitchel A, Reiners C, Schneider P (1995) European semianthropomorhic phantom for the cross-calibration of peripheral bone densitometers: assessment of precision, accuracy and stability. Bone Miner 27:109–120

23. Rüegsegger P, Kalender W (1993) A phantom for standardization and quality control in peripheral bone measurements by pQCT and DEXA. Phys Med Biol 38:1963–1970
24. Takada M, Engelke K, Hagiwara S, Grampp S, Genant HK (1996) Accuracy and precision study in vitro for peripheral quantitative computed tomography. Osteoporosis Int 6:307–312
25. Hangartner TN, Overton TR, Harley CH, van den Berg L, Crockford PM (1985) Skeletal challenge: an experimental study of pharmacologically induced changes in bone density in the distal radius, using gamma-ray computed tomography. Calcif Tissue Int 37:19–24
26. Medici TC, Rüegsegger P (1990) Does alternate-day cloprednol therapy prevent bone loss? A longitudinal double-blind, controlled clinical study. Clin Pharmacol Ther 48:455–466
27. Dambacher MA, Ittner J, Rüegsegger P (1986) Long-term fluoride therapy of postmenopausal osteoporosis. Bone 7:199–203
28. Müller A, Rüegsegger E, Rüegsegger P (1989) Peripheral QCT: a low-risk procedure to identify women predisposed to osteoporosis. Phys Med Biol 34:741–749
29. Rüegsegger P, Dambacher M A, Rüegsegger E, Fischer JA, Anliker M (1984) Bone loss in premenopausal and postmenopausal woman. J Bone Joint Surg 66A:1015
30. Hesp R, Tellez M, Davidson L, Elton A, Reeve J (1987) Trabecular and cortical bone in the radii of women with parathyroid adenomata: a greater trabecular deficit, with a preliminary assessment of recovery after parathyroidectomy. Bone Miner 2:301–310
31. Smith DAS, Hosie CJ, Deacon AD, Hamblen DL (1990) Quantitative g-ray computed tomography of the radius in normal subjects and osteoporotic patients. Br J Radiol 63:776–782
32. Schneider P, Börner W, Rendl J, Eilles C, Schlisske K, Scheubeck M (1992) Stellenwert zweier unterschiedlicher Knochendichtemessmethoden zur Bestimmung des Minergehalts am peripheren und axialen Skelett. Z Orthop 130:16–21
33. Hesp R, Klenerman L, Page L (1984) Decreased radial bone mass in Colles' fracture. Acta Orthop Scand 55:573–575
34. Dequeker J, Reeve J, Pearson J, Bright J, Felsenberg D, Kalender W, Langton C, Laval-Jeantet AM, Rüegsegger P, Van der Perre G (1993) Multicentre European COMAC-BME study on the standardisation of bone densitometry procedures. Technol Health Care 1:127–131
35. Reeve J, Kröger H, Nijs J, Pearson J, Felsenberg D, Reiners C, Schneider P, Mitchell A, Rüegsegger P, Zander C, Dequeker J (1996) Radial cortical and trabecular bone densities standardized with the European forearm phantom. Calcif Tissue Int 58:135–143
36. Schneider P, Butz S, Allolio B, Börner W, Klein K, Lehmann R, Petermann K, Tysarczyk-Niemeyer G, Wüster C, Zander C, Ziegler R, Reiners C (1995) Mul-

ticenter German reference data base for peripheral quantiative computer tomography. Technol Health Care 3:69–73

37. Kröger H, Lunt M, Reeve J, Dequeker J, Adams JE, Birkenhager JC, Diaz-Curiel M, Felsenberg D, Hyldstrup L, Laval-Jeantet AM, Lips P, Louis O, Perez Cano R, Reiners C, Ribot C, Rüegsegger P, Schneider P, Braillon P, Pearson J (1997) Bone density reduction in various measurement sites in osteoporosis with fracture of spine and hip. The European Quantitation of Osteoporosis Study. Osteoporosis Int (submitted)

38. Schneider P, Börner W (1990) Ability of peripheral QCT at the radius in comparson to DEXA of the spine to diagnose vertebral fractures in postmenopausal women. In: Christiansen C, Overgaard K (eds) Osteoporosis 1990. Osteopress, Kopenhagen, pp 921–924

39. Fujii Y, Miyauchi A, Takagi Y, Goto B, Fujita T (1994) Quantitative computed tomography of radius in Japanese patients with osteoporosis. J Bone Miner Res 9:S296

40. Schlamp D, Schneider P, Krahl A, Trott GE, Warnke A (1994) Untersuchungen zur Knochendichte bei Anorexia nervosa-mit Anmerkungen zur Prophylaxe und Therapie der Osteoporose. Z Kinder-Jugendpsychiat 22:183–188

41. Kruse K, Süss A, Büsse M, Schneider P (1987) Normal spongiosa density despite decreased secretion of monomeric calcitonin in children under anticonvulsant treatment with diphenylhydantoin and primidone. Acta Endocrinol 114:53–54

42. Schönau E, Wentzlik U, Michalk D, Scheidhauer K, Klein K (1993) Is there an increase of bone density in children? Lancet 342:689–690

43. Lettgen B, Jeken C, Reiners C (1994) Influence of steroid medication on bone mineral density in children with nephrotic syndrome. Pediatr Nehrol 8:667–670

44. Lettgen B, Rasche P, Reiners C (1995) Knochenmineralgehalt bei Kindern und Jugendlichen mit Hyperkalziurie. Monatsschr Kinderheilkd 143:46–49

45. Lettgen B, Hauffa B, Möhlmann C, Jeken C, Reiners C: Bone mineral density in children and adolescents with juvenile diabetes: selective measurement of bone mineral density of trabecular and cortical bone using peripheral quantitative computed tomography. Horm Res 43:173–175

46. Hageman WE, Westover L, Sanchez T, Jordan J, Minor L, Cini J, Demarest KT (1994) Chronic administration of methyl-prednisolone in adult ewes decreases radial bone density measured by peripheral quantitative computer tomography (pQCT). J Bone Miner Res 9:S404

47. Han B, Triantafillou J, Rahn-Bahrfield C, Baer PG (1994) Effect of ovariectomy on rat tibia trabecular bone mineral density as measured by DEXA and pQCT. J Bone Miner Res 9:S258

48. Rosen HN, Chen V, Cittadini A, Greenspan SL, Douglas PS, Mosese AC, Beamer WG (1995) Treatment with growth hormone and IGF-I in growing rats increases bone mineral content but not bone mineral density. J Bone Miner Res 10:1352–1358

49. Sauls HR, Bajin H, Triantafillou J, Morris DC, Baer PG (1994) Plasma PTH levels after minimal doses causing increased bone mineral density in osteopenic rats. J Bone Miner Res 9:S325

50. Shen V, Birchman R, Liang XG, Walliser J, Otter M, Wu DD, Dempster DW, Lindsay R (1994) Long term effects of estrogen and dietary calcium deficiencies on bone mass and mechanical strength in long bones of mature rats. J Bone Miner Res 9:S261

51. Gasser JA (1996) Assessing bone quantity by pQCT. Bone 17:145S–154S

52. Sato M (1996) Comparative X-ray densitometry of bones from ovariectomized rats. Bone 17:157S–162S

53. Jerome CP, Johnson CS, Lees CJ (1995) Effect of treatment for 3 months with human parathyroid hormone 1-34 pepetide in ovariectomized cynomolgus monkeys (Macaca fascicularis). Bone 17:415S–420S

54. Faulkner KG, Glüer CC, Majumdar S, Lang P, Engelke K, Genant HK (1991) Non invasive measurements of bone mass, structure and strength. Current methods and experimental techniques. Am J Roentgenol 157:1229–1237

55. Müller R, Hildebrand T, Rüegsegger P (1994) Non-invasive bone biopsy: a new method to analyse and display the three-dimensional structure of trabecular bone. Phys Med Biol 39:145–164

56. Ferretti JL, Capozza RF, Mondelo N, Zanchetta JR (1993) Interrelationships between densitometric, geometric and mechanical properties of rat femora: Inferences concerning mechanical regulation of bone modeling. J Bone Miner Res 8:1389–1396

57. Augat P, Reeb H, Claes LE (1996) Prediction of fracture load at different skeletal sites by geometric properties of the cortical shell. J Bone Miner Res 11:1356–1363

58. Schneider P, Börner W, Reiners C (1995) Mechanical properties of the radius in patients with distal radius fracture and with spinal osteoporosis. Radiology 197:S362

59. Schneider P, Ferretti JL, Capozza RF, Braun M, Reiners C (1996) Bone densitometric and biomechanical properties of the distal radius by noninvasive assessment. Eur Radiol 6:C17

60. Ma YF, Ferretti JL, Capozza RF, Cointry G, Alippi R, Zanchetta J, Jee WSS (1995) Effects of on/off anabolic hPTH and remodelling inhibitors on metaphyseal bone of immobilized rat femurs. Tomographical (pQCT) description and correlation with histomorphometric changes in tibial cancellous bone. Bone 17:321S–327S

61. Ferretti JL, Gaffuri O, Capozza RF, Cointry G, Bozzini C, Olivera AM, Zanchetta JR, Bozzini CE (1995) Dexamethasone effects on mechanical, geometric and densitometric properties of rat femur diaphyses as described by peripheral quantitative computerized tomography and bending tests. Bone 16:119–124

62. Ferretti JL, Scheinsohn V, Machi M, Zanchetta JR (1992) Biological determination of diaphyseal thickness according to mechanical quality of bone material in several vertebrate species. Bone Miner 17:S133

63. Liberman UA, Weiss SR, Bröll J et al (1995) Effect of oral alendronate on bone mineral density and the incidence of fractures in postmenopausal osteoporosis. N Engl J Med 333:1437–1443
64. Reiners C, Arnold B, Brust AS, Sonnenschein W (1990) Precision of bone mineral measurement with the new QCT scanner Stratec SCT 900. J Nucl Med 31:856
65. Zander CC (1995) Die periphere quantitative Computertomographie (pQCT) zur Osteodensitometrie am distalen Radius: Qualitätskontrolle, Referenzbereiche und Einflussfaktoren. Thesis, University of Essen
66. Wapniarz M, Lehmann R, Randerath R, Baedecker RO, Baedecker S, John W, Klein K, Allolio B (1994) Precision of Dual-X-ray absorptiometry and peripheral computed tomography using mobile densitometry units. Calcif Tissue Int 54:219–223
67. Lehmann R, Wapniarz M, Kvasnicka HM, Baedecker S, Klein K, Allolio B (1992) Reproduzierbarkeit von Knochendichtemessungen am distalen Radius mit einem hochauflösenden Spezialscanner für periphere quantitative Computertomographie. Radiologe 32:177–181
68. Grampp S, Lang P, Jergas M et al (1995) Assessment of the skeletal status by quantitative peripheral computed tomography: short-term precision in-vivo and comparison to dual X-ray absorptiometry. J Bone Miner Res 10:1566–576
69. Guglielmi G, Giannatempo GM, Willnecker J, Cammisa M (1996) Precision of peripheral QCT: impact on quality assurance. Osteoporosis Int 6:S81

18 Comparison of Quantitative Computed Tomography and Dual X-Ray Absorptiometry at the Lumbar Spine in the Diagnosis of Osteoporosis

T. Fuerst, G. Guglielmi, M. Cammisa, and H. K. Genant

Introduction

The noninvasive measurement of bone mass is an essential tool in the clinical diagnosis of osteoporosis. Bone mineral density (BMD) is an established, important predictor of risk of osteoporotic fracture. Various methods to quantify spinal BMD are currently in use to obtain an early diagnosis of osteoporosis and to follow its development or, alternatively, to evaluate the success of a particular therapy. The two methods of noninvasive spinal BMD assessment most widely used are quantitative computed tomography (QCT) and dual X-ray absorptiometry (DXA). Both methods offer specific inherent qualities.

Quantitative Computed Tomography

QCT uses general-purpose CT scanners to provide true volumetric BMD generally of purely trabecular bone of the midvertebral body (Fig. 18-1). The quanti-

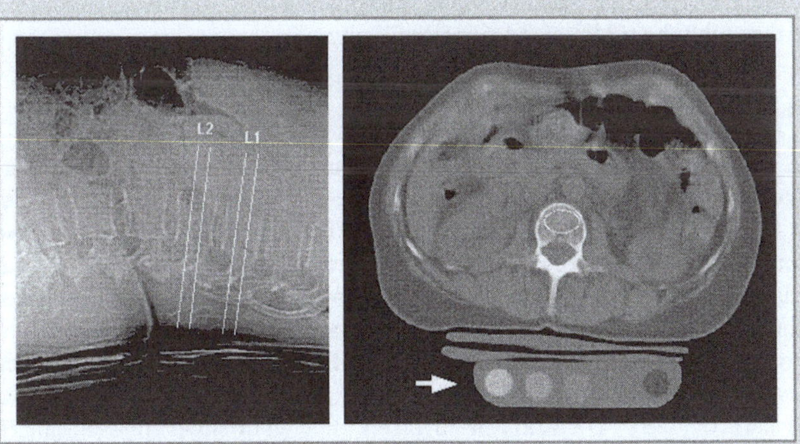

Fig. 18-1 Scout view (*left*) and axial slice (*right*) through middle of L2 vertebral body. Scout view shows location of slices through bodies of first (L1) and second (L2) vertebral bodies. The elliptical region of interest measuring purely trabecular bone of the vertebral body is shown in the axial slice along with the QCT calibration phantom (*arrow*) used to convert Hounsfield units to mg/cm^3 of calcium hydroxyapatite

tation of the image is achieved by calibration of the Hounsfield units with a phantom positioned under the patient during scanning. QCT is unique among methods of mass measurement in providing separate estimates of trabecular and cortical bone BMD as a true volumetric mineral density (mass/volume in milligrams per cubic centimeter). Clinical results indicate that QCT can reliably evaluate and monitor the many forms of osteoporosis and its various treatments. The greatest advantages of spinal QCT for noninvasive bone mineral measurement lie in the high precision of the technique (1.5%–2%) [1], the high sensitivity of the vertebral spongiosa for fracture risk assessment, and the potential for widespread use. QCT has the ability to measure selectively the trabecular compartment of the vertebral body, which is eight times more metabolically active than cortical bone. Since trabecular bone is the first to respond to menopausal changes, spinal QCT has been recognized as a sensitive method with which to assess BMD changes in patients with osteoporosis [1–3]. QCT trabecular density measurements are independent of anthropometric parameters. However, it requires a high radiation dose and longer imaging time, and its accuracy is substantially influenced by bone marrow fat [4].

Variants to the QCT approach include dual-energy QCT (DE-QCT) which combines QCT scans of different X-ray energy (typically 80 and 140 kVp) to correct for errors resulting from marrow fat changes. The cost of this technique is higher radiation dose and lower precision than with the more common single-energy approach. It is used primarily in research applications where accuracy is required. Recently there has been increased interest in volumetric QCT using multiple contiguous slices or spiral acquisition. These techniques promise to improve precision by examining a larger volume of bone and using anatomical landmarks to reproducibly define the volume of interest on sequential visits. However, almost all clinical QCT examinations employ the single-energy approach, and a single slice through the middle of the vertebral body.

Dual X-Ray Absorptiometry

DXA has gained widespread acceptance because of its low radiation exposure, low cost, high precision, and ability to measure bone density at different skeletal sites [5, 6]. DXA is less sensitive to changes in marrow fat and uses relatively uncomplicated equipment and procedures, ensuring ease of operation. DXA uses specially designed instruments to provide a projectional measurement of bone mineral content (BMC in grams), area (in square centimeters), and areal density (mass/area, BMD in grams per square centimeter); volume is not measured. However, the two-dimensional measurement of integral bone (trabecular and cortical) provided by DXA may be adversely affected by superimposed calcified tissues, particularly for posteroanterior DXA (PA-DXA) of the lumbar spine.

To increase the sensitivity of DXA it has been suggested to measure BMD of the spine in the lateral projection [7–11]. There are several advantages to measuring bone mineral content in the vertebral body from a lateral projection. First, bone loss with age or disease differs in trabecular and cortical bone, being substantially larger in the more metabolically active trabecular bone of the vertebral body. With 40%–60% of vertebral body bone mass being trabecular bone [12,13], a lateral approach which excludes the predominantly cortical bone of the posterior elements is more sensitive to changes in bone mass. Second, the biomechanics of the spine are such that most of the weight is borne by the vertebral body. Thus a technique which can isolate bone of the vertebral body is likely to have greater ability to assess vertebral strength and fracture risk. Finally, extraskeletal calcium (calcification of the abdominal aorta) and degenerative changes (such as osteophytes and sclerosis) of the vertebral body endplates and facet joints of the posterior elements can mask bone loss when measured in the PA projection. A lateral projection can remove these artifacts from the region of interest, allowing more accurate assessment of vertebral bone loss move below.

Lateral spine DXA studies were initially performed using the decubitus lateral position (Fig. 18-2) [7–9]. From these scans lateral BMD results can be obtained for the whole vertebral body (L-DXA) or for a region of interest limited to the midvertebral body (mL-DXA). The midvertebral body region excludes the dense cortical bone of the endplates and most of the cortical shell allowing a nearly selective assessment of trabecular bone. This midlateral region can further minimize the affect of degenerative changes. BMD measurements derived from the lateral projection have exhibited poorer precision with the coefficient of variation (CV) in the range of 2%–4% [7–10,14,15], compared to about 1% for the PA spine. The poor precision of the decubitus scan is partly the result of the difficulty in reproducing subjects' position on follow-up scans which leads to variations in the position of the vertebrae and in the thickness and composition of the surrounding soft tissue.

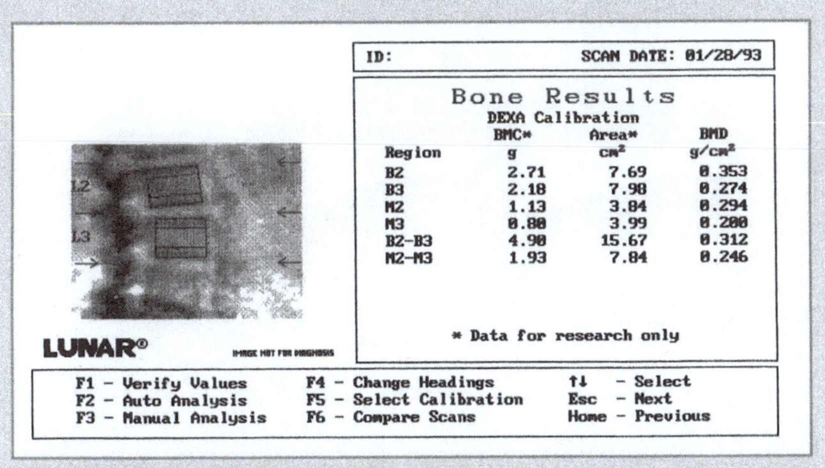

Region	BMC* g	Area* cm²	BMD g/cm²
B2	2.71	7.69	0.353
B3	2.18	7.98	0.274
M2	1.13	3.84	0.294
M3	0.80	3.99	0.200
B2-B3	4.90	15.67	0.312
M2-M3	1.93	7.84	0.246

Fig. 18-2 Lateral DXA from a Lunar densitometer with subject in decubitus position. L2 and L3 are evaluated for total vertebral body and mid-slice regions of interest. Iliac crest is seen overlying the L4 vertebral body

The development of bone densitometers with rotating C-arms (Hologic QDR 2000 and 4500 and Lunar Expert-XL) has allowed the lateral scan to be performed in the supine postion, overcoming some of the difficulties of the lateral decubitus scan. On Hologic scanners [11, 16, 17] PA and lateral scans of the lumbar spine are acquired in matched pairs with the patient in the standard supine position (Fig. 18-3). After completion of the PA scan the scanning arm with X-ray tube and detectors is rotated 90°, and a lateral scan is performed without the subject moving. The principal advantage is the greater ease, comfort, and reproducibility of patient positioning than in the decubitus position. Moreover, the spatial registration between the paired PA- and L-DXA scans allows two additional improvements in the lateral measurement. The first is baseline compensation [11]. Baseline compensation is a technique by which the data from the PA scan are used to compensate for changes in the soft tissue baseline of the lateral scan. The result is marked improvement in the precision of the measurement. Supine lateral BMD has a CV of about 2% [11, 16–18], compared to 3% or higher for decubitus lateral scanning. The second advantage of pairing the PA and lateral scans is for accurate assessments of volumetric BMD (in grams per cubic centimeter). The average width of vertebra measured from the PA projection is combined with the lateral measurement to estimate the volume of the vertebral body and calculate volumetric BMD with good accuracy [19]. L-DXA in either the decubitus or supine position is hindered by overlapping bone from the ribs (overlying L2) and pelvis (overly-

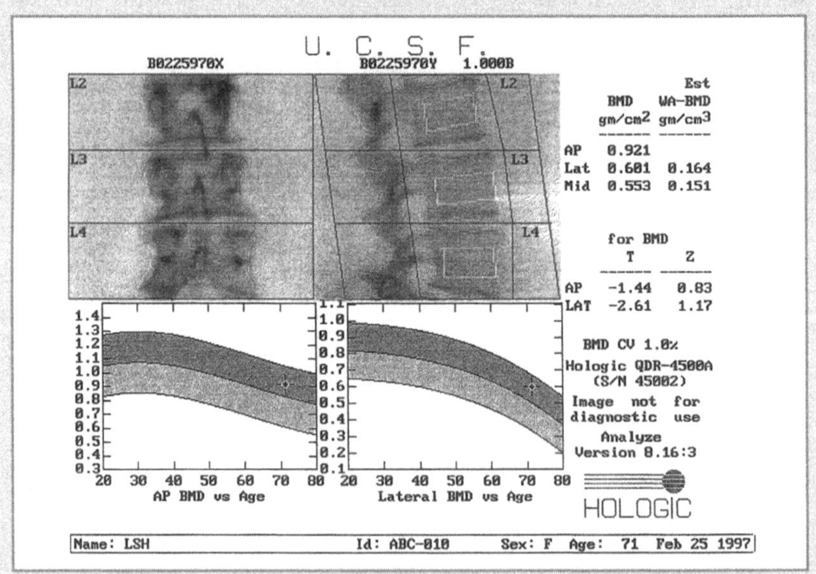

Fig. 18-3 Paired PA-/L-DXA study from a Hologic QDR 4500 showing the analysis for L2-L4. Because of the use of the supine lateral technique with a rotating C-arm there is an exact line-by-line match between the two scans. Evidence of osteophytes and/or sclerosis is seen in the PA view at the superior portion of L2. mL-DXA regions of interest are shown as *white rectangles* within the vertebral bodies

ing L4) [20]. Jergas et al. investigated the question of which vertebrae to measure in the lateral projection [18]. They demonstrated a marked improvement in measurement precision (2%) when three lumbar vertebrae (L2–L4) were combined compared to individual vertebra (3%–5%). This contributed to better diagnostic sensitivity. However, they recommended excluding L4 from the results if there is overlap with the pelvic bone.

Comparison of QCT and DXA

There is an ongoing scientific discussion about the most suitable method for measuring BMD, assessing changes with aging or treatment and evaluating the risk of osteoporotic fracture for individual patients. The first consideration for measuring BMD is the skeletal site to assess. The spine with its large proportion of cancellous bone is an attractive site for bone mass measurement. Moreover, it is a common site of osteoporotic fracture. Consequently both DXA and QCT have been used extensively at the spine. The success of these techniques for the evaluation of osteoporosis depends on their respective precision and accuracy. The instrument stability, patient positioning, the thickness and heterogeneity of surrounding soft tissue, changing marrow composition, and other factors affect both techniques. Diagnostic accuracy of DXA is also influenced by the degree of osteoarthritic changes present. Many studies have investigated the relative merits of DXA and QCT for measurement of bone density.

The predictive value of DXA has been established in several prospective studies. QCT has been tested in several cross-sectional studies and in at least one prospective study [21]. Cross-sectional studies yield information on fracture association, not risk of fracture. Still, when properly designed, cross-sectional and longitudinal studies yield similar results. QCT has generally shown better ability than DXA to discriminate between fracture and nonfracture subjects [3, 22–25]. This is in part due to the nature of postmenopausal bone loss where a disproportionate loss of trabecular bone is typically observed. It has been demonstrated that the rate of loss in trabecular bone of the vertebral body measured with QCT is approximately twice that observed in the total vertebra [26, 27]. Thus QCT, which can selectively measure trabecular density, is a more sensitive measure of bone loss in early postmenopausal women.

Age-Related Changes and Response to Treatment

The dynamics of bone loss have been studied in cross-sectional and longitudinal studies. Typically accelerated loss occurs in the first years after menopause, with slower loss later in life. BMD measurements derived from the lateral projection have been shown to be more sensitive for detection of age-related bone loss than the PA projection (1.0% versus 0.6% per annum, respectively) [8, 9, 16, 22, 28, 29]. The rate of postmenopausal loss of trabecular bone measured by QCT is about 2% per year, greater than that found for DXA. Bone density changes in the spine resulting from various treatment options depend on the potency of the treatment and population studied. Changes in spine BMD by PA-DXA of +1%–2% per year have been reported for estrogen and etidronate treatment [30, 31]. L-DXA changes with etidronate treatment were reported to be +1.5%–2% per year depending on the parameter (vertebral body, midregion or volumetric estimates). Changes in trabecular spine BMD by QCT have been reported for estrogen to range from +2%–5% [32, 33] per year. Similar to the greater losses observed with aging, larger percentage increases in density following treatment are measured by L-DXA and QCT.

While L-DXA and QCT have demonstrated greater changes with aging and treatment than PA-DXA, these results must be considered in the context of the precision of these measurements. Doing so allows better comparison of the ability of these techniques to diagnose disease and detect changes in BMD in the individual. L-DXA has exhibited less precision than PA-DXA, having a CV in the range of 2%–4% [8, 9, 11, 14] with supine measurements at the lower end of this range (2%–3%) and decubitus at the upper end (3% or more). This compares to about 1%–1.5% for the PA spine in postmenopausal women. Precision of the QCT measurement using 10 mm slices through the middle of two vertebral bodies is roughly 1.5%–2% [1]. Thus some of the enhanced changes measured by L-DXA and QCT are offset by the poorer precision of these techniques. L-DXA is comparable to PA-DXA while QCT appears to maintain some advantage. Blake et al. recently reported a comparison of PA-DXA and supine L-DXA for the monitoring of longitudinal changes with cyclical etidronate treatment [31]. Examining women 1–10 years after the menopause, they found a 4% increase in BMD by PA-DXA in the treatment group compared to placebo and a 5%–8% increase in the L-DXA measurement. However, when these changes were normalized for long-term precision of the measurement technique, PA-DXA was demonstrated to be superior to all lateral techniques although these differences were not statistically significant for lateral measurement of the whole vertebral body. These results imply the equivalence of PA-DXA and L-DXA for monitoring changes in spine BMD. While no direct comparisons of DXA and QCT for measuring treatment response have been reported, the greater response reported with QCT and comparable precision to DXA suggests that there is some advantage for QCT.

Influence of Degenerative Joint Disease on BMD Assessed by DXA and QCT

A common finding in the spine of the elderly is degenerative joint disease (DJD) which refers to the deterioration of articular structures resulting from mechanical stress. Also known as osteoarthrosis and osteoarthritis, DJD causes changes in the spine that can be detected radiographically. DJD changes in the spine such as disc space narrowing, sclerosis, and osteophytosis can influence BMD measurements. Several studies have investigated the impact of vertebral osteophytes on BMD measurements [34–39], each showing that the presence of osteophytes increased the measured BMD. DJD includes not only osteophytes at vertebrae, but also other changes at vertebral bodies, spinal processes, and facet joints. BMD results may be influenced when any of these changes occur within the region of BMD measurement. For this reason QCT may have an advantage in the assessment of BMD because it can evaluate the trabecular bone of the vertebral body which should not be influenced by DJD. Likewise, L-DXA may be superior to PA-DXA because it avoids measurement of the posterior elements of the spine where DJD changes often occur.

A recent study by Yu et al. confirmed the impact of vertebral osteophytes but also found that disc narrowing, sclerosis, and osteophytes at other sites in the spine elevated PA-DXA BMD compared to women without DJD changes [39]. They also evaluated the impact of DJD on L-DXA using the global region of interest and the midlateral region (mL-DXA) and QCT. In the lateral projection DJD continued to affect L-DXA results although to a lesser extent than observed for PA-DXA. However, BMD measured by either mL-DXA or trabecular QCT was not affected by DJD changes. This result is to be expected as spinal DJD changes frequently occur at the edges of vertebral bodies, and this area is not included in the regions evaluated by QCT or mL-DXA. However, PA-DXA, which measures the entire vertebral body and the posterior elements, was significantly affected by the presence of DJD changes. The percentage difference in PA-DXA BMD between women with DJD and controls ranged from 6% to 33%. L-DXA BMD was significantly increased (+4.5%) only among women with vertebral body osteophytes. DJD has been shown to influence BMD measurements in several other reports [34–38]. Reid et al. reported that vertebral osteophytes increased BMD measured by PA-DXA in the lumbar spine [35]. Ito et al. reported that PA-DXA BMD and cortical BMD (QCT) were higher in a group of men with osteophytes whereas trabecular BMD measured by QCT was unaffected [37].

Although osteoporosis and DJD are two different disease entities, there may be a relationship between them. Osteoporosis and DJD are diseases whose prevalence increases with age and are known to coexist in the elderly [40]. Whether patients with DJD are protected against fracture has been debated in the literature [40]. Evidence has been reported suggesting that an antagonism exists between osteoporosis and osteophytosis of the vertebral spine. In contrast, the reports from Yu et al. indicated that spinal DJD did not protect against osteoporotic fractures, nor did low BMD protect against DJD [39]. Thus when DJD changes were present, PA-DXA, and to a lesser extent L-DXA, tended to underestimate the osteopenic status of a subject. For assessment of osteoporotic fracture risk, a spine BMD measurement technique that is insensitive to degenerative changes, such as mL-DXA or QCT, is preferred.

Fracture Association

Many studies have demonstrated in vitro the correlation between vertebral strength and bone mass measured with DXA or QCT [41–47]. However, varying results have been reported depending on the mechanical [ultimate force or stress (force per area)] and bone mass (BMC, area BMD, volumetric BMD) parameters evaluated and it remains unclear what advantages there may be for L-DXA or QCT. For example Myers et al. have reported better association between vertebral body strength and BMD measured in vitro by L-DXA compared to PA-DXA [41]. In contrast, Bjarnason et al. showed no advantage for L-DXA when measured in situ [44]. Furthermore Tabensky et al. found that BMC, area BMD and volumetric BMD by DXA were equivalent predictors of vertebral body strength [43]. Similar questions about QCT exist (single versus dual energy, trabecular compared to integral BMD).

Given the difficulties in executing and interpreting the results of in vitro studies, it seems appropriate to investigate the merits of these different techniques in vivo with cross-sectional and prospective studies. Early investigations of L-DXA in the decubitus position demonstrated larger percentage decrements in BMD values than in PA-DXA but similar Z and T scores [15, 48, 49]. Receiver-operating characteristic (ROC) analysis also found no advantage for L-DXA. Some reports of supine lateral scanning have indicated similar results [17, 18, 25] while others have shown L-DXA to be superior to PA-DXA but not as good as QCT [22–24, 50, 51]. In these latter studies Z or T scores tended to be significantly lower for L-DXA but not as low as for QCT. Also the area under ROC curves was significantly larger for L-DXA but, again, not as good as QCT [22, 24, 50]. Finally, several authors performed age-adjusted logistic regression analysis and found standardized odds ratios for vertebral fracture to be lowest for PA-DXA (odds ratios 1.5–2.4) and higher for L-DXA (2.0–2.9) but highest for QCT (3.2–4.3) [23, 24, 51]. Taken together these data suggest greater diagnositic sensitivity for BMD measurements of the spine in the lateral projection. However, QCT remains superior for discrimination of women with prevalent fracture from age-matched controls.

When evaluating the individual patient the apparent better performance of L-DXA must be interpreted in the context of the accuracy errors of this measurement. Given the greater thickness of soft tissue and inhomogeneity in the lateral projection, the accuracy error of the L-DXA measurement is larger [52, 53]. This is illustrated in the study of Bjarnason et al. [44] who showed that the correlation of lateral spine BMD with breaking strength was less when measured in situ ($r=0.45$) than in vitro ($r=0.71$). This degradation did not occur with PA-DXA ($r=0.48$ and 0.51, respectively). Thus while the studies discussed above indicate better diagnostic capability for L-DXA the chance of incorrectly assessing the risk of the individual is higher with the lateral measurement. Of course, this error must be weighed against the errors due to degenerative changes in the spine as well as other error sources in PA-DXA and QCT.

Estimates of Volumetric Bone Density from DXA

With DXA, BMD is calculated as the quotient of the bone mineral content (BMC, in grams) and the projected area (in square centimeters). This normalization has been shown to reduce the influence of the skeletal size. However, since areal density does not take vertebral depth into account, a dependence on bone size remains. For a constant volumetric bone density, a larger vertebra would yield higher area BMD results than a small vertebra. Several estimates of volumetric density have been proposed with the intention of reducing the effect of body size on area BMD measurements, some of which are derived from PA-DXA measurements and some from paired PA- and L-DXA measurements of the lumbar spine [16, 24]. In this section we discuss the utility of various estimates of volumetric bone density from projectional PA and L-DXA measurements of the lumbar spine compared to a measurement of true volumetric trabecular bone density by QCT.

Jergas et al. evaluated six volumetric estimates of spinal BMD as derived from the DXA scan [24]. From PA-DXA measurements a bone mineral apparent density was calculated as BMD divided by the square root of the projected area [54]. In addition, two other parameters which correspond to PA-BMD measurements corrected for vertebral body width were investigated. From the paired PA- and L-DXA measurements three highly correlated width-adjusted estimates of volumetric BMD were evaluated. All models used corrections based on vertebral dimensions and are given in grams per cubic centimeter. These estimates were based on simplified models since they take into account neither the true vertebral shape nor its specific structural composition of cortical and trabecular bone, and thus they do not reflect "volumetric density" as accurately as QCT. The data presented in the study of Jergas et al. showed that estimated volumetric BMD from paired PA-/L-DXA scans eliminated the body size dependence seen for areal BMD. Similar results were reported by Duboeuf and colleagues [16]. Furthermore, volumetric estimates of BMD were found to be superior for discrimination of women with prevalent vertebral fracture from those without. Using logistic regression analysis to determine odds ratios for vertebral fracture, Jergas et al. [24] demonstrated that estimated volumetric measures of BMD based on paired PA and L-DXA scans are more strongly correlated with the presence of vertebral fractures (odds ratios OR = 2.8–2.9) than BMD by L-DXA alone (OR = 1.9), PA-DXA (OR = 1.5), or volumetric estimates of bone density that are solely based on PA-DXA scans (OR = 1.7–2.0). The results from paired PA/lateral scans compared well to QCT (OR = 3.2). Thus both L-DXA and estimated volumetric BMD from the PA-DXA scan had significantly better discriminatory power than simple PA-DXA. Moreover, volumetric estimates based on paired PA/lateral scans offered further significant improvements that rivaled QCT. These findings are in contrast to the results of Guglielmi et al. who did not find width adjusted spine BMD measurements given by the Hologic software to be superior to lateral measurements of the spine [22].

Volumetric estimates of BMD from projectional measurements may provide useful additional information that results in better discrimination of osteoporotic from nonosteoporotic populations and less dependence on body size parameters in comparison with the projectional measurements from which they are derived. As such volumetric estimates represent an interesting option for the study of bone density differences in dissimilar populations (age, gender, race, ethnicity) where bone size may play a confounding role. Volumetric BMD estimates from DXA are a useful diagnostic test but accuracy and precision of the measurement should be considered when applied to the individual.

Conclusions

QCT is highly sensitive in detecting age-related bone loss and in differentiating normal from osteoporotic patients. BMD measurement by QCT has advantages over DXA (including PA-DXA and L-DXA) in detecting bone loss in postmenopausal women, since QCT BMD is not susceptible to accuracy errors due to DJD. However DJD may represent a major source of accuracy errors for PA-DXA, leading to overestimation of BMD when DJD is present. The diagnostic sensitivity of L-DXA is between that of PA-DXA and QCT. The lower radiation exposure and cost of L-DXA compared with QCT suggest that L-DXA is a valid alternative to QCT in the clinical setting. Because of these reasons QCT or DXA in either projection can be recommended for diagnosing osteoporosis, with the caveat that PA-DXA is inappropriate for use in individuals with advanced DJD. All techniques can be used for longitudinal follow-up although the supine scanning technique is recommended for L-DXA because of the large precision errors associated with the decubitus measurement.

References

1. Steiger P, Block JE, Steiger S, Heuck A, Friedlander A, Ettinger B, Harris ST, Gluer CC, Genant HK (1990) Spinal bone mineral density measured with quantitative CT: effect of region of interest, vertebral level, and technique. Radiology 175:537–543
2. Genant HK, Faulkner KG, Gluer CC (1991) Measurements of bone mineral density: current status. Am J Med 91 [Suppl 5B]:49–53
3. Pacifici R, Rupich RC, Griffin MG, Chines A, Susman N, Avioli LV (1990) Dual energy radiography versus quantitative computer tomography for the diagnosis of osteoporosis. J Clin Endocrinol Metab 70:705–710
4. Gluer CC, Genant HK (1989) Impact of marrow fat on accuracy of quantitative CT. J Comp Assist Tomogr 13:1023–1035
5. Sartoris DJ, Resnick D (1989) Dual energy radiographic absorptiometry for bone densitometry: current status and prospective. AJR 152:241–246
6. Wahner HW, Fogelman I (1994) The evaluation of osteoporosis: dual energy X-ray absorptiometry in clinical practice. Dunitz, London
7. Uebelhart D, Duboeuf F, Meunier PJ, Delmas PD (1990) Lateral dual-photon absorptiometry: a new technique to measure the bone mineral density at the lumbar spine. J Bone Miner Res 5:525–531
8. Slosman DO, Rizzoli R, Donath A, Bonjour JP (1990) Vertebral bone mineral density measured laterally by dual-energy X-ray absorptiometry. Osteoporos Int 1:23–29

9. Rupich R, Pacifici R, Griffin M, Vered I, Susman N, Avioli LV (1990) Lateral dual energy radiography: a new method for measuring vertebral bone density: a preliminary study. J Clin Endocrin Metabol 70:1768–1770

10. Mazess RB, Gifford CA, Bisek JP, Barden HS, Hanson JA (1991) DEXA measurement of spine density in the lateral projection. I. methodology. Calcif Tissue Int 49:235–239

11. Blake GM, Jagathesan T, Herd RJM, Fogelman I (1994) Dual X-ray absorptiometry of the lumbar spine: the precision of paired anteroposterior/lateral studies. Br J Radiol 67:624–630

12. Nottestad SY, Baumel JJ, Kimmel DB, Recker RR, Heaney RP (1987) The proportion of trabecular bone in human vertebrae. J Bone Miner Res 2:221–229

13. Eastell R, Mosekilde L, Hodgson SF, Riggs BL (1990) Proportion of human vertebral body bone that is cancellous. J Bone Miner Res 5:1237–1241

14. Larnach TA, Boyd SJ, Smart RC, Butler SP, Rohl PG, Diamond TH (1992) Reproducibility of lateral spine scans using dual energy X-ray absorptiometry. Calcif Tissue Int 51:255–258

15. Del Rio L, Pons F, Huguet M, Setoain FJ, Setoain J (1995) Anteroposterior versus lateral bone mineral density of spine assessed by dual X-ray absorptiometry. Eur J Nucl Med 22:407–412

16. Duboeuf F, Pommet R, Meunier PJ, Delmas PD (1994) Dual energy X-ray absorptiometry of the spine in anteroposterior and lateral projection. Osteoporos Int 4:110–116

17. Finkelstein JS, Cleary RL, Butler JP, Antonelli R, Mitlak BH, Deraska DJ, Zamora-Quezada JC, Neer RM (1994) A comparison of lateral versus anterior-posterior spine dual energy X-ray absorptiometry for the diagnosis of osteopenia. J Clin Endocrinol Metab 78:724–730

18. Jergas M, Breitenseher M, Gluer CC, Black D, Lang P, Grampp S, Engelke K, Genant HK (1995) Which vertebrae should be assessed using lateral dual-energy X-ray absorptiometry of the lumbar spine. Osteoporosis Int 5:196–204

19. Sabin MA, Blake GM, MacLaughlin-Black SM, Fogelman I (1995) The accuracy of volumetric bone density measurements in dual X-ray absorptiometry. Calcif Tissue Int 56:210–214

20. Rupich RC, Griffin MG, Pacifici R, Avioli LV, Susman N (1992) Lateral dual-energy radiography: artifact error from rib and pelvic bone. J Bone Miner Res 7:97–101

21. Ross PD, Genant HK, Davis JW, Miller PD, Wasnich RD (1993) Predicting vertebral fracture incidence from prevalent fractures and bone density among non-black, osteoporotic women. Osteoporosis Int 3:120–126

22. Guglielmi G, Grimston SK, Fischer KC, Pacifici R (1994) Osteoporosis: diagnosis with lateral and posteroanterior dual X-ray absorptiometry compared with quantitative CT. Radiology 192:845–850

23. Yu W, Gluer CC, Grampp S, Jergas M, Wu CY, Genant HK (1995) Spinal bone mineral assessment in postmenopausal women: a comparison between dual X-ray absorptiometry and quantitative computed tomography. Osteoporosis Int 5:433–439

24. Jergas M, Breitenseher M, Gluer CC, Yu W, Genant HK (1995) Estimates of volumetric bone density from projectional measurements improve the discriminatory capability of dual X-ray absorptiometry. J Bone Miner Res 10:1101–1110

25. Duboeuf F, Jergas M, Schott AM, Wu CY, Gluer CC, Genant HK (1995) A comparison of bone densitometry measurements of the central skeleton in postmenopausal women with and without vertebral fracture. Br J Radiol 68:747–753

26. Cann CE, Genant HK, Ettinger B, Gordan GS (1980) Spinal mineral loss in oophorectomized women. Determination by quantitative computed tomography. JAMA 244:2056–2059

27. Sandor T, Felsenberg D, Kalender WA, Glain A, Brown E (1992) Compact and trabecular components of the spine using quantitative computed tomography. Calcif Tissue Int 50:502–506

28. Mazess RB, Barden HS, Eberle RW, Drue Denton M (1995) Age changes of spine density in postero-anterior and lateral projections in normal women. Calcif Tissue Int 56:201–205

29. Hui S, Slemenda C, Johnston C, Appledorn C (1987) Effects of age and menopause on vertebral bone density. Bone Miner 2:141–146

30. Wimalawansa SJ (1995) Combined therapy with estrogen and etidronate has an additive effect on bone mineral density in the hip and vertebrae: four-year randomized study. Am J Med 99:36–42

31. Blake GM, Herd RJM, Fogelman I (1996) A longitudinal study of supine lateral DXA of the lumbar spine: a comparison with posteroanterior spine, hip and total-body DXA. Osteoporosis Int 6:462–470

32. Villareal DT, Rupich RC, Pacifici R, Griffin MG, Maggio D, Avioli LV, Civitelli R (1992) Effect of estrogen and calcitonin on vertebral bone density and vertebral height in osteoporotic women. Osteoporosis Int 2:70–73

33. Genant HK, Symons J, Rowan J, Speroff L (1996) The effect of continuous HRT on spinal trabecular bone mineral density. Osteoporosis Int 6 [Suppl 1]:227

34. Orwoll E, Oviatt S, Mann T (1990) The impact of osteophytic and vascular calcifications on vertebral mineral density measurements in men. J Clin Endocrinol Metab 70:1202–1207

35. Reid I, Evans M, Ames R, Wattie D (1991) The influence of osteophytes and aortic calcification on spinal mineral density in postmenopausal women. J Clin Endocrinol Metab 72:1372–1374

36. Drinka PJ, DeSmet AA, Bauwens SF, Rogot A (1992) The effect of overlying calcification on lumbar bone densitometry. Calcif Tissue Int 50:507–510

37. Ito M, Hayashi K, Yamada M, Uetani M, Nakamura T (1993) Relationship of osteophytes to bone mineral density and spinal fracture in men. Radiology 189:497–502

38. Franck H, Munz M, Scherrer M (1995) Evaluation of dual-energy X-ray absorptiometry bone mineral measurement – comparison of a single-beam and fan-beam design: the effect of osteophytic calcification on spine bone mineral density. Calcif Tissue Int 56:192–195

39. Yu W, Gluer CC, Fuerst T, Grampp S, Li J, Lu Y, Genant HK (1995) Influence of degenerative joint disease on spinal bone mineral measurements in postmenopausal women. Calcif Tissue Int 57:169–174

40. Dequeker J (1985) The relationship between osteoporosis and osteoarthritis. Clin Rheum Dis 11:271–296

41. Myers BS, Arbogast KB, Lobaugh B, Harper KD, Richardson WJ, Drezner MK (1994) Improved assessment of lumbar vertebral body strength using supine lateral dual-energy X-ray absorptiometry. J Bone Miner Res 9:687–693

42. Moro M, Hecker AT, Bouxsein ML, Myers ER (1995) Failure load of thoracic vertebrae correlates with lumbar bone mineral density measured by DXA. Calcif Tissue Int 56:206–209

43. Tabensky AD, Williams J, Deluca V, Briganti E, Seeman E (1996) Bone mass, areal, and volumetric bone density are equally accurate, sensitive and specific surrogates of the breaking strength of the vertebral body: an in vitro study. J Bone Miner Res 11:1981–1988

44. Bjarnason K, Hassager C, Svendsen OL, Stang H, Christiansen C (1996) Anteroposterior and lateral spinal DXA for the assessment of vertebral body strength: comparison with hip and forearm measurement. Osteoporosis Int 6:37–42

45. Eriksson SA, Isberg BO, Lindgren JU (1989) Prediction of vertebral strength by dual photon absorptiometry and quantitative computed tomography. Calcif Tissue Int 44:243–250

46. Mosekilde L, Bentzen SM, Ortoft G, Jorgensen J (1989) The predictive value of quantitative computed tomography for vertebral body compressive strength and ash density. Bone 10:465–470

47. Singer K, Edmondston S, Day R, Breidahl P, Price R (1995) Prediction of thoracic and lumbar vertebral body compressive strength: correlations with bone mineral density and vertebral region. Bone 17:167–174

48. Peel NFA, Eastell R (1994) Diagnostic value of estimated volumetric bone mineral density of the lumbar spine in osteoporosis. J Bone Miner Res 9:317–320

49. Bjarnason K, Nilas L, Hassager C, Christiansen C (1995) Dual energy X-ray absorptiometry of the spine-decubitus lateral versus anteroposterior projection in osteoporotic women: comparison to single energy X-ray absorptiometry of the forearm. Bone 16:255–260

50. Lafferty FW, Rowland DY (1996) Correlations of dual-energy X-ray absorptiometry, quantitative computed tomography, and single photon absorptiometry with spinal and non-spinal fractures. Osteoporosis Int 6:407–415

51. Grampp S, Genant HK, Mathur A, Lang P, Jergas M, Takada M, Glüer CC, Lu Y, Chavez M (1997) Comparisons of non-invasive bone mineral measurements in assessing age-related loss, fracture discrimination, and diagnostic classification. J Bone Miner Res (in press)

52. Tothill P, Pye DW (1992) Errors due to non-uniform distribution of fat in dual X-ray absorptiometry of the lumbar spine. Br J Radiol 65:807–813

53. Tothill P, Avenell A (1994) Error in dual energy X-ray absorptiometry of the lumbar spine owing to fat distribution and soft tissue thickness during weight change. Br J Radiol 67:71–75

54. Carter DR, Bouxsein ML, Marcus R (1992) New approaches for interpreting projected bone densitometry data. J Bone Miner Res 7:137–145

19 Quantitative Ultrasound for Assessing Bone Properties

D. Hans, T. Fuerst, G. Guglielmi, and H. K. Genant

Introduction

Osteoporosis is a systemic skeletal disease characterized by low bone mass and structural deterioration of bone tissue, with a consequent decrease in the mechanical competence of bone and thus an increase in the susceptibility to fracture [1]. It most commonly presents as vertebral fractures. Colle's fractures of the forearm and low-trauma fractures at other sites are also associated with this disease. However, the most severe complications of osteoporosis are hip fractures. Today the lifetime risk of hip fracture for a 50-year old woman is about 18% [2], and the continuing rise in life expectancy is expected to cause a threefold rise in worldwide fracture incidence over the next 60 years [2]. It is clear that osteoporosis represents a major worldwide public health problem that will grow in importance in the coming decades as the population ages. The associated increase in the financial burden to the public health system is an additional concern. In the United States alone the combined public health costs from osteoporosis were 10 billion dollars in 1989 [3–5]. Such forecasts have lead to the search for new, cost-effective methods for early detection, prevention, and treatment.

As fracture is the principal outcome of osteoporosis, understanding of the determinants of fracture risk is crucial. Intrinsic bone strength is one important determinant and is influenced by bone mineral density (BMD) and bone structure, which includes both bone size and shape and the microarchitectural characteristics of bone. In addition to these internal factors, the external forces applied to a bone are also important. For example, in the case of hip fracture the frequency and dynamics of falls is an important determinant of hip fracture risk [6–8]. Melton et al. [9] have shown that the incidence of hip fracture is inversely related to femoral bone density, and, in a recent prospective study, a decrease of 1 SD of the hip BMD was associated with a two- to three-fold increase in the risk of hip fractures. These data indicate that BMD is a strong predictor of hip fracture risk.

However, age-related bone loss does not completely explain the increasing incidence of hip fracture with age, since after the age of 65 years the BMD-adjusted risk of hip fracture increases by a factor of about two per decade [10]. Furthermore, although patients with hip fracture have a lower bone density than controls, there is a large overlap in bone density between women with fracture and age- and sex-matched controls [3, 9]. BMD explains only about 70%–75% of the variance in strength, while the remaining variance could be due to other factors such as accumulated fatigue damage, inferior bone microarchitecture and the state of bone remodeling [11, 12]. Bone architecture refers to the three-dimensional arrangement of trabecular struts. The architecture of bone may be defined by a combination of porosity (volume fraction), connectivity (degree of connection of trabecular fibers), and anisotropy (orientational dependence of connectivity) [13].

Because of the importance of BMD in determining bone strength, many non-invasive techniques based on the attenuation of ionizing radiation have been developed to quantify BMD in the axial and peripheral skeleton. These include single-photon absorptiometry (SPA), single X-ray absorptiometry (SXA), dual X-ray absorptiometry (DXA), quantitative computed tomography (QCT) and peripheral QCT (pQCT) [14]. These techniques vary in the source of ionizing radiation and in the skeletal site and bone envelope measured (cancellous or compact). While they are effective for determining BMD, they represent relatively expensive approaches that give limited information on bone structure [15]. Since microfractures and bone architectural changes may also play a role in the process of bone weakening [3, 16], it is possible that information on bone elasticity and structure combined with density will allow better discrimination of individuals at risk for osteoporotic fracture than techniques which measure density alone. An ideal diagnostic tool should detect fragility, whatever its basis, and not merely decreased bone mass and in addition should be inexpensive and free of ionizing radiation.

Ultrasound, which has been used with success in industry as a nondestructive test to evaluate structural integrity and mechanical competence, has recently been applied to bone assessment. Early experience suggested that ultrasound provides information not only about bone density but also about architecture and elasticity [17, 18]. This association with determinants of bone strength led to the development of several applications of ultrasound to the assessment of bone. Collectively these techniques are referred to as quantitative ultrasound (QUS). The clinical application of this technology to osteoporosis with the specific goal of predicting fracture risk is being investigated. While several devices are now commercially available, registration with the United States Food and Drug Administration is still pending. This technique is thus used for research in the United States, and most of the devices in clinical use are distributed throughout Europe, Asia, and other countries of the Pacific Rim.

Quantitative Ultrasound Parameters

As with sound itself, ultrasound is a mechanical wave. The difference is that the ultrasound frequencies (extending from 20 kHz to 100 MHz) lie above the human audible range. The mechanical energy is transmitted through the specimen and reaches the opposite side. As the mechanical energy of the ultrasound wave interacts with the bone, the cortex and the trabecular network vibrate on a microscale. The shape, intensity, and speed of the wave are progressively altered during its propagation through the bone. The bone tissue may therefore be characterized in terms of ultrasound velocity and attenuation. Because the material and structural properties of bone affect the velocity and attenuation of ultrasound signals, the assessment of QUS parameters should allow one to deduce the mechanical properties of bone which in turn are important determinants of whole bone stiffness, failure load, and consequently fracture risk [19–23].

Attenuation and Broadband Ultrasound Attenuation

As an ultrasound beam passes through a material, some of its energy is lost. This phenomenon is known as attenuation. The intensity of a plane wave decreases with distance exponentially in much the same way as ionizing radiation. Moreover, the attenuation of ultrasound signal depends not only on the properties of the transmission medium but also on the frequency of the ultrasound wave. Thus analogous to the equation used to describe X-ray attenuation, we can describe ultrasound attenuation by:

$$I(x) = I_0 e^{-\mu(f)\,x}$$

where $\mu(f)$ is the frequency (f) dependent attenuation coefficient (dB/cm), I_0 is the incident signal intensity, and $I(x)$ is the intensity at a distance x.

The decrease in ultrasound beam intensity results from classical wave phenomena such as diffraction (beam spreading), scattering, energy absorption, and mode conversion [24, 25]. The predominant attenuation mechanism in cancellous bone is scattering, while absorption predominates in cortical bone. Absorption is the dissipation of ultrasound energy in the medium via conversion to heat, due main-

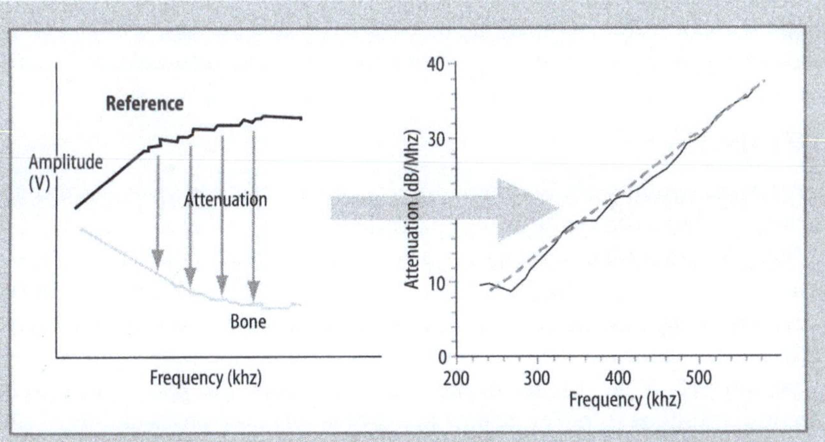

Fig. 19-1 BUA measurement by the substitution method described by Langton et al. The increase in attenuation as a function of frequency is measured by comparing the amplitude spectrum for a reference material with that for the measured sample. The slope of attenuation (BUA) in dB/MHz is given by linear regression of the spectral amplitude difference

ly to internal molecular friction. Scattering effects occur when particles absorb part of the ultrasound energy and reradiate it in new directions. The amount of scattering depends primarily on the ratio of ultrasound wavelength to the size of the scattering particle and on the acoustic impedance of the scattering particle [24, 26, 27].

In the frequency range of 0.1–1 MHz that is most useful for bone characterization, the total attenuation (expressed on a logarithmic scale) is linearly related to frequency. In clinical practice the slope of attenuation as a function of frequency has become known as broadband ultrasound attenuation (BUA). No theoretical relationship between ultrasound attenuation and the mechanical properties of cancellous bone has been established. The clinical systems that measure BUA have adopted the substitution method described by Langton et al. [28]. The relationship between attenuation and frequency is measured by comparing the amplitude spectrum for a reference medium with that for the measured sample. The slope of attenuation versus frequency (BUA) in dB/MHz is given by linear regression of the spectral amplitude difference (see Fig. 19-1).

Velocity of Ultrasound

The velocity of ultrasound wave propagation or speed of sound (SOS) through bone is determined by dividing the distance traversed (e.g., bone diameter or length) by the transit time. The resulting velocity is expressed in meters per second; this depends on the mechanical properties of the medium through which it is propagating and its mode of propagation. Longitudinal waves are the common mode of ultrasound propagation through tissue. High-elastic modulus materials such as bone can support additional propagation modes such as shear waves. The complex nature of bone (anisotropic, heterogeneous, dispersive) make it difficult to model the relationship between the mechanical properties of the bone and the velocity. Nevertheless, as a first approach and under certain conditions, SOS can be related to the mechanical properties of a material by the equation:

$$SOS = (E/\rho)^{1/2}$$

where E is the modulus of elasticity (a measure of resistance to deformation), and ρ is the physical density of the bone [24–26].

Clinically, velocity measurement may be achieved by either reflection or transmission techniques using large diameter (about 19 mm) piezoelectric transducers [25, 27]. The reflection technique uses a single transducer to transmit and receive the signal. The generated ultrasound pulse travels through the sample and is reflected at an interface to be detected by the same transducer. The disadvantage of the reflection technique is the low signal intensity of reflected waves and the resulting difficulty in making accurate measurements of velocity or attenuation. In the transmission method one transducer acts as the transmitter and the other as the receiver detecting ultrasound signals after transmission through bone. For application to the skeleton the transmission technique is most commonly used.

In the clinical application of ultrasound velocity measurements, there is no convention for the use of terms or for the velocity measurement method. For example, SOS, velocity of sound, apparent velocity of ultrasound (AVU) and ultrasound transmission velocity (UTV) all refer to the same generic ultrasound measurement. For the calcaneus three different methods of calculating velocity have been utilized, resulting in the limb (heel) velocity (calcaneus plus soft tissue), bone velocity (calcaneus only) and time-of-flight velocity (TOF; between transducers positioned at a fixed distance). In clinical measurements the TOF velocity method assumes a constant heel thickness and therefore the velocity measured depends upon heel width [28, 29]. The three velocity calculations yield slightly different values but are correlated strongly with each other. Miller et al. [30] showed that TOF had the best precision (coefficient of variation, CV=0.7 %) but the smallest dynamic range. On the other hand, bone velocity had the largest dynamic range, a factor that enhances its sensitivity, but suffered from the poorest precision (CV=2.7 %). Precision was reduced in the bone velocity measurement because of errors in the measurement of the width of the calcaneus.

Composite Parameter

BUA and SOS are moderately associated, with correlation coefficients around 0.7. This moderate correlation suggests they are influenced by somewhat different properties of bone. Two ultrasound equipment manufacturers, Lunar Corporation (Madison, Wisc.) and Hologic Inc. (Waltham, Mass.), have chosen to combine BUA and SOS mathematically to create a calculated variable named "stiffness" (which should not be confused with the biomechanical term) and quantitative ultrasound index (QUI), respectively. The goal in formulating these composite parameters was to combine the diagnositic information of each measurement into a single more powerful parameter and to improve the precision of the BUA measurement. From the point of view of clinical evaluation a single parameter such as "stiffness" or QUI which combines attenuation and velocity can simplify interpretation.

Quantitative Ultrasound Equipment

The first QUS devices were introduced in the late 1980s and measured velocity and attenuation in the heel. Since then more heel devices have been introduced, emulating the earlier designs and measuring equivalent parameters. With new models the manufacturers have introduced various improvements such as enhancing hardware performance, optimizing analysis algorithms or expanding capabilities (e.g., pediatric applications). Today the examination requires less time, and the initially poor reproducibility of BUA has been improved. However, precision is still the main limitation of the use of QUS in longitudinal studies. In addition to this variety of calcaneal devices, new systems have been developed to measure velocity at other skeletal sites including the tibia and phalanges. In general terms

Table 19-1 Different approaches and types of equipment for bone assessment with quantitative ultrasound

Device	Coupling medium	Parameter	Precision (CV, %)	Comments
Calcaneal single, scanning point QUS systems				
Walker Sonix UBA	Water	BUA	2.0%–5.0%	No longer in production
575+	Water	SOS	0.2%–0.6%	Bone velocity
Calcaneal single, fixed point QUS systems				
Lunar Achilles Plus	Heated Water	BUA	0.8%–2.5%	
	Heated Water	SOS	0.2%–0.4%	Time-of-flight velocity
	Heated Water	Stiffness	1.0%–2.0%	Heel width "constant"
McCue CUBA Clinical	Gel	BUA	1.5%–4.0%	Heel velocity
	Gel	SOS	0.2%–0.6%	
Hologic Sahara	Gel	BUA	0.8%–2.5%	
	Gel	SOS	0.2%–0.4%	
	Gel	QUI	1.0%–2.0%	Heel velocity
Calcaneal imaging QUS systems				
DMS UBIS 3000	Water	BUA	0.8%–2.5%	Imaging system
	Water	SOS	0.2%–0.4%	
Osteometer DTU-1	Water	BUA	0.8%–2.5%	Imaging system
	Water	SOS	0.2%–0.4%	
Tibial QUS system				
Myriad Soundscan 2000	Gel	SOS	0.2%–1.0%	Cortical Bone, soft tissue correction
Phalangeal QUS system				
IGEA DBM Sonic 1200	Gel	Ad-SOS	0.5%–1.0%	Amplitude dependent velocity

the commercial QUS devices introduced show a greater technological diversity than bone densitometry equipment. Furthermore, various ultrasound technologies assess different parameters [BUA, SOS, V_{bone}, stiffness, UBI, amplitude-dependent SOS (ad-SOS), and others] and may not measure the same anatomical site (heel, tibia, phalanges). This certainly reflects a strength of QUS but it also represents a challenge for the evaluation of the various devices. Positive results for fracture risk prediction obtained on one device cannot necessarily be directly translated into performance statements of other, technologically different QUS systems. The following groups of approaches and equipment have been developed into commercial systems [19] (see also Table 19-1).

Calcaneus

The calcaneus is the most popular QUS measurement site for several reasons. From a clinical perspective the calcaneus has a high proportion of cancellous bone, nearly 90%. Age-related changes in bone metabolism are first manifested in cancellous bone because of its higher metabolic turnover rate than compact bone [31]. Thus the calcaneus should be a sensitive indicator of skeletal status. Measurement of BMD in the calcaneus has been demonstrated to be a very good pre-

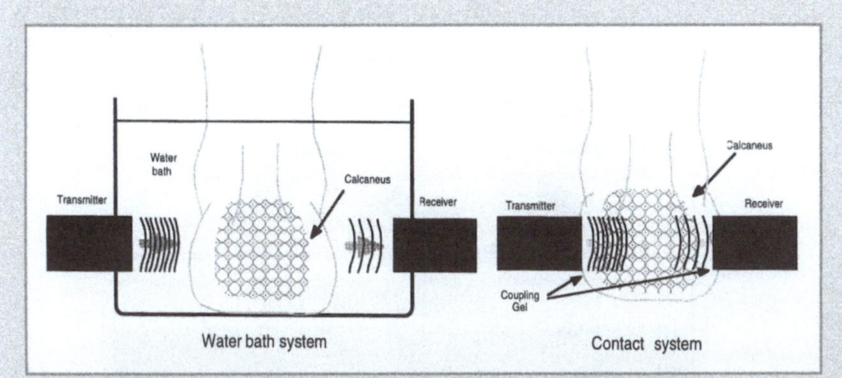

Fig. 19-2 Calcaneal fixed-single point transmission systems employing either water-based foot placement (left) or coupling by means of ultrasound gel (right)

dictor of fracture risk in perimenopausal [32] and older women [33], comparing well with measurement of the femur itself. From a technical perspective the calcaneus is easily accessible with little overlying soft tissue, an important requirement for accurate ultrasound evaluation. Furthermore, the mediolateral surfaces of the bone are fairly flat and parallel, providing good ultrasound transmission properties.

Calcaneal Single, Fixed-Point Systems. These represent the first generation in heel systems and measure BUA and SOS in the mediolateral direction by transmission at a single, fixed point in the calcaneus (See Fig. 19-2). These devices employ either a waterbath for acoustic coupling [34, 35] or couple to the heel by means of ultrasound gel [36]. The latter systems are sometimes called dry systems. The advantage of these single, fixed-point systems is that they are inexpensive, fast, and easy to use and are either portable or transportable. The disadvantages include being blind measurement, and that the point of measurement is not adjustable from subject to subject. Thus the region of interest evaluated may not be correct or comparable across all patients.

Calcaneal Imaging Devices. These second-generation heel devices operate in transmission mode and provide BUA images of the heel that are obtained using a pair of focused transducers immersed in a room temperature water bath [37, 38]. The ultrasound beam (3–5 mm diameter) is scanned across the heel in 1-mm steps to image the entire calcaneus. The advantage of the image is that it allows measurement artifacts to be identified and avoided. Moreover the image permits the evaluation of standardized regions of interest in all patients as well as the use of larger regions of interest which may improve precision.

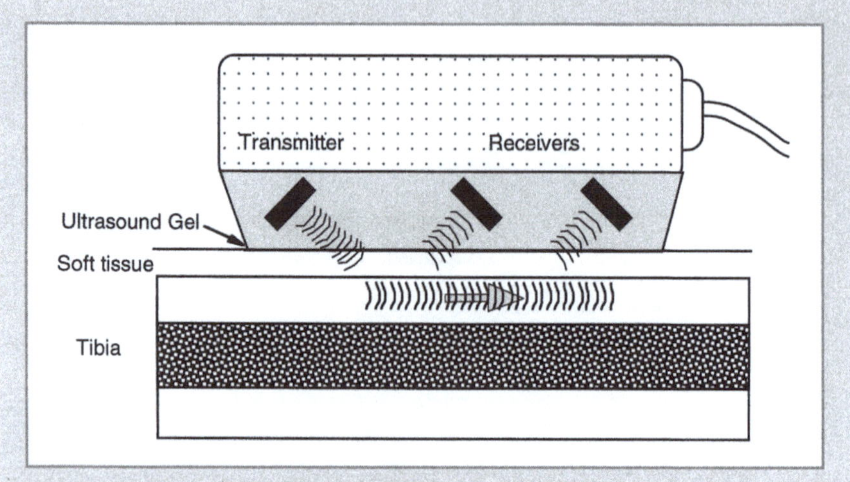

Fig. 19-3 Assessment of ultrasound velocity measurements of the tibial cortex using gel coupling. The system measures velocity longitudinally along the middle third of the anterior tibia

Tibia

Assessment of Ultrasound Velocity in the Tibial Cortex. This system differs from those previously mentioned in that it measures velocity longitudinally along the anterior aspect of the middle tibia [39–42]. The middle tibia was chosen because of its straight, smooth surface, again having little overlying tissue (see Fig. 19-3). Cortical bone accounts for 80% of the skeleton by mass. Osteoporosis manifests itself in both cortical and cancellous bone, although to a lesser degree. Nevertheless, cortical bone loss may play an important role in determining whole bone strength. This device is the only one which assesses a purely cortical site. The determinants of the velocity measurement (cortical density, thickness, or other property of bone) have not yet been established.

Finger Phalanges

Single-Point QUS Systems for Measurements at the Finger Phalanges. This method uses the transmission technique to measure amplitude dependent speed of sound (ad-SOS) through the proximal phalanges of the fingers [44–52] (See Fig. 19-4). The measurement site is the distal metaphysis of the first phalanx of the last four fingers. At this site the mediolateral surfaces are approximately parallel, reducing ultrasound scattering and allowing better transmission through the bone. In the metaphysis both cortical and trabecular bone are present. Both types of bone tissue are sensitive to age-related bone resorption. The number of trabeculae decreases and cortical bone becomes more porous with advancing age. In addition, the cortices of long bone become thinner because the rate of endosteal resorption

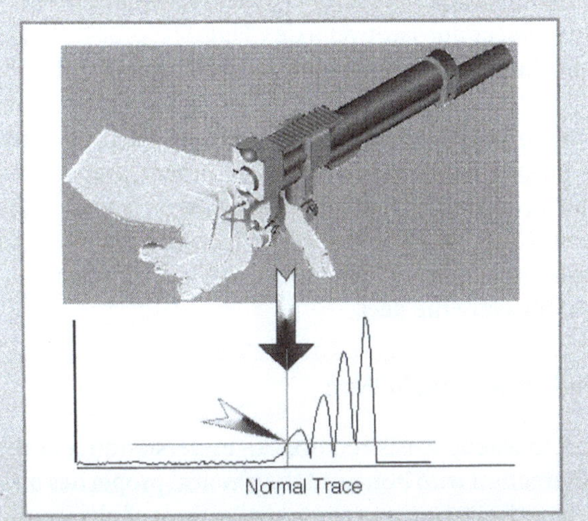

Fig. 19-4 Single-point QUS systems for measurements at the finger phalanges using gel coupling. This technique uses the transmission technique to measure amplitude-dependent ultrasound velocity through the proximal phalanges of the fingers. It is calculated by detecting the time of flight of the signal through the section of the finger. The related time instant corresponds to the first point of the signal overgoing the level of 2 mV

exceeds the rate of periosteal formation of bone. Taken together the age-related losses of cortical and cancellous bone substantially increase the fragility of bone. One study found that ad-SOS measurement in the phalanges of elderly women had greater percentage reduction from peak adult levels than other techniques such as QCT of the spine and DXA of the femoral neck and forearm and spine [53].

Other Skeletal Sites

In addition, a number of other ultrasound approaches including devices for measurements at the patella [54–56] and ulna (using a reflection technique) [57] have been described. Both approaches measured ultrasound velocity, by transmission at the patella and by reflection at the radius. While positive results were observed with both techniques, commercial systems are not currently available.

Quality Control of QUS Systems

As with radiation-based devices, QUS requires a strict quality control (QC) program. Typical changes in QUS parameters that occur with disease or treatment are small, only about 1% per year or less. As a result steps must be taken to ensure a device is accurate, precise, and stable. Each manufacturer has developed a QC program for its device and provides a test object for QC measurements. However, a universally applicable test object does not yet exist. Thus QC programs are specific to an instrument, and standardization across manufacturers is difficult to achieve.

Another aspect of QC is the proper training of the operator. Each operator should be well trained in the proper maintenance of the equipment, preparation of the patient, and patient positioning. Indeed, positioning error is one of the major sources of imprecision in QUS [58]. The devices to measure the tibia and phalanges require more operator training and experience to obtain precise measurements than the devices to measure the heel.

Investigation of Quantitative Ultrasound In Vitro

The application of ultrasound to osteoporosis requires an understanding of the mechanisms of ultrasound interaction with bone and the physical properties ultimately assessed. Theory and experience from previous applications of ultrasound indicate that QUS parameters are influenced by the mechanical properties of bone, which in turn are determined by bone's material (e.g., BMD) and structural properties (e.g., bone architecture). While these general statements can be made, the complexity of the interactions between sonic energy and bone tissue has prevented the development of useful theoretical models. Nevertheless many in vitro investigations have provided descriptive information offering some insight into the nature of ultrasound-bone interactions.

The first investigations of ultrasound applied to bone reported that attenuation and velocity parameters depend on BMD. Recent reports continue to confirm these initial findings [59–63]. Most investigations have been performed cross-sectionally, examining the QUS properties of specimens of trabecular bone with different density. However, from these studies it is unclear what role density and structure play in determining BUA and SOS. To answer this question two investigations used a demineralization technique to examine the relationship between QUS and BMD in the same specimens. Tavakoli and Evans [64] used acid to remove up to 20% of baseline bone mineral from sections of bovine trabecular bone in graded steps. They found a linear relationship between BMD and attenuation and velocity. Wu and coworkers [65] performed a similar study in cubes of bovine trabecular bone which they demineralized with formic acid. They measured BUA and BMD at various stages of demineralization. BUA was observed to decrease in a nonlinear fashion with continuing decalcification until all of the mineral had been removed. Differences in specimen geometry and degree of demineralization could account for the different results found in these investigations. Furthermore, it is unclear how well this demineralization procedure simulates the process which occurs in vivo. Despite these questions it is clear that BMD is positively related to both attenuation and velocity.

The strength of the relationship between QUS and density is reflected in the correlation coefficients reported by various investigators. In vitro studies of calcanei have reported correlations of R^2=0.59–0.88 between QUS and BMD measured by DXA or QCT [66–68]. Correlations are generally higher in vitro than in vivo, and this is perhaps due to the effects of soft tissue, acoustic coupling with the heel and differences in the regions of interest used for DXA and QUS. In vivo correlations with BMD are typically in the range of R^2=0.4–0.5 [69,70]. Thus only about half to three-quarters of the variance in BUA is explained by BMD. To varying degrees these studies suggest that some component of the QUS measurement is not explained by BMD and could reflect other properties of bone.

Evidence that these other properties may be structure related is found in the anisotropy of QUS parameters [71,72]. It has been shown that BUA measured in trabecular bone cubes depends on trabecular orientation, being 50% higher along the axis of compressive trabeculae, those principally responsible for weight bearing. This anistropy of BUA has been found in equine tarsal bones [73], bovine femora and radii [24,72,74], and human vertebrae [68] and calcanei [71]. Because the density of an individual cube is independent of the axis studied, any variation in ultrasound properties with orientation must be due to other factors. Trabecular structure is known to be anistropic and its relationship with QUS has been studied. Glüer et al. [74] measured in three orthogonal directions cubes of cancellous bone cut from fresh bovine proximal radii. The relative orientation of the trabeculae with respect to the direction of ultrasound beam was evaluated on high-resolution conventional radiographs employing a semiquantitative "alignment" score. They demonstrated that alignment shows significant association with BUA, indicating that BUA depends on trabecular orientation. Njeh et al. [24] have used permeability (a parameter that determines the rate of flow of fluid or gas through a porous medium such as cancellous bone) to quantify the structure of bovine and human cancellous samples. Two recent studies have used conventional histomorphometry to assess trabecular structure and its relationship to QUS. In agreement with the results described above, Bouxsein et al. [75] demonstrated an association between QUS and morphology in human calcaneal bone but did not test for independence from BMD. Hans et al. [76] reported similar results of a study of human calcanei in which they compared BMD, BUA, and SOS with histomorphometric parameters. However, Hans et al. found that after adjustment for BMD, none of the histomorphometric measures were related to BUA or SOS. This is in contrast to earlier work by Glüer et al. [72] who showed in bovine bone independent associations of SOS with trabecular separation and BUA with trabecular separation and connectivity. The use of a limited number of specimens, two-dimensional indices of bone architecture, and the severity of the statistical test used are potential criticisms of Hans' study, and additional investigation is required.

Attenuation and velocity are affected by the pathlength traversed in bone. Attenuation increases with pathlength as more energy is absorbed and scattered from the beam. Velocity should be independent of pathlength except when measured as TOF velocity. This is true even with the constant heel width adjustment made by the Lunar Achilles system. The effect of bone thickness has been investigated both in vitro [17, 24, 69, 77, 78] and in vivo [69, 79]. Serpe and Rho [77] and Njeh [24] reported a linear relationship between BUA and sample thickness in studies in vitro with bovine bone and phantoms, respectively. Wu et al. [69] investigated the impact of bone size using specimens of bovine trabecular bone. Comparison of attenuation in a whole specimen (width 24 mm) with the attenuation of the two halves (width 12 mm) showed that BUA was 32%–92% larger for the whole specimen than the mean of the corresponding halves. In addition, the BUA of the whole specimen was always less than the sum of the two halves, indicating that the association of bone size and BUA is complex and nonlinear. Other investigations have been performed in vivo. Hans et al. [28] investigated the relationship between QUS and various anthropometric parameters in 271 healthy women. After adjusting for age only heel width remained a significant predictor for SOS and weight for BUA. Wu et al. [69] measured BUA and the width of the calcaneus in 28 postmenopausal women and found a positive but statistically insignificant correlation between BUA and bone size. Kotzki et al. [29] found no significant correlation between heel width and BUA in situ. BUA therefore does not appear to depend substantially on bone size over the range of heel widths typically found in women. Moreover, an earlier study showed no improvement in the ability to discriminate women with vertebral fracture when BUA was normalized for calcaneus width [79]. Indeed, the impact of bone size on BUA in the clinical setting should be small, except where there is a marked variability of calcaneal bone width as in pediatric studies.

One of the promising charateristics of ultrasound as a mechanical wave is its relationship with the mechanical properties of bone. With the ultimate goal being the assessment of osteoporotic fracture risk, the relationship between QUS and bone strength is an important one. Several recent studies have investigated this relationship using mechanical testing [25, 75, 80, 81]. The results of these studies have shown that the mechanical properties (elastic modulus and ultimate strength) of trabecular bone specimens measured in vitro are well correlated with both BUA and SOS. The empirical data fit reasonably with the expected theoretical relationships. Moreover, the anisotropy of bone structure, which is detectable with ultrasound but not absorptiometry, is similarly reflected in the elastic modulus. In an important study of cadaveric specimens Bouxsein et al. [80] investigated the relationship between QUS at the heel and hip fracture. Their results showed that BUA and SOS in the calcaneus are good predictors of femoral failure loads (R^2=0.51 and 0.40, respectively). The QUS parameters were slightly inferior to those of calcaneus BMD (R^2=0.63) and femoral neck BMD (R^2=0.79). These studies confirm the validity of QUS for bone strength assessment and its utility for fracture risk prediction.

Investigation of Quantitative Ultrasound In Vivo

As an emerging alternative to photon absorptiometry techniques there is growing interest in the use of QUS measurements for the noninvasive assessment of osteoporotic fracture risk in the management of osteoporosis. If the relationships of

QUS with bone mass, structure, and strength are confirmed in vivo in a clinical population, there will be strong evidence that ultrasound is a useful tool in the clinical assessment of osteoporosis. Measurements in vivo have established normative data and the patterns of change in BUA and SOS that occur with aging. Studies have also been conducted to investigate the ability of ultrasound to discriminate patients with osteoporotic fracture from age-matched controls and to predict future fracture risk.

Precision and Sensitivity

Measurement precision varies depending upon the parameter measured, the site, and the system. Many authors have investigated short-term precision of QUS measurement [39, 82–87] (see Table 19-1). Precision of BUA measurements (expressed as percentage coefficient of variation) ranges from 2% to 5% while precision of velocity measured at the heel, tibia, phalanges, or patella is typically 0.5%–1.5%. The apparent superior precision of velocity may be misleading because it does not take into account the range of values seen across subjects or the sensitivity of velocity to skeletal changes [84–86]. Both precision and sensitivity are affected by the measurement site and the measurement technique. In an effort to standardize the precision of QUS devices and parameters two methods have been proposed. One method normalizes precision (CV) by dividing it by the percentage standard deviation of the variability across subjects (i.e., population standard deviation divided by the population mean). A larger population standard deviation suggests a larger difference between health and disease, making discrimination of patients easier. In assessing the suitability of a measurement technique to monitor changes the ratio of precision and sensitivity is important. This is a second method of standardizing precision; CV divided by the annual percentage change in the parameter with age or treatment. Using the first method of standardization, QUS parameters appear to be comparable and similar to but slightly poorer than DXA of the spine or femoral neck [41].

The relatively modest precision of QUS can be explained in part by the effect of soft tissue, acoustic coupling, and repositioning errors which affect the region of interest measured. Foot positioning is critical in the QUS measurement of the heel due to the inhomogeneity of the calcaneus. One study of the factors influencing precision has shown that rotation of the foot about the axis of the leg and translation in the heel-toe direction have the greatest effect on BUA measurement [58]. Other factors include immersion time of foot in the water bath, water depth, and water temperature.

QUS and Bone Mineral Density

Early investigations of QUS showed a dependence of attenuation and velocity parameters on BMD. Many investigators have reported the association of BUA and velocity with BMD measured by DXA or QCT at the spine, femur, forearm, and calcaneus. Investigators have reported only linear relationships, with correlation coefficients ranging from approximately 0.3 to 0.9 for both BUA and SOS [59–63, 88–90]. Site-matched comparisons of BMD and QUS measurements have produced correlations of about 0.7 [89, 90]. From these results it appears that only 50% of the variability of QUS measurements can be explained by BMD. The remainder may be determined by other properties of bone related to bone strength, which appears to be supported by in vitro investigations. The moderate correlation may also in part be due to measurement errors associated with both techniques.

Age-Related Change

Numerous cross-sectional studies of ultrasound normative data have been reported [62, 85–86, 91, 92]. These all show that QUS parameters are inversely correlated with age, showing a significant decrease in both BUA and SOS especially after the menopause. Before this age both BUA and SOS are relatively stable, although two studies have shown steady declines from the age of 20 years [87, 92]. Typical rates of change are 0.5–1.0 dB/MHz (0.5%–1.0%) per year for BUA and 1–5 m/s (0.1%–0.3%) per year for SOS at the heel, patella, and tibia. However, there are substantial differences between different devices. The first longitudinal study was performed by Schott et al. [93] on 140 healthy postmenopausal women measured at the calcaneus. The decrease that they observed over 2 years was 1.0% ± 4.3% for BUA and 0.8% ± 0.6% for SOS. The decrease in SOS was significantly greater soon after menopause compared to later in life. A similar trend was observed for BUA, but this did not reach statistical significance. Similar results have been found by Krieg et al. in institutionalized elderly women [94].

Quantitative Ultrasound and Osteoporotic Fracture Risk

The ultimate test of the clinical utility of QUS is its association with osteoporotic fracture risk. Many early cross-sectional [61, 63, 70, 83] studies have demonstrated that QUS can be used to discriminate normal from osteoporotic subject groups as well as traditional bone densitometry approaches. While these retrospective studies of cases and controls are useful, more important prospective studies [34–35, 54, 60, 95] of osteoporotic fracture have shown the ability of calcaneal, patellar, and tibial QUS to predict fracture risk. In the case of heel measurement this ability is of the same power as absorptiometric approaches and in some cases has been found to be independent of bone mass.

As the oldest technique, the majority of investigations have been made with QUS at the calcaneus. Associations with prevalent fracture have been found with the three most common osteoporotic fracture types: hip [63, 70, 82, 83, 96] vertebral [59–61, 70, 97–99], and forearm [100, 101] fractures. With the exception of the report by Stewart et al. [98] BUA and velocity have been reported to be as sensitive as spine or femur BMD to discriminate between normal subjects and patients with vertebral fracture. The results of logistic regression analyses indicate that risk of fracture (expressed as odds ratios) increases approximately 1.5- to 2.5-fold for each decrease of 1 SD in BUA or SOS at the calcaneus. This makes heel QUS comparable to but slightly lower than X-ray absorptiometry techniques which typically have odds ratios of 1.5–3.0 depending on the measurement site and the population studied.

Studies of similar design have found comparable results for velocity measurements at the patella [55, 56], tibia [39, 40, 42, 86, 102], and phalanges [44, 48, 103]. Association with prevalent vertebral fracture has been demonstrated for all three techniques. A large study of tibial SOS in 4175 women over age 65 found weak but significant associations with prevalent hip, vertebral, and forearm fractures (odds ratios of 1.1–1.2) [102]. This association disappeared after adjustment of SOS for spine or femoral neck BMD. Another study, conducted by Orgee et al. [39], reported a statistically significant difference in tibia velocity between normal patients and those with vertebral osteoporosis. In other studies the association between tibial SOS and prevalent vertebral fracture did not reach statistical significance [55, 62]. The study by Stegman et al. demonstrated that tibial SOS was significantly associated with low-energy appendicular fractures (odds ratios of 1.7 and 1.9 in women and men, respectively), performing as well as forearm bone densitometry [55]. In one report of 11 women with recent hip fracture, tibial SOS was significantly lower in fractured cases than in age-matched controls [86]. Velocity of ultrasound in the patella has been associated with low-energy appendicular fractures in men but not women [55]. Positive studies have also been reported at the phalanges. Guglielmi et al. [44] have highlighted the discrimination capability of ultrasound at phanlanges showing that both Z score and T score are lower in osteoporotic subjects than in controls. These results have been confirmed by Alenfeld et al. [48]. In general, few peer-reviewed data currently exist for velocity measured at these other skeletal sites, and larger prospective studies are needed to evaluate these methods more thoroughly.

Prospective studies are required to confirm the ability of a measurement to predict fracture risk. Porter et al. demonstrated for the first time the predictive power of BUA in a prospective study on hip fractures in postmenopausal women [95]. However, the statistical analysis did not quantify the fracture risk associated with decreased BUA. Recently two large prospective studies of hip fracture have been reported. The EPIDOS study conducted in France involved 7598 very elderly women (mean age 81 ± 4 years) who experienced 115 hip fractures during 2 years of follow-up [34]. Data from this study indicated that velocity and BUA measured at the calcaneus have the same diagnostic sensitivity as femoral neck BMD in predicting hip fractures in an age- and weight-adjusted model (see Table 19-2). In this population hip fracture risk increased 2.0-fold for each standard deviation decrease in femoral neck BMD or heel SOS. Relative risk was 2.2 per 1-SD reduction in heel BUA. After adjusting BUA and SOS for neck BMD logistic regression showed that both ultrasound parameters were still significant, independent predictors of hip fracture. In the Study of Osteoporotic Fractures (SOF) conducted in the US, Bauer et al. [35] followed 6183 elderly women (mean age 76±5) for an

Table 19-2 Relative risk (95% confidence interval) of hip fracture for a one standard deviation reduction in ultrasound and densitometric parameters according to the type of fracture in the EPIDOS and SOF studies

	All hip fracture	Cervical hip fracture	Trochanteric hip fracture
EPIDOS study			
BUA (dB/MHz)	2.0 (1.6–2.4)	1.6 (1.2–2.2)	2.9 (2.1–4.0)
SOS (m/s)	1.7 (1.4–2.1)	1.3 (1.0–1.7)	2.5 (1.8–3.5)
Femoral neck BMD (g/cm^2)	1.9 (1.6–2.4)	2.0 (1.5–2.7)	2.4 (1.7–3.4)
BUA adjusted by femoral neck BMD, age and center	1.7 (1.4–2.2)	1.4 (0.9, 1.8)	2.4 (1.6, 3.7)
SOF study			
BUA (dB/MHz)	2.0 (1.5, 2.7)	1.3 (0.9, 2.0)	3.3 (2.0, 5.5)
Calcaneal BMD (g/cm^2)	2.2 (1.9, 3.0)	1.4 (0.9, 2.1)	3.4 (2.1, 5.1)
Femoral neck BMD (g/cm^2)	2.6 (1.9, 3.8)	2.0 (1.2, 3.1)	3.9 (2.3, 6.8)
BUA adjusted by calcaneal BMD, age and clinic	1.3 (0.8, 2.1)	1.1 (0.6, 1.9)	1.8 (0.9, 3.7)
BUA adjusted by femoral neck BMD, age and clinic	1.5 (1.0, 2.1)	1.1 (0.7, 1.6)	2.7 (1.5, 5.0)

average of 2 years during which 54 women suffered a hip fracture. The age-adjusted relative risk of hip fracture was 2.0, 2.2, and 2.6 for heel BUA, heel BMD, and femoral neck BMD (see Table 19-2). As in the EPIDOS study, the associations between BUA and hip fracture remained significant after adjustment for hip BMD but were no longer significant after adjustment for calcaneal BMD. It is worth noting these two studies were carried out using two different ultrasound and DXA systems, the Lunar Achilles and DPX systems in the EPIDOS study and Walker Sonix UBA575 and Hologic QDR systems in the SOF study.

To our knowledge, only one prospective study of velocity at other skeletal sites besides the heel has been reported. Heaney et al. [54] confirmed the ability of ultrasound velocity at the patella to predict vertebral fractures in a 2-year prospective study.

QUS and Type of Hip Fracture

Two cross-sectional studies of hip fractures investigated the association of BUA with the type of fracture (trochanteric versus cervical). Both performed measurements within 2 weeks of the fracture event. Schott et al. [63] evaluated 43 hip fracture cases and 86 age-matched-controls. They reported significantly lower BUA in cases of trochanteric fracture than in those of cervical fracture, suggesting that the two types of fractures correspond to different processes. Because both the calcaneus and trochanter are composed primarily of trabecular bone, a better association with trochanteric fractures may be expected. In contrast, a study by Dretakis et al. showed no significant difference in BUA between 78 subjects with trochanteric (45) or cervical (33) hip fractures [96]. The two large prospective studies described above confirmed the results of Schott et al. In the EPIDOS study population (62 cervical and 53 trochanteric fractures) Hans et al. [104] found that for BUA and SOS of the heel the relative risk for trochanteric fracture was nearly twice that for cervical fractures (see Table 19-2). Relative risk predicted by femoral neck BMD did not differ significantly between fracture types. They also found that controlling for femoral neck or trochanteric BMD did not affect the significance of the associations between BUA parameters and the risk of cervical or trochanteric fracture whereas SOS was no longer significant for cervical fracture. This confirmed earlier studies by Bauer et al. [35] who found that the association between BUA and trochanteric fractures is stronger (RR=3.3, CI: 2.0, 5.5) than that observed between BUA and femoral neck fractures (RR=1.3, CI: 0.9, 2.0). In models with both femoral neck BMD and BUA each remained significantly associated with the risk of trochanteric fracture (RR=2.4, CI: 1.3, 4.2 for BUA, and RR=2.7, CI: 1.5, 5.0 for femoral neck BMD; see Table 19-2). These findings suggest that the principle subtypes of hip fractures have different causes, but the physiological and clinical significance of these differences remains uncertain.

Combining QUS and DXA to Improve Fracture Prediction

Whether combining QUS and DXA improves fracture prediction is still unclear and needs further analysis and studies. The studies which have attempted to answer this question have reported some conflicting results.

With regard to hip fracture Hans et al. [34] combined calcaneal BUA identified as the most density-independent parameter with femoral neck BMD (Fig. 19-5). They found that the incidence of hip fracture among women who were above the median for both BUA and femoral neck BMD was 2.7 per 1000 woman-years compared to 19.6 per 1000 woman-years among women who were below the median for both measurements. When only BUA or BMD was low, hip fracture incidence was 6.2 and 11.8 per 1000 woman-years, respectively. They also investigated the combination of both BUA and BMD according to the type of fracture [104]. These results showed that combination of femoral neck BMD and BUA did not improve the detection of women at high risk of cervical fracture whereas this combination is beneficial for predicting trochanteric fracture. They concluded that the use of both methods slightly increases the identification of women at very high risk only of trochanteric hip fracture (see Fig. 19-5). In the other hand, Bauer et al. [35], reported from the SOF study that for BUA alone the relative risk of hip fracture comparing the highest risk quartile to the lower three quartiles was 2.5 (95% CI: 1.3, 4.9), for femoral neck BMD alone the relative risk was 4.5 (CI: 2.4, 8.4), and for the combination of BUA and femoral neck BMD the relative risk was 5.0 (CI: 2.7, 9.5). They concluded the combination of BUA and BMD has little or no important clinical advantage over femoral neck BMD alone (see Fig. 19-6).

Two studies have examined improving vertebral fracture prediction by combining QUS with DXA. Bauer et al. [70] revealed an increased risk of vertebral fracture across tertiles of both BUA and BMD spine. The prevalence of vertebral

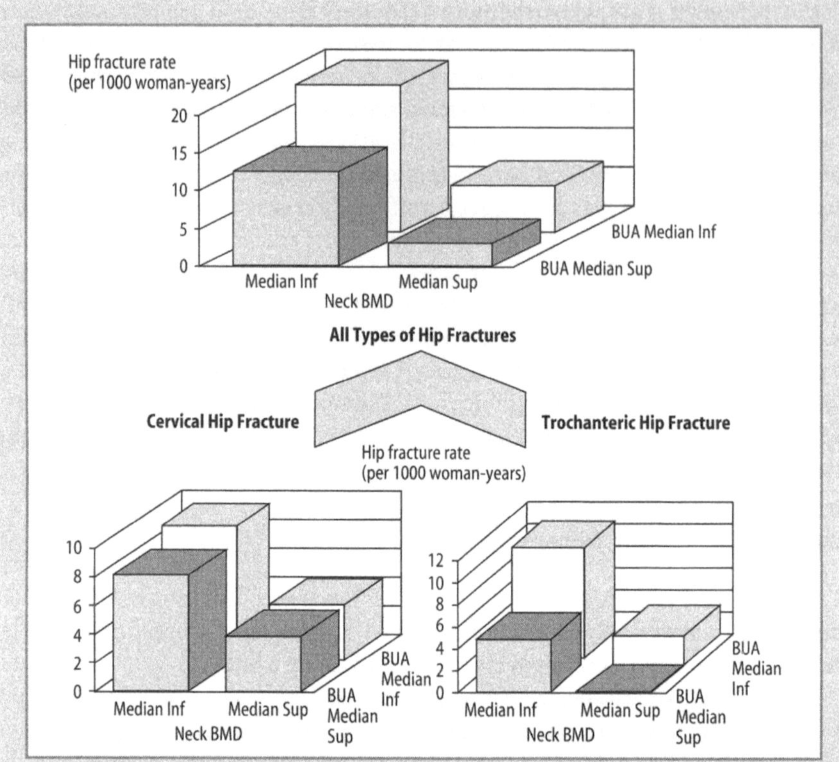

Fig. 19-5 Incidence of hip fracture (per 1000 woman-years) as a function of calcaneal BUA and femoral neck BMD median according to the type of fracture

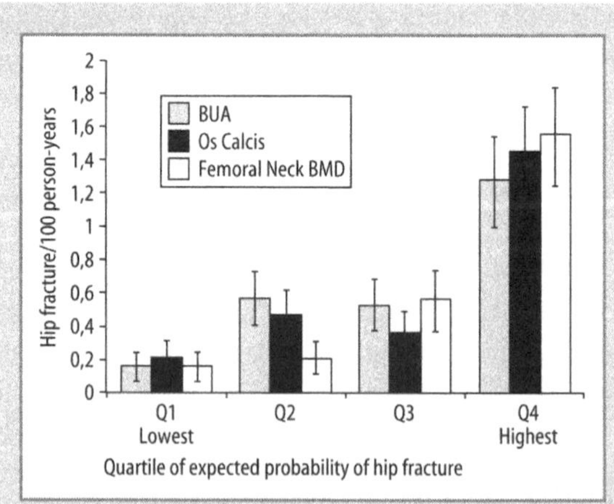

Fig. 19-6 Risk of hip fracture in the SOF study predicted by measurement of BUA, BMD of the os calcis, and femoral neck BMD. The total number of hip fractures is 48

fracture was four times higher among women in the lowest tertile of both BUA and spine BMD than among those in the highest tertile for this measurement. Similarly, Glüer et al. [105], using receiver-operating characteristic curve analysis on cross-sectional data concluded that combined measurements improved sensitivity and specificity.

QUS and Longitudinal Monitoring During Intervention

Another application of QUS is for the monitoring of changes in the skeleton that occur with disease or result from various interventions. Because of the relationship between QUS and bone density, interventions which affect BMD can also be expected to influence attenuation and velocity. Only a few studies documenting longitudinal changes in QUS parameters have been reported. The study by Schott et al. [93] discussed above followed 140 women for 2 years to measure changes in BUA and SOS that occur with aging and observed annual decreases of 0.5% and 0.4%, respectively. Jones et al. [106] examined the affect of an exercise walking program on BUA. Forty volunteers (mean age 44 years) were separated into exercise (25) and control (15) groups. Following a year of brisk walking (16–18 km/week) a 12% increase in BUA was observed in the exercise group, significantly different from the controls whose BUA decreased 6% ($p < 0.05$). These are very large changes, significantly larger than those that can be expected due to BMD changes alone. The 6% loss in the control group was more than three times the annual rate of loss in postmenopausal women. The results of this exercise intervention study have not been confirmed by other researchers.

To date few studies have reported drug effects [107–111] or addressed the usefulness of ultrasound to monitor treatment of osteoporosis. Hence further longitudinal studies are required. Four studies with 2-year follow-up measurements have shown positive changes in QUS parameters between controls and women treated with calcitonin (+4.2% for BUA and +0.8% for SOS) compared to controls [107], hormone replacement therapy (HRT; +3.6% for BUA and +0.7% for SOS) [111], and alendronate (+3.4% for BUA) [109]. These changes were statistically significant for treatment with calcitonin, HRT, and alendronate. Another study of pamidronate also showed increases in BUA but was limited by very small sample size ($n=12$) [110]. These results suggest some utility for QUS to monitor patients longitudinally. However, the imprecision of the measurement makes evaluation of changes in the individual more difficult. What remains to be determined is the extent to which the changes in QUS parameters are due to increased BMD in the calcaneus versus other properties of bone, like structure or quality, which also influence bone strength. More studies are required to answer this question.

Conclusions

The absence of ionizing radiation, the portability of the equipment, and its cost effectiveness make ultrasound assessment an attractive option for managing osteoporosis and it may be suited as a screening tool for osteoporosis. However, general screening for this disease is still controversial and must be evaluated not only on the diagnostic accuracy and cost effectiveness of the screening measurement but also the availability of effective, economic treatment options.

Although there is a growing body of evidence particularly from prospective studies and from in vitro studies that quantitative ultrasound is useful for the assessment of bone, there is still a need to determine which features of ultrasound velocity and attenuation are related to bone density, which reflect architecture, and how they combine to estimate mechanical competence. In addition, we do not know yet whether the current technology used in QUS is by any measure optimal. Indeed further investigations need to be carried out to test modified QUS techniques (e. g., reflection mode techniques or different frequency ranges) and to provide directions to improve existing technology (e. g., assessment of error sources) [19]. From the clinical perspective the situation is somewhat more complex since there is a conflict between the currently incomplete understanding of QUS and the fact that there are already several thousand QUS units in use around the world. A conservative approach would be to say we need a greater understanding of the physics of the measurement as well as more prospective fracture studies in younger populations and more clinical experience with the technology for longitudinal monitoring of disease progression in various forms of primary and secondary osteoporosis. A more pragmatic direction for the future would acknowledge the growing clinical market and establish guidelines for the use of ultrasound in osteoporosis while at the same time addressing the research questions which remain. For example, an appropriate use of QUS appears to be the assessment of fracture risk in women over 65 years old with fixed point calcaneal ultrasound systems. Furthermore, establishing criteria for the diagnosis of osteoporosis with QUS in a manner similar to that carried out for BMD by the World Health Organization study group [1] would clarify the role of QUS in the management of this disease. Taking these steps will avoid incorrect application of QUS and confusion of clinicians and regulatory agencies over this new technology. In this way quantitative ultrasound can be brought to the clinical realm for the benefit of the public while the remaining scientific questions are answered.

References

1. Consensus Development Conference (1993) Diagnosis, prophylaxis, and treatment of osteoporosis. Am J Med 94:646–650
2. Melton LJ, Chrischilles EA, Cooper C, Lane AW, Riggs BL (1992) Perspective: how many women have osteoporosis? J Bone Miner Res 7:1005–1010
3. Cummings SR, Kelsey JL, Nevitt MC, O'Dowd KJ (1985) Epidemiology of osteoporosis and osteoporotic fractures. Epidemiol Rev 7:178–208
4. Cummings SR, Rubin MPH, Black D (1990) The future of hip fractures in the United States. Clin Orthop Relat Res 252:163–166
5. Cooper C, Campion G, Melton LJ III (1992) Hip fractures in the elderly: a worldwide projection. Osteoporosis Int 2:285–289

6. Chevalley T, Rizzoli R, Nydegger V et al (1991) Preferential low bone mineral density of the femoral neck in patients with a recent fracture of the proximal femur. Osteoporosis Int 1:147–154

7. Duboeuf F, Braillon P, Chapuy MC et al (1991) Bone mineral density of the hip measured with dual-energy X-ray absorptiometry in normal elderly women and in patients with hip fracture. Osteoporosis Int 1:242–249

8. Cummings SR, Black DM, Nevitt MC et al (1993) Bone density at various sites for prediction of hip fractures. Lancet 341:72–75

9. Melton LJ, Wahner HW, Richelson LS et al (1986) Osteoporosis and the risk of hip fracture. Am J Epidemiol 124:254–261

10. Cummings SR, Black DM, Nevitt MC et al (1990) Appendicular bone density and age predict hip fracture in women. JAMA 263:665–668

11. Kleerekoper M, Villaneuva AR, Stanciu J, Rao DS, Parfitt AM (1985) The role of three-dimensional trabecular microstructure in the pathogenesis of vertebral compression fracture. Calcif Tissue Int 37:594–597

12. Mosekilde L (1989) Sex differences in age-related loss of vertebral trabecular bone mass and structure – biomechanical consequences. Bone 10:425–432

13. Langton CM (1992) Recent advances in the ultrasonic assessment of bone. Proceeding of current research in osteoporosis and bone mineral measurement II. Bath conference, p 44

14. Genant HK, Engelke K, Fuerst T et al (1996) Noninvasive assessment of bone mineral and structure: state of the art. J Bone Miner Res 11:707–730

15. Mosekilde L, Bentzen SM, Ortoft G, Jorgensen J (1989) The predictive value of quantitative computed tomography for vertebral body compressive strength and ash density. Bone 10:465–470

16. Melton LJ, Riggs BL (1985) Risk factors for injury after a fall. Clin Geriatr Med 1(3):525–536

17. Kaufman JJ, Einhorn TA (1993) Perspective: ultrasound assessment of bone. Osteoporosis Int 8:517–525

18. Hans D, Schott, Meunier PJ (1993) Ultrasonic assessment of bone: a review. Eur J Med 2:157–163

19. Glüer C, Genant H, Hans D, Langton C, the Consensus Group (1997) Quantitative ultrasound techniques for the assessment of osteoporosis: consensus on current status. J Bone Miner Res (submitted)

20. Abendschein W, Hyatt GW (1970) Ultrasonics and selected physical properties of bone. Clin Orthop Relat Res 69:294–301

21. Ashman RB, Corin JD, Turner CH (1987) Elastic properties of cancellous bone: measurement by an ultrasonic technique. J Biomech 20:979–986

22. Grimm MJ, Williams JL (1993) Use of ultrasound attenuation and velocity to estimate Young's modulus in trabecular bone. Proceedings of the IEEE 19th Northeast Bioengineering Conference, pp 62–63

23. Ashman B, Cowin SC, Van Buskirk WC, Rice JC (1984) A continuous wave technique for the measurement of the elastic properties of cortical bone. J Biomech 17:349–361

24. Njeh CF (1995) The dependence of ultrasound velocity and attenuation on the material properties of cancellous bone. PhD thesis, Sheffield Hallam University

25. Rho JY, Ashman RB, Turner CH (1993) Young's modulus of trabecular and cortical bone material: ultrasonic and microtensile measurements. J Biomech 26:111–119

26. Kinsler LE, Frey AR, Coppens AB, Sanders JV (1992) Fundamentals of acoustics. Wiley, New York

27. Bamber JC, Tristam M (1988) Diagnostic ultrasound. In: Webb S (ed) The physics of medical imaging. Hilger, Bristol, pp 319–386

28. Langton CM, Palmer SB, Porter RW (1984) The measurement of broadband ultrasound attenuation in cancellous bone. Eng Med 13:89–91

28. Hans D, Schott A M, Arlot ME, Sornay E, Delmas PD, Meunier PJ (1995) Influence of anthropometric parameters on ultrasound measurements of calcaneus. Osteoporosis Int 5:371–376

29. Kotzki PO, Buyck D, Hans D, Thomas E, Bonnel F, Favier F, Meunier PJ, Rossi M (1994) Influence of fat on ultrasound measurements of the calcaneus. Calcif Tissue Int 54:91–95

30. Miller CG, Herd RJM, Ramalingarn T, Fogelman I Blake GM (1993) Ultrasonic velocity measurements through the calcaneus: which velocity should be measured? Osteoporosis Int 3:31–35

31. Vogel JM, Wasnich RD, Ross PD (1988) The clinical relevance of calcaneus bone mineral measurements: a review. Bone Miner 5:35–58

32. Wasnich RD, Ross PD, Heilbrun LK, Vogel JM (1987) Selection of the Optimal skeletal site for fracture prediction. Clin Orthop Relat Res 216:262–269

33. Black DM, Cummings SR, Genant H K, Nevitt M C, Palermo L, Browner W (1992) Axial and appendicular bone density predict fractures in older women. J Bone Miner Res 7(6):633–638

34. Hans D, Dargent P, Schott AM et al (1996) Ultrasonographic heel measurements to predict hip fracture in elderly women: the EPIDOS prospective study. Lancet 348:511–514

35. Bauer DC, Gluer CC, Cauley JA et al (1997) Bone ultrasound predicts fractures strongly and independently of densitometry in older women: a prospective study. Arch Intern Med 157:629–634

36. Langton CM, Ali AV, Riggs CM, Evans GP, Bonfield W (1990) A contact method for the assessment of ultrasonic velocity and broadband attenuation in cortical and cancellous bone. Clin Phys Physiol Metab11:243–249

37. Laugier P, Giat P, Berger G (1994) Broadband ultrasonic attenuation imaging: a new imaging technique of the os calcis. Calcif Tissue Int 54:83–86

38. Roux C, Fournier B, Laugier P et al (1996) Ultrasound bone imaging: clinical evaluation of skeletal status. Osteoporosis Int 6:84

39. Orgee JM, Foster H, McCloskey EV, Khan S, Coombes G, Kanis JA (1996) A precise method for the assessment of tibial ultrasound velocity. Osteoporosis Int 6:1–7

40. Foldes AJ, Rimon A, Keinan DD, Popovtzer MM (1995) Quantitative ultrasound of the tibia: a novel approach for assessment of bone status. Bone 17:363–367

41. Fan B, Zucconi F, Fuerst T, Glüer CC, Genant HK (1995) Precision assessment: ultrasonic velocity measurement of the mid-tibia versus other techniques. J Bone Miner Res 10 [Suppl 1]:S368

42. Stegman MR, Heaney RP, Travers-Gustafson D, Leist J (1995) Cortical ultrasound velocity as an indicator of bone status. Osteoporosis Int 5:349–353

44. Guglielmi G, Giannantempo GM, Scillitani A, Chiodini I, Liuzzi A, Cammisa M (1996) Phalangeal QUS and computed X-ray images of hand radiographs. Osteoporosis Int 6 [Suppl 1]:493

45. Cadossi R, Cané V (1996) Pathways of transmission of ultrasound energy through the distal metaphysis of the second phalanx of pigs: an in vitro study. Osteoporosis Int 6(3):196–206

46. Mauloni M, Mura M, Paltrinieri F, Ventura V, Isani R (1995) Bone health evaluated in the female population by an ultrasound instrument on proximal phalanxes. J Bone Miner Res 10 [Suppl 1]:S471

47. Duboeuf F, Hans D, Dchott A, Giraud S, Delmas PD, Meunier PJ (1996) Ultrasound velocity measured at the proximal phalanges: precision and age related changes in normal females. Rev Rhum 63 (6):427–434

48. Alenfeld FE, Wüster C, Beck C, Meeder P-J, Ziegler R (1995) Quantitative Ultrasound at the phalanges: separation of osteoporotic and non-osteoporotic fractures. J Bone Miner Res 10 [Suppl 1]:S273

49. Benitez CL, Schneider DL (1996) QUS assessment of bone in normal and osteoporotic subjects: ability to distinguish between those with and without HRT. Osteoporosis Int 6 [Suppl 1]:184

50. Alenfeld FE, Eggens U, Diessel E, Müller C, Braun J, Sieper J, Gowin W, Felsenberg D (1996) Quantitative ultrasound and bone mineral density measurements at the proximal phalanges in rheumatoid arthritis. Osteoporosis Int 6 [Suppl 1]:347

51. Ventura V, Mauloni M, Mura M, Patrinieri F, de Aloysio D (1996) Ultrasound velocity changes at the proximal phalanges of the hand in pre-, peri-, and postmenopausal women. Osteoporosis Int 6:368–375

52. Rico H, Aguado F, Revilla M et al (1994) Ultrasound bone velocity and metacarpal radiogrammetry in hemodialyzed patients. Miner Electrolyte Metab 20:103–106

53. Kleerekoper M, Nelson DA, Flynn MJ, Pawluszka AS, Jacobsen G, Peterson EL (1994) Comparison of radiographic absorptiometry with dual-energy X-ray absorptiometry and quantitative computed tomography in normal older white and black women. J Bone Miner Res 9(11):1745–1749

54. Heaney RP, Avioli LV, Chesnut CH, Lappe J, Recker RR, Brandenburger GH (1995) Ultrasound velocity through bone predicts incident vertebral deformity. J Bone Miner Res 10:341–345

55. Stegman MR, Heaney RP, Recker RR (1995) Comparison of speed of sound

ultrasound with single photon absorptiometry for determining odds ratio. J Bone Miner Res 10(3):346–352

56. Lehmann R, Wapniarz M, Kvasnicka HM, Klein K, Allolio B (1993) Velocity of ultrasound at the patella: Influence of age, menopause and estrogen replacement therapy. Osteoporosis Int 3:308–313

57. Zerwekh JE, Antich PP, Sakhaee K, Gonzales J, Gottschalk F, Pak CYC (1991) Assessment by reflection ultrasound method of the effect of intermittent slow-release sodium fluoride-calcium citrate therapy on material strengh of bone. J Bone Min Res 6:239–244

58. Evans WD, Jones EA, Owen GM (1995) Factors affecting the in vivo precision of broadband ultrasonic attenuation. Phys Med Biol 40:407–151

59. Gnudi S, Malavolta N, Ripamonti C, Caudarella R (1995) Ultrasound in the evaluation of osteoporosis: a comparison with bone mineral density at distal radius. Br J Radiol 68:476–480

60. Ross P, Huang C, Davis J et al (1995) Predicting vertebral deformity using bone densitometry at various skeletal sites and calcaneus ultrasound. Bone 16:325–332

61. Funke M, Kopka L, Vosshenrich R, Fischer U, Ueberschaer A, Oestmann JW, Grabbe E (1995) Broadband ultrasound attenuation in the diagnosis of osteoporosis: correlation with osteodensitometry and fracture. Radiology 194:77–81

62. Rosenthall L, Tenenhouse A, Caminis J (1995) A correlative study of ultrasound calcaneal and dual-energy X-ray absorptiometry bone measurements of the lumbar spine and femur in 100 women. Eur J Nucl Med 22:402–406

63. Schott AM, Weill-Engerer S, Hans D, Duboeuf F, Delmas PD, Meunier PJ (1995) Ultrasound discriminates patients with hip fracture equally well as dual energy X-ray absorptiometry and independently of bone mineral density. J Bone Miner Res 10:243–249

64. Tavakoli MB, Evans JA (1991) Dependence of the velocity and attenuation of ultrasound in bone on the mineral content. Phys Med Biol 36:1529–1537

65. Wu C, Glüer CC, Fuerst T, Gindele A, Genant HK (1995) Ultrasound characterization of bone demineralization. J Bone Miner Res 10 [Suppl 1]:S374

66. Smeets AJ, Kuiper JW, Slis HW (1995) A comparison of site-matched ultrasound, QDR and DXA measurements in the os calcis in vitro: a pilot study. Osteoporosis Int 5:303

67. Droin P, Laugier P, Laval-Jeantet AM, Berger G (1995) Relationships between acoustic parameters and BMD assessed in vitro ultrasound parametric imaging. Program and abstracts of the 11th International Bone Densitometry Workshop, p 28

68. Nicholson PHF, Haddaway MJ, Davie MW (1994) The dependence of ultrasonic properties on orientation in human vertebral bone. Phys Med Biol 39:1013–1024

69. Wu C, Glüer C-C, Jergas M, Bendavid E, Genant HK (1995) The impact of bone size on broadband ultrasound attenuation. Bone 16:137–141

70. Bauer DC, Gluer CC, Genant HK, Stone K (1995) Quantitative ultrasound and vertebral fracture in postmenopausal women. J Bone Miner Res 10:353–358

71. Bouxsein ML, Radloff SE, Hayes WC (1995) Quantitative ultrasound reflects the anisotropy of calcaneal trabecular bone. Program and abstracts of the 11th International Bone Densitometry Workshop, p 29

72. Gluer CC, Wu CY, Jergas M, Goldstein SA, Genant HK (1994) Three quantitative ultrasound parameters reflect bone structure. Calcif Tissue Int 55:46–52

73. Langton CM, Evans GP, Hodgskinson R, Riggs CM (1990) Ultrasonic, elastic and structural properties of cancellous bone. In: Ring EFG (ed) Current research in osteoporosis and bone mineral measurement. British Institute of Radiology, Bath

74. Glüer CC, Wu CY, Genant HK (1993) Broadband ultrasound attenuation signals depend on trabecular orientation: an in vitro study. Osteoporosis Int 3:185–191

75. Bouxsein ML, Radloff SE, Hayes WC (1995) Quantitative ultrasound of the calcaneus reflects trabecular bone strength, modulus, and morphology. J Bone Miner Res 10 [Suppl 1]:S175

76. Hans D, Arlot ME, Schott AM, Roux JP, Kotzki PO, Meunier PJ (1995) Do ultrasound measurements on the os calcis reflect more the bone microarchitecture than the bone mass? A two-dimensional histomorphometric study. Bone 16:295–300

77. Serpe L, Rho J (1994) Broadband ultrasound attenuation values depend on bone path length: an in vitro study. J Bone Miner Res 9 [Suppl 1]:S278

78. Bouxsein ML, Radloff SE, Toledano TR, Hayes WC (1994) Calcaneal ultrasound measurements are moderately correlated with trabecular bone density and independent of foot geometry. J Bone Miner Res 9 [Suppl 1]:S208

79. Blake GM, Herd RJM, Miller CG, Fogelman I (1994) Should broadband ultrasonic attenuation be normalized for width of the calcaneus? Br J Radiol 67:1206–1209

80. Bouxsein ML, Courtney AC, Hayes WC (1995) Ultrasound and densitometry of the calcaneus correlate with the failure loads of cadaveric femurs. Calcif Tissue Int 56:99–103

81. Njeh CF, Langton CM (1995) Prediction of bone strength from ultrasound velocity and apparent density. Program and abstracts of the 11th International Bone Densitometry Workshop, p 30

82. Mautalen C, Vega E, Gonzales D, Carrilero P, Otano A, Silberman B (1995) Ultrasound and dual X-ray absorptiometry densitometry in women with hip fracture. Calcif Tissue Int 57:165–168

83. Turner CH, Peacock M, Timmerman L, Neal JM, Johnston CC Jr (1995) Calcaneal ultrasonic measurements discriminate hip fractures independently of bone mass. Osteoporosis Int 5:400–405

84. Naessen T, Mallmin H, Ljunghall S (1995) Heel ultrasound in women after long-term ERT compare with bone densities in the forearm, spine and hip. Osteoporosis Int 5:205–210

85. Van Daele PLA, Burger H, Algra D, Hofman A, Grobbee DE, Birkenhäger JC, Pols HAP (1994) Age-associated changes in ultrasound measurements of the calcaneus in men and women: the Rotterdam study. J Bone Miner Res 9:1751–1757

86. Funck C, Wuster C, Alenfeld FE, Pereira-Lima JSF, Fritz T, Meeder PJ, Gotz M, Ziegler R (1996) Ultrasound velocity of the tibia in normal German women and hip fracture patients. Calcif Tissue Int 58:390–394

87. Moris M, Peretz A, Tjeka R, Negaban N, Wouters M, Bergmann P (1995) Quantitative ultrasound bone measurements: normal values and comparison with bone mineral density by dual X-ray absorptiometry. Calcif Tissue Int 57:6–10

88. Faulkner KG, McClung MR, Coleman LJ, Kingston-Sandahl E (1994) Quantitative ultrasound of the heel: correlation with densitometric measurements at different skeletal sites. Osteoporosis Int 4:42–47

89. Gluer CC, Vahlensieck M, Faulkner KG, Engelke K, Black D, Genant HK (1992) Site-matched calcaneal measurement of broadband ultrasound attenuation and single X-ray absorptiometry: do they measure different skeletal properties? J Bone Miner Res 7(9):1071–1079

90. Salamone LM, Krall EA, Harris S, Dawson-Hughes B (1994) Comparison of broadband ultrasound attenuation to single X-ray absorptiometry measurements at the calcaneus in postmenopausal women. Calcif Tissue Int 54:87–90

91. Heaney RP, Avioli LV, Chestnut CH, Lappe J, Rescker RR, Brandenburger GH (1989) Osteoporotic bone fragility, detection by ultrasound transmission velocity. J Am Assoc 261:2986–2990

92. Schott AM, Hans D, Sornay-Rendu E, Delmas PD, Meunier PJ (1993) Ultrasound measurements on os calcis: precision and age-related changes in a normal female population. Osteoporosis Int 3:249–254

93. Schott AM, Hans D, Garnero P, Sornay E, Delmas PD, Meunier PJ (1995) Age-related changes in os calcis ultrasonic indices: a two-year prospective study. Osteoporosis Int 5:478–483

94. Krieg MA, Thiebaud D, Burckhardt P (1996) Quantitative ultrasound of bone in institutionalized elderly women: a cross-sectional and longitudinal study. Osteoporosis Int 6:189–195

95. Porter RW, Miller CG, Grainger D, Palmer SB (1990) Prediction of hip fracture in elderly women: a prospective study. BMJ 301:638–641

96. Dretakis EK, Kontakis GM, Steriopoulos K, Dretakis K, Kouvidis G (1995) Broadband ultrasound attenuation of the os calcis in female postmenopausal patients with cervical and trochanteric fracture. Calcif Tissue Int 57(6):419–421

97. Gluer CC, Fuerst T, Wu CY et al (1995) Diagnostic sensitivity of various quantitative ultrasound and dual X-ray absorptiometry approaches. J Bone Miner Res 10 [Suppl 1]:S373

98. Stewart A, Felsenberg D, Kalidis L, Reid DM (1995) Vertebral fractures in men and women: how discriminative are bone mass measurements? Br J Radiol 68:614–620

99. Wuster C, Paetzold W, Scheidt-Nave C, Brandt K, Ziegler R (1994) Equivalent

diagnostic validity of ultrasound and dual X-ray absorptiometry in a clinical case-comparison study of women with vertebral osteoporosis. J Bone Miner Res 9 [Suppl 1]:S211

100. Dretakis EC, Kontakis GM, Steriopoulos CA, Dretakis CE (1994) Decreased broadband ultrasound attenuation of the calcaneus in women with fragility fracture. Acta Orthop Scand 65:305–308

101. Kroger H, Jurvelin J, Amala I et al (1995) Ultrasound attenuation of the calcaneus in normal subjects and in patients with wrist fracture. Acta Orthop Scand 66:47–52

102. Uffmann M, Bauer DC, Fuerst TP et al (1996) Is tibial ultrasound velocity associated with previous fractures? J Bone Miner Res 11 [Suppl 1, S631]:247

103. Alenfeld F, Wüster C, Goetz M, Beck C, Ziegler R (1995) Diagnostic value of ultrasound measurements of bone mineral density on the metacarpals in healthy and osteoporotic subjects. Bone 16:147S

104. Hans D, Dargent P, Schott AM, Breart G, Meunier PJ, EPIDOS Group (1996) Ultrasound parameters are better predictors of trochanteric than cervical hip fracture: the EPIDOS Prospective Study. Osteoporosis Int 6 [Suppl 1]:24

105. Glueer CC, Cummings SR, Bauer DC et al (1996) Osteoporosis: association of recent fractures with quantitative US findings. Radiology 199:725–732

106. Jones PRM, Hardman AE, Hudson A, Norgan NG (1991) Influence of brisk walking on the broadband ultrasonic attenuation of the calcaneus in previously sedentary women aged 30–61 years. Calcif Tissue Int 49:112–115

107. Gonnelli S, Cepollaro C, Pondrelli C, Martini S, Rossi S, Gennari C (1996) Ultrasound parameters in osteoporotic patients treated with salmon calcitonin: a longitudinal study. Osteoporosis Int 6:303–307

108. Acotto C, Schott AM, Hans D, Njepomniszeze H, Mautalen CA, Meunier PJ (1995) Hyperthyroidism influences ultrasound bone measurements of the calcaneus. J Bone Miner Res 10 [Suppl 1]:S400

109. Giorgino R, Paparella P, Lorusso D, Mancuso S (1996) Effects of oral alendronate treatment and discontinuance on ultrasound measurements of the heel in postmenopausal osteoporosis. J Bone Miner Res 11 [Suppl 1]:M639

110. Ryan P, Herd R, Blake CC, Fogelman I (1996) Calcaneal BUA changes in a 2 year placebo controlled study of pamidronate in post menopausal osteoporosis. Osteoporosis Int 6 [Suppl 1]:516

111. Giorgino R, Lorusso D, Paparella P (1996) Ultrasound bone densitometry and 2-year hormonal replacement therapy efficacy in the prevention of early postmenopausal bone Loss. Osteoporosis Int 6 [Suppl 1]:569

20 Applications of Magnetic Resonance Imaging in the Study of Osteoporosis

S. Majumdar and H. K. Genant

Introduction

Studies have shown that changes in bone quality and structure affect both bone strength and individual risk of fracture independently of bone mineral density (BMD). The effect of these other factors is thought at least partially to explain the observed overlap in bone mineral measurements between patients with and those without osteoporotic fractures. Several new emerging techniques have therefore aimed at quantifying trabecular bone structure in addition to bone density. It is in the context of noninvasive assessment of trabecular bone architecture that recent efforts have focused on the development of imaging modalities such as magnetic resonance (MR) imaging.

Effect of Trabecular Bone on MR Relaxation Time T2*

MR is a complex technology which has evolved rapidly and is based upon the application of high magnetic fields, transmission of radiofrequency (RF) waves, and detection of RF signals from excited hydrogen protons. Most MR imaging techniques to date have been limited to studying soft tissue or gross skeletal structure because the presence of compact bone in MR images results in a total absence of signal. However, newly developed MR techniques have been used to study trabecular bone specifically. The presence of the trabecular bone matrix affects the signal intensity of bone marrow, an effect that is particularly enhanced in specific imaging sequences. The magnetic properties of trabecular bone and bone marrow differ significantly. These differences produce distortions of the magnetic lines of force which make the local magnetic field within the tissue inhomogeneous and alter the relaxation properties of tissue, such as the apparent transverse relaxation time T2*, in gradient-echo images. From theoretical considerations such changes in T2* should be related directly to the density of the surrounding trabecular network and its spatial geometry. The resultant shortening of relaxation time is greater with an increase in the concentration of trabecular bone in the surrounding homogeneous marrow tissue. Thus in a normal dense trabecular network T2* shortening should be more pronounced than in rarefied osteoporotic trabeculae.

Experimental studies have confirmed the theoretical predictions, suggesting MR as a promising tool for studying trabecular bone architecture and assessing osteoporosis. Davis et al. [1] have shown a reduction in the in vitro $T2^*$ of both water and cottonseed oil in the presence of bone powder at a magnetic field strength of 5.9 T. Rosenthal et al. [2] have measured a reduction in the $T2^*$ of water present in the trabecular spaces compared with extratrabecular water, using specimens of excised human vertebrae at 0.6 T. Majumdar et al. [3] used specimens of dried human vertebral bodies with varying bone densities and examined susceptibility-mediated relaxation effects. The mean trabecular bone density for each specimen as measured by QCT was significantly related to the overall relaxation rate $1/T2^*$ of intratrabecular saline. Similar relations in vivo have also been established in the forearm, distal femur, and proximal tibia sites at which the trabecular bone network shows significant variations as a function of the distance from the joint line, with the bone density and relaxation rate, $1/T2^*$, being greatest in the epiphysis and decreasing progressively towards the metaphysis and diaphysis [4,5]. In a similar fashion Wehrli et al. [6–8] have assessed variations in $T2^*$ between osteoporotic and normal subjects. In studies on the distal radius precision errors in measured $T2^*$ times were found to range from 1.3 to 2.9 ms, corresponding to 3.8%–9.5% CV [9].

High-Resolution Magnetic Resonance Imaging of Trabecular Bone Structure

In addition to the indirect measures of relaxation times, high-resolution MR imaging may be used to obtain images that depict trabecular bone structure. Images ranging in spatial resolutions of 78–200 μm in plane, and 300–1000 μm in slice thickness have been obtained in vivo, and considerably higher resolutions may be obtained in vitro at higher field strengths. In MR the trabecular bone appears as a signal void while bone marrow is the high intensity signal, unlike in X-ray based imaging modalities.

Two different classes of imaging sequences, spin-echo based and gradient-echo based sequences have been used to obtain images of trabecular bone structure. In spin-echo sequences a 180° RF pulse is applied to obtain an echo signal which is then used to generate an image, whereas in a gradient-echo sequence a reversal of the magnetic field gradient is used to generate such an echo. Due to the different physical principles that govern image contrast and appearance there are differences between two images obtained with the same resolution but different imaging sequences. In both spin-echo and gradient-echo images the susceptibility (the ability of a material to be magnetized) difference between bone and bone marrow affects the image appearance of trabecular bone. In both spin-echo and gradient-echo MR images the apparent size of trabeculae as depicted may show differences from their true dimensions [10, 11]. This amplification of trabecular dimensions is more pronounced in gradient-echo images (Fig. 20-1); however, it also depends on the echo time, TE, which is used to acquire the image. At short TE times the effect is not as marked and increases as the echo time increases.

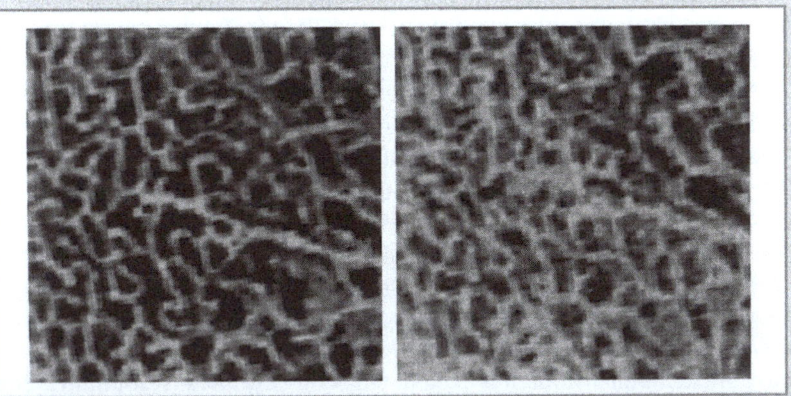

Fig. 20-1 Spin-echo and gradient-echo images of the same specimen from a human tibia. The spatial resolution is 128 mm isotropic

Factors such as the repetition time, TR, selected to obtain an MR image also affect the achievable signal to noise ratio (SNR). Increasing TR increases the SNR in an image; however, this increases the total scan time. The bandwidth or the total duration during which the MR signal is sampled also affects the SNR. The higher the bandwidth used to sample the MR signal, the shorter is the achievable echo time, TE. However, with a higher bandwidth the SNR achievable is also lower. Thus the choice of echo time, bandwidth, and scan parameters in MR imaging must be carefully weighed and adjusted because these factors interact in multiple ways and affect the image appearance, resolution, and quality.

In deriving quantitative parameters from images such as those shown in Fig. 20-1 one of the primary factors affecting the quantitative measures is the accurate segmentation of the bone and bone marrow components. As the image resolution is degraded, the segmentation of the bone and marrow phases becomes complicated due to partial volume-averaging effects. The observed density profile at the trabecular bone edge has a transition region between marrow and bone. When the image resolution is comparable to trabecular dimensions, the size of this transition zone is not negligible. As a result of this the intensity histogram in a region comprising trabecular bone and bone marrow may not be bimodal as one would expect in a two-phase model where pixels consist of a single component. In image processing there is no established technique for measuring the accuracy of any segmentation scheme. Every thresholding scheme has some associated subjectivity which may depend either on the operator or on the automated criteria that are specified in a algorithm. Several techniques may be applied when segmenting high-resolution images into bone and bone marrow. Intensity-based thresholding schemes based on the histogram of signal intensities [12] and internal calibration techniques [13] have been used, but because these schemes are based on a single value, it may lead to an apparent thickening of trabeculae or a loss of thinner trabeculae within the same image. An adaptive thresholding or an edge detection scheme in MR images may result in a detection of the heterogeneity of bone marrow in the trabecular spaces and thus inaccurately classify marrow components as bone. Recently proposed have also been Bayesian estimation techniques, the relative merits and resolution dependence of which remain to be evaluated [14]. After the images have been segmented into two phases, the MR images may be used to calculate standard histomorphometry measures of bone structure such as trabecular bone area fraction, trabecular width, trabecular number, and trabecular spacing using run length analysis methods [15].

Another factor that impacts the absolute quantitation of trabecular bone area fraction, trabecular width, and spacing is the image resolution, which if it is comparable to the dimension of the structure to be measured [16] can lead to errors in the estimated dimensions. It is evident that when the image resolution is equivalent to trabecular dimensions, the accuracy of measuring the dimensions of trabecular structure is prone to error, regardless of the segmentation scheme. For example, if the image resolution is 100 µm, and the trabecular dimensions are of the order of 100 µm, an error of 1 pixel may potentially be reflected as a 100% error in the estimated trabecular width. Similarly a trabeculum 50 µm thick is still detected as a 100-µm structure. Thus since the standard stereology measures derived from such MR images reflect an average over a finite resolution that the measures have been denoted as apparent measures such as the apparent trabecular bone area fraction (app-BV/TV), trabecular width (app-TbTh), trabecular number (app-TbN), and trabecular spacing (app-TbSp), etc. In addition to standard two-dimensional measures of trabecular bone architecture, the connectivity of the trabecular network, as determined from the Euler number [17] or the complexity of the network as determined from extensions of fractal based box-counting techniques [18] may also be used to characterize trabecular bone structure from MR images.

Specimen Studies

Hipp et al. [19] compared the MR derived stereology measures, determined from isotropic image voxels of 50 µm to those obtained using optical imaging and found good correlations, while Chung et al. [20] compared the apparent BV/TV determined from MR images to those determined using displacement techniques and also found good correlations between the two measures. In a recent study using high-resolution MR Antich et al. [21] confirmed that MR techniques may be used to monitor changes in trabecular bone structure after fluoride therapy using specimen from iliac crest biopsies. The relationship between the MR derived measures of trabecular structure obtained from images of distal radius cubes at resolutions comparable to those that may be obtained in vivo (156×156×300 µm) have been compared to those obtained from higher resolution three-dimensional X-ray tomographic microscopy (XTM) images obtained at an isotropic resolution of 18 µm using cubes from human radii [12] (Fig. 20-2).

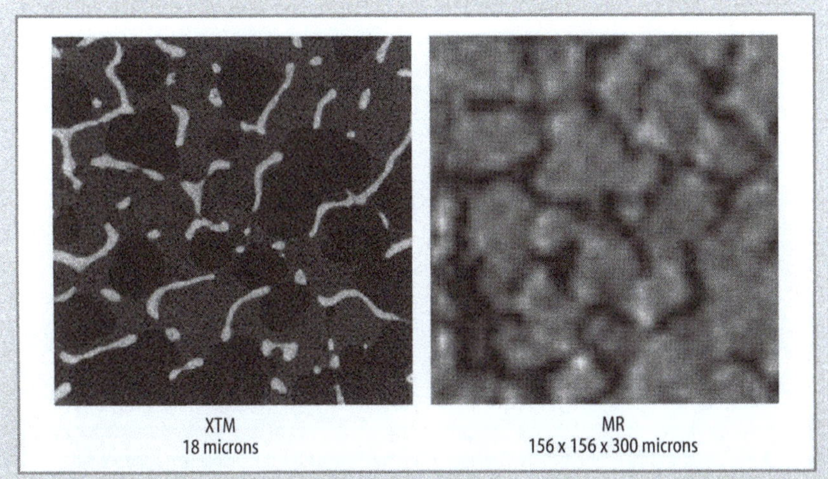

Fig. 20-2 Images of a radius cube obtained using X-ray tomographic microscopy at a spatial resolution of 18 mm, and using MR imaging at a resolution of 156 x156 x 300 mm

In the MR images partial volume effects result in an overestimation of trabecular bone area fraction, trabecular width (approx. 3 times), and an underestimation of trabecular spacing (approx. 1.6 times) compared to the 18-μm XTM images. A comparison of the MR-derived measures with the BMD measured using dual X-ray absorptiometry shows that trabecular width, area fraction, and number increases, while trabecular spacing decreases, as the BMD increases. The correlations between BMD and the measures of trabecular structure are also good. In the radius cubes the biomechanical elastic modulus in the three orthogonal directions corresponding to the anatomical distal-proximal (E_{D-P}), anterior posterior (E_{A-P}), and medial-lateral (E_{M-L}) correlated differently with the structural parameters. A preliminary bivariate analysis showed that the trabecular number and spacing contributed to an improvement in the prediction of the elastic modulus, compared to BMD alone.

Figure 20-3 presents reverse gray scale (bone shown in white) MR images at a spatial resolution of 117×117×300 μm for two specimens, one from the lumbar spine and the other from the proximal femur. The structural features of the trabecular bone at these two sites are quite different, as is clearly shown. In all specimens studied the primary orientation of the trabeculae was in the superior-inferior direction. This structural anisotropy was also reflected in the measured elastic modulus which was the highest in the superior-inferior (E_{S-I}) direction. The elastic modulus in the medial-lateral (E_{M-L}) and anterior-posterior (E_{A-P}) showed considerable variations. From such images the three-dimensional anisotropy of spine and femur have been determined. The binarized images can be used to determine the three-dimensional distribution of mean intercept lengths for such cubes. The mean intercept length in three dimensions generates an ellipsoid, the

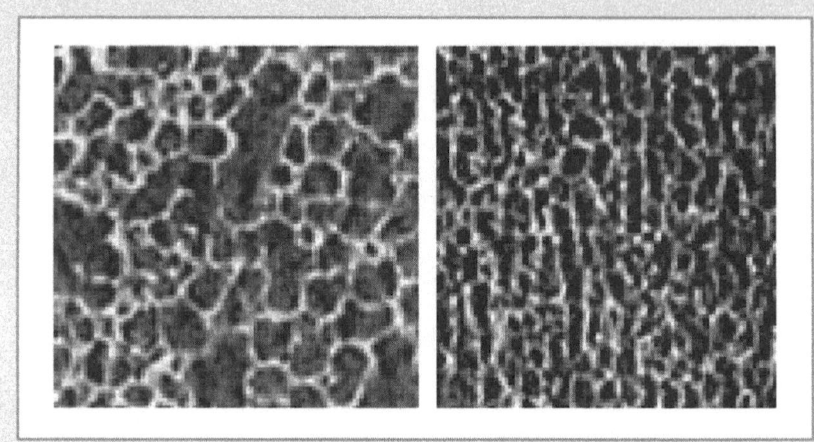

Fig. 20-3 Reverse gray scale (white, bone) MR images of two cubes, one from the lumbar spine, the second from the proximal femur showing differences in the pattern of trabecular bone structure

principal axis of which determines the primary trabecular orientation. The ratio of the principal axes gives the degree of anisotropy in the trabecular bone structure.

In Vivo Studies

A recent in vivo study obtained high-resolution MR images of the distal radius at 1.5 T in premenopausal normal (group I), postmenopausal normal (group II), and postmenopausal osteoporotic group (III) women. The women in groups II and III were also classified as being osteoporotic based on the T scores [22] of their distal radius BMD determined using peripheral quantitative computed tomography. Representative MR images are shown in Fig. 20-4. The MR images were used to derive measures of trabecular bone structure, which included apparent measures of trabecular bone area fraction, trabecular thickness, trabecular spacing, and trabecular number. The app-BV/TV decreased with age although it showed lower correlations with age, while the app-TbN showed moderate correlations and decreased with age. The app-TbSp showed the greatest increase and moderate correlation with age. The correlation coefficient and the level of significance for the relationship between age and app-TbTh was low, and the trend in variation of trabecular thickness with age was thus inconclusive.

Trabecular bone BMD in the distal radius, app-BV/TV, app-TbTh, app-TbN had the expected trend (Table 20-1), i.e., the mean values were the greatest in subjects in group I, decreased progressively in the postmenopausal group (group II), and were the lowest in the postmenopausal osteoporotic group (III). The app-TbSp was greatest in group III and lowest in group I. One tailed *t* tests were used to assess differences between the density and structure parameters in the post-

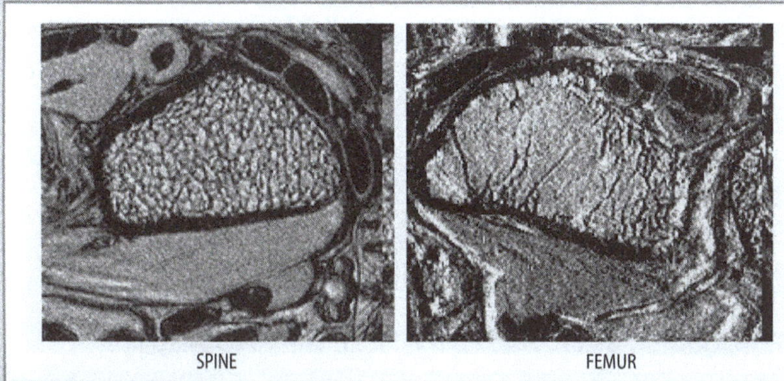

Fig. 20-4 MR images obtained in vivo through the distal radius of a normal premenopausal young subject and an osteoporotic 76-year-old postmenopausal subject

Table 20-1 Mean and standard deviation of trabecular bone structure parameters in the distal radius

	Group I: premenopausal normal	Group II: postmenopausal normal	Group III: postmenopausal osteoporotic
Trabecular BMD (mg/cm³)*	165.31±34.85	116.96±12.62	101.21±9.76
Cortical BMC (mg)*	201.98±23.46	186.56±42.19	147.23±60.91
app-BV/TV (%)*	34.0±10	34±9.0	26±8.5
app-Tb.Th (mm)*	0.36±0.08	0.35±0.08	0.33±0.07
app-Tb.Sp (mm)*	0.75±0.35	0.93 ±0.40	1.34±0.68
app-Tb.N (mm−1)*	0.96±0.20	0.84±0.34	0.66±0.22

* Fracture vs. nonfracture patients $p<0,05$

menopausal groups (II and III). Significant differences existed between the fracture and the nonfracture groups in the measured radial trabecular BMD, trabecular bone area fraction, trabecular spacing, and trabecular number.

Similarly, MR imaging applied to the quantitative measurement of age-related changes in calcaneal trabecular structure from MR images at a spatial resolution of approx. 200×200×1000 µm, showed that the trabecular structure parameters and age were significantly ($p<0.05$) correlated: app-BV/TV ($r=0.58$), app-Tb.Th ($r=0.52$), app-Tb.Sp ($r=0.54$) [13]. The annual rate of change in a normal population was −0.22%, −0.55%, and +1.37%, for app-BV/TV, app-Tb.Th, and app-Tb.Sp, respectively. Linear regression analysis also showed significant correlation between the MR-derived trabecular structure parameters and calcaneal BMD values. With improved phased-array coils the achievable image resolution in images of the calcaneus now may be as high as 156 µm in plane and 500 µm in slice thickness.

The heterogeneity of trabecular structure in the calcaneus is evident from the images. In the calcaneus the highest app-BV/TV is seen in the superior region and

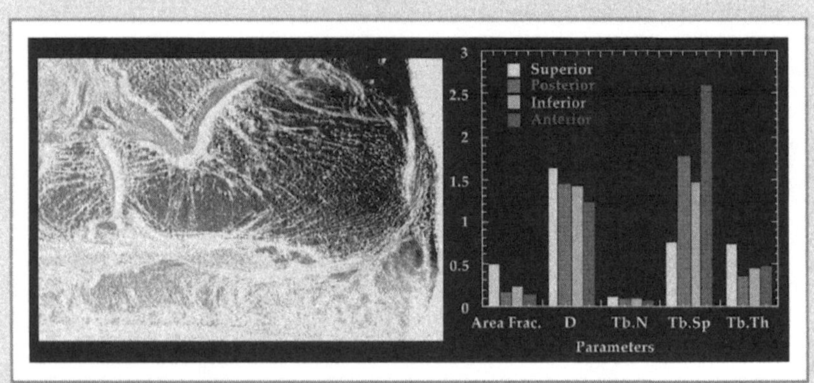

Fig. 20-5 High-resolution reverse gray scale image depicting trabecular bone structure, and measures of trabecular bone structure parameters in different anatomical regions

the lowest in the anterior region. App-Tb.N is highest in the posterior region and lowest in the anterior region. The highest app-Tb.Sp is in the anterior region and the lowest in the superior region. Conversely, app-Tb.Th is highest in the superior region and the lowest in the anterior region (Fig. 20-5). In the posterior part of the calcaneus the heterogeneity or percentage variation ($n=12$) was 41.7% for bone fraction while for trabecular number, trabecular spacing, and trabecular thickness it is 21.8%, 46.0%, and 42.5%, respectively. The percentage variation for BMD determined in the posterior part ($n=8$) of the calcaneus was considerably lower (approx. 11%).

Conclusion

The advances in MR imaging combined with image processing techniques have potential in vitro and in vivo applications in the study of trabecular bone architecture, its relationship to bone biomechanics, and applications to studies of osteoporosis and fracture risk prediction. The noninvasive, three-dimensional nature of MR, and its ability to predict bone marrow characteristics makes it particularly useful for in vivo studies.

References

1. Davis JW, Grove JS, Ross PD, Vogel JM, Wasnich RD (1992) Relationship between bone mass and rates of bone change at appendicular measurement sites. J Bone Miner Res 7:719–725
2. Rosenthal H, Thulborn KR, Rosenthal DI, Rosen BR (1990) Magnetic susceptibility effects of trabecular bone on magnetic resonance bone marrow imaging. Invest Radiol 25:173–178

3. Majumdar S, Thomasson D, Shimakawa A, Genant HK (1991) Quantitation of the susceptibility difference between trabecular bone and bone marrow: experimental studies. Magn Reson Med 22:111–127

4. Sebag GH, Moore SG (1990) Effect of trabecular bone on the appearance of marrow in gradient echo imaging of the appendicular skeleton. Radiology 174:855–859

5. Majumdar S, Genant HK (1992) In vivo relationship between marrow T2* and trabecular bone density determined with a chemical shift-selective asymmetric spin-echo sequence. J Magn Reson Imaging 2:209–219

6. Wehrli FW, Ford JC, Attie M, Kressel HY, Kaplan FS (1991) Trabecular structure: preliminary application of MR interferometry. Radiology 179:615–621

7. Wehrli FW, Hwang SN, Ford JC, Jara H (1994) Method for Image-based T2*. Measurement in bone marrow in Society of Magnetic Resonance, 2nd meeting, San Francisco, p 201

8. Wehrli FW, Ford JC, Haddad JG (1995) Osteoporosis: clinical assessment with quantitative MR imaging in diagnosis. Radiology 196:631–641

9. Grampp S, Majumdar S, Jergas M et al (1995) In vivo assessment of the distal radius by quantitative magnetic resonance imaging peripheral quantitative computed tomography and dual X-ray absorptiometry. Radiology 198:213–218

10. Bhagwandien R, Moerland MA, Bakker CJ, Beersma R, Lagendijk JJ (1994) Numerical analysis of the magnetic field for arbitrary magnetic susceptibility distribution in 3D. Magn Reson Imaging 12:101

11. Jara H, Wehrli FW (1994) Determination of background gradients with diffusion MR imaging. J Mag Reson Imag 4:787–799

12. Majumdar S, Newitt DC, Mathur A et al (1996) Magnetic resonance imaging of trabecular bone structure in the distal radius: relationship with X-ray tomographic microscopy and biomechanics. Osteoporosis Int 6:376–385

13. Ouyang X, Selby K, Lang P et al (1996) High resolution MR imaging of the calcaneus: age-related changes in trabecular structure and comparison with DXA measurements. Calcif Tissue Int (in press)

14. Wu Z, Chung H, Wehrli F (1993) Sub-voxel tissue classification in NMR microscopic images of trabecular bone. In: Proceedings of the Society of Magnetic Resonance in Medicine, New York, p 451

15. Goulet RW, Goldstein SA, Ciarelli MJ et al (1994) The relationship between the structural and orthogonal compressive properties of trabecular bone. J Biomech 27:375–389

16. Flynn MJ, Reimann DA (1994) 3D measurement of trabecular architecture with microtomography: dose and resolution. Bone Miner 25:S4

17. Feldkamp LA, Goldstein SA, Parfitt AM, Jesion G, Kleerekoper M (1989) The direct examination of three-dimensional bone architecture in vitro by computed tomography. J Bone Miner Res 4:3–11

18. Majumdar S, Genant HK, Grampp S et al (1994) Analysis of trabecular bone structure in the distal radius using high resolution MRI. Eur Radiol 4:517–524

19. Hipp JA, Jansujwicz A, Simmons CA, Snyder B (1996) Trabecular bone mor-

phology using micro-magnetic resonance imaging. J Bone Miner Res 11:286–
292
20. Chung H W Wehrli F W Williams JL, Wehrli SL (1995) Three dimensional
nuclear magnetic resonance micro-imaging of trabecular bone. J Bone Miner Res 10:1452–1461
21. Antich PP, Mason RP, McColl R, Zerwech J, Pak CYC (1994) Trabecular architecture studies by 3D MRI microscopy in bone biopsies. J Bone Miner Res
9S1:327
22. WHO Technical Report (1994) Assessment of fracture risk and its application to screening for postmenopausal osteoporosis: a report of a WHO study
group in World Health Organization, Geneva

21 Beyond Bone Densitometry: Assessment of Bone Architecture by X-Ray Computed Tomography at Various Levels of Resolution

K. Engelke and W. Kalender

Introduction

Osteoporosis is defined as a systemic skeletal disease characterized by low bone mass and microarchitectural deterioration of bone tissue. In analogy to well-known examples from mechanical engineering such as steel bridges, bone strength and fracture resistance are determined not only by the amount of material but also by its spatial distribution, i.e., by the architecture or structure of the trabecular network. Established methods of bone densitometry such as quantitative computed tomography (QCT) of the spine or forearm and dual X-ray absorptiometry (DXA) of spine, hip, and forearm focus on measurement of bone mass, i.e., on bone mineral content (BMC) or bone mineral density (BMD). Microarchitecture is generally assessed by histomorphometry of thin sections, a technique established for many years. While densitometry delivers accurate and precise results on the scale of individual bones, histomorphometry measures thickness and distance on the trabecular scale. Densitometry allows us to investigate the global picture in vivo while histomorphometry concentrates on fine details of trabecular structure, but it is destructive by nature and is generally applied only postmortem or to bone biopsies. Investigated volumes of interest range from several cubic centimeters in the case of densitometry to cubic millimeters in histomorphometry.

Despite their high degree of technical sophistication, current densitometric techniques of QCT and DXA show an insufficient discrimination between healthy and osteoporotic subjects as well as an unsatisfactory ability to predict further fractures which constitute the most severe manifestations of osteoporosis. As an example, Fig. 21-1 shows the large overlap in BMD values of normal women and women with diagnosed vertebral fractures. The problem is further illuminated by results from biomechanical experiments; while BMD is typically the single best predictor of trabecular bone strength, alone it can only explain 49%–93% in the variance of mechanical properties such as the modulus of elasticity or compressive strength [1–10]. Studies of the correlation between BMD and fracture threshold [11–14] show even lower associations.

Improving our knowledge of bone loss and its relationship to bone fragility and fracture requires that bone structure be taken more into consideration. We must fill the gap between in vivo densitometry and in vitro histomorphometry. This is the topic of the present chapter. We start with an investigation of techniques assess-

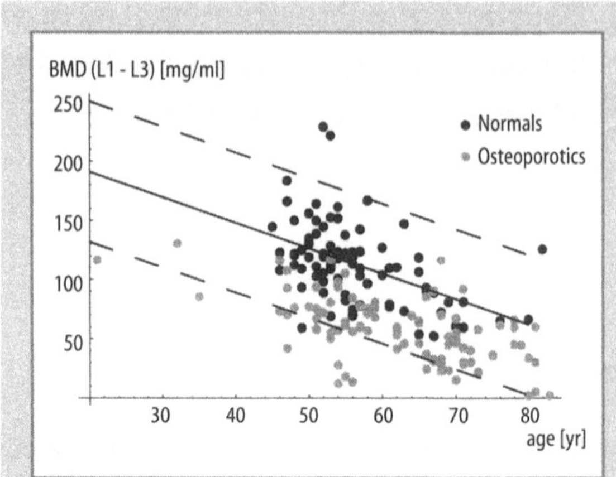

Fig. 21-1 Age-related changes in BMD among normal women and osteoporotic women with vertebral fractures as measured by spinal QCT, showing the large overlap of BMD values

ing the bone macrostructure, for example, an extended regional analysis using QCT and DXA images or the determination of geometrical parameters such as hip axis length. Recalling the steel bridge analogy, these methods investigate the main pillars in greater detail, and they also try to identify the regions that are most sensitive to changes and best allow predictions of failure.

We further discuss efforts to measure parameters of bone architecture in vivo. In recent years a variety of techniques using high-resolution computed tomography (CT) and magnetic resonance (MR) imaging have been developed. And we also present in vitro techniques of μCT and μMR which approach the spatial resolution of histomorphometry, but unlike it they assess bone structure in three dimensions. With these "μ methods" the topology of the trabecular network can be measured and a truly 3D analysis becomes available. They may be most useful in preclinical research and in the animal model. The emphasis of this chapter lies on X-ray based CT techniques. MR methods are introduced in broader detail in Chap. 20; they are mentioned here mainly for comparative purposes.

In discussing the potential of all the approaches aiming at bone structure we must keep in mind that the following criteria must be fullfilled: (a) the ability to measure age, disease, and treatment-related changes, (b) the capability to discriminate healthy from osteoporotic subjects, and (c) the power to predict future fractures. Bone mass and density may be merely surrogates of bone architecture, but it is unlikely that they will be completely replaced by techniques of structural analysis because they are strong predictors of bone fragility and structure, and because densitometry is easy to perform, cheap, and widely available. The question is therefore: will the new approaches for measuring structure improve the diagnostic capabilities of bone densitometry? Figure 21-1 indicates that there is substantial room for improvement.

Assessment of Bone Macrostructure

The best known examples of regional analysis are the differentiation of femoral DXA in neck and trochanteric regions and the selective assessment of trabecular and cortical bone in spinal QCT. Because the vertebral trabecular network shows a high bone turnover, it is a sensitive indicator of age- and disease-related BMD changes. Thus it is not surprising that QCT discriminates better between those with and those without vertebral fractures than does spinal DXA, which always includes cortical bone [15–19].

Several researchers have tried to further improve spinal QCT analysis by dividing the measured volume into small subregions because structural characteristics of trabecular architecture likely depend on the shape of the bone, the cortical thickness, and the distribution of applied forces. An interesting idea was introduced by Sandor and Kalender et al. [20] who divided the trabecular area of 8-mm thick CT scans in the form of a spider net (see Fig. 21-2). BMD was found to be distributed in a W-shaped pattern with maximum BMD in the lateral and anterior portions of the vertebral body. Regions with highest BMD showed the highest loss with age. This observation was confirmed in another CT study by Flynn et al. [21] who used 18 small cylindrical regions of interest (ROIs) in three contiguous 1-mm thick slices of the vertebral body. They found increased density in the inferior, posterior, and lateral regions.

A problem associated with an X-ray based analysis of small subregions is noise which scales inversely with the square of the area. Thus either the precision decreases or the radiation exposure must be increased. Flynn et al. estimated that their

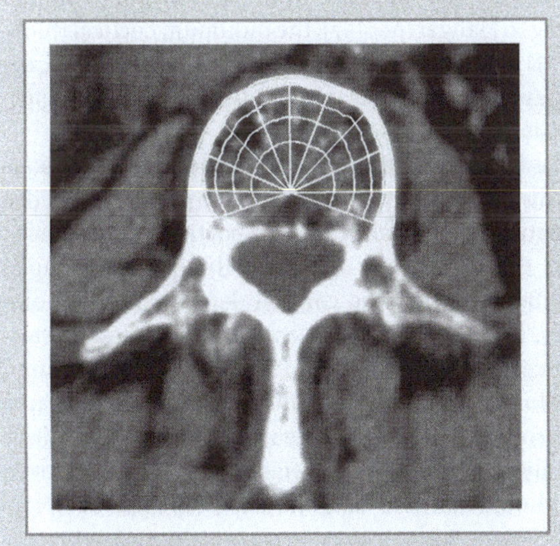

Fig. 21-2 Regional assessment of spinal BMD in standard QCT images. The spider net defines cortical and trabecular subregions [127]

thin-slice protocol (130 kV, 400 mAs) administered the same dose as diagnostic abdominal CT [22]. This means an increase of more than ten times over a low-dose QCT protocol (80 kV, 120 mAs). The dose issue may be one reason why these investigations have never been applied in many studies and have not been further pursued recently.

Although the high remodeling rate favors investigations of trabecular bone to detect changes in response to therapy or disease, there is also continued interest in assessing cortical bone which is an important contributor to bone strength [23–27]. Most extremity bone fractures due to falls originate in the former epiphyseal or metaphyseal cortex and not in the spongiosa or diaphyseal cortex [28]. However, accurate and precise in vivo measurements of the cortex are still difficult to perform mainly due to the limited spatial resolution of the applied QCT equipment. Early data generated by QCT showed an age-related decrease in spinal cortical BMD of 0.7%–1.0% for elderly women relative to age 50 and a decrease of 0%–0.32% for men [29–31]. However, these and similar [32] CT measurements were density oriented and overestimated cortical thickness because of partial volume effects [26]. This is in general also true for clinical peripheral QCT (pQCT) applied to the distal forearm.

Forearm pQCT studies investigating age-related changes and discriminative capabilities indicate that cortical thickness, area, or BMC may be more important parameters than cortical BMD [33,34]. Recent histomorphometric data [35] of the spine do not show gender-specific differences of cortical thickness, but they do reveal significant differences between healthy controls and subjects with osteoporotic fractures. There is also a significant age-related decrease in the cortical thickness for vertebrae below T8. For L3 cortical thickness decreases by approx. 0.5% annually relative to age 50. Cortical thickness of the spine varies from 180 to 600 µm [25,35,36]. According to Hangartner [37], the minimum cortical thickness for an accurate spinal BMD evaluation of the cortex using clinical CT scanners is 2–2.5 mm. Our own phantom-based measurements show that the determination of cortical thickness is accurate down to 1 mm.

The discrepancy between the accuracy of density and thickness measurements is illustrated in Fig. 21-3 which displays a profile perpendicular to the cortical ridge line. The step function schematically represents the true cortical bone density. Due to partial volume effects the CT scanner measures the gaussian-shaped curve which is a convolution between the true cortical density and the point spread function of the scanner. The thickness of the cortical bone can be determined by the horizontal distance between points A and B. However, the measured mass within the boundaries is lower than the true value because the shaded area does not contribute to the measured value. Despite accuracy problems repetitive measurements using this analysis technique are relatively precise. However, higher resolution techniques should increase discriminative capabilities of cortical measurements.

Considerably fewer methods exist to measure the macrostructure of the most important fracture site, the proximal femur, although several studies analyzing

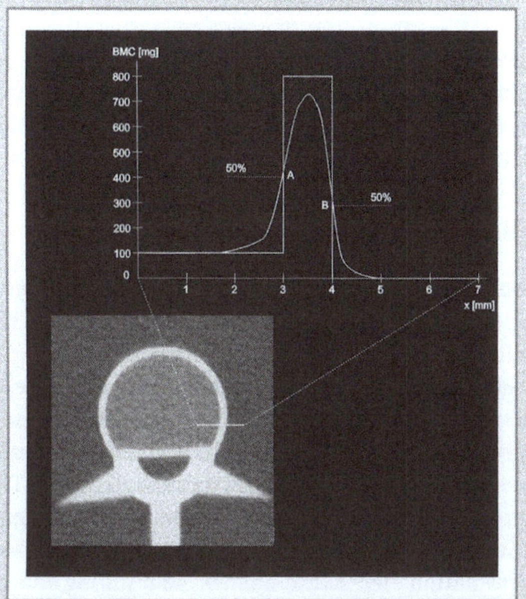

Fig. 21-3 Discrepancy between density and thickness determination of cortical bone. The cortex of the European spine phantom was analyzed along the horizontal line indicated in the L2 vertebra (nominal cortical thickness: 1 mm). The actual cortical density is represented by the box profile in the graph and the measured CT profile by the gaussian-shaped curve. Using the two 50% thresholds, the cortical thickness of 1 mm can be accurately measured, but the cortical density within the boundaries is underestimated by the integral of the shaded area

geometrical parameters from DXA scans indicate the importance of regional BMD variations [38–41]. However, imaging methods to obtain 3D datasets suitable for a quantitative analysis of the femur are not available. QCT of the femur has never progressed beyond an initial stage because earlier attempts [42–44] worked with multiple 2D slices. Experimental data for 3D hip QCT were reported only recently [45–47]. The definition of anatomically oriented coordinate systems greatly improves the alignment of 3D datasets obtained from serial measurements. For a further discussion of this subject see Chap. 16.

Ironically, a geometrical parameter determined from 2D projectional images such as DXA scans or X-rays, the so called hip axis length (HAL), has been established as a parameter to predict hip fractures independently of densitometry [48, 49]. A longer HAL is associated with an increased risk of femoral neck and trochanteric fractures. The HAL does not vary with age after midadolescence but appears to be largely influenced by genetic factors [50]. This supports the view that differences in HAL may at least partly explain racially related differences in fracture risk [51–53]. Part of the success story of the HAL was the fact that its value could be easily tested in the large prospective Study of Osteoporotic Fractures

(SOF) [54] confirming its predictive value immediately. This is typically not the case for parameters derived from CT because large prospective studies using QCT have not been undertaken. However, the HAL is also a good example that a more detailed macroscopic analysis of bone structure should be undertaken. Although HAL predicts fractures it is not well understood why it does so, and it is not unlikely that a more detailed 3D analysis could result in more powerful parameters.

In Vivo Assessment of Bone Microstructure

For the discussion below we use the following terminology: The discrete volume elements of a digital image are denoted as pixels (2D case) or voxels (3D case). The gray value of the pixel or voxel codes the information of the image, for example, the CT value. In gray-scale images the gray value can have a range of values (e.g., 0–255) whereas in binary (black and white) images the gray value can have only two. Spatial resolution in the physical sense should typically be given in line pairs per millimeter or as an 5% or 10% value of the modulation transfer function (MTF). It requires a measurement of the MTF or the point spread function of the imaging system. However, due to simplicity many authors give the pixel or voxel dimensions, or in the case of isotropic resolution their side lengths in the resulting images. This simplistic approach results in a "pseudo" resolution which typically overestimates the physically "correct" resolution by a factor of 2–4. Without going into details, the reader should keep in mind, however, that in order to image 50 μm thick structures the "correct" resolution must be 50 μm. Thus, according to the Nyquist theorem the pixel/voxel size must be 25 μm or smaller. In this section the term in vivo should always be read as "in vivo for humans." In vivo investigations of small animals can also be carried out with some of the μCT equipment introduced in the next section.

Table 21-1 gives an overview of high-resolution imaging techniques applied in vivo to determine structural parameters. As is discussed below, most of these are in the experimental phase and are not yet being used in clinical practice. Data are typically acquired slice by slice, and the slice thickness is most often larger than the in-plane pixel size. Currently MR methods are restricted to the peripheral skeleton whereas CT is applied to spine and forearm. However, radiation exposure limits spinal CT measurements to single slices of one or two vertebrae whereas in the periphery 3D data sets are acquired.

First attempts to extract structural information of the trabecular network in vitro were reported by Kalender et al. in 1986 [55–57]. They imaged vertebral specimens using a thin-slice (1 mm) CT technique and compared results to contact microradiography of the same specimen. This work revealed the principal difficulties of in vivo structural analysis techniques:
- In all X-ray based techniques the acceptable radiation dose limits the achievable spatial resolution and the signal to noise ratio. Theoretical considerations show that a spatial resolution of 100 μm is the approximate limit for human in vivo investigations [58].

Table 21-1 State of the art characteristics of high-resolution in vivo imaging techniques currently in use (typical values)

	Pixel size (μm^2)	Slice thickness (μm)	2D/3D data acquisition	Limits to spatial resolution
CT spine	150 x 150	1000	2D	Dose Technical factors limiting slice thickness
CT forearm	150 x 150	150	2D/3D	Dose and reproducibility
MRI calcaneus	150 x 150	500	3D	Scan time Field homogeneity
MRI forearm	150 x 150	700	3D	Scan time Field homogeneity
MRI finger	150 x 150	300	3D	Scan time Field homogeneity

– Before a structural analysis can be carried out, the image must be segmented to decide which image pixels represent bone and which background or marrow. Thus the structural analysis is typically based on binary images whereas a densitometric measurement is based on gray-scale images. The CT value of each pixel is converted to a BMD value by a linear transformation derived from a calibration measurement. Thus depending on the amount of bone within the pixel a lower or higher BMD value is associated with it.

– The decision of what is bone and what not is very sensitive to partial volume effects. We must remember that the thickness of individual trabeculae is smaller than 200 μm, and that their spacing typically ranges from 500 to 1000 μm. The parameters given in Table 21-1 make clear that partial volume effects are unavoidable in current in vivo techniques. While the in-plane pixel size approaches trabecular dimensions, the slice thickness most often is larger by a factor of 5–10 than the trabecular thickness. Thus many image pixels may contain some bone and some marrow, but in order to obtain a binary image we must assign them unequivocally to bone or marrow.

Figure 21-4 shows a series of CT images (Siemens Somatom Plus 4) derived from a human vertebral body embedded in a 15x15 cm^2 perspex block. All images show the midvertebral slice and are reconstructed with a field of view of 7.8 cm resulting in a pixel size of 152 x 152 μm^2. The images were not processed after reconstruction. Window level and width were adjusted to give the reader an impression of the noise present in the images. The black streaks in the spinal canal and in the transverse processes indicate embedding problems. The streaks are small air gaps in the otherwise homogeneous perspex. The streaks nicely demonstrate the effects of varying slice thickness. In Fig. 21-4a the low-dose standard osteodensitometry QCT protocol with a slice thickness of 10 mm was used. In Fig. 21-

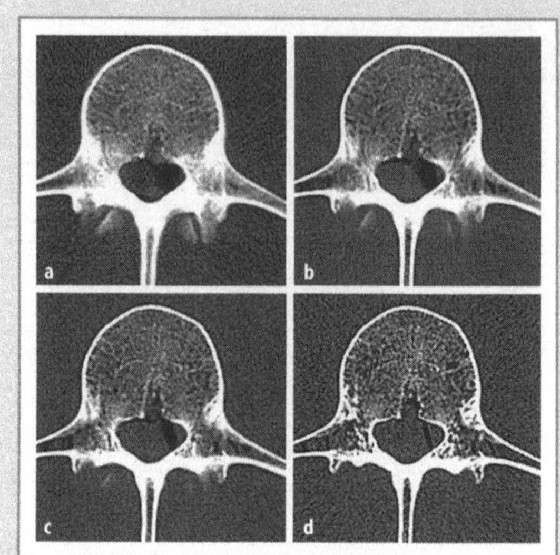

Fig. 21-4 CT images of a human vertebral body embedded in a 15x15 cm^2 perspex block (pixel size: 152 x152 mm^2; window width: 1380; window level: 780). **a** Low-dose standard osteodensitometry QCT protocol (80 kV; 146 mAs; slice thickness 10 mm). **b-d** Voltage and mAs settings (120 kV; 260 mAs) differed from **a** but were kept constant in **b-d**. Decrease in slice thickness to improve visualization of the trabecular network (**b** 5 mm; **c** 3 mm; **d** 1 mm)

4b–d voltage and mAs were increased to improve the visualization of the trabecular network. The slice thickness was gradually decreased from 5 to 1 mm.

The parameters of the scans along with noise and contrast-related results are given in Table 21-2. Features of the network are visible in all images, but the lower the slice thickness is, the clearer the image is. The image contrast of trabecular bone is highest in Fig. 21-4d. This is understandable because slice thickness-related partial volume effects are smaller. Thus the pixels representing trabecular bone are "filled" with a larger amount of bone and a smaller amount of marrow (actually perspex in the case of this phantom) which results in a higher trabecular contrast. However, this is only part of the story because noise must be considered as well. Table 2 also lists percentage background noise calculated as the standard deviation divided by the mean. The noise is relatively high in the standard low-dose QCT image (Fig. 21-4a). It is more than halved in Fig. 21-4b because a considerably higher dose is used. The reduction in slice thickness by a factor of 5 increases the noise again to an anticipated value of $47=22 \cdot \sqrt{5}$.

In order to combine the effects of image contrast and noise we also calculated the ratio of the highest contrast present in the trabecular bone to the background noise. The results demonstrate that with decreasing slice thickness the effect of higher trabecular image contrast is offset by higher noise. The clearer nature of Fig. 21-4c,d is a result of sharper structures due to thinner slices and not a result

Table 21-2 Characteristic parameters of images shown in Fig. 21-4. Background noise is given as standard coefficient of variation in %. Max. trabecular contrast: highest grayvalue within trabecular region subtracted by mean background CT value.

Fig.	Voltage (kV)	Current (mA)	Scan time (s)	Slice thickness (mm)	Background noise (%)	Max. trabecular image contrast/ background noise	Relative effective dose (approx. values)
4a	80	195	0,75	10	47	11.7	1
4b	120	130	2	5	22	14.5	4
4c	120	130	2	3	27	14.5	3
4d	120	130	2	1	47	14.2	1

of a better image contrast. It is desirable to further reduce the minimum slice thickness of clinical CT scanners below 1 mm. However, even then the increasing noise limits the detectability of finer details of the bone architecture, and only the larger structures or patterns can be determined. An increase in mAs is possible to compensate partly the increase in noise when thinner slices are investigated. The numbers in Table 2 show that the effective dose for the 1-mm thin-slice image is about the same as the dose for the standard QCT protocol used in Fig. 21-4a because a much thinner slice is used.

A texture related to the network architecture is clearly visible even in the 10-mm thick image (Fig. 21-4a). A major deterioration in the trabecular architecture probably changes this texture, and textural parameters even in relatively low-resolution images may supplement pure densitometric information. This idea was first tested by Braillon [59] using the calcium image derived from dual-energy QCT of the spine. He measured the coefficient of variation (CV) of the trabecular BMD in L2–L4. The CV, calculated as the standard deviation divided by the mean BMD value, is the simplest parameter characterizing texture. A high CV could indicate a high degree of gray-level variations in the image and thus a highly networked bone architecture. Indeed, CV values of trabecular BMD in osteoporotics were three to ten times higher than normals. In addition Braillon claimed a sensitivity of 96% at a specificity of 95% in using trabecular CV to separate normals from osteoporotics. However, CV analysis of a dataset of 214 women examined with a low-dose technique used for standard single-energy QCT did not confirm Braillon's results [60]. Nevertheless, it is tempting to apply this type of analysis to images with slightly higher resolution using higher dose protocols.

In order to further illustrate problems of limited spatial resolution in the in vivo assessment of bone architecture (see Fig. 21-5) we used stained grindings typically employed for histomorphometry. We started with a stack of 21 sagittal grindings (9×7 mm²) of a trabecular network from a human calcaneus. The thickness of each grinding was 5 μm and the distance between two adjacent grindings was 51 μm due to preparation requirements. All grindings were digitized resulting in a stack of binary images indicated in Fig. 21-5a (pixel area:

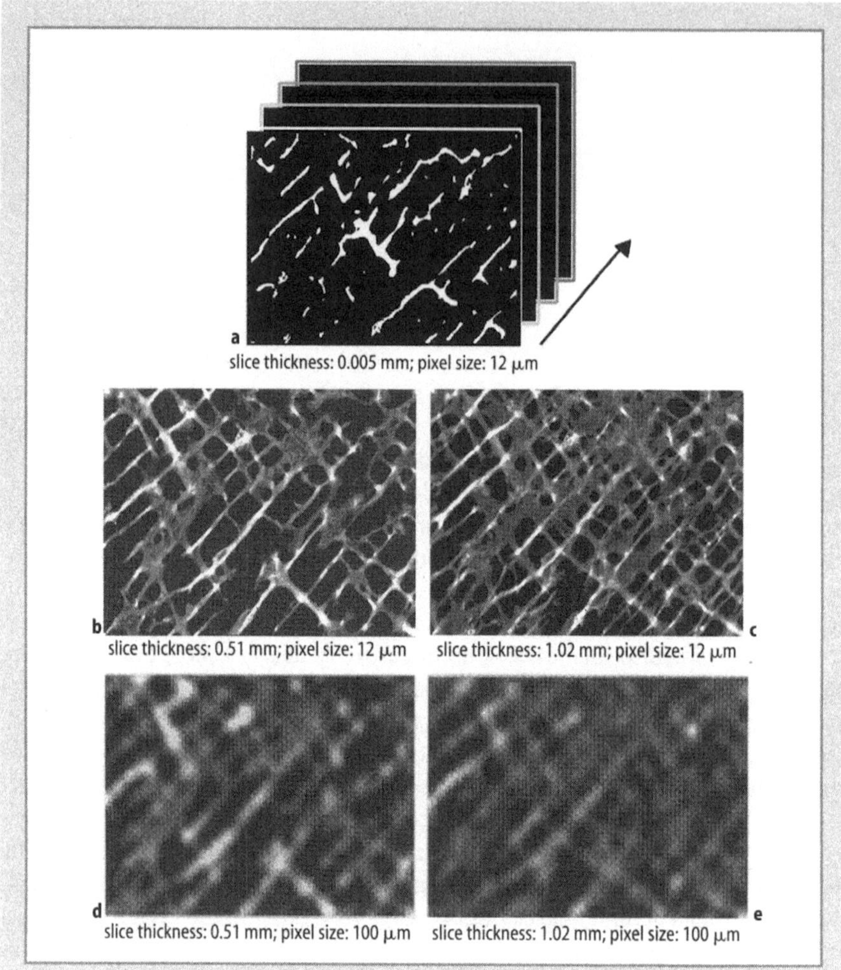

Fig. 21-5 Synthesis of typical radiographic and CT images from stained grindings. **a** Stack of 21 digitized grindings (courtesy of G. Delling and M. Hahn, University of Hamburg). **b** Half the stack was averaged in the direction indicated in a to obtain a "radiographylike image. **c** as **b**, but the complete stack was averaged. **d,e** Radiographic images in **c** and **d** were degraded in resolution to obtain "CT-like" images. Slice thicknesses and in plane pixel sizes are displayed under the images

12×12 μm²). Additional slices obtained by interpolation between adjacent binary images were added to simulate a slice thickness of 12 μm. Thus the final dataset consisted of isotropic voxels.

This dataset was then used to simulate high-resolution CT images. The images of the stack were averaged along the direction indicated in Fig. 21-5a. Two radiographic type images are displayed. One resulted by averaging half the stack (Fig. 21-5b) and the other by averaging all images of the stack (Fig. 21-5c). Thus a total slice thickness of 0.51 and 1.02 mm was simulated, respectively. The in-plane pixel area in these radiographic type images is still 12×12 μm^2. In particular in Fig. 21-5b there are still artificial discontinuities in the gray value variations. These would be avoided by averaging more images. Finally, an in-plane pixel size of 100 µm was simulated by degrading the resolution in the projected images in Fig. 21-5b,c by a factor of 8. The resolution-degraded images were blurred with a gaussian filter to give a more realistic impression of what can be expected in vivo. Results are shown in Fig. 21-5d,e. Compared to the images in Fig. 21-5b,c the side length of these two images should be reduced by a factor of 8, but for visualization purposes they were magnified.

These simulations again confirm conclusions drawn from Fig. 21-4: in the thin-slice CT-like images only the dominant structures are preserved; details of the trabecular network cannot be extracted. The textures in the CT-like and the radiography-like images are similar, and a major deterioration of the network is noticeable in the thin-slice CT images. However, a determination of parameters typically analyzed in histomorphometry is problematic. Even by visual comparison between the binarized grinding and the radiographylike images in Fig. 21-5b,c it is evident that parameters such as trabecular separation, trabecular thickness, trabecular number, and bone volume change drastically.

If thin-slice techniques are to be useful for structural analysis the following questions must be answered:
- What spatial resolution is required for a meaningful analysis of histomorphometric parameters?
- What segmentation methods can be used to obtain binary images?
- If a resolution adequate for histomorphometric analysis cannot be achieved, what textural or pattern analysis methods can be used to give information independent of BMD? What is the impact of analysis results on spatial resolution?
- Which sites are most suited for thin-slice techniques?

With the exception of the first of these questions none has been conclusively answered. The dependency of histomorphometric analysis results on spatial resolution has been investigated using µCT images (see next section for a more detailed discussion). A three-dimensional measurement of iliac crest biopsies showed that for a very precise analysis of histomorphometric parameters an isotropic spatial resolution of approximately 10 µm is required. Up to about 150 to 200 µm resolution dependent changes of these parameters could be described by a linear relationship, that is, appropriate calibration techniques can restore accurate values [61].

The answer to the second question depends on the image. The two major types of segmentation are threshold and edge based. The former depends on the absolute gray value of the pixel, i.e., in CT mainly on bone and marrow densities. Whereas global thresholds apply the same threshold to the whole image, local thresholds adapt this value to a neighborhood of a selectable size. Edge-based methods typically apply the first- or second-order derivative and thus detect changes in gray values. Global thresholds work well in high-resolution and high-contrast images, but often they fail in images such as those displayed in Figs. 21-4 and 21-5. In early approaches using thin-slice CT to analyze structure, global [62] and adaptive thresholds [63] and edge-based segmentation methods [56] were used. It is difficult to draw conclusions because none of the studies compared segmentation methods. We discuss this issue further in the last section of this chapter by introducing the idea of a digital model, which can serve as a standard to evaluate different segmentation and analysis schemes.

If the spatial resolution of the imaging system is too low to discriminate individual trabeculae, that is, if the resolution is worse than typically 200 μm, a structural analysis must concentrate on the dominant structures present in the image. Thus a pattern or texture analysis replaces a truly histomorphometric assessment. However, even a textural analysis is often used to determine histomorphometry-like parameters. After a segmentation step quantities such as mean structure width and separation can still be measured. Obviously these results are not accurate in the sense of measuring true trabecular thickness or width but age, disease, or treatment-related changes may nevertheless be quantifiable using these or similar parameters. Unfortunately, data are very sparse. In their study Klotz et al. [56] showed a relatively high correlation between CT and contact microradiography for bone volume ($r=0.8$) and for bone surface area ($r=0.8$). However, microradiography itself shows considerable partial volume artifacts [64]. Durand et al. demonstrated a separation of osteoporotics from normals using the slope from a linear regression of bone density versus bone surface area from thin-slice CT of the forearm, and Ito et al. [63] reported that this kind of texture analysis was helpful in assessing vertebral fractures. None of these studies was finally conclusive, in particular regarding the critical question of whether this type of analysis really improves the results of a purely densitometric measurement.

A textural analysis of thin-slice images can also be used to derive parameters describing the network character of the bone structure. This is seen, again, by inspecting Fig. 21-5. Although individual trabeculae are beautifully displayed in the digitized grinding, the image in Fig. 21-5a does not really give an impression of structure; the "network character" is lost. Thus, while classical methods of histomorphometry allow trabecular separation and thickness to be determined with high accuracy and precision, they fail to capture the impression present in the radiography-like images in Fig. 21-5b,c. Parameters such as connectivity of the network can potentially be better quantified if the images display a certain degree of "projectional" character. Interestingly, a number of textural analysis methods have been applied to plain X-ray films [65, 66], in particular to those of hands or fingers [67–70] where projectional artifacts are relatively small. Laval-Jeantet et al. [71] suggested analyzing the length of the skeletonized trabecular network in 1.5 mm thin spinal CT images. However, their approach did not separate postmenopausal osteoporotic women with vertebral fracture from a group of normal and osteopenic women without fractures.

Thin-slice CT applications in the spine so far have yielded ambiguous results mainly because a slice thickness of 1 mm is too large, and specific analysis algorithms are still missing. This may change with technological progress of clinical CT scanners such as the use of dual detector rings, but the radiation dose still limits the application to single slices. Thus the trabecular-rich ultradistal forearm has been used as an alternative site for the assessment of bone architecture. Compared to a tissue diameter of 40–80 cm at the spine, one of less than 10 cm must be imaged at the forearm. If the same scan parameters are used, this reduction in size can be translated to an increase in spatial resolution. The spatial resolution of specific clinical peripheral QCT (pQCT) scanners is comparable to thin-slice spinal CT, and resulting images have been used for textural analysis [62, 72]. Recently Rüegsegger and Müller et al. developed an in vivo pQCT system to obtain 3D datasets with an isotropic voxel size of 170 μm^3 [73, 74]. Figure 21-6 shows a section of a distal radius from a young healthy male volunteer measured with this system which currently defines the state of the art in X-ray based high-resolution in vivo CT systems.

The appendicular skeleton is also the target of high-resolution MR imaging. The underlying physical effect which is used to assess bone structure is the difference of the magnetic susceptibility between bone and bone marrow. This results in a modification of the apparent transverse relaxation time T2* which theoretically should be related directly to the density of the trabecular network and its spatial geometry. Experimental studies [75–78] and simulations [79, 80] have indeed confirmed the potential of this technique. As with BMD, T2* can be determined macroscopically within a larger ROI [78, 81, 82], but so far a distinction between the structural contributions and the density contributions of the T2* signal has not been evaluated. This could in principle give some information on a textural but not on an trabecular level.

Spin-echo [83] and gradient-echo sequences [84, 85] have been used to directly generate high-resolution images of bone structure. Gradient-echo techniques

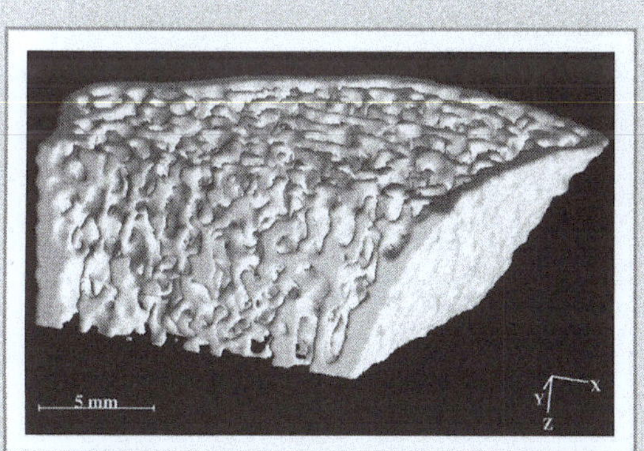

Fig. 21-6 Distal radius from a young healthy male volunteer measured with a state of the art pQCT system. The dataset was obtained with an isotropic voxel size of 170 mm³. (Courtesy of P. Rüegsegger, ETH Zurich) [128]

are currently in wider use because they require less sampling time and are therefore better suited for in vivo investigations. Sampling time and the requirement of highly homogeneous fields currently restrict high-resolution MR to the appendicular skeleton. The in-plane resolution is comparable to CT-based techniques, but the slice thickness does not yet match that of forearm pQCT (see Table 1). Thus, again, the segmentation to derive binary images for structural analysis is a major problem. Adaptive threshold- and edge-based methods do not work well in MR images because they tend to amplify susceptibility differences in the bone marrow, resulting in a misclassification of marrow as bone. Most often global thresholds based on the histogram of the gray-value distribution are used [85]. Alternatively, an internal calibration based on fat, air, tendon, and cortical bone has been proposed [86], but for both methods analysis results are strongly affected by operator-adjustable parameters. Thus within a given study typically the same segmentation scheme is applied to all patient or specimen scans.

Most publications in the field of high-resolution MR imaging are still concerned with technical issues. Only recently cross-sectional and longitudinal patient data were reported from two studies. Both derived histomorphometric parameters from textural analysis. In the calcaneus trabecular separation and thickness discriminated between pre- and postmenopausal healthy women but were correlated less strongly with age than calcaneal BMD [86]. Figure 21-7 shows as an example the MR image of a calcaneus from this study. The second publication concen-

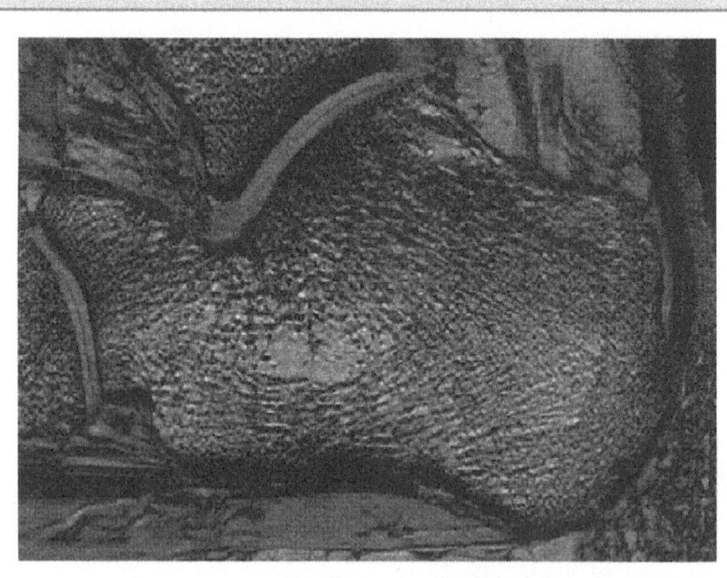

Fig. 21-7 In vivo high-resolution MR image of a human calcaneus. One slice out of a 3D dataset is displayed (slice thickness: 1 mm; pixel size: 200 mm²)

trated on the distal radius although spinal QCT was also included. Trabecular separation showed greater age-related changes but a lower correlation with age than spinal QCT. Trabecular separation, trabecular number, and bone volume discriminated between postmenopausal women with and those without spinal fractures whereas trabecular thickness did not [87]. These initial results look promising, but as discussed above it has not been investigated whether high-resolution MR results really improve results from bone densitometry.

A major issue with the advent of high-resolution in vivo imaging is the question of reproducibility in serial measurements. Even if the imaging equipment is stable patient repositioning is increasingly difficult. A reproducible analysis of identical ROIs in serial measurements is crucial to achieve high precision. Many image processing procedures such as selecting an analysis ROI require operator interaction and contribute to precision errors. With regard to MR based techniques precision errors of 4%–10% for $T2^*$ measurements of the distal radius [78] and of 3% and 5% for histomorphometric parameters of the calcaneus [86] have been reported for serial measurements several weeks apart. In the case of the calcaneus the patients' foot was held firmly in a custom-built frame to improve repositioning. In both studies the analysis ROIs were manually repositioned based on anatomical landmarks.

As manual repositioning of analysis ROIs is relatively coarse, a reduction of precision errors requires automated matching algorithms to align follow-up and baseline measurements. This is not a trivial task in 3D high-resolution images. The use of a highly sophisticated algorithm based on correlation techniques for serial measurements with the pQCT system developed by Münch et al. resulted in excellent precision errors of 0.5% for structural parameters [74, 88]. Obviously the size of the analysis ROI also determines the effort necessary to align serial measurements, but it should be kept in mind that even in standard spinal QCT measurements a reproducible placement of the analysis ROI relative to an anatomical coordinate system improves precision significantly [89, 90].

Ultrahigh-Resolution In Vitro Assessment of Bone Microstructure and In Vivo Examinations of Small Animals

The previous section dealt with techniques resolving structures in the range of 100–1000 µm. Here we review µCT and µMR techniques with resolution spanning the range from 100 down to 5–10 µm. Thus we enter the domain of histomorphometry, but the techniques that we discuss differ in two major aspects. Firstly, they are nondestructive in the sense that the sample, for example, the bone biopsy, remains intact and can be used for further investigations, such as mechanical testing. Secondly, they are inherently suited for 3D data acquisition and analysis whereas histomorphometry is principally a 2D technique. Serial sectioning of a volume resulting in a 3D stack of histomorphometric images has been successfully tried [91], but the intense preparation required renders this technique impractical for daily use. Other investigators have used scanning electron microscopy

[92] and stereo microscopy [93] to obtain 3D images. However, quantitative structural analysis strategies do not yet exist for images of this type.

Results of 2D analysis from histomorphometry of planar sections can be used to estimate 3D parameters such as bone volume or surface area. Also, assuming either a platelike or a rodlike trabecular network, other 2D histomorphometric parameters such as trabecular separation or thickness can be extrapolated into the third dimension [94]. However, a true assessment of many structural parameters such as the anisotropy and the topology describing connectivity and porosity can be performed only with a 3D assessment [91, 95]. Age-related vertebral bone loss seems to be associated with a transition from predominantly platelike trabeculae to a predominantly rodlike structure. Whole trabeculae are lost [96]. In contrast to the case in younger subjects, free ends and microcallus are frequently found in older patients. The mechanism of the transformation has been explained by perforations and progressive thinning [97]. Perforations, however, can be quantified only with 3D data.

Before we describe μCT techniques in more detail we briefly review some of the fundamental parameters impacting on structural analysis with μCT. There is a close relationship between sample size, resolution, radiation dose, and scan time. Unfortunately, not all parameters can be optimized simultaneously, and an application specific compromise must be found. To illustrate the principal factors we assume for simplicity a circular sample of diameter, d, which is scanned in contiguous slices with a slice thickness, h. The in-plane resolution is denoted by w:

- The applied surface dose, D, is affected by the resolution, w, and the slice thickness, h: $D \sim 1/w^3h$ [58]. Thus, if for a given object the resolution of the resulting image is to be increased by a factor of 2 without an increase in noise, the dose must be increased by a factor of 8 provided the slice thickness remains constant. Dose must be increased by a factor of 16 if the slice thickness is additionally reduced by a factor of 2.
- The scanning time depends in the same way on resolution and slice thickness as the dose. Thus high-intensity X-ray sources are required to complete datasets within time frames typically for clinical CT scanners. This is of particular importance for in vivo scans of small animals.
- Unfortunately, the requirement of high X-ray intensity contradicts the requirement of a small focus of the X-ray source in order to prevent geometrical unsharpness of the structures to be imaged.
- The sample size, d, depends on the sufficient matrix size m: $d = m \times w$. Thus for an image matrix of 512^2 pixels and a pixel size of 20 μm the sample diameter is then restricted to 1 cm; for a pixel size of 100 μm d is limited to 5 cm.

The development of μCT equipment during the past decade has progressed along two major avenues. Either fine- or microfocus X-ray tubes have been used for fan or cone beam projection tomography. Alternatively, synchrotron radiation (SR) from electron storage rings has been used as an X-ray source for parallel beam projection tomography. Both approaches have advantages and disadvantages: The X-ray intensity of SR is magnitudes higher than that of X-ray tubes. If scanning time matters, and for ultimate resolution below 1–5 μm, SR is the better choice. The continuous X-ray spectrum of SR furthermore allows the use of monochromatic radiation for an optimal adaptation of the X-ray energy to the sample. This procedure, again, may be important for in vivo investigations of small animals because it can be used to minimize radiation exposure. However, electron storage rings are stationary and cannot be operated in a small laboratory. Compared to systems with X-ray tubes the experimental effort to use SR for μCT is much larger, and there are only a few SR centers available worldwide. Further details can be extracted from the literature [58, 98].

3D μCT for structural investigation of bone biopsies was pioneered by Feldkamp and Goldstein using a cone beam set-up with a microfocus X-ray tube [3, 99, 100]. They also proposed applying morphological measures such as the Euler characteristic to quantify connectivity. Figure 21-8 illustrates the concept of connectivity; Fig 21-8a shows a small portion of a trabecular network and Fig. 21-8b a skeleton of the highlighted structure. Nodes A and B are multiply connected. Thus a removal of the branch AC does not disconnect node A from B as the connection ADB is still intact. Connectivity is a measure of the maximum number of branches which can be removed before the structure is divided into multiple pieces. For a better view a 2D representation was used in Fig. 21-8, but the discussion is equally valid for the 3D case. The connectivity c of a two-component system such as bone and marrow can be derived directly from the Euler characteristic e by $c=1-e$ [91]. This relationship is valid provided that all trabeculae are connected, and no isolated marrow cavities exist inside bone. The Euler characteristic can be determined in the μCT dataset without a prior skeletonization [91, 99]. The resulting connectivity is usually normalized to the investigated tissue volume and reported as connectivity density in $1/mm^3$. Results of connectivity measurements reported in the literature have not been consistent. In particular

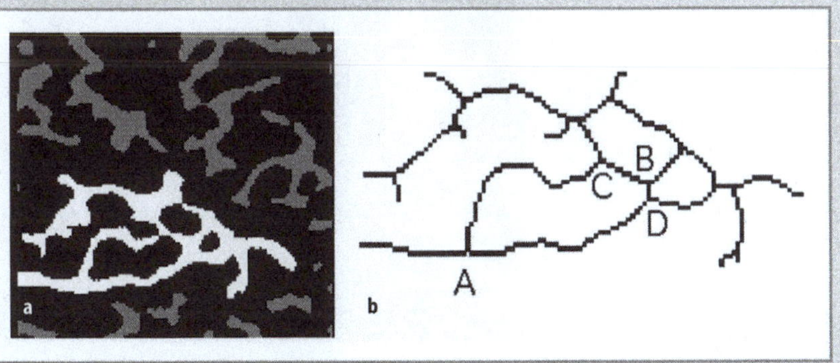

Fig. 21-8 Concept of connectivity of a trabecular network. **a** Binary image of a small portion of a trabecular network. **b** Skeleton of the highlighted structure. Removal of branch AC does not disconnect node A from B as the connection ADB is still intact but reduces connectivity and stability of the network (see text for details)

the comparison with bone volume has yielded disparate data, ranging from highly linear to nonlinear relationships [91, 99, 101, 102]. Part of this discrepancy may be due to the specifics of the data analysis involved and to the different specimen and sample sizes investigated.

Feldkamp et al. reported an isotropic spatial resolution of approx. 70 μm for their system. Further improvements in spatial resolution to 30 μm were recently achieved by Rüegsegger et al. [103, 104]. A μCT image of a lumbar spine biopsy taken from a 60-year-old woman is shown in Fig. 21-9. The image clearly reveals the mixture of rods and plates and gives a vivid impression of plate perforations of various sizes. As with Feldkamp's system this tomograph is also dedicated to the investigation of small specimens in vitro or of bone biopsies. Scanning time varies between 20 min for 50 μm resolution and 2 h for 30 μm resolution.

The determination of structural parameters in serial measurements is of substantial interest in preclinical research using small animals such as rats. The femur and the tibia are best suited for μCT. In the rat trabecular width is in the order of 50 μm and trabecular spacing around 150 μm or less. Thus in vivo imaging requires a resolution of 20–30 μm while scanning times should be less than 30–60 min due to anesthesia. Compared to the systems discussed in the previous paragraph, the X-ray intensity must be increased to shorten scan times. Consequently SR has been used for serial in vivo investigations of rats. Scans of the proximal tibia just prior to and 5 weeks after ovariectomy showed a high degree of absorption of platelike structures [102]; 60% of trabecular bone volume was lost. Scan-

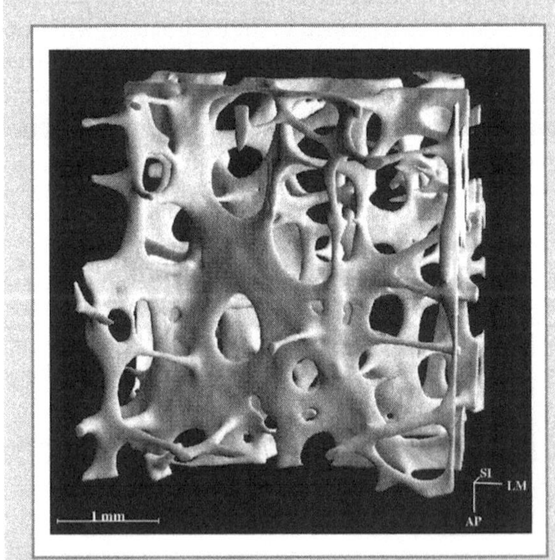

Fig. 21-9 3D surface rendered view of a lumbar spine biopsy from a 60-year-old woman imaged with μCT (spatial resolution: 30 mm; courtesy of P. Rüegsegger, ETH Zurich) [104]

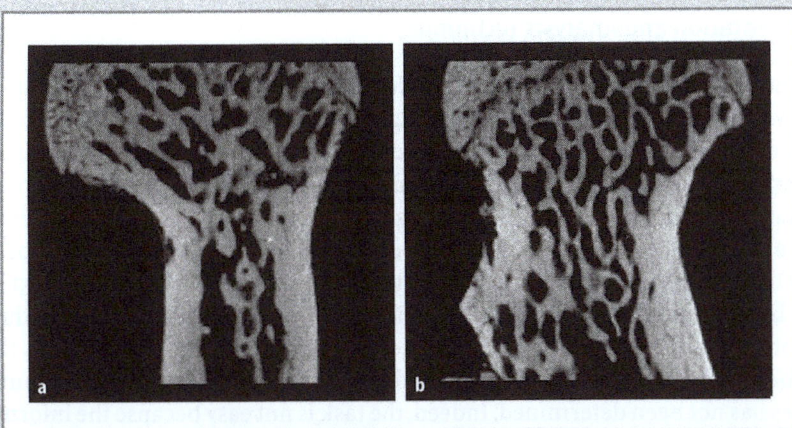

Fig. 21-10 In vitro µCT coronal **a** and sagittal slices **b** of a rat femur taken with an X-ray tube based cone beam system (spatial resolution: 30 mm; exposure time: 25 min; courtesy of ARACOR, Sunnyvale Calif., and OARG, University of California)

ning time for a 2 mm long section varied between 30 min using monochromatic X-rays and 2.5 min using the unmonochromatized so called "white" beam. A maximum surface dose of 0.9 Gy was administered.

Example images from a rat femur are shown in Fig. 21-10. However, these data were obtained in vitro from a cone beam system with an X-ray tube developed by ARACOR (Sunnyvale, Calif). A µCT system specific to in vitro investigations of small animals with somewhat lower resolution has also been developed by Stratec Medizintechnik (Pforzheim, Germany). In another system SR was used to investigate bone specimens three-dimensionally with ultrahigh resolution (voxel size 8 µm) [98, 105]. At this resolution microcallus formation could be identified which is not feasible at spatial resolutions around 50 µm.

Several researchers have also demonstrated the feasibility of µMR to image bone structure [106, 107]. High-field MR spectrometers with imaging possibilities or small-bore MR imaging scanners must be used to obtain ultrahigh spatial resolution. An isotropic resolution (pixel size 78 µm³) of small defatted bone samples has been reported [108] using a rapid spin-echo technique. Precision of structural parameters derived from µMR measurements was determined by Hipp et al. who compared their values to precision data for the µCT system developed by Feldkamp [100, 109]. Precision for bone volume was better for CT (3% versus 6%) while precision for trabecular number was better for µMR (1% versus 2.5%). In vivo experiments with µMR using small animals have not been reported, to our knowledge.

A Digital Bone Model as a Standard to Investigate Segmentation and Analysis Techniques

The need for reliable segmentation techniques is more obvious in lower resolution in vivo images than in μCT or μMR images because partial volume effects are a major source of image degradation. Also, most structural analysis concepts are either closely related to the ideas of histomorphometry, or they try to assess parameters such as connectivity. These strategies rely on the proper separation of individual trabeculae and do not work properly in in vivo images where most often only dominant structures result in a textural appearance. Differences in texture may be intuitively obvious, but the question remains of how to characterize them quantitatively. Textbooks on image processing present a wealth of methods that can be applied, but which strategies should be applied to in vivo images of human bones has not been determined. Indeed, the task is not easy because the information to be extracted should be independent of BMD. Therefore, if the segmentation step is strongly affected by density, it may not be surprising that the so-called structural parameters are closely correlated with BMD and thus do not provide independent information. Also, it is typically difficult to verify structural analysis results derived from in vivo measurements because a necessary μCT or histomorphometric analysis cannot be performed.

Inspired by this dilemma, we developed the concept of a trabecular bone model as a possibility to test analysis and segmentation strategies. However, instead of trying to construct a trabecular bone model from scratch [110] we started with a real 3D dataset imaged with the μCT scanner developed by Feldkamp. Bone was separated from marrow by a simple threshold, and further manipulation of the binary dataset ensured that (a) all voxels classified as bone were connected, and

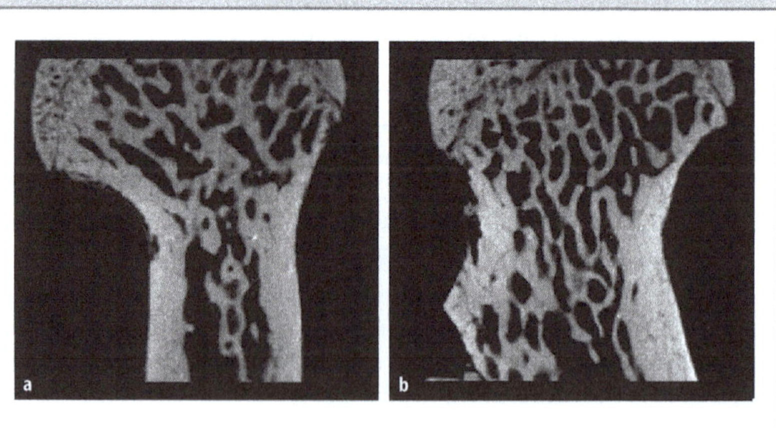

Fig. 21-10 In vitro μCT coronal **a** and sagittal slices **b** of a rat femur taken with an X-ray tube based cone beam system (spatial resolution: 30 mm; exposure time: 25 min; courtesy of ARACOR, Sunnyvale Calif., and OARG, University of California)

that (b) all voxels classified as marrow were connected. The resulting binary dataset was then defined as the standard. As the resolution of this standard is of course determined by the μCT system used for imaging (approx. 70 μm), it does not contain very fine trabeculae, but it is very realistic compared to the resolution of in vivo systems applicable to humans.

The advantage of the model lies in its generation which is based on a binary image. Thus, in contrast to data obtained in vivo, in the model the truth is known because it is defined what is bone and what is marrow. Realistic gray values within the bone voxels of the model (taken from the original μCT dataset) are restored afterwards. Further details can be found in [111]. Figure 21-11a shows a 3D surface rendered view of the model. This model can in principle be used to for example, separate the effects of segmentation and spatial resolution on the analysis of structural parameters. The appearance of texture to be expected in high-resolution in vivo images can be simulated by degrading the model resolution. Thus it should be possible to better investigate the relationship between structure and texture by varying the structure of the model in a controlled manner. Figure 21-11b shows as an example the result after one iteration of a gradual 3D thinning process. The approach to image processing problems with this or similar models is promising but still needs to be validated.

Conclusions and Outlook

During the past decade considerable progress has been achieved to assess bone structure in addition to bone mass. Both X-ray-CT and MR techniques are under experimental evaluation for in vivo applications down to 100 μm resolution and for in vitro or specimen investigations at resolution levels approaching 1–10 μm. Thus the gap between densitometry and histomorphometry seems to be closing. This is definitely true from a technical standpoint, although most of the equipment and the analytical techniques discussed in this chapter still a have prototypic character and have not been employed routinely in research or clinical practice. So far, however, insufficient data exist to evaluate these new techniques with regard to the three criteria mentioned in the introduction: assessment of relevant changes of bone structure, discriminative capabilities, and power to predict fractures. It is still unclear to what degree in vivo structural analysis of humans can complement bone densitometry to improve the diagnosis of osteoporosis, guide treatment decisions, and monitor therapy. The HAL may be an exception as it adds information to BMD and seems to be useful in cross-sectional investigations of risk factors for osteoporosis, but it has no value in longitudinal studies.

The new technical developments for 3D in vivo data acquisition offer exciting new possibilities. The lack of appropriate 3D scanning protocols has been the main obstacle for a more detailed investigation of the proximal femur. This will soon change as spiral CT ensures a faster acquisition and lower dose than the older multiple slice techniques. A 3D assessment of femoral macrostructure will be possible, but acceptable levels of radiation exposure will limit thin-slice investigations for the determination of the trabecular texture to single slices. This is also true for the spine, but due to the rapid turnover of vertebral trabecular BMD appropriate textural analysis techniques may yield useful information even from single slices. However, a slice thickness of less than 1 mm should be achieved.

The acquisition of high-resolution 3D in vivo data in humans is restricted to the appendicular skeleton. The distal forearm seems to be the favorite site because it is an important fracture site, and because a wealth of densitometric data exists. However, investigation of the phalanges should also be considered because phalangeal BMD measured by radiographic absorptiometry seems to better discriminate spinal fractures than radial DXA [112, 113]. As the diameter of the fingers is considerably smaller than that of the distal forearm, phalangeal trabecular structure can be determined with higher spatial resolution than the structure at the radius. Recently MR was also applied to image the trabecular structure of the phalanges [114]. Thin-slice 3D in vivo MR techniques will compete with thin-slice CT at appendicular sites. In MR the achievable spatial resolution is limited by the magnetic field strength and homogeneity; in X-ray based systems it is limited by radiation dose.

Segmentation and analysis of both MR and CT images are still problems. Currently available algorithms are too oriented towards individual trabeculae and insufficiently adapted to texture. Thus particularly in in vivo images, which are often heavily affected by partial volume artifacts, structural information may be obscured by improper analysis. Some textural measures such as the fractal dimension have been used. However, their meaning and results are still controversial when applied to bone structure [115–119]. A texture analysis using gray-scale morphology [120] is an interesting attempt to bypass the segmentation step necessary to obtain binary images. However, an adequate characterization and understanding of segmentation and analysis strategies requires a standard or phantom with known structure from which in vivo images can be measured or simulated. Such a model is introduced in the last section. Attempts are under way to transform the digital model into a real phantom using the rapid prototyping technique of stereolithography [121]. If successful, a spongiosa phantom with a realistic and known structure will become available which can be used to characterize high-resolution imaging equipment.

Ultrahigh-resolution μCT and μMR techniques providing spatial resolutions close to those of histomorphometry are opening new avenues of research. A true 3D assessment of the networked character of bone is possible and rod or plate model assumptions are no longer necessary. Apart from the extension into the third dimension the nondestructive character of these techniques is highly relevant. As the tedious sample preparation for histomorphometry is no longer required, and because measurement and analysis can be highly automated, greater numbers of samples can be investigated. Thus structural results can be determined with higher statistical significance, and more studies can be carried out. Although μCT and μMR systems are yet not in widespread use, a commercial market for these systems seems to be developing, promising a broader distribution in the future.

μCT has also demonstrated the ability to obtain in vivo serial measurements of small animals which is of the utmost importance in preclinical research. Longitudinal instead of cross-sectional studies can be used to investigate mechanisms of bone loss, reducing sample size requirements. Another field of application is the comparison of structure with biomechanical parameters and destructive testing. Finite element analysis of bones can be put on a new basis because the bone structure itself instead of density values averaged over a larger volume can be used as a starting point [122–126]. Potentially the interaction of the cortex with the trabecular structure, the transmission of forces inside the bone, and the contribution of the cortex to bone strength can be investigated in greater detail. Thus structural analysis based on CT and MR techniques will contribute to our understanding of osteoporosis and should finally benefit the patient suffering from this disease.

References

1. Hansson T, Roos B, Nachemson A (1980) The bone mineral content and ultimate compressive strength of lumbar vertebrae. Spine 5:46–55
2. McBroom RJ, Hayes WC, Edwards WT, Goldberg RP, White AA (1985) Prediction of vertebral body compressive fracture using quantitative computed tomography. J Bone Joint Surg Am 67:1206–1214
3. Goldstein SA (1987) The mechanical properties of trabecular bone: Dependence on anatomic location and function. J Biomech 20(11):1055–1061
4. Mosekilde L, Bentzen SM, Ørtoft G, Jørgensen J (1989) The predictive value of quantitative computed tomography for vertebral body compressive strength and ash density. Bone 10:465–470
5. Lang SM, Moyle DD, Berg EW, Detorie N, Gilpin AT, Pappan NJ Jr, Reynolds JC, Tkacik M, Waldron RL (1988) Correlation of mechanical properties of vertebral trabecular bone with equivalent mineral density as measured by computed tomography. J Bone Joint Surg Am 70:1531–1538
6. Brinckmann P, Biggemann M, Hilweg D (1989) Prediction of the compressive strength of human lumbar vertebrae. Clin Biomech 4 [Suppl 2]:S1–S27
7. Ciarelli MJ, Goldstein SA, Kuhn JL, Cody DD, Brown MB (1991) Evaluation of orthogonal mechanical properties and density of human trabecular bone from the major metaphyseal regions with materials testing and computed tomography. J Orthop Res 9:674–682
8. Hayes WC, Piazza SJ, Zysset PK (1991) Biomechanics of fracture risk prediction of the hip and spine by quantitative computed tomography. Rad Clin North Am 29:1–18
9. Lotz JC, Gerhart TN, Hayes WC (1990) Mechanical properties of trabecular bone from the proximal femur: a quantitative CT study. J Comput Assist Tomogr 14(1):107–114
10. Keaveny TM, Hayes WC (1993) A 20 year perspective on the mechanical properties of trabecular bone. J Biomech Eng 115:534–542

11. Smith MD, Dickie-Cody D, Goldstein SA, Cooperman AM, Matthews LS, Flynn MJ (1992) Proximal femoral bone density and its correlation to fracture load and hip-screw penetration load. Clin Orthop Relat Res 283:244–251

12. Alho A, Husby T, Høiseth A (1988) Bone mineral content and mechanical strength. Clin Orthop Relat Res 227:292–297

13. Høiseth A, Strømsøe K, Alho A (1995) Comparison between femoral bone mineral parameters assessed by QCT and dual X-ray densitometry. Eur J Radiol 5:264–268

14. Felsenberg D (1992) Klinische Anwendung der quantitativen Computertomographie. In: Schild HH, Heller M (eds) Osteoporose. Thieme, Stuttgart, pp 100–126

15. Heuck A, Block J, Glüer CC, Steiger P, Genant HK (1989) Mild versus definite osteoporosis: comparison of bone densitometry techniques using different statistical models J Bone Miner Res 4(6):891–900

16. Pacifici R, Rupich RC, Griffin M, Chines A, Susman N, Avioli LV (1990) Dual energy radiography versus quantitative computer tomography for the diagnosis of osteoporosis. J Clin Endocrinol Metab 70(3):705–710

17. Ott S (1991) Methods of determining bone mass. J Bone Miner Res 6 [Suppl 2]:S71–S75

18. Yu W, Glüer C-C, Grampp S, Jergas M, Fuerst T, Wu CY, Lu Y, Fan B, Genant HK (1995) Spinal bone mineral assessment in postmenopausal women: a comparison between dual X-ray absorptiometry and quantitative computed tomography. Osteoporosis Int 5:433–439

19. Ito M, Hayashi K, Ishida Y, Uetani M, Yamada M, Ohki M, Nakamura T (1997) Discrimination of spinal fracture with various bone mineral measurements. Calcif Tissue Int 60:11–15

20. Sandor T, Felsenberg D, Kalender W, Brown E (1991) Global and regional variations in the spinal trabecular bone: single and dual energy examinations. J Clin Endocrinol Metab 72:1157–1168

21. Flynn MJ, Cody DD, Peterson E, Wang DC, Kleerekoper M (1992) Recognition of lower lumbar vertebral architecture patterns in osteoporosis. Radiology 185(P):126

22. Dickie-Cody D, Flynn MJ, Vickers DS (1989) A technique for measuring regional bone mineral density in human lumbar vertebral bodies. Med Phys 16(5):766–772

23. Mazess RB (1990) Fracture risk: a role for compact bone. Calcif Tissue Int 47:191–193

24. Snyder SM, Schneider E (1991) Estimation of mechanical properties of cortical bone by computed tomography. J Orthop Res 9:422–431

25. Vesterby A, Mosekilde L, Gunderson HJG, Melsen F, Mosekilde L, Holme K, Sorenson S (1991) Biologically meaningful determinants of the in vitro strength of lumbar vertebrae. Bone 12:219–224

26. Louis O, Van den Winkel P, Covens P, Schoutens A, Osteaux M (1993) Size of cortical bone and relationship to bone mineral density assessed by quantitative computed tomography image segmentation. Invest Radiol 28:802–805

27. Spadaro JA, Werner FW, Brenner RA, Fortino MD, Fay LA, Edwards WT (1994) Cortical and trabecular bone contribute strength to the osteopenic distal radius. J Orthop Res 12:211–218

28. Ferretti JL, Frost HM, Gasser JA, High WB, Jee WS, Jerome C, Mosekilde L, Thompson DD (1995) Perspectives on osteoporosis research: its focus and some insights from a new paradigm. Calcif Tissue Int 57:399–404

29. Kalender WA, Felsenberg D, Louis O, Lopez P, Klotz E, Osteaux M, Fraga J (1989) Reference values for trabecular and cortical vertebral bone density in single and dual-energy quantitative computed tomography. Eur J Radiol 9:75–80

30. Pacifici R, Rupich RC, Avioli LV (1990) Vertebral cortical bone mass measurement by a new quantitative computed a tomography method: correlations with vertebral trabecular bone measurements. Calcif Tissue Int 47:215–220

31. Sandor T, Felsenberg D, Kalender WA, Clain A, Broen E (1992) Compact and trabecular components of the spine using quantitative computed tomography. Calcif Tissue Int 50:502–506

32. Sumner DR, Olson CL, Freeman PM, Lobick JJ, Andriacchi TP (1989) Computed tomography measurement of cortical bone geometry. J Biomech 22:649–653

33. Rüegsegger P, Durand E, Dambacher MA (1991) Localization of regional forearm bone loss from high resolution computed tomographic images. Osteoporosis Int1(2):76–80

34. Grampp S, Lang P, Jergas M, Glüer CC, Mathur A, Engelke K, Genant HK (1995) Assessment of the skeletal status by peripheral quantitative computed tomography of the forearm: short-term precision in vivo and comparison to dual X-ray absorptiometry. J Bone Miner Res 10:1566–1576

35. Ritzel H, Amling M, Pösl M, Hahn M (1997) The thickness of human vertebral cortical bone and its changes in aging and osteoporosis: a histomorphometric analysis of the complete spinal column from thirty-seven autopsy cases. J Bone Miner Res 12:89–95

36. Silva MJ, Wang C, Keaveny TM, Hayes WC (1994) Direct and computed tomography thickness measurements of the human, lumbar vertebral shell and endplate. Bone 4:409–414

37. Hangartner TN, Gilsanz V (1996) Evaluation of cortical bone by computed tomography. J Bone Miner Res 11:1518–1525

38. Courtney AC, Wachtel EF, Myers ER, Hayes WC (1994) Effects of loading rate on strength of the proximal femur. Calcif Tissue Int 55:53–58

39. Beck TJ, Christopher BR, Warden KE, Scott WW, Rao GU (1990) Predicting femoral neck strength from bone mineral data: a structural approach. Invest Radiol 25:6–18

40. Yoshikawa T, Turner CH, Peacock M, Slemenda CW, Weaver CM, Teegarden D, Markwardt P, Burr DB (1994) Geometric structure of the femoral neck measured using dual-energy X-ray absorptiometry. J Bone Miner Res 9(7): 1053–1064

41. Beck TJ, Ruff CB, Bisseur K (1993) Age-related changes in femoral neck geometry: Implications for bone strength. Calcif Tissue Int 53 [Suppl 1]:S41–S46

42. Bhasin S, Sartoris DJ, Fellingham L, Zlatkin MB, Andre M, Resnick D (1988) Three-dimensional quantitative CT of the proximal femur: relationship to vertebral trabecular bone density in postmenopausal women. Radiology 167:145–149

43. Glüer CC, Genant HK (1987) Quantitative computed tomography of the hip. In: Genant HK (ed) Osteoporosis Update 1987. University of California Printing Services, San Francisco, pp 187–196

44. Sartoris DJ, Andre M, Resnick C, Resnick D (1986) Trabecular bone density in the proximal femur: quantitative CT assessment. Radiology 160:707–712

45. Heitz M, Kalender WA (1994) Evaluation of femoral mineral density and strength using volumetric CT and anatomical coordinate systems. 10th International Bone Densitometry Workshop 1994, Venice, Italy. Bone Miner 25 [Suppl 2]:S11

46. Genant HK, Engelke K, Fuerst T, Glüer CC, Grampp S, Harris ST, Jergas M, Lang T, Lu Y, Majumdar S et al (1996) Noninvasive assessment of bone mineral and structure: state of the art. J Bone Min Res 11:707–730

47. Prevrhal S, Heitz M, Lowet G, Engelke K, Kalender WA (1997) Quantitative CT am proximalen Femur: in vitro-Studie. Z Med Phys (submitted)

48. Faulkner KG, Cummings SR, Glüer CC, Palermo L, Black D, Genant HK (1993) Simple measurement of femoral geometry predicts hip fracture: the study of osteopotic fractures. J Bone Min Res 8:1211–1217

49. Glüer CC, Cummings SR, Pressman A, Li J, Glüer K, Faulkner KG, Grampp S, Genant HK (1994) Prediction of hip fractures from pelvic radiographs: the study of osteoporotic fractures. J Bone Miner Res 9:671–677

50. Flicker L, Faulkner KG, Hopper JL, Green RM, Kaymacki B, Nowson CA, Young D, Wark JD (1996) Determinants of hip axis length in women aged 10–89: a twin study. Bone 18:41–45

51. Cummings SR, Cauley JA, Palermo L, Ross PD, Wasnich RD, Black D, Faulkner KG (1994) Racial differences in hip axis lengths might explain racial differences in rates of hip fractures. Osteoporosis Int 4:226–229

52. Nelson DA, Jacobsen F, Barondess DA, Parfit AM (1995) Ethnic differences in regional bone density, hip axis length and lifestyle variables among healthy balck and white men. J Bone Miner Res 10:782–787

53. Mikhail MB, Vaswani AN, Aloia JF (1996) Racial differences in femoral dimensions and their relation to hip fracture. Osteoporosis Int 6:22–24

54. Cummings SR, Black DM, Nevitt MC et al (1990) Appendicular bone density and age predict hip fracture in women. JAMA 263(5):665–668

55. Klotz E, Kalender W, Henschke F, Bayer T (1985) Dual energy CT and morphometric analysis of high resolution CT images for the diagnosis of bone mineral diseases in CAR. Springer, Berlin Heidelberg New York, pp 438–442

56. Klotz E, Henschke F, Kalender W (1986) Morphometrische Analyse hochauf-

lösender CT-Bilder der Wirbelsäule. In: 17th meeting of the Deutsche Gesellschaft für Medizinische Physik (DGMP), Lübeck, pp 45–51

57. Kalender W, Klotz E, Brestowsky H (1989) Automatische Auswertung von CT Bildern in der Diagnose der Osteoporose. Electromedica 57:20–24

58. Graeff W, Engelke K (1991) Microradiography and microtomography. In: Ebashi S, Koch M, Rubenstein E (eds) Handbook on synchrotron radiation. North-Holland, Amsterdam, pp 361–405

59. Braillon PM, Bochu M, Meunier PJ (1993) Quantitative computed tomography (QCT). A new analysis of bone quality in osteoporosis and osteomalacia. 9th International Workshop of Bone Densitometry, Traverse City. Calcif Tissue Int 52:166

60. Engelke K, Grampp S, Glüer CC, Jergas M, Yang S-O, Genant HK (1995) significance of QCT bone mineral density and its standard deviation as parameters to evaluate osteoporosis. J Comput Assist Tomogr 19:111–116

61. Müller R, Koller B, Hildebrand T, Laib A, Gianolini S, Rüegsegger P (1996) Resolution dependency of microstructural properties of cancellous bone based on three-dimensional μ-tomography. Technol Health Care 4:113–119

62. Durand EP, Rüegsegger P (1991) Cancellous bone structure: analysis of high-resolution CT images with the run-length method. J Comput Assist Tomogr 15(1):133–139

63. Ito M, Ohki M, Hayashi K, Yamada M, Uetani M, Nakamura T (1995) Trabecular texture analysis of CT images in the relationship with spinal fracture. Radiology 194:55–59

64. Engelke K, Graeff W, Meiss L, Hahn M, Delling G (1993) High spatial resolution imaging of bone mineral using computed microtomography. Invest Radiol 28:341–349

65. Caligiuri PC, Giger ML, Favus MJ, Jia H, Doi K, Dixon LB (1993) Computerized radiographic analysis of osteoporosis: preliminary evaluation. Radiology 186:471–474

66. Caldwell CB, Willett K, Cuncins AV, Hearn TC (1995) Characterization of vertebral strength using digital radiographic analysis of bone structure. Med Phys 22:611–615

67. Chang C-L, Chan H-P, Niklason LT, Cobby M, Crabbe J, Adler RS (1993) Computer-aided diagnosis: detection and characterization of hyperparathyroidism in digital hand radiographs. Med Phys 20:983–992

68. Cheng SNC, Chan H-P, Niklason LT, Adler RS (1994) Automated segmentation of regions of interest on hand radiographs. Med Phys 21(8):1293–1300

69. Geraets WGM, Van der Stelt PF, Elders PJM (1993) The radiographic trabecular bone pattern during menopause. Bone 14:859–864

70. Korstjens CM, Geraets WGM, van Ginkel FC, Prahl-Andersen B, van der Stelt PF, Burger EH (1995) Longitudinal analysis of radiographic trabecular pattern by image processing. Bone 17:527–532

71. Chevalier F, Laval-Jeantet AM, Laval-Jeantet M, Bergot C (1992) CT image analysis of the vertebral trabecular network in vivo. Calcif Tissue Int 51:8–13

72. Durand EP, Rüegsegger P (1992) High-contrast resolution of CT images for bone structure analysis. Med Phys 19:569–573
73. Müller R, Hildebrand T, Rüegsegger P (1994) Non-invasive bone biopsy: a new method to analyze and display the three-dimensional structure of trabecular bone. Phys Med Biol 39:145–164
74. Müller R, Hildebrand T, Häuselmann HJ, Rüegsegger P (1996) In vivo reproducibility of noninvasive bone biopsies using 3d-pQCT. J Bone Miner Res 11:1745–1750
75. Rosenthal H, Thulborn KR, Rosenthal DI, Rosen BR (1990) Magnetic susceptibility effects of trabecular bone on magnetic resonance bone marrow imaging. Invest Radiol 25(2):173–178
76. Majumdar S (1991) Magnetic field inhomogeneity effects induced by inherent tissue susceptibility differences in gradient echo magnetic resonance imaging: computer simulations. Magn Reson Med 22:101–110
77. Majumdar S, Genant HK (1992) In vivo relationship between marrow T2* and trabecular bone density determined with a chemical shift-selective asymmetric spin-echo sequence. J Magn Res Imaging 2:209–219
78. Grampp S, Majumdar S, Jergas M, Lang P, Gies A, Genant HK (1995) MRI of bone marrow in the distal radius: in vivo precision of effective transverse relaxation times. Eur Radiol 5(1):43–48
79. Ford JC, Wehrli FW, Chung H (1993) Magnetic field distribution in models of trabecular bone. Magn Reson Med 30:373–379
80. Engelke K, Majumdar S, Genant HK (1994) Impact of trabecular structure on marrow relaxation time, T2*: phantom studies. Magn Reson Med 31:380–387
81. Majumdar S, Genant HK (1992) In vivo relationship between marrow relaxation time T2* and trabecular bone density using a chemical shift selective asymmetric spin-echo sequence. J Magn Res Imaging 2:209–219
82. Sugimoto H, Kimura T, Ohsawa T (1993) Susceptibility effects of bone trabeculae quantification in vivo using an asymmetric spin-echo technique. Invest Radiol 28(3):208–213
83. Jara H, Wehrli FW, Chung H, Ford JC (1993) High-resolution variable flip angle 3D MR imaging of trabecular microstructure in vivo. Magn Reson Med 29:528–539
84. Foo TKF, Shellock FG, Hayes CE, Schenck JF, Slayman BE (1992) High-resolution MR imaging of the wrist and eye with short TR, short TE, and partial-echo acqusition. Radiology 183:227–281
85. Majumdar S, Newitt D, Jergas M, Gies A, Chiu D, Osman D, Keltner J, Keyak J, Genant H (1995) Evaluation of technical factors affecting the quantification of trabecular bone structure using magnetic resonance imaging. Bone 17:417–430
86. Ouyang X, Selby K, Lang P, Engelke K, Klifa C, Fan B, Zucconi F, Hottya G, Chen M, Majumdar S et al (1997) High resolution magnetic resonance imaging of the calcaneus: age related changes in trabecular structure and com-

parision with dual X-ray absorptiometry measurements. Calcif Tissue Int 60:139–147

87. Majumdar S, Genant HK, Grampp S, Newitt DC, Truong V-H, Lin JC, Mathur A (1997) Correlation of trabecular bone structure with age, bone mineral density and osteoporotic status: in vivo studies in the distal radius using high resolution magnetic resonance imaging. J Bone Miner Res 12:111–118

88. Münch B, Rüegsegger P (1993) 3-D repositioning and differential images of volumetric CT measurements. IEEE Trans Med Imaging 12:509–514

89. Kalender WA, Klotz E, Süss C (1987) Vertebral bone mineral analysis: an integrated approach with CT. Radiology 164:419–423

90. Steiger P, Block JE, Steiger S, Heuck A, Friedlander A, Ettinger B, Harris ST, Glüer CC, Genant HK (1990) Spinal bone mineral density by quantitative computed tomography: effect of region of interest, vertebral level, and technique. Radiology 175:537–543

91. Odgaard A, Gundersen HJG (1993) Quantification of connectivity in cancellous bone, with special emphasis on 3-D reconstructions. Bone 14:173–182

92. Boyde A, Jones SJ (1996) Scanning electron microscopy of bone: instrument, specimen, and issues. Microsc Res Techn 33:92–120

93. Hahn M, Vogel M, Pompesius-Kempa M, Delling G (1991) Undecalcified preparation of bone tissue: report of technical experience and development of new methods. Virchows Arch [A] 418:1–7

94. Parfitt AM (1983) Stereologic basis of bone histomorphometry; theory of quantitative microscopy and reconstruction of the third dimension. In: Recker R (ed) Bone histomerphometry: techniques and interpretations. CRC, Boca Raton, pp 53–87

95. Compston JE (1994) Connectivity of cancellous bone: assessment and mechanical implications. Bone 15:463–466

96. Amling M, Grote HJ, Pösl M, Hahn M, Delling G (1994) Polyostotic heterogeneity of the spine in osteoporosis. Quantitative analysis and three dimensional morphology. Bone Miner 27:193–208

97. Parfitt AM, Matthews C, Villanueva A (1983) Relationships between surface, volume, and thickness of iliac trabecular bone in aging and in osteoporosis. J Clin Invest 72:1396–1409

98. Bonse U, Busch F (1996) X-ray computed microtomography (µCT) using synchrotron radiation (SR). Prog Biophys Mol Biol 65:133–169

99. Feldkamp LA, Goldstein SA, Parfitt AM, Jesion G, Kleerekoper M (1989) The direct examination of three-dimensional bone architecture in vitro by computed tomography. J Bone Miner Res 4(1):3–11

100. Kuhn JL, Goldstein SA, Feldkamp LA, Goulet RW, Jesion G (1990) Evaluation of a microcomputed tomography system to study trabecular bone structure. J Orthop Res 8:833–842

101. Goldstein SA, Goulet R, McCubbrey D (1993) Measurement and significance of three-dimensional architecture in the mechanical integrity of trabecular bone. Calcif Tissue Int 53(S1):S127–133

102. Kinney JH, Lane NE, Haupt DL (1995) In vivo, three-dimensional microscopy of trabecular bone. J Bone Miner Res 10(2):264–270

103. Rüegsegger P, Koller B, Müller R (1996) A microtomographic system for the nondestructive evaluation of bone architecture. Calcif Tissue Int 58:24–29

104. Hildebrand T, Rüegsegger P (1997) A new method for the model independent assessment of thickness in three-dimensional images. J Microsc 185:67–75

105. Bonse U, Busch F, Günnewig O, Beckman F, Delling G, Hahn M, Graeff W (1994) 3D computed X-ray tomography of human cancellous bone at 8 µm spatial and 10^{-4} energy resolution. Bone Miner 25:25–38

106. Wehrli FW, Ford JC, Chung H-W, Wehrli SL, Williams JL, Grimm MJ, Kugelmass SD, Jara H (1993) Potential role of nuclear magnetic resonance for the evaluation of trabecular bone quality. Calcif Tissue 53 [Suppl 1]:S162–S169

107. Chung H, Wehrli FW, Williams JL, Kugelmass SD (1993) Relationship between NMR transverse relaxation, trabecular bone architecture, and strength. Proc Natl Acad Sci USA 90:10250–10254

108. Chung H, Wehrli FW, Williams JL, Wehrli SL (1995) Three-dimensional nuclear magnetic resonance microimaging of trabecular bone. J Bone Miner Res 10:1452–1461

109. Hipp JA, Jansujwicz A, Simmons CA, Snyder BD (1996) Trabecular bone morphology from micro-magnetic resonance imaging. J Bone Miner Res 11:286–292

110. Jensen KS, Mosekilde L, Mosekilde L (1990) A model of vertebral trabecular bone architecture and its mechanical properties. Bone 11:417–423

111. Engelke K, Song SM, Glüer CC, Genant HK (1996) A digital model of trabecular bone. J Bone Miner Res 11:480–489

112. Takada M, Engelke K, Hagiwara S, Grampp S, Jergas M, Glüer CC, Genant HK (1997) Assessment of Osteoporosis: Comparison of radiographic absorptiometry of the phalanges and dual X-ray absorptiometry of the radius and lumbar spine. Radiology 202:759–763

113. Ross P, Huang C, Davis J, Imose K, Yates J, Vogel J, Wasnich R (1995) Predicting vertebral deformity using bone densitometry at various skeletal sites and calcaneus ultrasound. Bone 16:325–332

114. Kühn B, Stampa B, Heller M, Glüer C-C (1997) High spatial resolution magnetic resonance imaging of the phalangeal bone structure. In: European Congress of Radiology. Springer, Vienna New York, p 137

115. Majumdar S, Weinstein RS, Prasad RR (1993) Application of fractal geometry techniques to the study of trabecular bone. Med Phys 20:1611–1619

116. Benhamou CL, Lespessailles E, Jacquet G, Harba R, Jennane R, Loussot T, Tourliere D, Ohley W (1994) Fractal organization of trabecular bone images on calcaneus radiographs. J Bone Miner Res 9(12):1909–1918

117. Buckland-Wright JC, Lynch JA, Rymer J, Fogelman I (1994) Fractal signature analysis of macroradiographs measures trabecular organization in lumbar vertebrae of postmenopausal women. Calcif Tissue Int 54:106–112

118. Rogers S, Silcocks PB, Gross SS, Cotton DWK (1993) Trabecular bone does not have a fractal structure on light microscopic examination. J Pathol 170:311–313

119. Chung HW, Chu C-C, Underweiser M, Wehrli FW (1994) On the fractal nature of trabecular structure. Med Phys 21:1535–1540

120. Chen Y, Dougherty ER, Totterman SM, Hornak JP (1993) Classification of trabecular structure in magnetic resonance images based on morphological granulometries. Magn Reson Med 29:358–370

121. Engelke K, Prevrhal S, Coman J, Süß C, Kalender W (1997) A 3D stereolithographic spongiosa model to quantify the potential if high resolution QCT and MR in the analysis of structural parameters of trabecular bone. In: European Congress of Radiology. Springer, Vienna New York

122. Faulkner KG, Cann CE, Hasegawa BH (1991) Effect of bone distribution on vertebral strength: assessment with patient-specific nonlinear finite element analysis. Radiology 179:669–674

123. Keyak JH, Skinner HB (1992) Three-dimensional finite element modelling of bone: effects of element size. J Biomech Eng 14:483–489

124. Lotz JC, Cheal EJ, Hayes WC (1991) Fracture predicion for the proximal femur using finite element models. I. Linear analysis. J Biomech Eng 113:353–360

125. Müller R, Rüegsegger P (1995) Three-dimensional finite element modelling of non-invasively assessed trabecular bone structures. Med Eng Phys 17:126–133

126. von Rietbergen B, Weinans H, Huiskes R, Odgaard A (1995) A new method to determine trabecular bone elastic properties and loading using micromechanical finite-element models. J Biomech 28:69–81

127. Sandor T, Kalender WA, Hanlon WB, Weissman BN, Rumbaugh C (1985) Spinal bone mineral determination using automated contour detection: application to single and dual energy CT. SPIE Med Imaging Instrum 555:188–194

128. Laib A, Hildebrand T, Rüegsegger P (1996) In vivo assessment of trabecular bone structure with 3D computed tomography and local reconstruction. Bone 19:147S

22 Which Site, Which Method? Dilemmas in Bone Densitometry

Y. Lu, A. Mathur, and H. K. Genant

Introduction

The previous chapters of this volume discuss many noninvasive techniques to measure bone quality/quantity, including radiographic absorptiometry, single and dual X-ray absorptiometry (DXA), quantitative computed tomography (QCT), peripheral quantitative computed tomography (pQCT), and quantitative ultrasound (QUS). Each of these techniques measures multiple anatomic sites and gives multiple parameters for each body part. As has been widely observed, there are many choices available, not only with respect to the technique, but with respect to the anatomic site and the parameter that should be measured. In addition to these choices, we are faced with the dilemmas of how often the measurements should be made, and how to interpret the measurements effectively to optimize patient care and treatment. To address these issues and dilemmas we need to know (a) whether these techniques (including anatomic sites and parameters) "agree" with each other, and thus (b) whether there are advantages in using multiple techniques to measure multiple anatomic sites for clinical diagnosis, treatment, and prevention of osteoporosis. In addition, for effective use of these techniques we also need to know (c) what classification criterion should be used so that the patients are classified more consistently with respect to osteoporosis.

In this chapter we aim to provide the readers with (a) an overview of the relationships between various noninvasive bone measurement techniques, (b) the dilemmas that we face in choosing the technique, measurement sites, and appropriate classification rules, and (c) some guidelines on when such decisions are to be made.

To address the issues we refer to studies that have been conducted in the past by various researchers. In addition, we use various datasets available to us to address the same issues. One of these datasets is the Multi-Modality (MM) dataset [1], collected on about 120 women and including young normal, postmenopausal healthy, and postmenopausal osteoporotic women. Most of these women were measured once by each of the commonly used techniques/modalities and as such provide us with data to address some of the issues raised above. The other dataset is from a large community-based prospective study known as the Study of Osteoporotic Fractures (SOF) [2,3]. This covers approximately 10 000 women followed over time with respect to their bone mineral density (BMD) and fracture status.

The modalities used in this study were not as numerous as in the MM study but are sufficient to address some of the issues encountered in bone densitometry. One factor which currently limits the usefulness of this dataset is that we have only the baseline measurements (as opposed to longitudinal bone measurements) and follow-up fracture information from this longitudinal cohort study. In addition to these studies, we have access to the data of various longitudinal clinical trials which our group have helped to conduct. Typically these include only DXA data. A point to be noted regarding these datasets is that we were blinded to the drug being received by each patient. We refer to this dataset as the drug trial dataset.

Dilemmas in Bone Densitometry

Low bone densities and ultrasound parameters at various skeletal sites are significantly associated with the risk of osteoporotic fractures, including fractures of hip and spine. The risk of fracture is significantly associated not only with the bone mass and density at the skeletal site of the fractures but also other remote body sites. However, all these parameters are correlated to each other. The relationships of these measurements have been studied in many natural history cohort and cross-sectional studies, and substantial knowledge has been accumulated [4–15] and has been reviewed by Genant et al. [16].

Correlations Between Techniques for Measuring BMD

Typically the correlations between different techniques and measurement sites are statistically significant and average about $r=0.5-0.7$. In the MM study the correlations ranged from 0.11 to 0.94 depending on the anatomic site and the technique used (See Table 22-1). The strongest correlation across techniques was between the integral BMD of the spine measured by QCT and BMD of the lateral spine measured by DXA, and the weakest correlation within a technique was between trabecular BMD and cortical BMC at the wrist measured by pQCT. Generally correlations between measurements at the lumbar spine including QCT and DXA were moderate to strong. Correlations between the various measurements at the femur using DXA were modest. Those between the various calcaneal measurements using QUS ranged from weak to moderate. At the radius measurements performed with pQCT and DXA did not show strong correlations, and the trabecular and cortical bone parameters by pQCT were only weakly correlated. The correlation between X-ray based methods and ultrasound measurements were only marginally lower than those between X-ray based methods alone.

All these observations point to the fact that even though the correlations are statistically significant, they are not strong enough to allow prediction of one measure from the other. This problem is reflected in the so-called root mean square error (RMSE), which measures the spread of data around the regression line. The RMSE is directly proportional to the error in prediction. This has been shown and addressed in many studies, especially in a report of the WHO panel experts

Table 22-1 Correlation coefficients (r, upper row), %SEE (CV, middle row), and statistical significance (p[a], lower row) between measurement techniques and sites

r CV p	QCT TRAB BMD	QCT INTG BMD	DXA PA BMD	DXA LAT BMD	DXA FEM NECK BMD	DXA FEM TROC BMD	DXA UD RAD BMD	pQCT TRAB RAD BMD	pQCT CORT RAD BMC	RA CH METC BMD	RA CO PHAL BMD	BUA WS CALC db/MHz	SOS WS CALC m/s	BUA LA CALC db/MHz	SOS LA CALC m/s
QCT TRAB BMD	1	0.94 8.8 -4	0.72 12.1 -4	0.87 9.2 -4	0.71 14.2 -4	0.77 12.1 -4	0.76 11.0 -4	0.40 23.0 -4	0.64 28.7 -4	0.71 12.1 -4	0.81 9.8 -4	0.64 19.9 -4	0.40 1.1 -4	0.40 11.5 -4	0.79 1.7 -4
QCT INTG BMD	0.94 15.1 -4	1	0.83 9.6 -4	0.88 8.9 -4	0.77 12.8 -4	0.83 10.7 -4	0.76 11.0 -4	0.41 22.8 -4	0.62 29.4 -4	0.72 11.9 -4	0.80 10.1 -4	0.60 20.7 -4	0.37 1.1 -4	0.41 11.4 -4	0.76 1.9 -4
DXA PA BMD	0.72 30.2 -4	0.83 14.0 -4	1	0.74 12.8 -4	0.76 13.1 -4	0.76 12.3 -4	0.62 13.3 -4	0.36 23.2 -4	0.48 32.8 -4	0.57 14.0 -4	0.61 13.5 -4	0.50 22.4 -4	0.31 1.1 -3	0.34 11.8 -3	0.58 2.3 -4
DXA LAT BMD	0.87 21.0 -4	0.88 11.9 -4	0.74 11.7 -4	1	0.71 14.2 -4	0.81 11.3 -4	0.67 12.5 -4	0.40 22.9 -4	0.55 31.2 -4	0.66 12.8 -4	0.75 11.3 -4	0.61 20.5 -4	0.41 1.1 -4	0.35 11.7 -4	0.74 1.9 -4
DXA FEM NECK BMD	0.71 30.6 -4	0.77 16.1 -4	0.76 11.3 -4	0.71 13.3 -4	1	0.84 10.4 -4	0.67 12.5 -4	0.40 22.9 -4	0.53 31.8 -4	0.60 13.7 -4	0.62 13.3 -4	0.54 21.8 -4	0.37 1.1 -4	0.34 11.8 -3	0.67 2.1 -4
DXA FEM TROC BMD	0.77 27.5 -4	0.83 14.2 -4	0.76 11.2 -4	0.81 11.2 -4	0.84 11.0 -4	1	0.65 12.8 -4	0.45 22.2 -4	0.49 32.6 -4	0.60 13.7 -4	0.69 12.3 -4	0.55 21.6 -4	0.34 1.1 -3	0.29 12.0 -2	0.72 2.0 -4
DXA UD RAD BMD	0.76 27.9 -4	0.76 16.3 -4	0.62 13.5 -4	0.67 13.8 -4	0.67 14.8 -4	0.65 14.4 -4	1	0.62 19.7 -4	0.69 25.9 -4	0.74 11.4 -4	0.77 10.8 -4	0.56 21.3 -4	0.42 1.1 -4	0.24 11.1 -1	0.66 2.1 -4
pQCT TRAB RAD BMD	0.40 40.3 -4	0.41 23.2 -4	0.36 16.0 -4	0.40 17.2 -4	0.40 19.1 -4	0.45 17.5 -4	0.62 13.3 -4	1	0.25 36.3 -1	0.38 15.5 -4	0.52 14.5 -4	0.41 23.3 -4	0.29 1.2 -2	0.11 11.8 NS	0.46 2.6 -4
pQCT CORT RAD BMC	0.64 33.8 -4	0.62 20.0 -4	0.48 15.1 -4	0.55 15.6 -4	0.53 17.7 -4	0.49 17.1 -4	0.69 12.1 -4	0.25 24.2 -1	1	0.62 13.2 -4	0.63 13.2 -4	0.42 23.2 -4	0.27 1.2 -2	0.30 11.3 -2	0.42 2.6 -4
RA CH METC BMD	0.71 32.7 -4	0.72 18.5 -4	0.57 14.9 -4	0.66 14.7 -4	0.60 16.5 -4	0.60 16.1 -4	0.74 12.2 -4	0.38 23.5 -4	0.62 30.3 -4	1	0.73 11.6 -4	0.51 23.7 -4	0.28 1.2 -2	0.26 12.0 -1	0.60 2.4 -4
RA CO PHAL BMD	0.81 27.1 -4	0.80 16.0 -4	0.61 14.5 -4	0.75 13.1 -4	0.62 16.2 -4	0.69 14.6 -4	0.77 11.6 -4	0.52 21.8 -4	0.63 29.9 -4	0.73 11.8 -4	1	0.62 21.5 -4	0.45 1.1 -4	0.38 11.4 -4	0.75 2.0 -4
BUA WS CALC db/MHz	0.64 33.3 -4	0.60 20.2 -4	0.50 15.0 -4	0.61 15.0 -4	0.54 16.9 -4	0.55 15.9 -4	0.56 14.0 -4	0.41 22.8 -4	0.42 33.9 -4	0.51 14.8 -4	0.62 13.2 -4	1	0.52 1.0 -4	0.41 11.4 -4	0.83 1.6 -4
SOS WS CALC m/s	0.40 39.2 -4	0.37 23.3 -4	0.31 16.3 -2	0.41 17.2 -4	0.37 18.6 -4	0.34 18.1 -3	0.42 15.1 -4	0.29 23.9 -2	0.27 36.0 -2	0.28 16.2 -2	0.45 14.9 -4	0.52 22.2 -4	1	0.24 12.1 -2	0.56 2.4 -4
BUA LA CALC db/MHz	0.40 38.9 -4	0.41 23.2 -4	0.34 16.3 -3	0.35 17.7 -4	0.34 19.1 -3	0.29 18.5 -2	0.24 16.3 -1	0.11 25.2 NS	0.30 35.1 -2	0.26 16.3 -1	0.38 15.4 -4	0.41 23.8 -4	0.24 1.1 -2	1	0.42 2.6 -4
SOS LA CALC m/s	0.79 26.1 -4	0.76 16.6 -4	0.58 14.2 -4	0.74 12.7 -4	0.67 15.1 -4	0.72 13.4 -4	0.66 12.6 -4	0.46 22.5 -4	0.42 33.4 -4	0.60 13.6 -4	0.75 10.9 -4	0.83 14.5 -4	0.56 1.0 -4	0.42 11.4 -4	1

[a] -1, $p \leq 0{,}05$; -2, $p \leq 0{,}01$; -3, $p \leq 0{,}001$; -4, $p \leq 0{,}0001$.

[17], as well as a number of others which have addressed these issues [1, 11, 12, 17–20].

In addition to the moderate overall correlations between the techniques, the correlations between the techniques are not constant over the various age groups. For example, based on the SOF data the correlation of femoral neck BMD and posteroanterior (PA) spine BMD measured by DXA was 0.65 for 65- to 69-year-olds but only 0.49 in those aged 85 or older [19]. This can be due to the fact that error sources (spinal degenerative diseases) may change as a function of age, and that the rates of bone loss differ at different sites as the bone loss occurs, and as a result the correlations between bone density measurement decrease with increasing age. This also raises the question of the validity of overall correlations and the possibility of using an age-dependent measurement technique.

Correlation Between the Techniques in Monitoring Age- and Menopause-Related BMD Loss

A related but different issue is whether the bone changes, as measured by the different techniques, either loss or gain, are correlated. This is important in the development of new drug therapies because the clinical trials for treatment efficacy and safety should choose the most effective technique to monitor the most sensitive parameters. Monitoring of bone changes is also important in the prevention of osteoporosis since the right technique is able to detect excessive bone loss precisely over time. To answer these questions an appropriate longitudinal follow-up of subjects for their serial bone changes is required, which in turn make these studies expensive and hard to carry out. As a result we have less knowledge about the comparison between the techniques for longitudinal performance than for one-time comparisons. However, it has been reported that regarding X-ray absorptiometry the annual percentage of BMD loss at PA spine and at the femur (including the subregions at femoral neck, Ward's triangle, trochanter and total BMD) are correlated, albeit only moderately. A 21-month follow-up study of postmenopausal women [21] found the correlations of 0.34–0.69 between the losses at PA spine and total femur BMD and 0.44–0.61 between the losses at various femur measurements.

On the other hand, the various drug trial datasets available to us show that the changes in BMD at PA spine and ultradistal wrist are not significantly correlated (correlations ranging from –0.01 to +0.06). This lack of significance was observed regardless of the length of patient follow-up. The same data reveal correlations of changes at PA spine versus femur measurements that are poor (0.03–0.2) for short-term follow-up (around one year) and are slightly improved for long term follow-ups (ranging from –0.07 to 0.45 for around two years). In agreement with Pouilles, the correlations between changes at various femur measurements were better both in the short-term follow-up (correlations of 0.1–0.7) and long-term follow-up (correlations of 0.2–0.8). Without knowledge of treatment codes our short-term and long-term correlations for clinical trials may be biased because of the unknown effect of interventions. In another study of 37 oophorectomized women in a 2-year clinical trial [22] Genant et al. reported a 0.58 correlation coefficient between mean peripheral cortical bone loss (average of several methods) and vertebral cancellous bone loss using QCT. Overall the above numbers suggest, again, that the techniques do not agree very well with each other in the relatively short term. Since short-term change in normal bone mineral density is relatively small for an individual compared to the precision errors of the techniques, only a modest correlation between short-term BMD changes should be expected. The correlations, however, should be improved by increasing the length of follow-up and/or increasing the frequency of measurements [23–25].

Another way to see the problems in "agreement" between the various techniques based on rate of BMD loss was pointed out by Pouilles. His group looked at the "disagreement" between techniques from another perspective. They defined a woman as a fast loser if her annual percentage bone loss was within the 25th percentile of the distribution of the individual values. Based on this categorization 48%–67% of women with a rapid PA spine BMD loss were normal according to their various femur BMD measurements. On the other hand, among 21 women classified as fast losers based on femoral neck BMD, 48% were normal at the PA spine BMD, and 67% at Ward's triangle and trochanteric BMD. We could not repeat these analyses on our datasets since we do not have the longitudinal datasets that are needed. Neither the MM nor the SOF dataset is longitudinal, while the drug trial datasets do not have the drug code for each patient, thus biasing such analyses and making the results possibly misleading. Despite this the study by Pouilles again points to the lack of complete "agreement" between the techniques, and even between various anatomic sites measured by the same technique.

Discrimination of Osteoporotic Women

Another important question with regard to "agreement" between techniques is how well the technique discriminates osteoporotic women from healthy women. Here the focus is on the use of a single bone measurement for the diagnosis of osteoporosis and prediction of oteoporotic fractures. This issue has also been addressed by various authors. In a report on 744 women from the Hawaii Osteoporosis Study, Davis and colleagues [26, 27] noticed discordance in BMDs measured at the spine, calcaneus, distal radius, and proximal radius after adjusting for age. Only 13.6% of women were consistently in the lower tertiles for all four sites. Among women who had at least one of the bone mass sites in the lower tertile 42.7% were in the middle or higher tertile groups according to other measured sites. About 15% of women had bone mass in both lower and higher tertile groups. Less than one-third (31.3%) of women were consistently in the same tertile groups for all four sites.

We addressed the same issue based on the SOF data and using a cutoff value. Since discriminating osteoporotic women from healthy women is of importance, classification methods based on single cutoff points/threshold levels are often advocated. A method of classifying individuals as osteopenic and/or osteoporotic based on the their T scores being less than a constant value (-0.1 for osteopenia and -2.5 for osteoporosis) has been suggested [17]. Based on these suggestions and the T scores from the manufacturer's peak bone mass reference data we found the following. By grouping individuals in the SOF study according to their T score being greater or less than -2.5, we found that the proportion of agreement ranged from 36% ($\kappa=0.08$) to 76% ($\kappa=0.44$) between disparate sites of spine, femur, and wrist and from 44% ($\kappa=0.14$) to 70% ($\kappa=0.40$) between hip sites [3]. When we used the SOF women aged 65 as the reference group in the T score calculations, the agreement between the sites improved. The proportion of agreement in this case ranged from 70% ($\kappa=0.36$) to 76% ($\kappa=0.49$) between disparate sites while among the femur sites it ranged from 73% ($\kappa=0.41$) to 85%

(κ=0.66). However, the magnitude of disagreement was still substantial and demonstrates the problem of different manufacturers using different normative populations.

This is one of the many potential sources causing inconsistencies in classification based on T scores. The disagreement can be reduced by using a unified normative population. The international DXA standardization committee has suggested using the third National Health and Nutrition Examination Survey (NHANES III, 1988–1994) as the standardized reference population for white women for DXA measurements. A universal reference population for all the bone measurements would be difficult to achieve, if not impossible. The use of a single reference population would reduce the disagreement between techniques, but Genant's findings also suggest that even if we use the same reference population, we will find inconsistencies in classification based on T scores from different body sites due to the biological variations among the sites. Black et al. [28] and Lu et al. [29] have suggested avoiding T scores as a classification tool. These findings of ours and other researchers point to various sources which can cause a disagreement between the techniques and demonstrate the magnitude of the dilemmas.

Further complicating the problem is the issue of using multiple techniques/ sites. If the clinical management of osteopenia/osteoporosis is based on bone measurement from only one site, a substantial number of patients could be misdiagnosed or mistreated. The Hawaii study by Ross and Wasnich and the French study by Pouilles [21, 30] (both discussed earlier) support the concept that measurements of bone density at several different sites are helpful in assessing the risk of osteopenia. They do not, however, provide the risk of osteoporotic fracture associated with the respective measurements, and since individuals with low bone measurements do not necessarily have osteoporotic fractures, it is necessary to assess this risk associated with low bone density measurement. Although many studies have measured BMD at multiple anatomic sites and have evaluated the associated risk of fracture, only a few of them have assessed the independent contributions of these bone mass measurements by adjusting for the other measurements. In other words, few studies have assessed the risk associated with a technique after adjusting for the correlation between the technique and another measured technique.

One of the largest prospective studies, the SOF, does address this issue. This study [31] compared the effectiveness of BMD at the femur (including total, neck, intertrochanteric region, trochanter, Ward's triangle), PA spine, distal radius, and middle radius at the wrist and calcaneus in predicting hip fractures. They found that after adjusting for the effect of age, the relative risk of hip fracture with 1 SD decrease in femur measurements was about 70% greater than the relative risk using BMD of PA spine and wrist, while the relative risk related to calcaneus BMD was between the levels associated with femur and spine. The authors concluded that low hip femoral BMD is a stronger predictor of hip fracture than BMD at other sites, which is consistent with the findings of other studies [32, 33]. In a more recent analysis of the same data, Black and colleagues [34] examined the effectiveness of combining femoral neck and PA spine BMD to identify a high-risk group for hip fracture. They found that after adjusting for age and femoral neck BMD, the PA spine BMD is no longer significantly associated with the risk of hip fractures. Distinguishing individuals with femoral neck BMD less than various cutoff values has a higher sensitivity in predicting hip fractures than distinguishing individuals with either femur or PA spine BMD less than the same cutoff value. Therefore they concluded that using a combination of femoral neck and PA spine BMD measurements to identify elderly women at high risk of hip fracture is no better than using femoral neck BMD alone, and an additional PA spine measurement is unjustified.

In contrast to this important study, there have been others suggesting that additional measurements reduce misclassification for the individual patients. Since 1982 the Hawaii Osteoporosis Study has followed 1098 Japanese-American women with initial average age of 63.3 years. In an examination of 699 patients from this study Wasnich and colleagues [35] assessed the association of bone mineral content at calcaneus, distal radius, and proximal radius at the wrist and PA spine with incident vertebral fractures. The relative risks of incident vertebral fracture with a 1-SD decrease in BMC were lowest for PA spine and highest for calcaneus. Multivariate analysis showed that BMC values at calcaneus and distal radius were independently associated with the probability of vertebral fracture. When -2 SD was used as a cutoff point for each site, the predicted probability of vertebral fracture by combining the two measurements was 25%, compared to 20% using only one of the two measurements. In recent reports from this group [27, 36] 744 women were classified according to their tertiles of age-adjusted Z score of bone mass at the above four sites. They found that the number of low bone mass sites predicted the risk of new vertebral fractures with an odds ratio of 1.3 per increase in number of low bone sites after adjusting for age and the number of prevalent fractures (including vertebral and nonvertebral fractures). Other reported results from this study [37, 38] consistently suggest that measurement of BMD at multiple anatomic sites and combinations of the information helps to determine risk of vertebral fractures for the individual.

A preliminary analysis of the SOF data has further found that combining BMD at calcaneus, femoral neck, and spine improves the prediction of hip fractures [3]. As Fig. 22-1 demonstrates, with increasing number of low BMD sites the age-adjusted odds ratio for hip fractures increases in the SOF study; in this figure the x-axis represents the number of low BMD sites of T=2.5 or less according to manufacturer's references. The bars represent the percentages of women in each of the categories and dots the age-adjusted odds ratio for hip fractures. The 95% confidence bands of estimated odds ratios are also plotted. In an extreme case when the number of low BMD sites reaches 8, the odds ratio of hip fractures is 37!

Since there are nearly 750 000 nonhip, nonvertebral fractures each year in the United States alone [39], it is also important to study the risk of these other fractures. In a prospective study of 304 women in Rochester, Minnesota, with 8.3 years of median follow-up time, Melton and colleagues [40] found that after adjusting

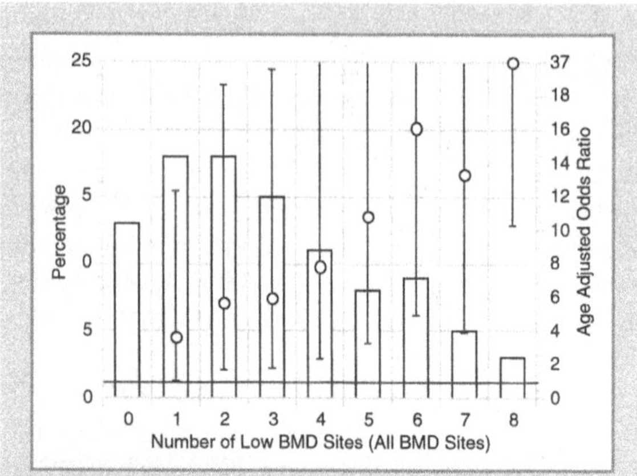

Fig. 22-1 Percentages of women with the number of low BMD sites and their correspodning age-adjusted odds ratio for hip fracture

for age, 1 SD decreases in BMD of PA spine, trochanteric region, and femoral neck were significantly related to the incidence rate of all fractures (relative hazards of 1.4, 1.2, and 1.3, respectively) and BMD values at the hip and spine were better individual predictors of fractures of all types than BMD at the forearm.

In the light of all these studies and contradictory results, the question of the effectiveness of combining BMD at various sites is still inconclusive. The results of the above studies depend on the variables used in their statistical analysis and can change when other risk variables (for example, the number of prevalent fractures, the vertebral dimension) [38, 41] and measurements using other modalities (ultrasound and QCT, etc.) are included [14]. The sample size of the study also affects the conclusion of the study [41]. In addition, different statistical methods such as logistic regression, discriminant analysis, Cox proportional hazards model, and classification and regression tree analysis [42] may produce different classification algorithms [43]. Furthermore, for studies involving vertebral fractures, the results may be inconsistent between various studies due to the use of different definitions of vertebral fractures.

Considerations in Choosing Measurement Sites and Methods

The measurements of bone quality/quantity are important in the diagnosis, prevention, and treatment of osteoporosis and their resulting osteoporotic fractures. Due to the proliferation of technological advances and biological/anatomic variations, we are facing dilemmas in choosing the method, site, and frequency of bone measurements. Since osteoporosis is a chronic and prevalent disease, the use of bone measurements actually has different purposes. In choosing the technique and the anatomic site for bone measurement we need to consider the purpose to which such measurements are to be put. While clinicians are concerned with the best diagnostic and treatment strategies for an *individual*, the epidemiological studies help us to select preventive strategies for the entire *population*, such as how to perform disease screening.

For prevention and epidemiological screening of osteoporosis, the purpose is to identify a group of individuals that have a high risk of femur, vertebral, or other fractures. Since such studies or interventions involve a large sample size, we must take into account the cost of conducting such studies. A minimum number of measurements that have the highest predictive power should be employed. For example, Black et al. [34] report that using either lower femoral neck BMD or PA spine BMD did not significantly increase the number of fractures per 1000 screened. Therefore an additional PA measurement after femur DXA scan is not necessary for population screening. Despite this finding consideration should be given to wrist BMD measurement or ultrasound measurement of the calcaneous because of their operational convenience. A potential multistage screening method based on the cost effectiveness of the strategy might be useful. This could be designed using a low cost but relatively less sensitive method for population screening and then using more costly measurements for those individuals who have neither very high BMD nor very low BMD to better define their risk.

For clinical use of bone measurements, the concern is to provide the best diagnostic and treatment strategies for an individual patient. Thus a physician wishes to know as much about the patient as possible. The additional cost of scanning both femur and spine in individual patients may be small compared to the cost of an incorrect therapeutic decision derived from only one BMD measurement.

Bone measurement in clinical trials differs from either epidemiological screening or clinical patient management. There are two major concerns in conducting clinical trials. To evaluate the efficacy of an intervention one would like to select the anatomic site that is most effected by the drug and the technique that is most sensitive for that anatomic site. For example, PA spine BMD is generally selected as a primary endpoint of clinical trials [44]. This choice of site and technique increases the power and reduces the length of a trial. On the other hand, safety monitoring of a clinical trial should take into account the discordant nature of bone density measurements as responses at different body sites. Thus monitoring multiple body sites using multiple techniques may still be necessary, but the frequency of the measurements may vary from site to site and from technique to technique.

Conclusions

The dilemmas in choosing the anatomic sites and the techniques used for bone densitometry do not disappear with advances in technology and by increasing the number of techniques. They provide us with both challenges and opportunities for using innovative approaches to integrate multidimensional information from bone densitometry. While most bone densitometry measurements are interrelated, they differ from one another and cannot replace each other. The choice of sites and methods depends on the purpose of performing the bone measurements. Further studies are needed to determine how best to use bone densitometry information. Cost-effectiveness studies to compare diagnostic and treatment strategies based on information of bone measurements from single or multiple sites are needed and will provide useful information that is unavailable from current clinical or epidemiological studies. Advances in these research areas will eventually lead to more precise guidelines in solving our current dilemmas.

References

1. Grampp S, Genant H, Mathur A, Lang P, Jergas M, Takada M, Gluer C, Lu Y, Chavez M (1997) Comparisons of non-invasive bone mineral measurements in assessing age-related loss, fracture discrimination, and diagnostic classification. J Bone Miner Res 12(5):697–711
2. Cummings S, Nevitt M, Browner W, Stone K, Fox K, Ensrud K, Cauley J, Black D, Vogt T et al (1995) Risk factors for hip fracture in white women. N Engl J Med 332:767–773
3. Genant H, Lu Y, Mathur A, Fuerst T, Cummings SR (1996) Classification based on DXA measurements for assessing the risk of hip fractures. J Bone Miner Res 11:S120
4. Seeley DG, Browner WS, Nevitt M, Cummings SR, Genant HK, Scott J, Cumming S (1997) Which fractures are predicted with measurement of bone mineral density? Ann Intern Med 115:837–842
5. Cummings SR, Rubin MPH, Black D (1990) The future of hip fractures in the United States. Clin Orthop Relat Res 252:163–166
6. Melton L, Atkinson E, O'Fallon W, Wahner H, Riggs B (1993) Long-term fracture prediction by bone mineral assessed at different sites. J Bone Miner Res 8:1227–1233
7. Hui SL, Slemenda CW, Johnston CC (1990) The contribution of bone loss to postmenopausal osteoporosis. Osteoporosis Int 1:30–34
8. Black D, Cummings SR, Melton LJ (1992) Appendicular bone mineral and a woman's lifetime risk of hip fracture. J Bone Miner Res 7:639–646
9. Black D, Nevitt M, Palermo L, Ensrud K, Genant H (1993) Prediction of new vertebral deformities. J Bone Miner Res 8 [Suppl 1]:S135
10. Smith DM, Khairi MRA, Johnston CC Jr (1975) The loss of bone mineral with aging and its relationship to risk of fracture. J Clin Invest 56:311–318
11. Mazess R, Barden H (1990) Interrelationships among bone densitometry sites in normal young women. Bone Miner 11:347–356
12. Grampp S, Jergas M, Lang P, Steiner E, Fuerst T, Gluer C, Mathur A, Genant H (1996) Quantitative CT assessment of the lumbar spine and radius in patients with osteoporosis. Am J Roentgenol 167:133–140
13. Gluer C, Cummings S, Bauer D, Stone K, Pressman A, Mathur A, Genant H (1996) Osteoporosis: association of recent fractures with quantitative US findings. Radiology 199:725–732

14. Hans D, Dargent-Molina D, Schott A, Sebert J, Cormier C, Kotzki P, Delmas P, Pouilles J, Breart G, Meunier P (1996) Ultrasonographic heel measurements to predict hip fracture in elderly women: the EPIDOS prospective study. Lancet 348:511–514

15. Genant H, Fuerst T, Faulkner K, Gluer C (1996) In evaluating bone density for osteoporosis, are any of the available methods clearly superior? Am J Roentgenol 167:1589–1590

16. Genant H, Engelke K, Fuerst T, Gluer C, Grampp S, Harris S, Jergas M, Lang T, Lu Y, Majumdar S, Mathur A, Takada M (1996) Noninvasive assessment of bone mineral and structure: state of the art. J Bone Miner Res 11:707–730

17. WHO (1994) Assessment of fracture risk and its application to screening for postmenopausal osteoporosis: report of a WHO study group. World Health Organization, Geneva

18. Steiger P, Genant HK, Black D, Cummings SR (1989) Bone mineral density in women over 65 as measured by single photon absorptiometry of the radius and os calcis. J Bone Miner Res 4:S376

19. Steiger P, Cummings SR, Black DM, Spencer NE, Genant HK (1992) Age-related decrements in bone mineral density in women over 65. J Bone Min Res 7:625–632

20. Guglielmi G, Grimston SK, Fischer KC, Pacifici R (1994) Osteoporosis: diagnosis with lateral and posteroanterior dual X-ray absorptiometry compared with quantitative CT. Radiology 192:845–850

21. Pouilles JM, Tremollieres F, Ribot C (1993) Spine and femur densitometry at the menopause: are both sites necessary in the assessment of the risk of osteoporosis? Calcif Tissue Int 52:344–347

22. Genant HK, Cann CE, Ettinger B, Gordan GS (1982) Quantitative computed tomography of vertebral spongiosa: a sensitive method for detecting early bone loss after oophorectomy. Ann Intern Med 97:699–705

23. He Y-F, Ross PD, Davis JW, Epstein RS, Vogel JM, Wasnich RD (1994) When should bone density measurements be repeated? Calcif Tissue Int 55:243–248

24. He Y, Davis J, Ross P, Wasnich R (1993) Declining bone loss rate variability with increasing follow-up time. Bone Miner 21:119–128

25. Nguyen T, Sambrook P, Eisman J (1997) Sources of variability in bone mineral density measurements: implications for study design and analysis of bone loss. J Bone Miner Res 12:124–135

26. Davis JW, Ross PD, Wasnich RD (1994) Evidence for both generalized and regional low bone mass among elderly women. J Bone Miner Res 9:305–309

27. Wasnich R (1993) Bone mass measurement: prediction of risk. Am J Med 95:65–105

28. Black D, Palermo L, Genant H, Cummings SR (1996) Four reasons to avoid the use of BMD T-scores in treatment decisions for osteoporosis. J Bone Miner Res 11:S118

29. Lu Y, Mathur A, Genant H (1995) Pitfalls of using Z-score, T-score for discriminant purpose. J Bone Miner Res 10:S264

30. Pouilles JM, Tremollieres F, Ribot C (1996) Variability of vertebra and femoral post-menopausal bone loss: a longitudinal study. Osteoporosis Int 6:320–324

31. Cummings SR, Black DM, Nevitt MC, Browner W, Cauley J, Ensrud K, Genant HK, Hulley SB, Palermo L, Scott J, Vogt TM (1993) Bone density at various sites for prediction of hip fractures: the study of osteoporotic fractures. Lancet 341:72–75

32. Mazess RB, Barden H, Ettinger M, Schultz E (1988) Bone density of the radius, spine, and proximal femur in osteoporosis. J Bone Miner Res 3:13–18

33. Riggs BL, Wahner HW, Seeman E et al (1982) Changes in bone mineral density of the proximal femur and spine with aging: differences between the post-menopausal and senile osteoporosis syndromes. J Clin Invest 70:716–723

34. Black D, Bauer D, Lu Y, Tabor H, Genant H, Cummings SR (1995) Should BMD be measured at multiple sites to predict fracture risk in elderly women? J Bone Miner Res 10:S7

35. Wasnich R, Ross P, Davis J, Vogel J (1989) A comparison of single and multi-site BMC measurements for assessment of spine fracture probability. J Nucl Med 30:1166–1171

36. Davis JW, Ross PD, Wasnich RD (1994) Evidence for both generalized and regional low bone mass among elderly women. J Bone Miner Res 9:305–309

37. Ross PD, Genant HK, Davis JW, Miller PD, Wasnich RD (1993) Predicting vertebral fracture incidence from prevalent fractures and bone density among non-black, osteoporotic women. Osteoporosis Int 3:120–126

38. Ross P, Huang C, Davis J, Imose K, Yates J, Vogel J, Wasnich R (1995) Predicting vertebral deformity using bone densitometry at various skeletal sites and calcaneous ultrasound. Bone 16:325–332

39. Johnston CJ, Slemenda CW (1993) Risk assessment: theoretical considerations. Am J Med 95(5A):25–55

40. Melton LD, Atkinson EJ, O'Fallon WM, Wahner HW, Riggs BL (1993) Long-term fracture prediction by bone mineral assessed at different skeletal sites. J Bone Miner Res 8:1227–1233

41. Ross P, Huang C, Davis J, Wasnich R (1995) Vertebral dimension measurements improve prediction of vertebral fracture incidence. Bone 16:257S–262S

42. Cooper C, Atkinson EJ, Jacobsen SJ, O'Fallon WM, Melton LD (1993) Population-based study of survival after osteoporotic fractures. Am J Epidemiol 137:1001–1005

43. Breiman L, Friedman JH, Olshen RA, Stone CJ (1984) Classification and regression trees. Wadsworth, Belmont

44. Lu Y, Mathur A, Black D, Fuerst T, Genant H (1996) Survival tree analysis for fracture risk. Osteoporosis Int 6:126

45. Faulkner K, McClung M, Ravn P, Hosking D, Wasnich R, Daley M, Yates A (1996) Monitoring skeletal response to therapy in early post-menopausal women: which bone to measure? J Bone Miner Res 11:S9

23 Quality Assurance in Bone Densitometry

T. Fuerst, Y. Lu, D. Hans, and H. K. Genant

Introduction

The validity of quantitative assessment of bone depends on the accuracy and precision with which the measurements are made. The two basic factors that affect accuracy and precision are the performance of (a) the operators who acquire and analyze the scans and (b) the instrument used to make the measurements. Most clinic staff claim a high level of quality in their work. However, performance of both instruments and operators needs to be carefully monitored and controlled to achieve reliable information on skeletal health. Consequently the principles of quality control (QC) that are often employed in manufacturing to monitor a process and ensure consistent quality have an important role in densitometry.

Quality assurance in bone densitometry is based on a program of formal and regular review of each component of the procedure to achieve accurate and precise measurements that can be used with confidence. The concept of quality assurance in clinical trials has been previously addressed [1]. This chapter reviews the various methodologies for QC of dual X-ray absorptiometry (DXA) with emphasis on the clinic. The QC procedures of the manufacturers of densitometers are reviewed and compared to alternative methods using third-party standards or test objects. Independently of the performance of the densitometer, artifacts during scanning and errors by the operator can invalidate the bone mineral density (BMD) results of a DXA examination. Therefore in addition to QC of the device, QC of the examination is discussed. While the details to be described are specific to measurements with DXA, the concepts are easily generalized to any other method of quantitative bone assessment.

Review of Techniques for Bone Mass Measurement

The recently introduced Lunar Expert [2] and Hologic QDR 4500 represent great advances in densitometer performance. Both systems are equipped with higher output X-ray tubes and multielement solid state detector arrays. These changes have provided improved image quality at higher resolution with large reductions in scan times. Radiation exposure has increased moderately but still remains extremely low, being on the same order as daily background exposure for most scan types. Both systems also boast mechanical, rotating gantries for lateral scanning of the spine. Many of the improvements in hardware have been driven by the desire to achieve high-quality lateral images of the spine for the purpose of vertebral fracture diagnosis. This capability has led to the use of the term imaging densitometer.

Densitometers using pencil beam geometry have also seen recent improvements in both image quality and scan speed. These densitometers are Norland's XR QuikScan and the Lunar DPX-IQ systems. The XR QuikScan system employs a more efficient scanning movement and has a PA spine scan time of 2 min, reduced from 4 min on earlier models. The DPX-IQ system benefits from similar strategies and has higher resolution than previous DPX systems.

All DXA densitometers have demonstrated linear response and long term stability. Accuracy has in general been good (5%–10%) and precision quite high (1%–2%) [3–5]. While there is some indication that pencil beam systems are more precise than fan beam, the precision realized in general clinical practice depends more on the skill and attention of the operator than on machine performance.

Monitoring Densitometer Performance

Standards for Quality Control

While the general mechanical and electrical integrity of a densitometer can be assessed with little difficulty, examination of the more subtle aspects of scanner performance requires an appropriate tool to test system operation. The manufacturers of DXA scanners provide proprietary standards or test objects to examine system stability. Lunar and Norland have developed test objects with simplified geometries which test various aspects of instrument performance and calibration. While this provides useful information which can alert the operator to significant failures, more subtle drifts or shifts may go undetected.

The ability to monitor densitometer performance accurately requires a more appropriate test object which provides a realistic approximation of the in vivo measurement. The ideal test object should simulate as closely as possible the conditions encountered during routine use. For densitometry this means a standard which resembles the human body or body part (spine, femur, forearm) and is composed of materials which approximate the density and attenuation properties of both mineralized and soft tissue. One can achieve close simulation of the in vivo measurement by using excised human vertebrae encased in tissue-equivalent material. However, the limited availability of specimens for this purpose, the questionable long-term stability of a phantom composed of organic material and the inevitable production variability (each phantom's nominal values are unique, depending on the vertebrae used) are disadvantages of this approach.

Lunar and Norland also provide calibration standards which must be scanned regularly to check and update the calibration of the system over time. The Hologic densitometers have an internal reference standard which continuously calibrates the instrument during a scan. The scanner manufacturers also provide with their densitometers a spine phantom for QC evaluations. To varying degrees the spine phantoms simulate the geometry and attenuation properties of the lumbar spine. The phantoms are scanned and analyzed using the same protocols employed for in vivo measurements and thus are capable of testing the algorithms used to find bone edges and determine soft tissue baselines.

Lunar Spine Phantom

Lunar provides a stylized spine phantom constructed of aluminum. Four lumbar vertebrae (L1–L4) are simulated, increasing in size and density between L1 and L4. The precisely machined phantom can be used to simulate the patient measurement. The aluminum spine phantom is scanned in 15 cm of water or uncooked rice to mimic the soft tissue thickness and attenuation characteristics of a typical patient and analyzed using the standard spine analysis protocol. An obvious shortcoming of the aluminum spine phantom is the limited anthropomorphic design. The phantom is formed from a flat piece of aluminum (approximately 1.0 cm thick) and each vertebra is a uniform density with sharp edges. Thus it does not provide a good test of the edge detection software. In addition, the flat profile of the phantom could cause anomalies when comparing systems that use pencil and fan beam geometries. However, the density of the phantom vertebrae does increase from L1 to L4, allowing a test of system linearity.

Norland Spine Phantom

The Norland spine phantom is more anthropomorphic than the Lunar phantom. It is constructed of calcium hydroxyapatite [$Ca_5(PO_4)_3OH$] embedded in acrylic. The hydroxyapatite is molded into a shape that resembles a three-dimensional relief map of a bone density scan of the lumbar vertebrae L2–L4. The thickness of the phantom is only 2 cm. This design provides a more appropriate test of the edge detection algorithms because the scan image has more realistic edge gradients. However, as with the aluminum phantom, the narrow profile is of limited usefulness measured with a fan beam scanner. The density of the three vertebrae are similar and linearity or calibration checks are not possible with the Norland spine phantom.

Hologic Spine Phantom

The standard provided with Hologic densitometers is more anthropomorphic than the previous phantoms. It is composed of four hydroxyapatite vertebrae embedded in a tissue mimicking epoxy-resin block 17.5 cm thick. The vertebrae are of homogeneous density but closely resemble true vertebrae in size and shape. When measuring this test object the standard protocols for spine scan acquisition and analysis are used. While the Hologic phantom is a closer approximation of the real spine, it has several documented limitations. The vertebrae are composed of hydroxyapatite of uniform density showing none of the heterogeneity of the real spine. As a consequence the edge finding algorithms of the software are still not adequately tested. However, the imaging geometry more closely resembles that of the spine in vivo than either the Lunar or Norland phantoms. Another limitation is that the vertebrae are all of similar density, thus the phantom does not allow testing of system linearity or calibration. Finally the surrounding and overlying epoxy (density=1.15 g/cm^3) representing soft tissue is uniform and does not represent the proportion of lean and fat tissue found in the typical patient. The epoxy represents approximately 78% lean tissue. The Lunar and Norland phantoms have the same limitation.

European Spine Phantom

As another approximation to the lumbar spine a phantom has been developed with support from the European Union under its organization Committee d'Actions Concertés–Biomedical Engineering (COMAC-BME) [6]. Commonly known as the European spine phantom (ESP), it was designed for use as a calibration standard and QC tool in both DXA and quantitative computed tomography (QCT). The ESP is constructed of water-equivalent plastics and epoxy resins (approx. 10% fat). Both cancellous and compact bone-equivalent tissues are simulated by adding calcium hydroxyapatite to the water-equivalent materials. The phantom was designed to be anthropomorphic yet is geometrically well defined to allow calculation of true values for all of the quantities to be measured. The phantom is composed of three vertebrae which vary in mineral density and cortical thickness. True values for BMD of each vertebra measured in the PA projection are 0.5, 1.0, and 1.5 g/cm^2. Thus the ESP can be used to evaluate linearity of the BMD measurement.

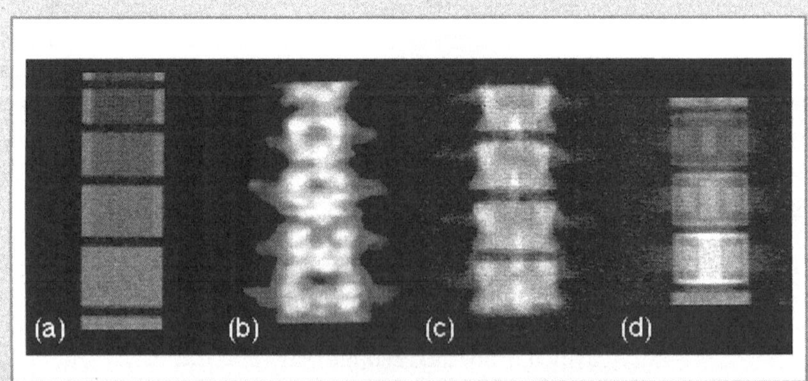

Fig. 23-1 DXA scan image of spine phantoms of various design. **a** Lunar aluminum spine phantom, L1–L4. **b** Norland spine phantom, L2–L4. **c** Hologic spine phantom, L1–L4. **d** European Spine Phantom (ESP), L2–L4

Table 23-1 Comparison of spine phantoms for DXA

Spine phantom	Anthropomorphic design	Linearity and calibration check	Suitable for cross-platform use	Cost and availability
Ex vivo spine	+++	-	+	-
Lunar	--	+	-	+
Norland	-	-	-	+
Hologic	+	-	+	+
ESP	++	++	++	-

COMAC-BME has also undertaken the development of a forearm phantom which is also designed to be used by DXA and peripheral QCT [7]. Using similar design concepts and construction materials a semianthropomorphic phantom to simulate the proximal and distal radius has been proposed. As with the ESP the COMAC-BME forearm phantom simulates both the compact and cancellous bone compartments of the radius. While this initial design has shown some promise, suggestions for improvements are being solicited to be incorporated into a second generation phantom.

Figure 23-1 shows the radiographic appearance of each of the spine phantoms discussed. The phantoms of Lunar and Norland are not widely distributed but are primarily restricted to use on densitometers from their respective manufacturers. The Hologic spine phantom has been adopted as the phantom of choice for daily instrument QC in multicenter clinical trials. It has been used for this purpose because of its anthropomorphic design, relatively low cost and ease of use on the various brands of densitometers. The Hologic spine phantom has also played a role in the cross-calibration of densitometers in multicenter studies. The ESP has benefited from the backing of COMAC-BME and the International Committee for Standards in Bone Measurement. Moreover, it is the only phantom to be endorsed by the scanner manufacturers. Compared to the Hologic spine phantom it is relatively expensive and has not come into widespread use as a QC standard. However, it has seen growing use for cross-calibration in multicenter studies, being used to standardize BMD measurements of both the spine [8] and femur [9]. Table 23-1 summarizes the relative merits of the phantoms developed for DXA.

In addition to these phantoms used to monitor performance for measurement of bone density, other phantoms are required if densitometers are used to measure soft tissue composition (e.g., percentage body fat) or vertebral morphometry by lateral imaging of the entire spine in a process called morphometric X-ray absorptiometry. Today there are no commercially available phantoms to test performance in these areas although soft tissue phantoms have been described in the literature [10].

Daily Quality Control Procedures of the DXA Manufacturers

Each of the manufacturers of bone densitometers has developed test objects and procedures for regular QC of their systems. These tests are designed to be run daily to assure the correct operation of the instrument before scanning patients. The results of these tests are checked against established limits of performance, and a report is printed. Failure to pass a test requires repeating the QC procedures. If the system fails again, it is necessary to contact the service department of the manufacturer for interpretation and potentially to schedule a service visit. The results of these tests are also reviewed during regular maintenance visits to detect trends in machine performance which may indicate failing components.

The standard tests of the Lunar DPX and Norland systems require daily checks of mechanical and electrical operation and verification of instrument calibration. Both manufacturers use a proprietary test object containing different filters which mimic the absorption characteristics of tissue and bone. The daily QC test of Hologic densitometers employs a semianthropomorphic spine phantom as test object. The Hologic QC test checks the primary measurement endpoints: BMD, bone mineral content (BMC), and area. The BMD of the spine phantom measured on a Hologic instrument is approximately 1.0 g/cm^2, the typical spine BMD of young, normal adult women. The Hologic QC program involves scanning this phantom once every day before patients are scanned. The scan is analyzed by the operator using the standard analysis protocol and results are compared to historical data by plotting the QC data against time. The results of the phantom measurement are evaluated by various methods and checked by the operator against limits for acceptable performance. A similar QC check is applied to Lunar and Norland densitometers using proprietary spine phantoms. This test is not a required component of the Lunar QC program. It is usually performed less frequently (weekly), and some owners choose not to perform this test at all.

Analysis of Longitudinal Quality Control Data

After choosing an appropriate test tool and establishing a procedure for routine measurements the next step is the interpretation of the longitudinal data collected. As described above the manufacturers use visual inspection and various analytical tests to evaluate QC data. Visual inspection is universally available but is subject to the experience of the inspector; as such, objective tests are more attractive. Shewhart charts represent one class of tests which have been applied in DXA [11, 12]. Shewhart charts are based on a set of rules which can be used to detect systematic deviation from normal performance. One set of rules which have been applied to scanner QC data are the following (from Faulkner and McClung [15]):

- 1.5% rule: one measurement more than 1.5% from the established baseline value

- 1.0% rule: two consecutive measurements more than 1.0% above or below the established baseline value
- 0.5% rule: four consecutive measurements more than 0.5% above or below the established baseline value
- Mean×10 rule: ten consecutive measurements either above or below the established baseline value

These rules can be applied prospectively or retrospectively and provide an objective, reproducible evaluation of scanner performance. A drawback of standard Shewhart rules is that they tend to be overly sensitive and result in many false positive alarms when applied to DXA. Sensitizing rules have been developed to reduce the false alarm rate of Shewhart charts.

Other tests have been proposed including cumulative sum (CUSUM) charts [13]. The tabular CUSUM charts which have been used in DXA represent a running sum of the deviations of each day's BMD measurement from the established mean BMD. Mathematically the cumulative sum can be represented by the equation:

$$S_H(i) = \max\left[0,\ S_H(i-1) + \left(\frac{x_i - \mu}{\sigma} - k \right) \right]$$

where S_H is the cumulative sum, x_i the current measurement, m is the established baseline, s the measurement standard deviation (often taken to be 0.005 g/cm^2), and k is a tuning parameter which equals 0.5. This is the equation for evaluating positive deviations from the baseline. A similar equation with ($\mu-x_i$) replacing the numerator in parentheses is used to detect deviations below the baseline. For an instrument that is in control, normal deviation above and below the mean keeps the sum near zero. However, systematic departure from the mean BMD or a single large deviation results in a large sum. An alarm is raised when the cumulative sum exceeds a predefined threshold (a threshold of five has been suggested [13]). After each alarm a new mean is established from the first data points after the discontinuity, and the process continues. An advantage of the CUSUM chart is that it provides an accurate estimate of the date of failure which facilitates the investigation of cause and the application of correction factors when desired.

These QC tests have been compared by Lu et al. [13] using actual data from densitometers as well as simulated data sets. They found CUSUM charts to have the best performance, demonstrating high sensitivity and specificity, giving estimates of the time of failure with near zero bias and second only to Shewhart in time to detect a change. Visual inspection also performed well but was less sensitive to small yet statistically significant drifts and shifts. In contrast, Shewhart charts were overly sensitive and gave many false positive alarms. Figure 23-2 compares these two methods using QC data collected from a densitometer.

Currently these automated and objective methods of evaluating longitudinal QC data are not routinely used in the clinic environment. However, visual inspec-

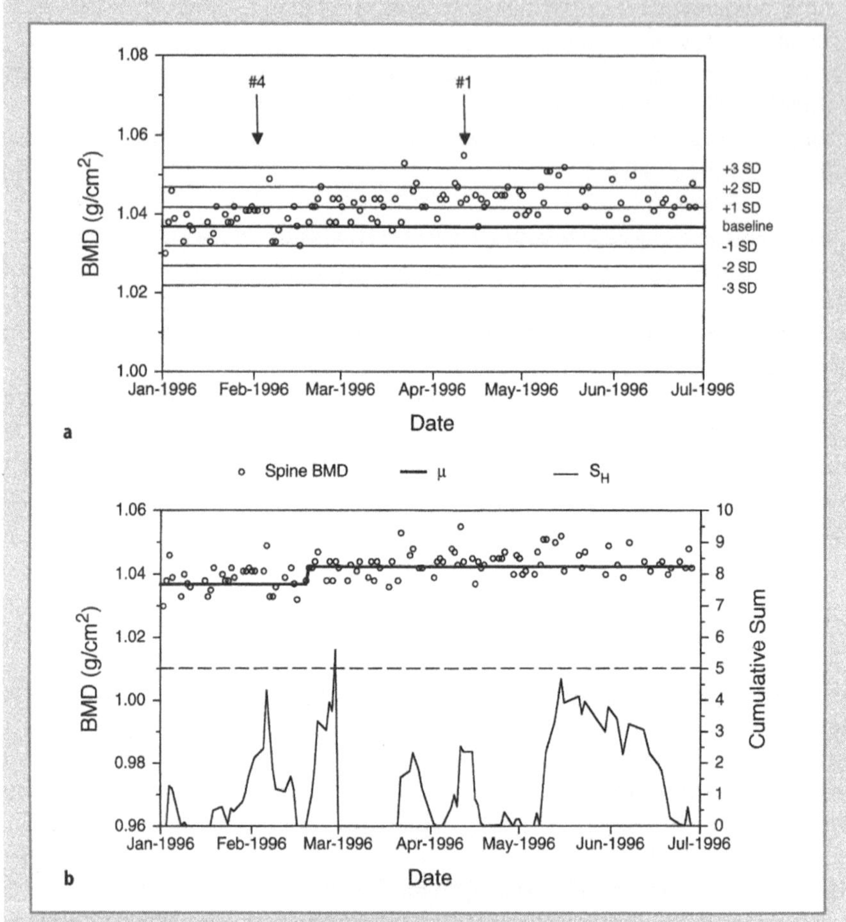

Fig. 23-2 Shewhart **a** and CUSUM **b** chart rules applied to QC data from a densitometer. The Shewhart chart detected two break points (Rule #4 on February 2 and Rule #1 on April 11) during this period while the CUSUM chart found only one (February 20). The Shewhart graph does not show the new baseline and limits established after the first break point

tion is actually very effective in identifying changes in scanner performance that are clinically significant and warrant a service visit. Analytic tests would be able to detect smaller changes, but these may not have a clear, assignable cause and thus cannot be corrected by service. Moreover, excessive false alarms could desensitize the clinic staff and respective service departments. Automated analysis with QC charts would clearly benefit from filters designed to reduce the number of alarms to those representing clinically significant performance changes. For example Shewhart charts combined with visual inspection may complement each other and provide effective evaluation of QC data.

While some QC charts are overly sensitive, visual inspection can be overly sensitive as well. This demonstrates another important purpose of objective QC charts such as Shewhart and CUSUM. Not only are they able to detect when equipment is operating incorrectly, but they also confirm proper operation. Some variation in performance is expected even when a densitometer is operating within specifications. QC charts verify that these variations are within acceptable ranges and prevent well-intentioned but unnecessary service interventions which themselves could cause performance changes.

While small changes in performance are of minimal importance in routine clinical use, they may have relevance in the context of clinical trials that use BMD as an endpoint for evaluating drug efficacy. In this case objective analytical tests with sufficient sensitivity to detect these changes are required. Given the magnitude of data associated with trials (some trials involve up to 200 densitometers), the QC tests also need to have high specificity to reduce the time spent investigating false alarms. Finally, the test should provide the information necessary to allow data correction when deemed necessary.

Replacing Old Densitometers with New Equipment

When replacing a densitometer with new equipment it is important to consider the impact of potential differences in calibration. If measurements of patients on the new scanner are expected to be compared to earlier measurements made on the original equipment, a careful investigation of systematic differences in calibration is warranted. Even when the new instrument is of the same make and model as the old, calibration differences can exist. There are many reports of comparisons of scanners [14–19]. Most have used the Hologic spine phantom to show that scanners of the same make and model provide similar results. However, differences between equivalent scanners can be as great as 2%–3%. Disagreement between the scanners of different manufacturers is also well documented, and the observed differences are much larger. PA spine BMD measured on a Lunar scanner is about 13% higher than on Hologic or Norland scanners [17]. Thus careful comparison of the new and old scanners is required for consistency of results. This comparison can be achieved by cross-calibration experiments performed with phantoms or with volunteers. An experiment using in vivo measurements is more difficult to execute and requires additional resources but ultimately provides more accurate results.

Each manufacturer makes great effort to ensure the consistency of the calibration of each densitometer produced. These steps have proven to be effective in keeping calibration differences to 1% or less for the majority of systems. Figure 23-3 compares intermachine calibration differences for 83 Hologic densitometers. The calibration of these scanners was measured as part of the interscanner cross-calibration for a clinical drug trial. A single traveling Hologic spine phantom which was shipped to each clinic and scanned ten times on the local densitometer. The mean of the ten scans at each site was compared to the overall mean and percent-

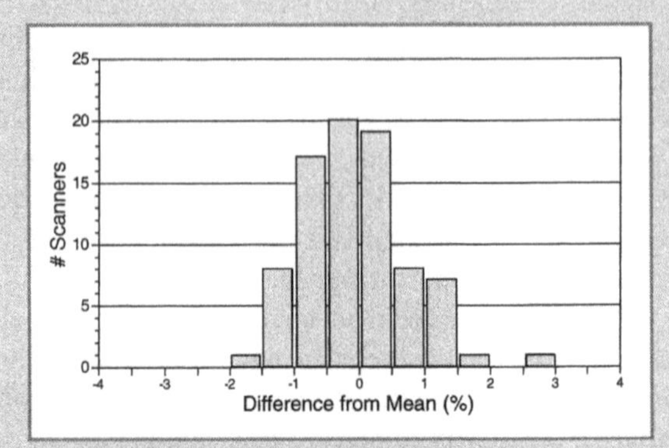

Fig. 23-3 Histogram of calibration differences between 83 Hologic densitometers. Data show the percentage difference from the overall mean of the measured BMD of a traveling Hologic spine phantom scanned on all densitometers. Three quarters of scanners have a calibration within ±1% of the overall mean

age difference calculated. These data show that about half of densitometers have a calibration within 0.5% of average Hologic scanner calibration and three-quarters are within 1%. Similar distributions have been observed for Lunar and Norland densitometers. Given this close agreement, each manufacturer uses the same normative data on all scanner models it produces. These small differences in calibration are on the order of the measurement precision and have negligible impact on diagnosis. Nevertheless any two scanners can have calibrations which differ by 1% or more. These systematic differences after a scanner change can be important when comparing longitudinal measurements made in the clinic or as part of a research protocol.

The nature of the upgrade determines what cross-calibration measurements are required. With the arrival of third-generation scanners with significant differences in design, the possibility for greater differences in calibration exist. In these instances more extensive comparisons are required to assure equivalent performance. An upgrade can be arbitrarily classified into one of three types. A lateral upgrade involves replacing a scanner with a system of the same make and model, a step upgrade is a change to another model of the same manufacturer, and a cross-platform upgrade involves changing to the equipment of another manufacturer. Table 23-2 shows the recommended phantom cross-calibration procedures for these upgrades. In general phantom cross-calibration is imperfect [18]. However, it can provide agreement to within about 1% for lateral upgrades and 2% for step upgrades. This may be sufficient in a clinical setting but research involving longitudinal evaluations will require in vivo measurements to obtain closer agreement. In vivo cross-calibration experiments should involve at least 20–30 volunteers spanning the clinical range of bone densities. Scans for each volunteer should be made within a few weeks of each other, preferably on the same day.

Table 23-2 Recommended cross-calibration procedures when replacing DXA densitometers

Upgrade type	Cross-calibration procedures	
	In vitro measurements	In vivo measurements[a]
Lateral (same manufacturer and model)	10 scans on each machine of the ESP or Hologic spine phantom	10–20 volunteers scanned on both machines at the spine (other skeletal sites if desired)[b]
Step (different model)	10 scans on each machine of the ESP or Hologic spine phantom and linearity phantom if available	20–30 volunteers scanned on both machines at the spine (other skeletal sites if desired)[b]
Cross-platform (different manufacturer)	10 scans on each machine of the ESP or Hologic spine phantom and linearity phantom if available	All research participants scanned on both machines at all anatomical sites being measured

[a] In vivo measurements are optional and provide greater accuracy in the cross-calibration and are strongly recommended for scanner changes during research studies.
[b] Scanning other skeletal sites is recommended for scanners used in research protocols with longitudinal evaluation of BMD changes.

Patient positioning and region of interest (ROI) placement should be matched for each pair of scans. When upgrading a scanner that has been used only for clinical patients, scans of the PA spine are sufficient. Research scanner upgrades should scan volunteers at all relevant skeletal sites as a calibration match at the spine does not guarantee a match at other skeletal sites.

Many older scanners using pencil beam scanning are replaced with new scanners that employ a fan-beam geometry. The influence of magnification due to the fan beam has been investigated [19]. Systematic differences in BMC and area that are correlated with body habitus have been observed. However, BMC and area scale similarly with magnification and the effect on the clinically relevant variable BMD is insignificant. Figure 23-4 shows in vivo cross-calibration results comparing a Hologic QDR 1000 (pencil beam) with a Hologic QDR 4500A (fan beam). Close agreement in BMD measured with these instruments is apparent. Data follow the line of identity, and the root mean square error is 1%–2%, similar to the measurement precision.

When changing to a densitometer of the same manufacturer, it is always desirable to compare the two instruments and adjust the calibration of the new system to match the old. In this way comparison of follow-up patient data to historical results is transparent. This can be best achieved by comparing the two systems with phantoms and adjusting the calibration of the new equipment as necessary. If desired, subsequent in vivo measurements can be used to confirm the calibration match or fine tune it for better agreement. Execution of an in vivo cross-calibration experiment can be simplified if the two scanners can be in service simultaneously. However, space limitations sometimes prohibit this.

Changing to another manufacturer's equipment raises several additional questions. Differences in absolute mineral calibration, patient positioning techniques,

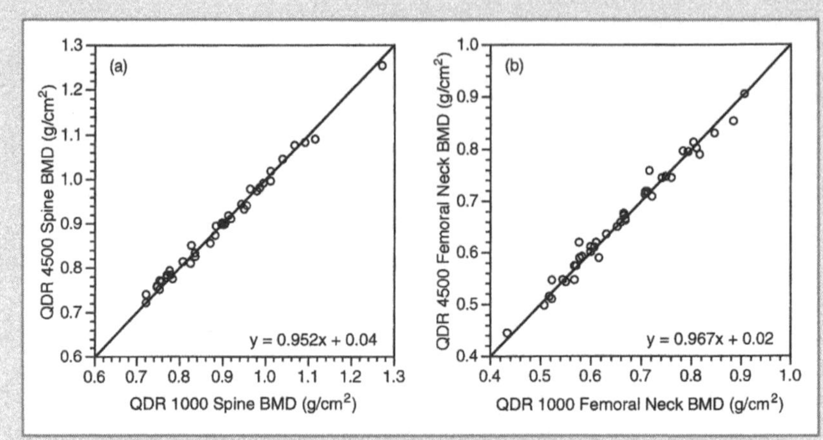

Fig. 23-4 Comparison of AP spine (L1–L4, a) and femoral neck BMD (b) measured in 41 women on a Hologic QDR 1000 (pencil beam) and QDR 4500 (fan beam). These data are typical of agreement between two scanners from the same manufacturer. The line of identity is shown

ROI definition, and edge detection algorithms make comparison of results between manufacturers difficult. While published reports comparing Lunar, Norland, and Hologic scanners have shown good correlation, prediction of an individual's BMD across scanners of different manufacture can have errors of 3%–4%, more than double the errors expected when the two scanners are the same brand. In general cross-calibration equations such as those produced by the International Committee for Standards in Bone Measurement can be used to standardize the BMD measurements from different manufacturers [17]. However, care should be exercised when comparing an individual patient's measurements from different scanners of different manufacture. For research studies this type of upgrade should be avoided. However, if it is unavoidable, all research participants should be scanned in duplicate on the old and new instruments and corrections generated.

Quality Control of the DXA Examination

The discussion above centers on procedures for monitoring DXA systems to assure their accurate and precise operation. However, even when data are collected on a properly functioning scanner the results can be compromised by poor performance of the operator responsible for scanning and analyzing the data. Errors due to scan artifacts, poor positioning, or incorrect analysis can be as greater or greater than the those likely to result from changing scanner performance. A recent investigation of the sources of variability in DXA has shown that error sources related to operator performance and in vivo factors in the patient are more important than those relating to the equipment [20, 21].

Correct patient preparation and positioning are required to ensure valid scan data. Inconsistent positioning on follow-up can confound patient evaluation. Several authors have investigated the effect of patient positioning in scanning the proximal femur and have demonstrated the importance of leg rotation on femoral neck BMD [22]. Careful attention to this aspect of patient positioning can lead to greatly improved results. A positioning aid has been developed to facilitate consistent abduction and rotation of the femur. Use of the device has been shown to provide significant improvement in the reproducibility of the measurement of femoral neck BMD [23]. However, conscientious adherence to the procedures recommended by the manufacturers can also yield quite good results.

Likewise, proper scan analysis technique is crucial, and inconsistent technique results in poor quality data [24–26]. Bendavid et al. [24] reported the results of a review of DXA scans collected as part of a clinical trial. More than 6000 scans of the AP and lateral spine, proximal femur, forearm, and whole body were reviewed at the DXA Quality Assurance Center at the University of California. Scan analysis technique was critiqued, and the frequency and magnitude of errors were summarized. Figure 23-5 shows the observed frequency of analysis errors by scan type. Error rates were highest for scans of the proximal femur. This result is in agreement with intuition, which would predict that the scan type with the highest error rates are those with more intricate analysis procedures, and which require more operator interaction in the placement of the various lines and regions. This figure also shows the effect of these errors on BMD. Average errors are on the order of a few percentage points, which can interfere with the measurement of changes in BMD. However, errors for the individual can be quite large and can lead to possible misdiagnosis.

Efforts to ensure the correct acquisition and analysis of quantitative data begins with proper training and certification of the operators. Operator training should

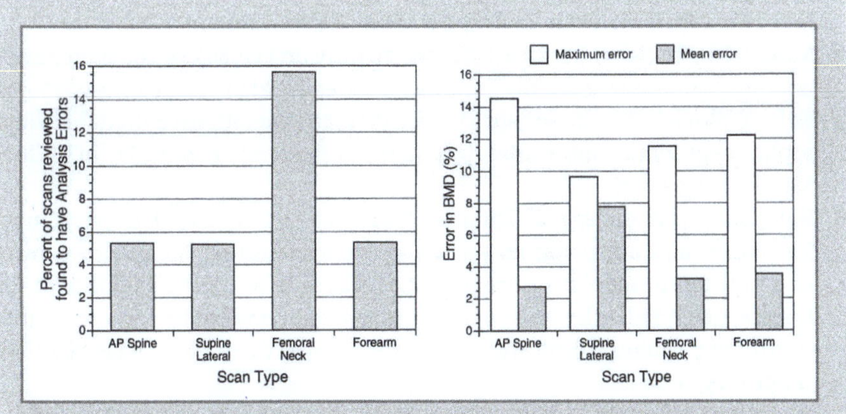

Fig. 23-5 Investigation of analysis errors in DXA scans in a multicenter clinical trial showing the frequency **a** and magnitude **b** of errors in BMD measurement at four skeletal sites

be provided by the manufacturer of the instrument at the time of installation. Typically the training involves 1–2 days of instruction and hands-on exercises in acquisition and analysis. For already installed systems the training of new staff is often handled in house with experienced operators training the new personnel. This has varying degrees of success and depends on the expertise of the mentors and the amount of time that they can devote to the training. Peer-to-peer training opens the possibility of bad habits being passed on to the next generation. Retraining by the manufacturer is generally more reliable. Another alternative is to obtain training from other organizations such as the International Society for Clinical Densitometry which provide certification of densitometer operators and physicians.

A second important step in operator quality assurance is peer review of measurements. This can be performed by an experienced operator or by the physician responsible for interpretation of the exams. This procedure is effective in catching most mistakes that result from carelessness or haste. It also requires the interpreting physician to have the knowledge necessary to evaluate the quality of the examination and to be familiar with those factors that can lead to measurement errors (e.g., patient positioning errors, image artifacts, incorrect ROI placement). This knowledge is critical to the correct assessment of the DXA scan.

References

1. Gluer CC, Faulkner KG, Estilo MJ, Engelke K, Rosin J, Genant HK (1993) Quality assurance for bone densitometry research studies: concept and impact. Osteoporosis Int 3:227–235
2. Lang T, Takada M, Gee R, Wu C, Li J, Hayashi-Clark C, Schoen S, March V, Genant HK (1997) A preliminary evaluation of the Lunar Expert-XL for bone densitometry and vertebral morphometry. J Bone Miner Res 12:136–143
3. Wahner HW, Fogelman I (1994) The evaluation of osteoporosis: dual energy X-ray absorptiometry in clinical practice. Dunitz, London
4. Mazess RB, Collick B, Trempe J, Barden H, Hanson J (1989) Performance evaluation of a dual energy X-ray bone densitometer. Calcif Tissue Int 44:228–232
5. Kelly T, Slovick D, Schoenfield D, Neer R (1988) Quantitative digital radiography versus dual photon absorptiometry of the lumbar spine. J Clin Endocr Metab 67:839–844
6. Kalender W, Felsenberg D, Genant HK, Fischer M, Dequeker J, Reeve J (1995) The European spine phantom – a tool for standardization and quality control in spine bone mineral measurements by DXA and QCT. Eur J Radiol 20:83–92
7. Rüegsegger P, Kalender W (1993) A phantom for standardization and quality control in peripheral bone measurements by pQCT and DXA. Phys Med Biol 38:1963–1970
8. Dequeker J, Pearson J, Reeve J, Henley M, Bright J, Felsenberg D, Kalender W, Rüegsegger P, Adams J, Laval-Jeantet AM, Diaz Curiel M, Fischer M, Galan F, Geusens P, Hyldstrup L, Jaeger P, Kotzki P, Kröger H, Lips P, Mitchell A,

Louis O, Perez Cano R, Pols H, Reid DM, Ribot C, Schneider P, Lunt M (1995) Dual X-ray absorptiometry-cross-calibration and normative reference ranges for the spine: results of a European community concerted action. Bone 17:247–254

9. Pearson J, Dequeker J, Reeve J, Felsenberg D, Henley M, Bright J, Lunt M, Adams J, Diaz Curiel M, Galan F, Geusens P, Jaeger P, Kröger H, Lips P, Mitchell A, Perez Cano R, Pols H, Rapado A, Reid DM, Ribot C, Schneider P, Rüegsegger P, Laval-Jeantet AM, Kalender W (1995) Dual X-ray absorptiometry of the proximal femur: normal European values standardized with the European spine phantom. J Bone Miner Res 10:315–324

10. Goodsitt MM (1992) Evaluation of a new set of calibration standards for the measurement of fat content via DPA and DXA. Med Phys 19:35–44

11. Orwoll ES, Oviatt SK, Biddle JA (1993) Precision of dual-energy X-ray absorptiometry: development of quality control rules and their application in longitudinal studies. J Bone Miner Res 8:693–699

12. Faulkner KG, McClung MR (1995) Quality control of DXA instruments in multicenter trials. Osteoporosis Int 5:218–227

13. Lu Y, Mathur AK, Blunt B, Glüer C-C, Will AS, Fuerst TP, Jergas MD, Andriano KN, Cummings SR, Genant HK (1996) Comparison of visual examination and process-control charts to detect change points in longitudinal dual X-ray absorptiometry quality control data. J Bone Miner Res 11:626–637

14. Blake GM, Tong M, Fogelman I (1991) Intersite comparison of the Hologic QDR-1000 dual energy X-ray bone densitometer. Br J Radiol 64:440–446

15. Faulkner KG, Glüer C, Estilo M, Genant HK (1993) Cross-calibration of DXA equipment: upgrading from a Hologic QDR 1000/W to a QDR 2000. Calcif Tissue Int 52:79–84

16. Finkelstein J, Butler JP, Cleary RL, Neer RM (1994) Comparison of four methods for cross-calibrating dual-energy X-ray absorptiometers to eliminate systematic errors when upgrading equipment. J Bone Miner Res 12:1945–1952

17. Genant HK, Grampp S, Glüer CC, Faulkner KG, Jergas M, Engelke K, Hagiwara S, van Kuijk C (1994) Universal standardization for dual X-ray absorptiometry: patient and phantom cross-calibration results. J Bone Miner Res 9:1503–1514

18. Blake GM (1996) Replacing DXA scanners: cross-calibration with phantoms may be misleading. Calcif Tissue Int 59:1–5

19. Blake GM, Parker JC, Buxton FM, Fogelman I (1993) Dual X-ray absorptiometry: a comparison between fan beam and pencil beam scans. Br J Radiol 66:902–906

20. Fuleihan GE, Testa MA, Angell JE, Porrino N, Leboff MS (1995) Reproducibility of DXA absorptiometry: a model for bone loss estimates. J Bone Miner Res 10:1004–1014

21. Nguyen TV, Sambrook PN, Eisman JA (1997) Sources of variability in bone mineral density measurements: implications for study design and analysis of bone loss. J Bone Miner Res 12:124–135

22. Wilson CR, Fogleman I, Blake GM, Rodin A (1991) The effect of positioning on dual X-ray bone densitometry of the proximal femur. Bone Miner 12:63–76
23. Hans D, Duboeuf F, Schott AM, Horn S, Avioli LV, Drezner MK, Meunier PJ (1997) Effects of a new positioner on the precision of hip bone mineral density measurements. J Bone Miner Res 12:1289–1294
24. Bendavid EJ, Young KC, Glüer CC, Genant HK (1992) Frequency and magnitude of analysis errors of bone density results assessed by dual X-ray absorptiometry. J Bone Miner Res 7:373–382
25. Trevisan C, Gandolini GG, Sibilla P, Penotti M, Caraceni MP, Ortolani S (1992) Bone mass measurement by DXA: influence of analysis procedures and interunit variation. J Bone Miner Res 7:373–382
26. Wahner HW, Looker A, Dunn WL, Walters L, Hauser MF (1993) Precision of bone mineral measurement (BMD) at the proximal femur in a multicenter study using three mobile examination centers (NHANES III). J Bone Miner Res 8 [Suppl 1]:S354

24 Clinical Application of Bone Densitometry

P. D. Miller and S. T. Harris

Osteoporosis has been defined empirically as "a systemic skeletal disease characterized by low bone mass and microarchitectural deterioration of bone tissue, with a consequent increase in bone fragility and susceptibility to fracture" (Consensus Development Conference 1993). Implicit in this definition is the observation that bone loss is universal: it occurs in everyone, both men and women, past the peak of skeletal maturity at approximately the age of 30 years. The bone loss of osteoporosis is itself painless and as a consequence is quite insidious clinically because there are no obvious signs or symptoms to suggest that the bone loss is occurring. Because the bone loss is asymptomatic, however, it is also in a sense clinically irrelevant; bone loss per se is not of clinical importance, but it is the increased fracture risk associated with that bone loss that is the true concern.

The clinical interest in quantitative bone density measurements has been based upon two important assumptions: (a) that bone density is in fact related to fracture risk, and (b) that treatments to affect bone density can be developed. There is now reasonable evidence to support both assumptions:

Bone density is related to fracture risk. A number of studies have demonstrated that bone density measurements at baseline are related to the subsequent risk of fracture at diverse skeletal sites (Hui et al. 1989; Cummings et al. 1990, 1993; Ross et al. 1990; Black et al. 1992). As a rough approximation it appears that each decrease of 1 SD in bone density is associated with a relative risk of around 1.5 for fracture. As a consequence a bone density at the "lower limits of normal for age," i.e., 2 SD below the mean, is associated with a several-fold increased risk of fracture, despite being "normal" statistically. Interestingly, there is surprisingly weak evidence for site specificity. In the Study of Osteoporotic Fractures, measurement of hip density was a strong predictor of subsequent hip fracture – women in the lowest quartile of hip density had a 8.5-fold greater risk of hip fracture than women in the highest quartile – but measurements of density at the spine, radius, and calcaneus were only slightly weaker predictors of hip fracture (Cummings et al. 1993). The diagnosis of osteoporosis in otherwise healthy individuals who are at risk for an osteoporotic (fragility) fracture is important for the prevention of the first fracture. At this time, a quantitative measurement of bone density is the only objective method available to identify the individual patient at risk of fracture.

Treatments to affect bone density can be developed. The importance of bone density measurements would be diminished were there no clinically useful treatments capable of affecting bone density and the consequent risk of fracture. There is an extensive literature surrounding the effect of various treatments upon bone density, but much less literature surrounding fracture risk. Prospective, randomized, controlled trials have demonstrated both a beneficial effect upon bone density and a decrease in fracture rate for treatment with bisphosphonates such as alendronate and etidronate (Black et al. 1996; Liberman et al. 1995; Storm et al. 1990; Watts et al. 1990), as well as estrogen (Lindsay et al. 1980; Lufkin et al. 1992).

Until recently the diagnosis of osteoporosis was based largely upon history and clinical presentation. Although plain radiographs often suggested the diagnosis in asymptomatic individuals, most clinical attention focused upon the patient who presented with a fracture. With the advent of the quantitative techniques of bone densitometry, however, the diagnosis of osteoporosis has broadened to encompass asymptomatic patients with reductions in bone density by statistical criteria. The diagnosis of osteoporosis is now often analogous to the diagnosis of high blood pressure or hyperlipidemia in asymptomatic individuals. Objective measures of blood pressure and cholesterol are strongly related to the risk of subsequent cardiovascular disease. Similarly, low bone density is the most important predictor of fragility fracture (Black et al. 1992).

The clinical application of bone densitometry requires a knowledge of the strengths and weaknesses of central bone density measurement techniques versus peripheral bone density measurement techniques (Miller and McClung 1996; Genant et al. 1996a,b). The selection of the measurement technique and the proper interpretation of the results are largely determined by the intended application (Miller et al. 1995; Consensus Development Conference 1993; Johnston et al. 1991). Three clinical applications of bone density measurements are: (a) to establish a diagnosis of osteopenia (low bone density), (b) to predict fragility fractures, as noted above, and (b) to monitor serial changes in the skeleton over time.

Considering the first application, various techniques are now used to diagnose low bone density. Two important clinical considerations for the choice of measurement technique and/or skeletal site for this application are: (a) the presence of discordance at various skeletal sites, and/or (b) the presence of false elevations in bone density at specific skeletal sites. Bone density is not homogeneous throughout the skeleton, i.e., the relative bone densities of the spine, wrist, and hip may be different in an individual patient (Melton et al. 1992). This discordance is more apparent in early menopausal women than in elderly women. It may be related to the higher bone turnover rate and loss of trabecular bone observed in the perimenopausal population than in the elderly population (Genant et al. 1982). Because of this accelerated trabecular bone loss, a higher proportion of early postmenopausal women may be diagnosed with low bone density by measuring the spine by dual energy X-ray absorptiometry (DXA) or quantitative computed tomography (QCT) than by measuring the wrist or hip (Melton et al. 1992; Eastell 1995). For these reasons it is ideal to measure more than one skeletal site in order not to miss the diagnosis of low bone density (Pouilles et al. 1993; Davis et al. 1994; Genant et al. 1996a,b). This is more easily accomplished, from a practical point of view, with the fan-beam or rapid pencil-beam DXA systems.

After the age of 65 years the discordance among skeletal sites is less, and the diagnosis of low bone density can therefore be made using the hip measurement (Looker et al. 1995) or other peripheral measurements (wrist, heel, hand). In fact, in the elderly these peripheral measurements may be more accurate than spinal DXA measurements, which may be artifactually elevated by sclerosis of posterior spinal elements (Black et al. 1992; Nordin et al. 1996). Because of facet joint sclerosis, the measurement of spinal density in the elderly by the posteroanterior DXA technique frequently underestimates the severity of osteoporosis (Greenspan et al. 1996; Peel et al. 1993; Genant et al. 1984). Hence in the elderly population it may be preferable to measure spinal trabecular density by QCT or lateral spinal density by DXA. Alternatively, hip and/or peripheral densities can be measured in the elderly, although rarely the hip density is also falsely elevated due to sclerotic processes. The diagnosis of osteoporosis in the elderly may therefore be missed by DXA measurements of both the posteroanterior spine and the hip, although the latter measure is generally the strongest predictor of hip fracture.

In conclusion, in those clinical circumstances in which the bone density should be low but is found to be "normal," consider that discordance may be present, or that false elevations of the measurement may obscure the diagnosis. It may be necessary to measure other skeletal sites or to use other bone density measurement techniques to secure an accurate diagnosis. The clinical circumstances in which bone density might be expected to be reduced include: (a) late postmenopausal women not receiving estrogen replacement therapy, (b) patients with fragility fractures, and (c) patients receiving chronic glucocorticoids or other medications which may negatively affect bone density. Other techniques or skeletal sites to consider in these patients include (Genant et al. 1996a,b; Baran et al. 1991; Kleerekoper et al. 1994):
- Spinal density by QCT or lateral DXA
- Wrist density by peripheral DXA or peripheral QCT (pQCT)
- Heel density by single X-ray absorptiometry or ultrasound
- Hand X-rays by radiographic absorptiometry

The second intention of bone density measurement is to predict fragility fractures. Again, the age of the patient should be considered in the determination of the appropriate technique and the interpretation of the resulting density. The vast majority of data relating bone density to the relative risk, annual risk, and absolute risk of fracture have been derived from studies of women over the age of 65 (Ross et al. 1991; Hui et al. 1988; Melton et al. 1993; Cummings et al. 1993). Very few fracture data exist for the younger perimenopausal population (Parkkari et al. 1994; Matkovic et al. 1979). Hence the relative risk or annual risk of fracture attributed to a 70-year-old woman with a given bone density should not be attributed to a 50-year-old woman with the same bone density. In fact, since age is such an important independent risk factor for fracture prediction, the elderly woman clearly has a higher short-term fracture risk at equivalent bone density (Hui et al. 1988; Cummings et al. 1995). This difference in fracture predictability according to age is an important concept for clinicians to embrace. In younger women health-promoting measures such as exercise, the avoidance of tobacco use, and the optimization of calcium intake seem clinically reasonable. It may be unnecessary, however, to advise wholesale changes in life-style in order to avoid fragility fractures.

The issue of fracture risk is evolving further in the concept of remaining life-time fracture probability (RLFP). This concept entails an estimation of the probability of a fracture within a patient's lifetime, based on the patient's present age, current bone mineral density, probable rate of bone loss, and life expectancy (Wasnich 1993). Because the fracture projections in the RLFP model are indirectly calculated, it remains a potentially important, yet untested, method of fracture prediction in the younger population.

A third clinical application of bone density measurement is the monitoring of serial skeletal changes over time. In clinical medicine serial measurements of bone density might be used to monitor natural changes with aging, changes caused by disorders known to influence bone, or changes due to pharmacological intervention. These potential uses depend, however, both on the precision of the measurement technique and the true biological change at the target skeletal site. The precision error [coefficient of variation (CV)] of density measurement techniques is very low, typically 1%–2%. However, from a statistical perspective the bone density change must exceed 2.8 times the CV to distinguish with 95% confidence a true change in bone density from random "noise" due to measurement variability (Christiansen 1994; Gluer et al. 1995).

As noted, the expected rate of change in bone density at the particular skeletal site must also be considered. For example, if the natural density loss with aging at the femoral neck is 1% per year, and the CV measurement error at the femoral neck is 2% with a particular densitometer, nearly 6 years of observation is required to detect the 6% change with 95% confidence. Alternatively, if the change in bone density is expected to be 3% per year, as is often seen in the spine at menopause or in response to pharmacological therapy, and the measurement CV% is 1%, one can reasonably measure a serial change over 1 year. Hence for the clinical interpretation of bone density measurement results both the precision error of the measurement technique and the expected rate of change at the particular skeletal site must be known prior to determining that a serial change is likely due to a true biological change rather than measurement error.

These considerations have led to the conclusion that bone density measurements might reasonably be employed in several different clinical situations (Johnston et al. 1991):

1. In estrogen deficient women, to diagnose significantly low bone mass in order to help make decisions about hormone replacement therapy (or an alternative therapy). If treatment for osteoporosis prevention were inexpensive, universally effective, and absolutely nontoxic, screening for treatment would be unnec-

essary because everyone would be treated. In the absence of such an ideal treatment, however, it seems reasonable to use bone densitometry to identify those patients in greatest need of preventive treatment – if the test results influence treatment. For many women undecided about treatment, bone densitometry results may help to shape a decision, a "low" density leading to the start of therapy (Rubin and Cummings 1992).

2. In patients with vertebral abnormalities or radiographic osteopenia. Plain radiographs may be described as showing "osteopenia" – which may in fact be an artifact related to film technique – or various vertebral deformities which may be related to old trauma or epiphysitis. Bone density measurements may be helpful in determining the need for further evaluation.

3. In patients with disorders known to influence the risk of bone loss. To the extent that clinical decision-making is influenced, bone density measurements – both screening and follow-up – may be justifiable in patients with a variety of disorders known to influence bone. These disorders include primary hyperparathyroidism, Cushing's syndrome, chronic steroid treatment, organ transplantation, testosterone deficiency, amenorrhea, eating disorders, treatment with suppressive doses of thyroid hormone, alcoholism, disuse, treatment with multiple anticonvulsants, treatment with heparin, and renal osteodystrophy. In most of these disorders the loss of trabecular bone outstrips the loss of cortical bone, making the measurement of a site rich in trabecular bone, such as the spine, desirable. In hyperparathyroidism, however, the loss of cortical bone may exceed that of trabecular bone, making measurement of the radius and/ or hip desirable. Parathyroidectomy has been proven to lead to augmentation of bone density in asymptomatic patients with primary hyperparathyroidism (Silverberg et al. 1995). As interventions to blunt or reverse steroid-induced osteoporosis evolve (Diamond et al. 1995; Adachi et al. 1994; Mulder and Struys 1994; Ringe and Welzel 1987), guidelines will follow regarding the appropriate time to perform and repeat bone density measurements in patients receiving glucocorticoids (Eastell 1995).

4. In patients on treatment, to monitor the efficacy of such treatment. Treatment intended to prevent bone loss would ideally be shown to do so. As noted above, the precision of contemporary measurement techniques permits an assessment of treatment efficacy in individual patients. Among postmenopausal patients there appear to be relatively few "nonresponders," who continue to lose bone density despite consistent therapy with estrogen or alendronate. Nevertheless, serial bone density measurements could help provide reassurance to physician and patient alike and improve long-term compliance with therapy. This possibility, however, requires more rigorous confirmation. It is nearly impossible to treat asymptomatic patients without providing an objective measure of the effect of the often expensive medication over time. This is, again, analogous to the treatment of hypertension or hyperlipidemia. The need for "positive feedback" from serial density results may be especially important for women receiving estrogen replacement therapy because long-term compli-

ance with therapy is low (Ravnikar 1987), and age-related bone loss may overwhelm the otherwise bone-sparing effects of estrogen in some patients (Ensrud et al. 1995).

The frequency with which serial bone density measurements should be performed is still debated. In women who are "responders" to estrogen therapy – as established by two annual bone density measurements – the frequency of future testing might be reduced to every 3–5 years. This suggestion may not be appropriate for the monitoring of new non-estrogen pharmacological therapies for which the response rate in the general population is not well known. In these cases annual or every other year bone density measurements may be necessary.

Although there is some degree of unanimity in the metabolic bone community regarding the "selective" applications of bone density testing described above, considerations of the accessibility and cost of "universal bone density screening" are still under debate. There are important medicoeconomic concerns regarding the identification of large groups of individuals at risk for fragility fractures. However, for the clinician caring for an individual patient, the only certain way to diagnose low bone density is by direct bone density measurement. Risk factor analysis for the detection of low bone density or for the prediction of fragility fractures is an important tool to assist health care economists in projecting cost effectiveness and reducing unnecessary overutilization of bone testing services. However, risk factor analysis is inadequate for the identification of individual patients with low bone density (Slemenda et al. 1990). Thus the individual practitioner must select which patients should have bone density testing in the current health care environment.

Presently, unselected density bone density screening cannot be endorsed due to the high cost and limited accessibility of most bone density measurement techniques. If a clinician agrees, however, that the diagnosis of osteoporosis prior to the first fracture is important in order to reduce the risk of subsequent fragility fractures (Ross et al. 1991), and that the only objective method to diagnose low bone density is to measure bone density, then unselected bone density testing is logical (Miller and McClung 1996). The ideal age at which to perform this testing is 50 years in women and 65 years in men. This age in women is based on the fact that most postmenopausal women lose bone density unless they receive estrogen replacement therapy or other pharmacological intervention beyond calcium and vitamin D, and that 15%–20% of perimenopausal women enter the menopause with bone mineral density which is more than 1 SD below the peak adult bone density.

Age-related bone loss in men begins around the age of 65 years in groups of patients (Greenspan et al. 1994). Men are currently living longer and actually have a higher age-adjusted mortality for hip fractures (Seeman 1993); therefore measuring bone density in otherwise healthy men at the age of 65 is appropriate.

Bone density measurement in women at the menopause may be justified particularly for the identification of those perimenopausal women who enter the menopause with low bone density. The rate of bone loss after the menopause has been shown to be variable (Hui et al. 1990; Slemenda et al. 1996). Since the rate of loss as well as the ultimate bone mineral density later in life are determinants of fragility fracture risk (Riis et al. 1996; Garnero et al. 1996), the identification of those women with a high rate of loss and a low bone density may facilitate intervention decisions for the prevention of the first fracture.

Some have suggested that the first bone density measurement in white women be performed at the age of 65 years (Ettinger and Grady 1994). This recommendation is based on the assumptions that all perimenopausal women enter the menopause with a "normal" bone density, that rates of bone loss are constant, and that estrogen replacement in late postmenopausal women is followed by an increase in bone density in all patients. These are three untested assumptions.

Models of cost-effectiveness to determine the timing of the first bone density measurement yield different suggestions than models based on the practitioner's perspective. Both models are important to consider and put into proper perspective.

In summary, the clinical application of bone densitometry provides the only objective means of diagnosing low bone density in nonfractured individuals, predicting fragility fracture risk, and monitoring disease progression or longitudinal response to therapy. The measurement of bone density adds valuable information to the practice of clinical medicine. The responsible utilization of bone density measurement can enhance the diagnosis and assessment of patients with suspected or established osteoporosis.

References

Adachi JD, Cranney A, Goldsmith CH, Bensen WG, Bianchi F, Cividino A, Craig GL, Kaminska E, Sebaldt RJ, Papaioannou A, Boratto M, Gordon M, Steele M (1994) Intermittent cyclic therapy with etidronate in the prevention of corticosteroid induced bone loss. J Rheumatol 21:1922–1926

Baran DT, McCarthy CK, Leahey D, Lew R (1991) Broadband ultrasound attenuation of the calcaneus predicts lumbar and femoral neck density in Caucasian women: a preliminary study. Osteoporos Int 1:110–113

Black DM, Cummings SR, Genant HK, Nevitt MC, Palermo L, Browner W (1992) Axial and appendicular bone density predict fractures in older women. J Bone Miner Res 7:633–638

Black DM, Cummings SR, Karpf DB, Cauley JA, Thompson DE, Nevitt MC, Bauer DC, Genant HK, Haskell WL, Marcus R, Ott SM, Torner JC, Quandt SA, Reiss TF, Ensrud KE (1996) Randomised trial of effect of alendronate on risk of fracture in women with existing vertebral fractures. Lancet 348:1535–1541

Christiansen C (1994) Postmenopausal bone loss and the risk of osteoporosis. Osteoporos Int 4 [Suppl 1]:47–51

Consensus Development Conference (1993) Diagnosis, prophylaxis, and treatment of osteoporosis. Am J Med 94:646–650

Cummings SR, Black DM, Nevitt MC, Browner WS, Cauley JA, Genant HK, Mascioli SR, Scott JC, Seeley DG, Steiger P, Vogt TM, Study of Osteoporotic Fractures Research Group (1990) Appendicular bone density and age predict hip fracture in women. J Am Med Assoc 263:665–668

Cummings SR, Black DM, Nevitt MC, Browner W, Cauley J, Ensrud K, Genant HK, Palermo L, Scott J, Vogt TM (1993) Bone density at various sites for prediction of hip fractures. Lancet 341:72–75

Cummings SR, Nevitt MC, Browner WS, Stone K, Fox KM, Ensrud KE, Cauley J, Black D, Vogt TM (1995) Risk factors for hip fracture in white women. N Engl J Med 332:767–773

Davis JW, Ross PD, Wasnich RD (1994) Evidence for both generalized and regional low bone mass among elderly women. J Bone Miner Res 9:305–309

Diamond T, McGuigan L, Barbagallo S, Bryant C (1995) Cyclical etidronate plus ergocalciferol prevents glucocorticoid-induced bone loss in postmenopausal women. Am J Med 98:459–463

Eastell R (1995) Management of corticosteroid-induced osteoporosis. UK Consensus Group Meeting on Osteoporosis. J Intern Med 237:439–447

Ensrud KE, Palermo L, Black DM, Cauley J, Jergas M, Orwoll ES, Nevitt MC, Fox KM, Cummings SR (1995) Hip and calcaneal bone loss increase with advancing age: longitudinal results from the study of osteoporotic fractures. J Bone Miner Res 10:1778–1787

Ettinger B, Grady D (1994) Maximizing the benefit of estrogen therapy for prevention of osteoporosis. Menopause 1:19–24

Garnero P, Hausherr E, Chapuy MC, Marcelli C, Grandjean H, Muller C, Cormier C, Bréart G, Meunier PJ, Delmas PD (1996) Markers of bone resorption predict hip fracture in elderly women: the EPIDOS prospective study. J Bone Miner Res 11:1531–1538

Genant HK, Cann CE, Ettinger B, Gordan GS (1982) Quantitative computed tomography of vertebral spongiosa: a sensitive method for detecting early bone loss after oophorectomy. Ann Intern Med 97:699–705

Genant HK, Powell MR, Cann CE, Stebler B, Rutt BK, Richardson ML, Kolb FO (1984) Comparison of methods for in vivo spinal bone mineral measurement. In: Christiansen C, Arnaud CD, Nordin BEC, Parfitt AM, Peck WA, Riggs BL (eds) Osteoporosis: proceedings of the Copenhagen international symposium on osteoporosis, 3–8 June 1984, vol 1. Aalborg Stiftsbogtrykkeri, Denmark, pp 97–102

Genant HK, Engelke K, Fuerst T, Glher CC, Grampp S, Harris ST, Jergas M, Lang T, Lu Y, Majumdar S, Mathur A, Takada M (1996a) Noninvasive assessment of bone mineral and structure: State of the art. J Bone Miner Res 11:707–730

Genant HK, Lu Y, Mathur AK, Fuerst TP, Cummings SR (1996b) Classification based on DXA measurements for assessing the risk of hip fractures. J Bone Miner Res 11:S120 (abstract)

Gluer CC, Blake G, Lu Y, Blunt BA, Jergas M, Genant HK (1995) Accurate assessment of precision errors: how to measure the reproducibility of bone densitometry techniques. Osteoporos Int 5:262–270

Greenspan SL, Myers ER, Maitland LA, Kido TH, Krasnow MB, Hayes WC (1994) Trochanteric bone mineral density is associated with type of hip fracture in the elderly. J Bone Miner Res 9:1889–1894

Greenspan SL, Maitland-Ramsey L, Myers E (1996) Classification of osteoporosis in the elderly is dependent on site-specific analysis. Calcif Tissue Int 58:409–414

Hui SL, Slemenda CW, Johnston CC (1988) Age and bone mass as predictors of fracture in a prospective study. J Clin Invest 81:1804–1809

Hui SL, Slemenda CW, Johnston CC Jr (1989) Baseline measurement of bone mass predicts fracture in white women. Ann Intern Med 111:355–361

Hui SL, Slemenda CW, Johnston CC (1990) The contribution of bone loss to postmenopausal osteoporosis. Osteoporos Int 1:30–34

Johnston CC Jr, Slemenda CW, Melton LJ III (1991) Clinical use of bone densitometry. N Engl J Med 324:1105–1109

Kleerekoper M, Nelson DA, Flynn MJ, Pawluszka AS, Jacobsen G, Peterson EL (1994) Comparison of radiographic absorptiometry with dual-energy X-ray absorptiometry and quantitative computed tomography in normal older white and black women. J Bone Miner Res 9:1745–1749

Liberman UA, Weiss SR, Bröll J, Minne HW, Quan H, Bell NH, Rodriguez-Portales J, Downs RW, Jr, Dequeker J, Favus M, Seeman E, Recker RR, Capizzi T, Santora AC, II, Lombardi A, Shah RV, Hirsch LJ, Karpf DB (1995) Effect of oral alendronate on bone mineral density and the incidence of fractures in postmenopausal osteoporosis. N Engl J Med 333:1437–1443

Lindsay R, Hart DM, Forrest C, Baird C (1980) Prevention of spinal osteoporosis in oophorectomised women. Lancet 2:1151–1154

Looker AC, Johnston CC Jr, Wahner HW, Dunn WL, Calvo MS, Harris TB, Heyse SP, Lindsay RL (1995) Prevalence of low femoral bone density in older US women from NHANES III. J Bone Miner Res 10:796–802

Lufkin EG, Wahner HW, O'Fallon WM, Hodgson SF, Kotowicz MA, Lane AW, Judd HL, Caplan RH, Riggs BL (1992) Treatment of postmenopausal osteoporosis with transdermal estrogen. Ann Intern Med 117:1–9

Matkovic V, Kostial K, Simonovic I, Buzina R, Brodarec A, Nordin BEC (1979) Bone status and fracture rates in two regions of Yugoslavia. Am J Clin Nutr 32:540–549

Melton LJ III, Chrischilles EA, Cooper C, Lane AW, Riggs BL (1992) Perspective: how many women have osteoporosis. J Bone Miner Res 7:1005–1010

Melton LJ III, Atkinson EJ, O'Fallon WM, Wahner HW, Riggs BL (1993) Long-term fracture prediction by bone mineral assessed at different skeletal sites. J Bone Miner Res 8:1227–1233

Miller PD, Bonnick SL, Rosen C, Altman RD, Avioli LV, Dequeker J, Felsenberg D, Genant HK, Gennari C, Harper KD, Hodsman AB, Kanis JA, Kleerekoper M, Mautalen CA, McClung MR, Meunier PJ, Nelson DA, Peel NFA, Raisz LG, Recker RR, Utian WH, Wasnich RD, Watts NB (1995) Guidelines for the clinical utilization of bone mass measurement in the adult population. Calcif Tissue Int 57:251–252

Miller PD, McClung M (1996) Prediction of fracture risk. I. Bone density. Am J Med Sci 312:257–259

Mulder H, Struys A (1994) Intermittent cyclical etidronate in the prevention of corticosteroid-induced bone loss. Br J Rheumatol 33:348–350

Nordin BEC, Chatterton BE, Schultz CG, Need AG, Horowitz M (1996) Regional bone mineral density interrelationships in normal and osteoporotic postmenopausal women. J Bone Miner Res 11:849–856

Parkkari J, Kannus P, Niemi S, Pasanen M, Järvinen M, Lüthje P, Vuori I (1994) Increasing age-adjusted incidence of hip fractures in Finland: the number and incidence of fractures in 1970–1991 and prediction for the future. Calcif Tissue Int 55:342–345

Peel NFA, Johnson A, Barrington NA, Smith TWD, Eastell R (1993) Impact of anomalous vertebral segmentation on measurements of bone mineral density. J Bone Miner Res 8:719–723

Pouilles JM, Tremollieres F, Ribot C (1993) Spine and femur densitometry at the menopause: are both sites necessary in the assessment of the risk of osteoporosis. Calcif Tissue Int 52:344–347

Ravnikar VA (1987) Compliance with hormone therapy. Am J Obstet Gynecol 156:1332–1334

Riis BJ, Hansen MA, Jensen AM, Overgaard K, Christiansen C (1996) Low bone mass and fast rate of bone loss at menopause: equal risk factors for future fracture: a 15-year follow-up study. Bone 19:9–12

Ringe JD, Welzel D (1987) Salmon calcitonin in the therapy of corticoid-induced osteoporosis. Eur J Clin Pharmacol 33:35–39

Ross PD, Davis JW, Vogel JM, Wasnich RD (1990) A critical review of bone mass and the risk of fractures in osteoporosis. Calcif Tissue Int 46:149–161

Ross PD, Davis JW, Epstein RS, Wasnich RD (1991) Pre-existing fractures and bone mass predict vertebral fracture incidence in women. Ann Intern Med 114:919–923

Rubin SM, Cummings SR (1992) Results of bone densitometry affect women's decisions about taking measures to prevent fractures. Ann Intern Med 116:990–995

Seeman E (1993) Osteoporosis in men: epidemiology, pathophysiology, and treatment possibilities. Am J Med 95:22S–28S

Silverberg SJ, Gartenberg F, Jacobs TP, Shane E, Siris E, Staron RB, McMahon DJ, Bilezikian JP (1995) Increased bone mineral density after parathyroidectomy in primary hyperparathyroidism. J Clin Endocrinol Metab 80:729–734

Slemenda CW, Hui SL, Longcope C, Wellman H, Johnston CC (1990) Predictors of bone mass in perimenopausal women. A prospective study of clinical data using photon absorptiometry. Ann Intern Med 112:96–101

Slemenda C, Longcope C, Peacock M, Hui S, Johnston CC (1996) Sex steroids, bone mass, and bone loss – a prospective study of pre-, peri-, and postmenopausal women. J Clin Invest 97:14–21

Storm T, Thamsborg G, Steiniche T, Genant HK, Srensen OH (1990) Effect of intermittent cyclical etidronate therapy on bone mass and fracture rate in women with postmenopausal osteoporosis. N Engl J Med 322:1265–1271

Wasnich R (1993) Bone mass measurement: prediction of risk. Am J Med 95 [Suppl 5A]:6S–10S

Watts NB, Harris ST, Genant HK, Wasnich RD, Miller PD, Jackson RD, Licata AA, Ross P, Woodson GC, III, Yanover MJ, Mysiw WJ, Kohse L, Rao MB, Steiger P, Richmond B, Chesnut CH III (1990) Intermittent cyclical etidronate treatment of postmenopausal osteoporosis. N Engl J Med 323:73–79

25 Bone Densitometry in Children

S. Mora and V. Gilsanz

Introduction

The development of accurate, noninvasive methods for measuring bone mineral content (BMC) during the past decade has significantly improved our ability to assess changes in bone mass. Regrettably, whereas the rate of bone loss in elderly postmenopausal women has justifiably received much attention, less attention has been paid to the analysis of how much bone is gained with growth. However, it is becoming increasingly clear that the amount of bone gained during growth is an important determinant of future susceptibility to fractures, and measuring BMC in children will improve our understanding of the childhood antecedents of a condition that manifests in adulthood: osteoporosis. Moreover, bone measurements in children help to diagnose and quantify the loss of bone mineral associated with the various pediatric disorders that cause osteopenia.

Several techniques have been used for bone mass measurements for both research and clinical purposes in pediatrics. Single- and dual-photon absorptiometry have been used extensively in the past but have been superseded. Magnetic resonance imaging is a promising technique for the analysis of cancellous bone, but it is still under investigation, and its applications in pediatrics are yet to be defined. In this chapter, we describe the advantages and disadvantages of the three current modalities employed in pediatrics: the most widely used, dual-energy X-ray absorptiometry (DXA), the most versatile, quantitative computed tomography (QCT), and the newest technique, quantitative ultrasound (QUS). Comparison between these techniques, which are totally dissimilar in the way in which they acquire data, is difficult and, more often than not, judgment regarding their value has been, at least partially, subjective.

Dual-Energy X-Ray Absorptiometry

DXA has become the most commonly employed technique for the assessment of BMC worldwide [45]. Bone mineral measurements by DXA rely on the attenuation (absorption) of energy that occurs as the beam of X-ray photons scan across the region of interest. Two different energy photons are used; the low-energy photons penetrate only the soft tissue surrounding the bone, whereas the high-energy photons penetrate both the soft tissue and the bone. A detector measures the exiting photons from the region of interest and a computer subtracts the low-energy values from the high energy measurements. The attenuation values are converted into measurements of mass of mineral with the use of calibration materials, and the results are expressed as BMC. Frequently, BMC values are divided by the projected area of the bone analyzed, and the resulting measurements are conventionally referred to as an "areal" bone mineral density (BMD).

The preferred anatomic sites for DXA measurements of bone mineral include the lumbar spine, the proximal femur and the whole body, but peripheral sites such as the forearm and the hand can also be scanned. With the initial DXA devices the examination procedure took 6–15 min, but newly developed devices using enhanced generators or a fan-beam instead of a pencil-beam X-ray source have shortened the examination time to 2 min. Radiation exposure involved in DXA examinations is extremely low. The subject's effective dose has been estimated to be about 1 µSv for lumbar spine measurements [28] and about 4 µSv for whole skeleton scans (Table 25-1) [37]. In children, the precision of DXA measurements ranges from 0.8% to 2.5% in most studies [4, 8, 30, 33, 51, 53].

Several limitations of DXA must be stressed with reference to bone measurements during childhood, when major changes in body composition, body size and skeletal mass occur. DXA is a projectional technique, and its measurements are based on the two-dimensional projection of a three-dimensional structure. Thus DXA values are a function of three skeletal parameters: the size of the bone being examined, the volume of the bone, and its mineral density [6]. These values are frequently expressed as measurements of the bone content per surface area

Table 25-1 Whole-body equivalent doses in millirems for children at different ages (adapted from [5, 28, 37])

	Age (years)		
Exam	5	10	20
Chest X-ray	4.4	3.9	3.2
Lumbar spine			
Anteroposterior	2.1	2.0	1.8
Lateral	13.1	12.1	11.2
DXA			
Posteroanterior spine	0.1	0.1	0.1
Lateral spine	0.3	0.3	0.3
Proximal femur	0.1	0.1	0.1
Whole body	0.4	0.4	0.4
QCT spine			
Scout view	4.8	4.5	4.1
Axial scan	0.9	0.9	0.8
Natural background (per month)	22	18	11
Transcontinental flight	4	3	2

(gm/cm²), as determined by scan radiographs. However, scan radiographs provide only an approximation of the size of the bone, and any correction based on these radiographs is only a very rough estimate of the "density." Attempts to overcome this disadvantage with the use of correction factors, i. e., the square root of the projected area, the height of the subject, the width of the bone, assuming the cross-sectional area of the vertebrae is a square, a circle or an ellipse, or that the femur can be modeled as a cylinder, etc. [29, 33, 34, 41, 43], are subject to error, as there is no closed formula that defines the size of the vertebrae or the femur. While the inability of DXA to account for bone size is not of great concern when studying the mature skeleton, in growing children longitudinal DXA values are subject to considerable error as they reflect both the changes in skeletal size and in bone mass.

Inaccuracies in DXA values can also result from the unknown composition of the soft tissues adjacent to the bone being analyzed. Because corrections for soft tissues are based on a homogeneous distribution of fat around the bone, changes in DXA measurements are observed if fat is distributed inhomogeneously around the bone measured. It has been calculated that inhomogeneous fat distribution in soft tissues, resulting in a difference of 2 cm fat layer between soft tissue area and bone area, influences DXA measurements by 10% [25]. While this is not of concern when studying subjects whose weight and body size remain constant, longitudinal DXA values in children are subject to considerable error, and measurements may reflect the changes in body size and composition that occur with growth more than true changes in bone density. This disadvantage especially limits the use of DXA in studies of children with eating disorders, such as obesity and anorexia nervosa.

It should also be noted that the standard software from most DXA manufacturers was designed for adults. Although several manufacturers have developed special software to be used in pediatrics, this software requires longer scanning time, which makes cooperation from children difficult. Lack of cooperation results in motion and the presence of artifacts, which may alter DXA values markedly [31], and children have been restrained [8, 30], sedated [4, 35], or studied while asleep [7] to overcome these errors. Correct positioning is also of the utmost importance in studies of children. Lumbar studies may be inaccurate with even the mildest bending of the trunk, and exact positioning of the foot is required for proper assessment of the proximal femur.

Normative data for DXA values in pediatrics is available in the literature and is included in most DXA software packages. It should be noted, however, that different DXA manufacturers display substantial variation in BMD values of the same bone. Therefore, caution is advised before using published normative data for clinical use, and institutional and device-specific norms are preferable to published references. Recently, leading manufacturers of DXA equipment have proposed a standardization of BMD for measurements in the lumbar spine (Fig. 25-1) [12]. To provide similar standardization at other sites will require substantial changes in the specifications of the equipment.

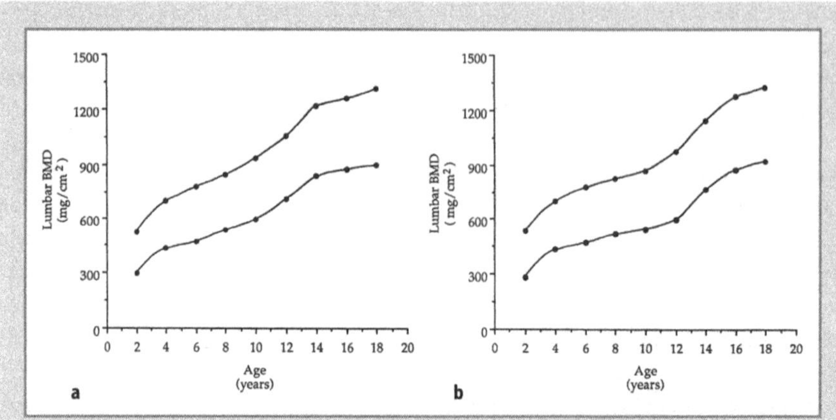

Fig. 25-1 DXA values for the lumbar spine in healthy girls **a** and boys **b** obtained with a Lunar DPX-L absorptiometer (Lunar, Madison, Wisc., USA) [8], and standardized according to the method of Genant [12]. Values represent 95% confidence limits and are expressed as mg/cm²

Bone determinations in children with DXA have been performed at all ages, including newborns [4, 35, 51] and infants [7, 30, 44]. In general, values measured at different skeletal sites increase from infancy to adulthood [3, 8, 10, 11, 22, 34, 38, 40, 43, 48, 50, 53]. The relationship between age and BMD in the lumbar spine appears to be represented by a segmented polynomial curve [8, 10, 22, 38, 52]; a rapid increase during childhood is followed by an even greater increase during puberty that ends in the third decade of life [3, 8, 22, 29, 33, 38, 43, 49, 52]. Similar relationships may be seen in the femoral neck [3, 10, 38, 52] and the entire skeleton [10, 11, 38, 52]. However, radial DXA values in children have not been found to be influenced by puberty [52].

The majority of the studies on gender differences, using DXA, indicate that by the age of 12 or 13 years girls have greater BMD than boys in the lumbar spine [3, 8, 22, 34, 40]. Most [3, 10, 34, 52], but not all [38, 41], of the studies in the femoral neck have found greater BMD in boys than in girls 14–16 years of age. Measurements in the radius have yielded discrepant results; one study found no gender differences [52], while boys had greater values than girls in another study [40].

Studies examining racial differences in bone mass in children have also yielded conflicting results. While some investigators have found no differences in bone measurements between African-American and white girls [43, 48], others report higher values for African-American girls at all ages [1]. A recent study found that Asian-American children have lower spine, femur, and whole body DXA values than white children and suggested the difference to be size related [2].

In summary, the relatively low cost, availability, and ease of use are the main advantages of DXA. While this technique is unable to measure cancellous and cortical bone independently, it does provide an accurate and precise quantitation of bone mass in the mature skeleton. Unfortunately, the inability of DXA to account for the large changes in body and skeletal size that occur during growth limits its use in longitudinal studies in children.

Quantitative Computed Tomography

QCT bone measurements can be obtained at any skeletal site with a standard clinical CT scanner using an external bone mineral reference phantom for calibration and specially developed software. The ability of QCT to assess both the volume and the density of bone in the axial and appendicular skeletons, without influence from body or skeletal size, is the major advantage of this modality when used in children. Unfortunately, CT scanners are expensive, large, nonportable machines that require costly maintenance and considerable technological expertise for proper function. Moreover, this equipment is usually located in the radiology department and is under constant clinical demand, creating a lack of accessibility. These disadvantages have partially been overcome by the recent development of smaller, mobile, less expensive peripheral QCT scanners designed exclusively for bone measurements. These scanners, however, can assess only the bones of the appendicular skeleton.

The radiation exposure from QCT measurements is related to the technique employed and can be as low as 150 mrem (1.5 mSv) localized to the region of interest in the appendicular or axial skeleton. The total-body equivalent dose of radiation is approximately 4–9 mrem (40–90 μSv), and this figure includes the radiation associated with screening digital radiographs used to localize the site of measurement [5, 28]. This amount of radiation is far lower than that associated with other CT imaging procedures, accounting for the wide range of published figures for the radiation dose associated with CT measurements. It is also less than many other commonly used radiographic diagnostic tests. By comparison, a round-trip transcontinental flight in North America exposes a child to roughly 6–8 mrems (60–80 μSv) of ionizing radiation (Table 25-1) [5, 28]. Therefore bone measurement determinations using QCT, as those using DXA, do not expose children to amounts of ionizing radiation that deviate from the amount that constitutes part of their normal life experience.

In the axial skeleton QCT has principally been employed to determine cancellous bone density (mg/cm^3) in the vertebral bodies and, less frequently, the dimensions of the vertebrae. It should be noted that because the vertebrae of children contains proportionally more bone and less fat than those of elderly subjects, both the precision and accuracy of QCT cancellous bone density determinations in children are far better than that reported for adults. Coefficients of variation for determinations of cancellous bone density, vertebral body height, and vertebral cross-sectional area have been calculated as 1.5%, 1.3%, and 0.8%, respectively [15, 17].

Differences in morphology of cancellous and cortical bone must be considered for the appropriate understanding of QCT measurements of these two compartments. Cancellous bone exists as a three dimensional lattice of plates and columns (trabeculae). The trabeculae divide interior volume of the bone into inter-communicating pores, which are filled with a variable mixture of red and yellow marrow [9]. Because of the relatively small size of the trabeculae when compared to the pixel, the CT unit of measurement, QCT values for cancellous bone density reflect not only the amount of mineralized bone and osteoid but also the amount of marrow per pixel [13]. Similar limitations apply to in vitro determinations of the volumetric density of trabecular bone which are obtained by washing the marrow from the pores of a specimen of cancellous bone, weighing it, and dividing the weight by the volume of the specimen, including the pores [9]. Both QCT and in vitro bone density determinations of cancellous bone are therefore directly proportional to the bone volume fraction and inversely proportional to the porosity of the bone. The relatively large coefficient of variation for values of cancellous bone density reflect the considerable variations in the dimensions of the pores throughout the vertebral body.

In the appendicular skeleton three bone parameters can be measured by QCT, the cross-sectional area (cm^2) of the bone, the cortical bone area (cm^2), and the cortical bone density [26, 32]. To this effect, the outer and inner boundaries of the cortex are identified by specially developed software at the place of the maximum slope of the profile through the bone. The area within the outer cortical shell represents the cross-sectional area, while the area between the outer and inner shells represents the cortical bone area. The mean CT numbers of the pixels within the inner and outer cortical shells provide the average density of the bone. The coefficients of variation for repeated QCT measurements of cortical bone density, cortical bone area, and cross-sectional area of the femur range between 0.6% and 1.5% [20].

In children, the material density of cortical bone (the amount of collagen and mineral in a given volume of bone), when measured by QCT, remains fairly constant, 1180 ± 50 g/cm^3 (Fig. 25-2) [26]. Because of the relative lack of porosity in cortical bone, QCT measurements of its density circumvent volume-averaging errors and reflect the material density of the bone if the cortex is thicker than 2–2.5 mm [26]. Above this thickness the measured pixel represents the combination of the attenuation coefficients defined by the densities and concentrations of osteoid and mineral. While the nonmineral fraction may contribute to minor fluctuations in measurements of cortical bone density, QCT numbers are based primarily on the calcified bone fraction, which has a high attenuation coefficient [26]. These measurements are analogous to in vitro determinations of the intrinsic mineral density of bone, which are commonly expressed as the ash weight per unit volume of bone [24].

Studies in healthy children using QCT have shown that events during puberty are the major determinants of the increases in cancellous bone density during growth [39], and that the density of cancellous bone reaches its peak around the time of cessation of longitudinal growth and epiphyseal closure [18, 26]. QCT studies have also found a greater increase in vertebral cancellous bone density in African-American girls than in white girls during the later stages of puberty

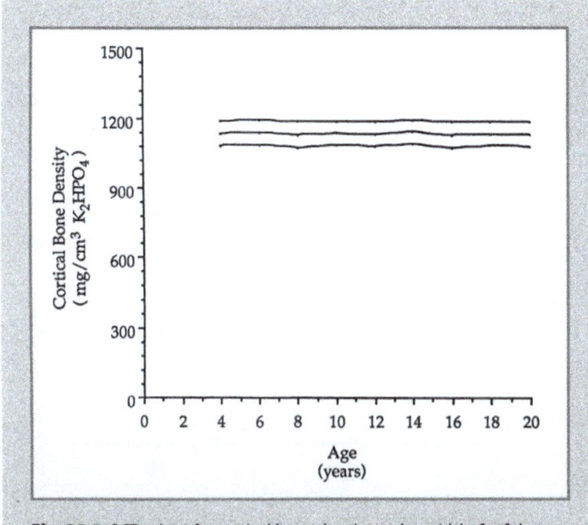

Fig. 25-2 QCT values for cortical bone density at the midshaft of the femur in healthy children. Values represent the mean±1 SD [26]

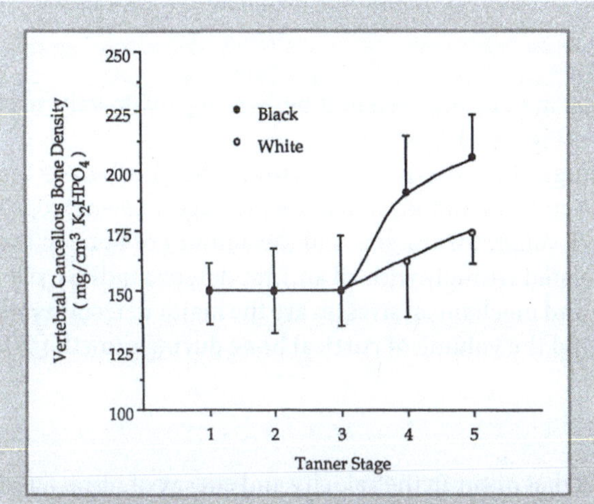

Fig. 25-3 values for cancellous vertebral bone density in healthy white and African-American children in relation to Tanner stage of sexual development. Values represent the mean±1 SD and are valid for both boys and girls [19, 21]

(Fig. 25-3) [19, 21]. Other studies have analyzed the influence of gender on the amount of bone that is gained during childhood and adolescence [16, 17]. QCT has helped establish that the lower vertebral bone mass of females when compared to males results from early gender differences in the size of the bones rather than differences in cancellous bone density. Even after accounting for differences in

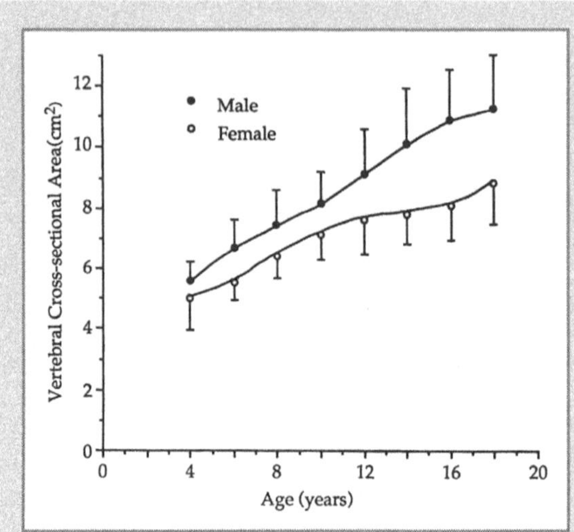

Fig. 25-4 QCT values for cross-sectional area of the midportion of the vertebral body in healthy white boys and girls in relation to age. Values represent the mean±1 SD [17, 20]

body size, the cross-sectional area of the vertebral body is approximately 20% smaller in girls than in boys (Fig. 25-4) [17].

In contrast to these findings, the cross-sectional area at the midshaft of the femur does not differ between boys and girls matched for age and anthropometric parameters [20]. QCT values for the size and the amount of bone in the appendicular skeleton correlated strongly with all anthropometric indices, suggesting that weight bearing and mechanical stresses are the major determinants of the increases in the size and the volume of cortical bone during growth [39].

Ultrasound

Measurement of the changes that occur in the velocity and energy of ultrasound waves as they pass through bone are the basis of QUS. Ultrasound equipment consists of two transducers, a transmitter, and a receiver that are placed on opposite sides of the bone of interest, most commonly the calcaneus, patella, tibia, and phalanges. The ultrasound transmission velocity (UTV) is obtained by dividing the width of the region of interest by the transit time and is expressed in meters per second. The loss of acoustic energy that occurs when the ultrasound wave is absorbed or scattered by the medium through which it is being propagated results in a reduction in the amplitude of the wave and is referred to as broadband ultrasound attenuation (BUA). BUA is defined as the slope of attenuation versus the frequency in the range of 200–600 kHz and is expressed in decibels per megahertz.

Ultrasound measurements are influenced by the number, thickness, and mineral content of the trabeculae, as well as by their three-dimensional arrangement. BUA values are known to vary as much as 50% depending upon the principle orientation of the trabeculae [13]. Moreover, both UTV and BUA values are also influenced by soft tissues in the path of the ultrasound waves and the amount and composition of marrow in the bone [13]. In adults, the poor precision of ultrasound has limited its usefulness for longitudinal monitoring of disease progression or response to treatment [14]. However, because ultrasound is able to predict fracture risk in adults with osteoporosis independently of bone mass determinations, QUS measurements must be related to some aspects of bone strength [23]. Nevertheless, numerous studies comparing QUS with other bone measurement techniques have failed to find a strong correlation, and therefore ultrasound should not be used as a substitute for other modalities [13].

Several technical issues need to be addressed when applying QUS to the study of children. It should be stressed that all commercially available ultrasound equipment for bone measurements are designed for adults and use relatively large transducers. Smaller transducers are required when studying children to allow closer contact with the region of interest to be scanned without interference from air. On average the diameter of the specially designed transducers for pediatric studies has been 1 cm [27,36,42,46]. As in adults, ultrasound studies in children require a coupling medium (a water bath or gel) between the transducers and the skin overlying the bone. The temperature of the coupling medium must be maintained constant to avoid inaccuracies in the velocity and attenuation of ultrasound measurements. Moreover, when examining children, specially developed foot pads or calipers for small feet are needed to maintain the correct position of the transducer near the bone to be scanned.

In children, UTV values have been obtained at the calcaneus, patella, and phalanges of the thumb, whereas BUA is determined mainly in the calcaneus, although no device has been used to measure more than one skeletal site [27, 36, 42, 46]. UTV and BUA values in children have been found to increase with age, but they exhibit considerable variability [27, 46]. The influence of puberty on ultrasound indices has been investigated with the findings that UTV values increase substantially between the second and third Tanner stages of sexual development in girls, while the increase is constant throughout all stages of puberty in boys [42]. Recent studies in children have reported intra-observer coefficients of variation for UTV of 0.64% for the calcaneus, 1.2% for the patella, and 0.5% for the thumb [27, 36, 46] while those for BUA range from 2.9% to 5% for the calcaneus [27, 42].

The attractiveness of QUS for bone measurements in children lies in its low cost, portability, ease of use, and lack of ionizing radiation. Unfortunately, ultrasound values depend on so many structural parameters which are not yet fully understood that it is difficult to use this information in a meaningful way in children. These measurements seem to be correlated more with bone size than with changes in the amount, density, or geometry of bone [47]. Therefore increases in BUA measurements during childhood and adolescence may be related to changes in skeletal size associated with growth.

References

1. Bell NH, Shary J, Stevens J, Garza M, Gordon L, Edwards J (1991) Demonstration that bone mass is greater in black than in white children. J Bone Miner Res 6:719–723
2. Bhudhikanok GS, Wang M-C, Eckert K, Matkin C, Marcus R, Bachrach LK (1996) Differences in bone mineral in young Asian and Caucasian Americans may reflect differences in bone size. J Bone Miner Res 11:1545–1556
3. Bonjour J-P, Theintz G, Buchs B, Slosman D, Rizzoli R (1991) Critical years and stages of puberty for spinal and femoral bone mass accumulation during adolescence. J Clin Endocrinol Metab 73:555–563
4. Braillon PM, Salle BL, Brunet J, Glorieux FH, Delmas PD, Meunier PJ (1992) Dual energy X-ray absorptiometry measurement of bone mineral content in newborns: validation of the technique. Pediatr Res 32:77–80
5. Cann CE (1991) Why, when and how to measure bone mass: a guide for the beginning user. In: Frey GD, Yester MV (eds) Expanding the role of medical physics in nuclear medicine. American Physics Institute Washington DC, pp 250–279
6. Carter DR, Bouxsein ML, Marcus R (1992) New approaches for interpreting projected bone densitometry data. J Bone Miner Res 7:137–145
7. Chan GM (1992) Performance of dual-energy X-ray absorptiometry in evaluating bone, lean body mass, and fat in pediatric subjects. J Bone Miner Res 7:369–374
8. del Rio L, Carrascosa A, Pons F, Gusinyé M, Yeste D, Domenech FM (1994) Bone mineral density of the lumbar spine in white Mediterranean Spanish children and adolescents: changes related to age, sex, and puberty. Pediatr Res 35:362–366
9. Dyson ED, Jackson CK, Whitehouse WJ (1970) Scanning electron microscope studies of human trabecular bone. Nature 225:957–959
10. Faulkner RA, Bailey DA, Drinkwater DT, McKay HA, Arnold C, Wilkinson AA (1996) Bone densitometry in Canadian children 8–17 years of age. Calcif Tissue Int 59:344–351
11. Faulkner RA, Bailey DA, Drinkwater DT, Wilkinson AA, Houston CS, McKay HA (1993) Regional and total body bone mineral content, bone mineral density, and total body tissue composition in children 8–16 years of age. Calcif Tissue Int 53:7–12
12. Genant HK (1995) Letter to the editor: universal standardization for dual X-ray absorptiometry: patient and phantom cross-calibration results. J Bone Miner Res 10:997–998
13. Genant HK, Engelke K, Fuerst T, Glüer CC, Grampp S, Harris ST, Jergas M, Lang T, Lu Y, Majumdar S, Mathur A, Takada M (1996) Noninvasive assess-

ment of bone mineral and structure: state of the art. J Bone Miner Res 11:707– 730

14. Genant HK, Faulkner KG, Fuerst T, Glüer CC (1996) Controversies in the diagnosis of osteoporosis. Radiology 201:28

15. Gilsanz V (1988) Quantitative computed tomography. In: Siegel M (ed) Pediatric body CT. Churchill Livingstone New York, pp 349–369

16. Gilsanz V, Boechat MI, Gilsanz R, Loro ML, Roe TF, Goodman WG (1994) Gender differences in vertebral sizes in adults: biomechanical implications. Radiology 190:678–682

17. Gilsanz V, Boechat MI, Roe TF, Loro ML, Sayre JW, Goodman WG (1994) Gender differences in vertebral body sizes in children and adolescents. Radiology 190:673–677

18. Gilsanz V, Gibbens DT, Carlson M, Boechat MI, Cann CE, Schulz EE (1988) Peak trabecular vertebral density: a comparison of adolescent and adult females. Calcif Tissue Int 43:260–262

19. Gilsanz V, Gibbens DT, Roe TF, Carlson M, Senac MO, Boechat MI, Huang HK, Schulz EE, Libanati CR, Cann CC (1988) Vertebral bone density in children: effect of puberty. Radiology 166:847–850

20. Gilsanz V, Kovanlikaya A, Costin G, Roe TF, Sayre J, Kaufman F (1997) Differential effect of gender on the size of the bones in the axial and appendicular skeletons. J Clin Endocrinol Metab 82:1603–1607

21. Gilsanz V, Roe TF, Mora S, Costin G, Goodman WG (1991) Changes in vertebral bone density in black girls and white girls during childhood and puberty. N Engl J Med 325:1597–1600

22. Glastre C, Braillon P, David L, Cochat P, Meunier PJ, Delmas PD (1990) Measurement of bone mineral content of the lumbar spine by dual energy X-ray absorptiometry in normal children: correlations with growth parameters. J Clin Endocrinol Metab 70:1330–1333

23. Glüer CC, Cummings SR, Bauer DC, Stone K, Pressman A, Mathur A, Genant HK (1996) Osteoporosis: association of recent fractures with quantitative US findings. Radiology 199:725–732

24. Gong JK, Arnold JS, Cohn SH (1964) Composition of trabecular and cortical bone. Anat Rec 149:325–331

25. Hangartner T (1990) Influence of fat on bone measurements with dual-energy absorptiometry. Bone Miner 9:71–78

26. Hangartner T, Gilsanz V (1996) Evaluation of cortical bone by computed tomography. J Bone Miner Res 11:1518–1525

27. Jaworski M, Lebiedowski M, Lorenc RS, Trempe J (1995) Ultrasound bone measurement in pediatric subjects. Calcif Tissue Int 56:368–371

28. Kalender WA (1992) Effective dose values in bone mineral measurements by photon absorptiometry and computed tomography. Osteoporosis Int 2:82–87

29. Katzman DK, Bachrach LK, Carter DR, Marcus R (1991) Clinical and anthropometric correlates of bone mineral acquisition in healthy adolescent girls. J Clin Endocrinol Metab 73:1332–1339
30. Koo WW, Walters J, Bush AJ (1995) Technical considerations of dual-energy X-ray absorptiometry-based bone mineral measurements for pediatric subjects. J Bone Miner Res 10:1998–2004
31. Koo WW, Massom LR, Walters J (1995) Validation of accuracy and precision of dual energy X-ray absorptiometry for infants. J Bone Miner Res 10:1111–1115
32. Kovanlikaya A, Loro ML, Hangartner TN, Reynolds RA, Roe TF, Gilsanz V (1996) Osteopenia in children: CT assessment. Radiology 198:781–784
33. Kroger H, Kotaniemi A, Kroger L, Alhava E (1993) Development of bone mass and bone density of the spine and femoral neck – a prospective study of 65 children and adolescents. Bone Miner 23:171–182
34. Kroger H, Kotaniemi A, Vainio P, Alhava E (1992) Bone densitometry of the spine and femur in children by dual-energy X-ray absorptiometry. Bone Miner 17:75–85
35. Lapillonne AA, Glorieux FH, Salle BL, Braillon PM, Chambon M, Rigo J, Putet G, Senterre J (1994) Mineral balance and whole body bone mineral content in very low-birth- weight infants. Acta Paediatr [Suppl] 405:117–122
36. Lappe JM, Recker RR, Malleck MK, Stegmane MR, Packard PP, Heaney RP (1995) Patellar ultrasound transmission velocity in healthy children and adolescents. Bone 16:251S–256S
37. Lewis MK, Blake GM, Fogelman I (1994) Patient dose in dual X-ray absorptiometry. Osteoporosis Int 4:11–15
38. Lu PW, Briody JN, Ogle GD, Morley K, Humphries IRJ, Allen J, Howman-Giles R, Sillence D, Cowell CT (1994) Bone mineral density of total body, spine, and femoral neck in children and young adults: a cross-sectional and longitudinal study. J Bone Miner Res 9:1451–1458
39. Mora S, Goodman WG, Loro ML, Roe TF, Sayre J, Gilsanz V (1994) Age-related changes in cortical and cancellous vertebral bone density in girls: assessment with quantitative CT. Am J Roentgenol 162:405–409
40. Moreira-Andrés MN, Cañizo FJ, Papapietro K, Rejas J, Hawkins FG (1995) Comparison between spinal and radial bone mineral density in children measured by X-ray absorptiometry. J Pediatr Endocrinol Metab 8:35–41
41. Moro M, van der Meulen MCH, Kiratli BJ, Marcus R, Bachrach LK, Carter DR (1996) Body mass is the primary determinant of midfemoral bone acquisition during adolescent growth. Bone 19:519–526
42. Mughal MZ, Langton CM, Utretch G, Morrison J, Specker BL (1996) Comparison between broad-band ultrasound attenuation of the calcaneum and total body bone mineral density in children. Acta Paediatr 85:663–665
43. Plotkin H, Núñez M, Alvarez Filgueira ML, Zanchetta JR (1996) Lumbar spine bone density in Argentine children. Calcif Tissue Int 58:144–149
44. Rupich RC, Specker BL, Lieuw-A-Fa M, Ho M (1996) Gender and race differences in bone mass during infancy. Calcif Tissue Int 58:395–397

45. Sartoris DJ, Resnick D (1989) Dual-energy radiographic absorptiometry for bone densitometry: current status and perspective. Am J Roentgenol 152:241– 246
46. Schonau E, Radermacher A, Wentzlik U, Klein K, Michalk D (1994) The determination of ultrasound velocity in the os calcis, thumb and patella during childhood. Eur J Pediatr 153:252–256
47. Serpe L, Rho J (1996) Broadband ultrasound attenuation value dependence on bone width in vitro. Phys Med Biol 41:197–202
48. Southard RN, Morris JD, Mahan JD, Hayes JR, Torch MA, Sommer A, Zipf WB (1991) Bone mass in healthy children: measurement with quantitative DXA. Radiology 179:735–738
49. Theintz G, Buchs B, Rizzoli R, Slosman D, Clavien H, Sizonenko PC, Bonjour JP (1992) Longitudinal monitoring of bone mass accumulation in healthy adolescents: evidence for a marked reduction after 16 years of age at the levels of lumbar spine and femoral neck in female subjects. J Clin Endocrinol Metab 75:1060–1065
50. Tsukahara H, Sudo M, Umezaki M, Hiraoka M, Yamamoto K, Ishii Y, Haruki S (1992) Dual-energy X-ray absorptiometry in the lumbar spine, proximal femur and distal radius in children. Pediatr Radiol 22:560–562
51. Venkataraman P, Ahluwalia BW (1992) Total bone mineral content and body composition by X-ray densitometry in newborns. Pediatrics 90:767–770
52. Zanchetta JR, Plotkin H, Alvarez Filgueira ML (1995) Bone mass in children: normative values for the 2–20-year-old population. Bone 16:393S–399S

26 Bone Mass and Bone Loss in Secondary Osteoporosis

R. Nuti, G. Martini, and C. Gennari

Introduction

The term secondary osteoporosis is generally used when bone loss is induced by specific and well-defined conditions. These conditions include the following:
- Drug-related
    - Glucocorticoids
    - Heparin
    - Oral anticoagulants
    - Thyroid hormone
    - Methotrexate
    - Lithium
    - Gonadotrophin-releasing analogs
    - Anticonvulsants (?)
- Endocrine disorders
    - Hyperthyroidism
    - Hypercorticolism
    - Diabetes mellitus
    - Hypogonadism
    - Hyperparathyroidism
- Gastrointestinal disorders
    - Gastrectomy
    - Inflammatory bowel disease
    - Malabsorption syndrome
- Marrow disorders
    - Leukemia
    - Lymphomas
    - Systemic mastocytosis
    - Plasma cell dyscrasia
    - Anemias
- Connective tissue disorders
    - Osteogenesis imperfecta
    - Ehlers-Danlos syndrome
    - Marfan syndrome
    - Rheumatoid arthritis

- Miscellaneous
  - Immobilization
  - Alcohol abuse
  - Anorexia nervosa
  - Pregnancy, lactation
  - Chronic neurological disease
  - Hyperphosphatasia
  - Malignancy
  - Cadmium poisoning

According to the statement provided by two consensus conferences, osteoporosis may be defined as a disease characterized by low bone mass and microarchitectural deterioration of bone tissue, leading to enhanced bone fragility and a consequent increase in fracture risk [1, 2]. From a practical point of view, diagnostic criteria for osteoporosis for clinical use include the presence of fractures (spine, distal forearm, hip) or a value for bone mineral density (BMD) or bone mineral content (BMC) that is more than 2.5 SD below the young adult mean value [3]. Certainly not all disorders listed above are able to give rise to a condition of osteoporosis but may cause only osteopenia or low bone mass, with BMD or BMC 1–2.5 SD below the young adult mean value [3]. In this chapter we describe the features of bone loss of the most common types of secondary osteoporosis.

Glucocorticoids

The association between glucocorticoid excess and osteoporosis was first described by Cushing in a patient with adrenal hyperfunction secondary to pituitary adenoma [4]. Very shortly after the introduction of cortisone as a therapeutic agent it appeared that patients receiving prolonged glucocorticoid therapy develop significant bone loss and atraumatic vertebral fractures [5]. Exogenous hypercortisolism is undoubtedly an important risk factor for secondary osteoporosis in the community, and glucocorticoid-induced osteoporosis is probably the most common type of secondary osteoporosis. The main clinical manifestations of steroid-induced osteoporosis are bone pain, pathological fractures in the axial and appendicular skeleton, and skeletal deformities [6]. Glucocorticoids have a number of effects on calcium metabolism and bone cell function. Histological and histomorphometric studies of bone from patients exposed to long-term glucocorticoid therapy have demonstrated decreased bone formation and increased bone resorption [7, 8], both contributing to a progressive decrease in trabecular bone volume [9, 10]. Glucocorticoid receptors have been identified both in osteoblast like bone cells and in cells of the osteoclast series [11].

The decrease in the rate of bone formation has been attributed to direct inhibitory effects of steroids on osteoblast function [12]. An indirect decrease in bone formation is also caused by a decrease in gonadal steroid secretion [13, 14]. The increase in bone resorption was documented by increased bone resorption surfaces, a trend toward increased osteoclast number, and increased eroded surfaces [7]; this was confirmed by studies using radiotracer kinetics [15]. It has been proposed that these changes in bone turnover result in large part from secondary hyperparathyroidism [16]; however, the role of parathyroid hormone has been recently challenged [17]. Corticosteroids may also influence the production and action of many cytokines and growth factors [18]. It is accepted that glucocorticoids decrease intestinal calcium absorption [14, 19, 20]. The mechanisms responsible for glucocorticoid-induced inhibition of the active transport of calcium in the duodenum include decreased synthesis of calcium-binding protein, vitamin D deficiency, and accelerated breakdown of $1,25(OH)_2D$ at the mucosal receptor site [13].

There is some evidence that there is also decreased tubular reabsorption of calcium and phosphorus [13, 15, 21]. It has generally been considered that bone loss due to glucocorticoid excess is diffuse, affecting both the appendicular and axial skeleton. However, the adverse effects appear to be more severe in regions of the skeleton with a higher proportion of trabecular bone [22]. In fact, marked bone loss was found at lumbar spine site and to a lesser extent at the distal radius [23]. Moreover, a significantly reduced distal radius BMD was observed in steroid-treated asthmatics, but no reduction at the proximal radius site [24]. In patients on long-term prednisone treatment the bone decay rate was 5.3%/year for the forearm, and 12.5%/year for the lumbar spine [22]. Sequential measurements of lumbar spine BMD carried out in women with bronchial asthma treated for 3–4 years with prednisone (15 mg daily) demonstrated that the highest rate of glucocorticoid-induced bone loss occurs during the first year of treatment, with a plateau in bone loss during the second year of treatment [26]. These data have been subsequently confirmed in a study in which bone loss from the lumbar spine was significantly less in patients receiving chronic corticosteroid therapy than in those followed from the start of corticosteroid therapy, suggesting that steroid-induced osteoporosis is characterized by rapid early bone loss [27].

Evidence has recently been reported that the bone loss seems to be partially reversible after discontinuation of steroid treatment [28]. As regards the effects of steroids on the hip, while earlier studies indicated that bone loss was greater in the lumbar spine than in the femur [29, 30], more recent results of a cross-sectional study demonstrated that there is no significant difference between the proximal femur and lumbar spine BMD in patients on long-term corticosteroid treatment [27]. However, a differential effect of steroids on cortical bone has been reported; the anterior cortical rim of the vertebral body was found to be more susceptible to the effects of glucocorticoids than the cortical bone in the forearm [31]. On the other hand, by measuring vertebral BMD using a lateral spine densitometry it has been stressed that the degree of osteopenia estimated by DXA in the anteroposterior projection is substantially less than that found when the vertebral body alone is assessed [32].

The extent to which corticosteroid-induced bone-loss is dose related is controversial. Some studies report that the degree of bone loss is dose dependent [33–35] although others failed to find a relationship between bone loss and corticosteroid dose [27]. In any case the nature of the underlying disease for which the patients received corticosteroids may also influence BMD. The exact threshold required for glucocorticoid dose to avoid detrimental effects on bone has not been established. Results of cross-sectional studies suggest that bone loss with corticosteroids is more likely with doses above 10 mg prednisone per day [30,36,37]. More recently in a study population of elderly Japanese-Americans 5 mg/day prednisone promoted bone loss rates at the calcaneus, distal radius, and proximal radius among women, approximately double than those of the controls, and bone loss rates among males during glucocorticoid use were two to three times that of controls for the calcaneus and radius sites [38]. High-dose inhaled corticosteroids for treatment of respiratory disease may have similar effects on bone density and bone turnover as orally administered corticosteroids [36].

The earliest attempts to establish the rate of glucocorticoid-induced fractures reported an incidence of approximately 3%–15% of vertebral crush fractures [40]. A population-based study of limb fractures reported that the relative risk of the hip, distal forearm, and proximal humerus fractures was twice as high in a group of patients with rheumatoid arthritis treated with steroids as in patients with rheumatoid arthritis alone [41]. Subsequent data confirmed that corticosteroid users are characterized by a twofold risk for hip fractures [42]. On the other hand, the prevalence of vertebral fractures was reported to be four-to fivefold increased in patients with rheumatoid arthritis treated with corticosteroids [43].

Heparin

Osteoporosis is considered one of the potentially serious side effects of heparin therapy. A number of studies during the past 10 years indicated that long-term heparin administration can cause osteoporosis in both laboratory animals and humans [44–46].

The occurrence of heparin-induced osteoporosis appeared to be strictly related to the length of treatment (over 4–5 months) and to the dose (15 000 U or more daily) [47,48]. Low BMD values were found rarely with short-term low-dose therapy [49]. It has been suggested that low molecular weight heparins (LMWH) have a lower potential to cause osteoporosis than the unfractionated preparations (UFH) or high molecular weight heparin (HMWH) [50,51]. In rabbits a reduction in cortical and trabecular BMD and a significant increase in femoral fragility were seen with UFH and HMWH but not with LMWH [52]. However, a recent case report demonstrated development of osteoporosis and pathological fracture of lumbar vertebrae following treatment with low-dose LMWH for 3 months [53].

During pregnancy heparin is the anticoagulant of choice in patients requiring thromboembolic prophylaxis. Fewer than 15 cases of heparin-induced fractures have been reported in the literature, and the majority of the patients were exposed to a minimum daily dose of 15 000 U for more than 3 months [54,55]. A recent series of 184 women receiving heparin prophylaxis found symptomatic vertebral fractures in only 2.2% [56]. Significant reductions in the metacarpal and phalangeal cortical areas were observed after long-term therapy (>25 weeks) in pregnant patients receiving 20 000 U daily, and cortical bone deficits were found to be persistent after 24 weeks after stopping the drug [57]. On the other hand, in a single pregnant woman who had received heparin for 7 months histomorphometric findings of elevated prevalence of osteoid surfaces were explained as an index of reversibility of osteoporotic bone loss [58]. In a prospective controlled study including 14 pregnant women the mean heparin dose was 12 000–21 000 U/day in one group and 23 000–50 000 U/day in the other one: 36% of patients had a 10% decrease from the baseline proximal femur BMD to immediate postpartum value, and no dose-response relationship was observed [59].

The pathogenesis of heparin-induced osteoporosis is poorly understood. Several mechanisms have been proposed. It has been suggested that heparin could causes an increase in bone resorption by increasing the number of differentiated osteoclasts and by enhancing the activity of individual osteoclasts [60]. The stimulatory effect of heparin on bone resorption was also related to its ability to bind and potentiate an osteoclast resorption-stimulating factor present in serum [61]. In vitro it was shown to have an inhibitory effect on DNA and collagen synthesis in rat calvarial cultures, suggesting decreased bone formation [62]. A secondary hyperparathyroidism evoked by the calcium binding properties of heparin has been also hypothesized [63]. From the observation that mast cell prevalence was higher in the bone marrow of osteoporotic patients than in control specimens it was speculated that heparin, a major secretory product of mast cells, plays a role in the pathogenesis of primary osteoporosis [64]. On the other hand, systemic mastocytosis, an abnormal proliferation of mast cells, may result in generalized osteoporosis [65, 66]. In osteoporotic patients with systemic mastocytosis a high-turnover state and an imbalance of remodeling activity were reported [67, 68].

Hyperthyroidism

It has been well documented that hyperthyroidism is associated with loss of trabecular and cortical bone [69, 70]. The enhanced bone turnover that develops in thyrotoxicosis is characterized by an increased number of osteoclasts and resorption sites and an increased ratio of resorptive to formative bone surfaces, with the net result of bone loss [71, 72]. Triiodothyronine and tetraiodothyronine were observed to stimulate directly bone resorption in vitro at concentrations approaching those that occurr in thyrotoxicosis [73]. Also, osteoblastic activity was demonstrated to be enhanced in hyperthyroid patients by elevated serum osteocalcin concentrations [74]. From a metabolic point of view, the increase in bone resorption has been considered in hyperthyroidism to be responsible for increased serum calcium, decreased serum parathyroid hormone and calcitriol, and decreased intestinal calcium absorption [75–77]. On the other hand, the defect of intestinal calcium transport was found to be reversible when thyroid function became normal after therapy [78].

Early absorptiometric studies of the appendicular skeleton of patients with hyperthyroidism have shown only marginal decrease in BMD [79]. In a group of 96 untreated hyperthyroid patients a significant decrease in forearm BMD was observed only in women, with no correlation between BMD and duration and severity of the disease [80]. Measuring lumbar spine BMD by dual-photon absorptiometry in patients with diffuse toxic goiter spinal bone loss was found to be more marked: the explanation for this apparent discrepancy is that the excess of thyroid hormone causes greater bone loss from the axial than from the appendicular skeleton [23]. In a relatively small group of thyrotoxic patients median BMD values for the lumbar spine were 12.6% lower with respect to a age-matched control group [81]. Despite these findings the occurrence of pathological fractures in patients with hyperthyroidism is relatively low [82, 83]. It is probably due to the fact that deficiences in bone mass may be reversed by treatment of thyroid disease [80, 81]. Indeed there have been some reports that indicated increased BMD values after correction of hyperthyroidism [79, 80]. On the other hand, midradius BMD values of patients with Graves' disease, which were 17% lower than those of a control group prior to treatment, were not modified by 2 years of successful therapy of the thyrotoxicosis [84]. More recently a 5-year study and a prospective follow-up trial over 2 years reported that successful treatment of hyperthyroidism produced a significant increase in the lumbar and in the distal forearm BMD [85, 86].

Several recent reports have generated considerable concern regarding the potential adverse effects of even mildly excessive doses of L-thyroxine (L-T_4) therapy on skeletal integrity. A 9% reduction in forearm BMD was demonstrated in women who had taken L-T_4 for 10 years or longer [87]. Premenopausal, clinically euthyroid women receiving L-T_4 therapy for a minimum of 5 years were found to have a 12.8% lower BMD at the femoral neck and 10.1% lower BMD at the femoral trochanter than matched controls; in contrast, lumbar spine BMD was similar in the two groups [88]. Similar results were achieved in premenopausal women with Hashimoto's thyroiditis receiving long-term physiological doses of L-T_4. These patients were characterized by BMD values at the femoral areas, both arms, and pelvis significantly lower than those of control healthy women, while total body and lumbar spine BMD levels were similar in the two groups [89].

A significant but clinically minimal decrement in spinal and hip BMD was demonstrated in both premenopausal and postmenopausal women receiving for 12–15 years L-T_4 that maintained the fT_4I in the physiological range, and the data suggest that the changes in BMD on long-term L-T_4 therapy are at most minimal and should not be a contraindication to therapy [90]. Indeed, in recent years several reports have been published showing that thyroxine therapy alone does not represent a significant risk factor for bone loss [91–93]. The negative effects of L-T_4 on bone can be furthermore minimized if the dose is carefully adjusted on a normal serum concentration of thyroid-stimulating hormone [94]. Indeed postmenopausal women who received thyroid hormone replacement therapy and had low thyroid-stimulating hormone levels showed more rapid rates of BMD loss from the spine and a trend toward greater bone loss at the radius and hip than women without known thyroid disease [95]. Recently a cross-sectional community-based study demonstrated that long-term thyroid hormone use at thyroxine-equivalent doses of 1.6 mg/kg or greater was associated with significant osteopenia at the forearm, hip, and lumbar spine, and that estrogen use appeared to negate thyroid hormone induced bone loss in postmenopausal women [96].

Diabetes Mellitus

Osteoporosis has been often reported as a consequence of diabetes. In humans two distinct types of diabetes are known: insulin-dependent diabetes mellitus (IDDM) which is associated with total lack of insulin and occurs usually in young, lean persons, and non-insulin-dependent diabetes mellitus (NIDDM) which develops gradually in later life, usually in obese patients. Most but not all studies performed in IDDM report an association with osteopenia. Using X-ray radiogrammometry and single- or dual-photon absorptiometry, a decrease in bone mass has been frequently reported both in young and adult patients [97–102]. The reductions in bone mass observed in these studies were generally small, and the bone loss was not necessarily associated with a decrease below the fracture threshold.

In a recent study BMD of whole body, lumbar spine, and femoral neck was measured by X-ray absorptiometry in postmenopausal women with IDDM [103]. Total-body BMD, lean mass, and fat mass were found to be similar in the diabetic patients and in control women, and BMD values at all sites were within the reference range in all examined patients. However, while there was no significant difference between the two groups in lumbar spine density, BMD values of the femoral neck and trochanter were lower in the diabetic women than in control group. No significant correlations were found between duration or control of diabetes and bone mass at any sites. These data confirm that in IDDM bone loss is usually of little extent and contribute to explain the discrepancy between the frequency of decreased BMD and the frequency of osteoporotic fractures in long-standing diabetes.

Regarding diabetic children the amount of bone loss has been estimated ranging from 5% to as much a 21% [99, 104]. In 48 white children (aged 5.2–19.6 years) with uncomplicated IDDM, decreased vertebral BMD was found to be a minor abnormality that only affects cortical bone [105]. There is also disagreement as to whether the duration of the IDDM and/or the quality of metabolic control influence BMC. Some but not all studies found a relationship between bone loss and poor blood glucose control, and suggested that the bone mass declined after several years of diabetes [99, 106].

Contradictory results have been obtained in NIDDM patients. Among older adult diabetics bone mass has been shown to be either elevated [107, 108] or decreased [109]. In a total of 36 NIDDM subjects a tendency to higher bone mass was found than in normal controls [110]. Positive significant correlations observed between fat mass and lean body mass with total-body BMD suggest that body mass is a more important determinant of BMD than hyperinsulinemia or insulin resistance in diabetic women [110]. The incidence of bone fracture is reported to be higher in diabetic patients than in a healthy population, with an approximately twofold increased risk. However, the presence of diabetic complications such as neuropathy, hypoglycemia or vascular disease that predispose to fall should be considered [111]. In a large multicenter prospective study of osteoporotic fractures in older women, NIDDM was strongly and independently associated with higher bone mass [112]. Recently the Rotterdam study carried out in 243 women and 335 men with NIDDM confirmed these data showing that both males and females had substantially higher mean BMD values at the lumbar spine and proximal femur than those with normal glucose tolerance. This increase was found not to be related to differences in age, body mass index, current use of medication known to influence bone metabolism, smoking, osteoarthritis, or impairment in activities of daily living. In addition, women with NIDDM reported having had fewer fractures in the 5 preceding years than women without this condition, while the frequency of fractures in men was similar in those with and those without NIDDM [113].

Several hypotheses have been proposed as pathogenetic mechanisms of diabetic osteopenia. Insulin deficiency itself probably influences bone cells directly or through its effects on other bone growth factors. Osteocalcin levels were reported lower in male and female NIDDM and in male IDDM, suggesting that deficient osteoblast function reduces bone formation [114, 115]. Hypercalciuria is frequent in both human and experimental diabetes [116] and may be partially explained by osmotic diuresis [111]. Intestinal calcium malabsorption has been also documented in diabetic animals [117] and in human diabetes [118]. This condition has been related to abnormalities in vitamin D metabolism. $1,25(OH)_2D$ levels were observed to be normal in most reports [118, 119], but serum $1,25(OH)_2D$ concentrations were usually depressed. Low $1,25(OH)_2D$ levels were found particularly in children and in adolescents during poor diabetes control or ketoacidosis [120]. The abnormality may be justified by decreased concentrations of the serum vitamin D binding protein, and by decreased renal synthesis of $1,25(OH)_2D$ [111, 117]. The concentration of vitamin D receptors has been also found to be markedly decreased in the duodenal mucosa of diabetic rats [117, 121]. In spite of hypercalciuria, reduced intestinal calcium absorption, and decreased $1,25(OH)_2D$ levels, no signs of secondary hyperparathyroidism or vitamin D deficiency were observed on bone histology of diabetic patients; on the other hand, dynamic bone histology studies indicated decreased bone formation [122, 123].

Gastrointestinal Disorders and Alcohol Abuse

Gastrectomy represents a risk factor for secondary osteoporosis. Increased rates of bone loss were demonstrated at the radius and lumbar spine in patients with two-thirds gastric resection and Billroth II reconstruction and in those with one-third resection and Billroth I anastomosis. [124–126]. In a case-control study BMD in the right calcaneus measured by DPA was 20% lower in men with Billroth II operation and 8% lower in those with a Billroth I operation [127]. In this report the incidence of vertebral fractures was 19% in men with previous partial gastrectomy and 4% in the control population. High prevalence of hip fracture was also found in gastrectomy patients [128, 129]. The long-term metabolic effects of partial gastrectomy still do not seem to be fully understood. Impaired intestinal calcium absorption was demonstrated in patients who underwent partial gastrectomy [130, 131]. Contradictory results have been reported concerning the role of gastric acid secretion in the absorption of dietary calcium [132, 133]. On the other hand, there may be effects related not only to calcium but also to magnesium [134]. Other studies indicate that gastrectomy may lead to phosphate depletion and decreased absorption of dietary vitamin D, with or without steathorrea [135].

In reality, the metabolic bone disease following gastrectomy may consist also of osteomalacia or mixed pattern of osteoporosis-osteomalacia, with secondary hyperparathyroidism [125, 136]. Patients with inflammatory bowel disease are also at risk of osteopenia; quantitative computed tomography or forearm absorptiometry demonstrated increased rates of bone loss [137, 138]. In cross-sectional studies low BMD values have beeen reported: the percentage of patients with osteopenia was found to be 31%–59% [139, 140]. A recent prospective study confirms these data, showing mean annual declines for lumbar and femoral neck BMD of 6.4% and 3.1% for patients with ulcerative colitis, and 6.9% and 5.6% for those with Crohn's disease [141]. However, in patients without steroid treatment the mean annual changes for lumbar and femur BMD were 0.87% and 0.20%, respectively. The pathogenesis of osteopenia associated with inflammatory bowel disease is incompletely understood. Intestinal calcium malabsorption, malnutrition, vitamin D deficiency, and high circulating levels of inflammatory factors such as interleukin 1, interleukin 6, and tumor necrosis factor have been proposed as pathogenetic mechanisms [142, 143]. In any case corticosteroid therapy is a likely contributory factor.

Histomorphometric and absorptiometric studies indicate that alcohol abuse may induce osteoporosis [144–146]. Bone loss was found to be significantly related to the length of alcohol abuse [147]. Moreover, increased incidence of skeletal fractures have been described in chronic alcoholism [148–150]. Although men are more prone to alcohol-induced osteoporosis than women, negative effects of alcohol intake have also been reported on bone mass in women [151, 152]. However, the role of alcohol as an osteoporosis-inducing agent was recently challenged in a study carried out in young or middle-aged women [153]. The mechanism by which alcohol abuse leads to osteopenia is not fully understood. There is suggestive evidence that ethanol directly inhibits osteoblast function [154, 155]. The rapid increase from low baseline values in serum osteocalcin concentrations following ethanol withdrawal may indicate a direct toxic effect of ethanol on osteoblastic function [156]. Furthermore, alterations in calcium and vitamin D metabolism, liver function, gonadal function, and nutrition have been advocated [147, 149, 157, 158].

Immobilization

It is generally recognized that rapid and diffuse bone loss may be a consequence of prolonged immobilization. Early studies in patients with paralytic poliomyelitis [159], and subsequent observations in patients with hemiplegia or hemiparesis demonstrated increased incidence of hip fractures [160, 161]. The development of diffuse osteoporosis appeared to be strictly related to the duration of hemiplegia [162]. In patients hospitalized for intervertebral disc disease the lumbar spine BMD decreased about 0.9% per week [163]. In a group of six healthy men placed in horizontal bed rest for a period of 17 weeks total body, lumbar spine, femoral neck, and trochanter BMD decreased significantly: expressed as the percentage change from baseline, these were 1.4%, 3.9%, 3.6%, and 4.6%, respectively. On the other hand, during deambulation the majority of the regions demonstrated positive slopes [164]. To stress the importance of muscle mass and weight-bearing activity in preserving bone, several studies showed that fractures occurred more frequently on the hemiplegic side [165, 166]. Immobilization osteopenia is characterized by an increase in remodeling dynamics. In patients with spinal cord injuries an increase in trabecular osteoclastic resorption surfaces and an early depression of osteoblastic bone formation were found [167]. Hypercalciuria and hyperphosphatasemia associated to low levels of immunoreactive parathyroid hormone and $1,25(OH)_2D$ were described as the main hormonal and metabolic consequences of immobilization [168].

As carefully demonstrated in long-duration space flights, gravitational stress plays a role of critical importance in the maintenance of bone mass [169]. Significant BMD decreases were reported for calcaneus during several missions in the Skylab and Soyuz-Salyut programs, in spite of the use of various exercise regimens [170]. Bone loss was found to be more pronounced after more prolonged missions. On the other hand, after space flights of relatively brief duration astronauts recovered bone mass after resumption of physical activity.

Disuse osteoporosis has also been described in patients after a stroke and in those with dementia [171, 172] and in those with Parkinson's disease [173, 174]. However, the increase fracture risk observed in these patients has been considered to be related also to the increased risk of falling.

Anorexia Nervosa

Anorexia nervosa is a chronic disease characterized by a fear of fatness, self-imposed semistarvation, and weight loss. It affects adolescent females and is fatal in 10%–15% of cases [175]. The disease is frequently associated with osteoporosis and consequently with a greater fracture risk. The most important factors contributing to the deficit in BMD in anorexia nervosa are hypogonadism and a profound reduction in body weight [176]. However, because anorexia nervosa occurs within the first three decades of life, a reduced peak bone mass may contribute to the development of osteoporosis in illness of earlier onset [177]. Indeed a study performed in 65 patients with anorexia nervosa demonstrated that in women with primary amenorrhea the reduction in BMD at the lumbar spine and femoral neck was greater than the reduction at the corresponding sites in the women with secondary amenorrhea [178]. In all patients lumbar spine and femoral BMD values diminished with increasing duration of amenorrhea. A 11.7-year follow-up examination of 51 subjects with anorexia nervosa showed a markedly reduced trabecular and cortical BMD, with a higher risk of fractures in patients with a chronically poor outcome: even in patients with good disease outcome a persistently reduced cortical and a slightly reduced trabecular BMD were observed [179].

Pregnancy and Lactation

Striking alterations in maternal calcium metabolism take place during pregnancy and lactation. There is a substantial calcium transfer from the mother to the fetus or infant. Consequently pregnancy and lactation may be considered risk factors for subsequent bone loss and osteoporosis.

In pregnancy the increased calcium needs are provided by the mother through adaptive mechanisms which may be summarized as a rise in the extent of maternal bone reabsorption and in a rise in intestinal calcium absorption associated with higher circulating levels of $1,25(OH)_2D$ and, probably parathyroid hormone [180]. Conflicting results have been reported in studies that examined the amount of BMD change with pregnancy. No changes in forearm BMD were reported in 13 pregnant women, without controls, examined three times during pregnancy and subsequently in the postpartum period [181]; these results were confirmed either at lumbar spine or at radius [182–184]. On the other hand, in a study performed with X-ray spectrophotometry in 14 pregnant women, with 9 controls, a loss in trabecular but not in cortical bone was found [185], and site-specific gain (tibia) and loss (femoral neck and radius) were even reported [186]. These controversies may be attribuitable at least in part to methodological and technical limitations.

During lactation calcium is transferred directly from serum to breast milk with increasing calcium demand with continued lactation. An estimated theoretical cost in minerals from the maternal skeleton with 6 months of full lactation would be approximately 4%–6% of the total minerals [180]. Indeed, prospective studies indicate substantial bone loss during lactation. A 10% midradial BMD decrease was reported in a teenaged group between 2 and 16 weeks of lactation [187]. In two additional studies a 7% BMD loss at forearm and 5% BMD loss at hip and spine were also demonstrated during the first 6 months of lactation, together with a recovery in each case from this loss with the reestablishment of menses [188,189]. Neverthless, other reports indicated very small bone loss or no changes of BMD values [184,186,190]. Conflicting results also arise from cross-sectional studies. Two large controlled studies performed in postmenopausal women (460 and 1100 subjects, respectively) reported no effect of lactation on BMD at radius, spine, and hip [191,192]. Similar results have also been achieved in premenopausal or perimenopausal women in spite of more precise lactation definitions. No significant association was demonstrated between breastfeeding duration and BMD measures, althought there were indications that women who had breast fed three to four children have lower bone mass than women who had breast fed one to two children [193–195]. No association of breast feeding with subsequent fracture was observed [196]. To explain the rapid bone loss during lactation decreased parathyroid hormone levels and elevated $1,25(OH)_2D$ concentrations have been suggested [197]. The rapid recovery of bone mineral after weaning has also been considered as being strictly related to the positive estrogen status after reestablishement of menses [184]. No association was found between either the calcium intake of well-nourished women, the amount of bone loss, or its recovery [189].

References

1. Consensus development conference (1991) Prophylaxis and treatment of osteoporosis. Am J Med 90:107–110
2. Consensus development conference (1993) Diagnosis, prophylaxis and treatment of osteoporosis. Am J Med 94:646–650
3. Kanis JA, Melton LJ III, Christiansen C, Johnston CC, Khaltaev N (1994) The diagnosis of osteoporosis. J Bone Miner Res 9:1137–1141
4. Cushing H (1932) Basophile adenomas. J Nerv Ment Dis 76:50
5. Curtiss PH, Clark WS, Hernddon CH (1954) Vertebral fractures resulting from prolonged cortisone and corticotrophin therapy. JAMA 156:467–469
6. Gennari C, Nuti R (1993) Complications of corticosteroid therapy. In: Christiansen C, Krane SM (eds) Advances in corticosteroids. Adis International. Langhorne, pA190047, USA, pp 39–51
7. Bressot C, Meunier PJ, Chapuy MC et al (1979) Histomorphometric profile, pathophysiology and reversiblity of corticosteroid-induced osteoporosis. Metab Bone Dis Relat Res 1:303–311
8. Lund B, Storm TL, Lund B (1985) Bone mineral loss, bone histomorphometry and vitamin D metabolism in patients with rheumatoid arthritis on long-term glucocorticoid treatment. Clin Rheumatol 4:143–149
9. Meunier PJ, Bressot C (1982) Endocrine influences on bone cells and bone remodeling evaluated by clinical histomorphometry. In: Parsons JA (ed) Endocrinology of calcium metabolism. Raven, New York, pp 445–465
10. Dempster DW, Arlot MA, Meunier PJ (1983) Mean wall thickness and formation periods of trabecular bone packets in corticosteroid-induced osteoporosis. Calcif Tissue Int 35:410–417
11. Peck WA (1984) Effects of glucocorticoids on bone cell metabolism and function. Adv Exp Med Biol 171:111–119
12. Bonucci E, Dearden LC, Mosier HD Jr (1984) Effects of glucocorticoid treatment on ultrastructure of cartilage and bone. Adv Exp Med Biol 171:269–278

13. Lukert BP, Raisz LG (1990) Glucocorticoid-induced osteoporosis: pathogenesis and management. Ann Intern Med 112:352–364

14. Adachi JD, Bensen WG Odsman AB (1993) Corticosteroid-induced osteoporosis. Semin Arthritis Rheum 22:375–384

15. Caniggia A, Nuti R, Lorè F, Vattimo A (1981) Pathophysiology of adverse effects of glucoactive corticosteroids on calcium metabolism in man. J Steroid Biochem 15:153–161

16. Reid IR (1989) Steroid osteoporosis. Calcif Tissue Int 45:63–67

17. Eastell R (1995) Management of corticosteroid-induded osteoporosis. J Intern Med 237:439–447

18. Reid IR, Gray AB (1993) Corticosteroid osteoporosis. In: Reidd DM (ed) Bailliere's clinical rheumatology, vol 7: osteoporosis. Baillière Tindall, London, pp 573–588

19. Klein RG, Arnaud SB, Gallagher JC, DeLuca HF, Riggs BL (1977) Intestinal calcium absorption in exogenous hypercortisolism. Role of 25-hydroxyvitamin D and corticosteroid dose. J Clin Invest 60:253–259

20. Gallagher JC, Aaron J, Horsman A, Wilkinson R, Nordin BE (1973) Corticosteroid osteoporosis. Clin Endocrinol Metab 2:355–368

21. Reid IR, Ibbertson HK (1987) Evidence for decreased tubular reabsorption of calcium in glucocorticoid-treatment asthmatics. Horm Res 27:200–204

22. Avioli LV (1984) Effects of chronic corticosteroid therapy on mineral metabolism and calcium absorption. Adv Exp Med Biol 171:81–89

23. Seeman E, Wahner HW, Offord KP, Kumar R, Johnson WJ, Riggs BL (1982) Differential effects of endocrine dysfunction on the axial and the appendicular skeleton. J Clin Invest 69:1302–1309

24. Adinof AD, Hollister JR (1983) Steroid-induced fractures and bone loss in patients with asthma. N Engl J Med 309:265–268

25. Olgaard K, Storm T, van Wowern N et al (1992) Glucocorticoid-induced osteoporosis in lumbar spine, forearm, and mandibole of nephrotic patients: a double blind study on the high dose, long-term effects of prednisone versus deflazacort. Calcif Tissue Int 50:490–497

26. Gennari C, Civitelli R (1987) Glucocorticoid-induced osteoporosis. In: Peck WA (ed) Clinics in rheumatic disease. Saunders, London, pp 637–654

27. Sambrook PN, Birmingham J, Kempler S et al (1990) Corticosteroid effects on proximal femur bone loss. J Bone Miner Res 5:1211–1216

28. Laan RF, van Riel PL, van de Putte LB, van Erning LJ, van't Hof MA, Lemmens JA (1993) Low-dose prednisone induces rapid reversible axial bone loss in patients with rheumatoid arthritis. Ann Intern Med 119:963–968

29. Shaadt O, Bohr H (1984) Bone mineral in lumbar spine, femoral neck and femoral shaft measured by dual-photon absorptiometry with 153-gadolinium in prednisone treatment. Adv Exp Med Biol 171:201–208

30. Sambrook PN, Eisman JA, Yeates MG, Pocock NA, Eberl S, Champion GD (1986) Osteoporosis in rheumatoid arthritis: safety of low dose corticosteroids. Ann Rheum Dis 45:950–953

31. Laan RFJM, Buijs WCAM, Van Erning LJTO et al (1992) Differential effect of glucocorticoids on appendicular and cortical vertebral mineral content. Calcif Tissue Int 52:5–9

32. Reid IR, Evans MC, Stapleton J (1992) Lateral spine densitometry is a more sensitive indicator of glucocorticoid-induced bone loss. J Bone Miner Res 7:1221–1225

33. Rickers H, Deding A, Christiansen G, Rodbro P (1984) Mineral loss in cortical and trabecular bone during high-dose prednisone treatment. Calcif Tissue Int 36:269–273

34. Reid DM, Kennedy NSJ, Smith MA, Tothill P, Nuki G (1982) Total body calcium in rheumatoid arthritis: effects of disease activity and corticosteroid treatment. BMJ 285:330–332

35. Gennari C, Civitelli R, Agnusdei D (1991) Corticosteroid-induced osteoporosis. In: Christiansen C, Overgaard K (eds) Osteoporosis 1990. Osteopress, Copenhagen, pp 1529–1538

36. Dykman TR, Gluck PS, Murphy WA, Hahn TJ, Hahn BH (1985) Evaluation of factors associated with glucocorticoid-induced osteopenia in patients with rheumatic diseases. Arthritis Rheum 28:361–368

37. Sambrook PN, Eisman JA, Champion GD, Yeates MG, Pocock NA, Eberl S (1987) Determinants of axial bone loss in rheumatoid arthritis. Arthritis Rheum 30:721–728

38. Saito JK, Davis JW, Wasnich RD, Ross PD (1995) Users of low-dose glucocorticoids have increased bone loss rates: a longitudinal study. Calcif Tissue Int 57:115–119

39. Packe GE, Douglas JG, McDonald AF, Robins SP, Reid DM (1992) Bone density in asthmatic patients taking high dose inhaled beclomethasone dipropionate and intermittent systemic corticosteroids. Thorax 47:414–417

40. Nordin BEC (1960) The systemic side effects of steroid therapy. Br J Dermatol 72:40–47

41. Hooyman JR, Melton LJ, Nelson AM, O'Fallon WM, Riggs BL (1984) Fracture after rheumatoid arthritis. A population-based study. Arthritis Rheum 27:1353–1361

42. Cooper C, Wickham C (1990) Rheumatoid arthritis, cortisteroid therapy and hip fracture. In: Christiansen C, Overgaard K (eds) Osteoporosis 1990. Osteopress, Copenhagen, pp 1578–1579

43. Verstraeten A, Dequeker J (1987) Vertebral and peripheral bone mineral content and fracture incidence in postmenopausal women with rheumatoid arthritis: effect of low dose of corticosteroids. Ann Rheum Dis 45:852–857

44. Goldhaber P (1965) Heparin enhancement of factors stimulating bone resorption in tissue culture. Science 147:407–408

45. Thompson RC (1973) Heparin osteoporosis: an experimental model using rats. J Bone Joint Surg Am 55:606–612

46. Rupp WM, McCarthy HB, Rohde TD, Blackshear PJ, Goldenberg FJ, Buchwald H (1982) Risk of osteoporosis in patient treated with long-term intravenous heparin therapy. Curr Surg 39:412–422

47. Squires JW, Puich LW (1979) Heparin induced spinal fractures. J Am Med Assoc 24:2417–2418

48. Burns ER (1987) Characteristic and use of antithrombotic drugs. In: Burns ER (ed) Clinical management of bleeding and thrombosis. Blackwell Science, Oxford, pp 175–185

49. Hirsh J, Dalen JE, Deykin D, Poller L (1992) Heparin: mechanism of action, pharmacokinetics, dosing considerations, monitoring, efficacy and safety. Chest 102:337–351

50. Monreal M, Vinas L, Monreal L, Lavin S, Lafoz E, Angles AM (1990) Heparin related osteoporosis in rats. A comparative study between unfractioned heparin and low molecular weight heparin. Haemostasis 20:204–207

51. Melissari E, Parker CJ, Wilson NV et al (1992) Use of low molecular weight heparin in pregnancy. Thromb Haemost 68:652–656

52. Murray WJG, Lindo VS; Kakkar VV, Melissari E (1995) Long term administration of heparin and heparin fractions and osteoporosis in experimental animals. Blood Coagul Fibrinolysis 6:113–118

53. Sivakumaran S, Ghosh K, Zaidi Y, Hutchinson RM (1996) Osteoporosis and vertebral collapse following low-dose, low molecular weight heparin therapy in a young patient. Clin Lab Haematol 18:55–57

54. Hellgren M, Nygards EB (1982) Long-term therapy with subcutaneus heparin during pregnancy. Gynecol Obstet Invest 13:76–89

55. Wise PH, Hall AJ (1980) Heparin-induced osteopenia in pregnancy. BMJ 3:110–111

56. Dahlman TC (1993) Osteoporotic fractures and the recurrence of thromboembolism during pregnancy and the puerperium in 184 women undergoing thromboprophylaxis with heparin. Am J Obstet Gynecol 168:1265–1270

57. DeSwiet M (1983) Prolonged heparin therapy in pregnancy causes bone demineralization. Br J Obstet Gynecol 90:1129–1134

58. Zimran A, Shilo S, Fisher D, Bab I (1986) Histomorphometric evaluation of reversible heparin-induced osteoporosis in pregnancy. Arch Intern Med 146:386–388

59. Barbour LA, Kick SD, Steiner JF et al (1994) A prospective study of heparin-induced osteoporosis in pregnancy using bone densitometry. Am J Obstet Gynecol 170:862–869

60. Chowdhury MH, Hamada C, Dempster DW (1992) Effects of heparin on osteoclast activity. J Bone Miner Res 7:771–777

61. Fuller K, Chambers TJ, Gallagher AC (1991) Heparin augments osteoclast resorption-stimulating activity in serum. J Cell Physiol 147:208–214

62. Hurley MM, Gronowicz G, Kream BE, Raisz LG (1990) Effect of heparin on bone formation in cultured fetal rat calvaria. Calcif Tissue Int 46:183–188

63. Mckenna MJ, Frame B (1985) The mast cell and bone. Clin Orthop 200:226–233

64. Frame B, Nixon RK (1968) Bone marrow mast cells in osteoporosis of aging. N Engl J Med 279:626–630

65. Fallon MD, Whyte MP, Teitlebaum SL (1981) Systemic mastocytosis associated with generalized osteoporosis. Hum Pathol 12:813–820
66. Harvey JA, Anderson HC, Borek D, Morris D, Lukert BP (1989) Osteoporosis associated with mastocytosis confined to bone: report of two cases. Bone 10:237–241
67. Lidor C, Frisch B, Gazit D, Gepstein R, Hallel T, Mekori YA (1990) Osteoporosis as the sole presentation of bone mastocytosis. J Bone Miner Res 5:871–876
68. Chines A, Pacifici R, Avioli LV, Teitlebaum SL, Korenblat PE (1991) Systemic mastocytosis presenting as osteoporosis: a clinical and histomorphometric study. J Clin Endocrinol Metab 72:140–144
69. Meunier PJ, Bianchi GGS, Edouard CM, Bernard JC, Courprou P, Vignou GE (1972) Bone manifestation of thyrotoxicosis. Orthop Clin North Am 3:745–774
70. Melsen F, Mosekilde L (1977) Morphometric and dynamic studies of bone change in hyperthyroidism. Acta Pathol Microbiol Scand 85:1676–1686
71. Fallon MD, Perry HM, Bergfeld M et al (1983) Exogenous hyperthyroidism with osteoporosis. Arch Intern Med 143:442–444
72. Jastrup B, Mosekilde L, Melsen F et al (1982) Serum levels of vitamin D metabolites and bone remodeling in hyperthyroidism. Metabolism 31:126–132
73. Mundy GR, Shapiro JL, Bandelin JG, Canalis EM, Raisz LG (1976) Direct stimulation of bone resorption. J Clin Invest 58:529–534
74. Garrel DR, Delmas PD, Malaval L, Tourniaire J (1986) Serum bone Gla protein: a marker of bone turnover in hyperthyroidism. J Clin Endocrinol Metab 62:1052–1055
75. Bouillon, Muls E, De Moor P (1980) Influence of thyroid function on the serum concentration of 1,25-dihydroxyvitamin D3. J Clin Endocrinol Metab 51:793–797
76. Haldimann B, Kaptein EM, Singer FR, Nioloff JT, Massry SG (1980) Intestinal calcium absorption in patients with hyperthyroidism. J Clin Endocrinol Metab 51:995–997
77. Nuti R, Martini G, Turchetti V et al (1987) Intestinal radiocalcium absorption in hyperthyroidism. Nuklearmedizin. Schattauer, Stuttgart, pp 696–700
78. Fraser SA, Anderson JB, Smith DA, Wilson GM (1971) Osteoporosis and fractures following thyrotoxicosis. Lancet 1:981–983
79. Peerenboom H, Keck E, Kruskemper HL, Strohmeyer G (1984) The defect of intestinal calcium transport in hyperthyroidism and its response to therapy. J Clin Endocrinol Metab 59:936–940
80. Linde J, Friis TH (1979) Osteoporosis in hyperthyroidism estimated by photon absorptiometry. Acta Endocrinol (Copenh) 91:437–448
81. Krolner B, Jorgensen JV, Nielsen SP (1983) Spinal bone mineral content in myxoedema and thyrotoxicosis: effect of thyroid hormones and antithyroid treatment. J Clin Endocrinol 18:439–446
82. Francis RM, Barnett MJ, Selby PL, Peacock M (1982) Thyrotoxicosis presenting as fracture of the femoral neck. BMJ 285:97–98
83. Solomon BL, Wartofsky L, Burman KD (1993) Prevalence of fractures in postmenopausal women with thyroid disease. Thyroid 3:17–23

84. Toh SH, Claunch BC, Brown PH (1985) Effect of hyperthyroidism and its treatment on bone mineral content. Arch Intern Med 145:883–886

85. Rosen CJ, Adler RA (1992) Longitudinal changes in lumbar bone density among thyrotoxic patient after attainment of euthyroidism. J Clin Endocrinol Metab 75:1531–1534

86. Mudde AH, Houbent AJHM, Krusemant ACN (1994) Bone metabolism during anti-thyroid drug treatment of endogenous subclinical hyperthyroidism. Clin Endocrinol (Oxf) 41:421–424

87. Ross DS, Neer RM, Ridgway EC, Daniels GH (1987) Subclinical hyperthyroidism and reduced bone density as a possible result of prolonged suppression of the pituitary-thyroid axis with L-thyroxine. Am J Med 82:1167–1170

88. Paul TL, Kerrigan J, Kelly AM, Braverman LE, Baran DT (1988) Long-term L-thyroxine therapy is associated with decreased hip bone density in premenopausal women. JAMA 3:3137–3141

89. Kung AWC, Pun KK (1991) Bone mineral density in premenopausal women receiving long-term physiological doses of levothyroxine. JAMA 265:2688–2691

90. Greenspan SL, Greenspan FS, Resnick NM, Block JE, Friedlander AL, Genant HK (1991) Skeletal integrity in premenopausal and postmenopausal women receiving long-term L-thyroxine therapy. Am J Med 91:5–14

91. Toh SH, Brown PH, (1990) Bone mineral content in hypothyroid male patients with hormone replacement: a 3-year study. J Bone Miner Res 5:463–467

92. Franklyn JA, Betteridge J, Daykin J et al (1992) Long-term thyroxine treatment and bone mineral density. Lancet 340:9–13

93. Franklyn J, Betteridge J, Holder R, Daykin J, Lilley J, Sheppard M (1994) Bone mineral density in thyroxine treated females with or without a previous history of thyrotoxicosis. Clin Endocrinol 41:425–432

94. Ross DS (1991) Monitoring L-thyroxine therapy: lessons from the effect of L-thyroxine on bone density. Am J Med 91:1–4

95. Stall GM, Harris S, Sokoll LJ, Dawson-Hughes B (1990) Accelerated bone loss in hypothyroid patients overtreated with L-thyroxine. Ann Intern Med 113:265–269

96. Schneider DL, Barret-Connor EL, Morton DJ (1994) Thyroid hormone use and bone mineral density in elderly women. JAMA 271:1245–1249

97. Ringe JD, Kunlencordt F, Kunhau J (1976) Mineralgehalt des Skeletts bei Langzeitdiabetikern. Densitometrischer Beitrag zu "Osteopathia diabetica." Dtsch Med Wochenschr 101:280–286

98. Santiago JV, McAlister WH, Ratzan SK et al (1977) Decreased cortical thickness and osteopenia in children with diabetes mellitus. J Clin Endocrinol Metab 45:845–848

99. McNair P, Madsbad S, Christiansen C et al (1979) Bone loss in diabetes: effects of metabolic state. Diabetologia 17:283–286

100. McNair P, Christiansen C, Christensen MS et al (1981) Development of bone mineral loss in insulin-treated diabetes: a $1^{1}/_{2}$ years follow-up study in sixty patients. Eur Clin Invest 11:55–59

101. Wiske PS, Wentworth SM, Norton JA, Epstein S, Johnston CC (1982) Evaluation of bone mass and growth in young diabetics. Metabolism 31:848–854
102. Hui SL, Epstein S, Johnston CC (1985) A prospective study of bone mass in patients with type I diabetes. J Clin Endocrinol Metab 60:74–80
103. Compston JE, Smith EM, Matthews C, Schofield P (1994) Whole body composition and regional bone mass in women with insulin-dependent diabetes mellitus. Clin Endocrinol (Oxf) 41:289–293
104. Rosenbloom AL, Lezotte DC, Weber FT et al (1977) Diminution of bone mass in childhood diabetes. Diabetes 26:1052–1055
105. Roe TF, Mora S, Costin G, Kaufman FF, Carlson ME, Glisanz V (1991) Vertebral bone density in insulin-dependent diabetic children. Metabolism 40:967–971
106. Weber G, Beccaria L, De Angelis M et al (1990) Bone mass in young patients in diabetes mellitus type I. Bone Miner 8:23–30
107. Weinstock RS, Goland RS, Shane E, Clemens TL, Lindsay R, Bilezikian JP (1989) Bone mineral density in women with type II diabetes mellitus. J Bone Miner Res 4:97–101
108. Barret-Connor E, Holbrook TL (1992) Sex difference osteoporosis in older adults with non-insulin-dependent diabetes mellitus. JAMA 268:3333–3337
109. Johnston CC, Hui SL, Longcope C (1985) Bone mass and sex steroid concentration in postmenopausal caucasian diabetics. Metabolism 34:544–550
110. Rishaug U, Birkeland KI, Falch A, Vaaler S (1995) Bone mass in non-insulin-dependent diabetes mellitus. Scand J Clin Lab Invest 55:257–262
111. Bouillon R (1991) Diabetic bone disease. Calcif Tissue Int 49:155–160
112. Bauer DC, Browner WS, Cauley JA et al (1993) Factors associated with appendicular bone mass in older women. Ann Intern Med 118:657–665
113. Van Daele PLA, Stolk RP, Burger H et al (1995) Bone density in non-insulin-dependent diabetes mellitus. Ann Intern Med 122:409–414
114. Pedrazzoni M, Ciotti G, Pioli G et al (1989) Osteocalcin levels in diabetic subjects. Calcif Tissue Int 45:331–336
115. Rico H, Hernandez R, Cabranes JA, Gomez-Castresana F (1989) Suggestion of a deficient osteoblastic function in diabetes mellitus: the possible cause of osteopenia in diabetics. Calcif Tissue Int 45:71–73
116. Raskin P, Stevenson MRM, Barilla DE, Pah CYC (1978) The hypercalciuria of diabetes mellitus: its amelioration with insulin. Clin Endocrinol (Oxf) 9:329–335
117. Nyomba BL, Verhaeghe J, Thomasset M, Lissens W, Bouillon R (1989) Bone mineral homeostasis in sponteneously diabetic BB rats. Abnormal vitamin D metabolism and impaired active intestinal calcium absorption. Endocrinology 124:565–572
118. Nuti R, Lorè F, Vattimo A, Di Cairano G, Turchetti V (1981) Bone mineral content, 25OH serum levels, 47Ca intestinal absorption in osteopenia of diabetes mellitus. Nuklearmedizin. Shattauer, Stuttgart, pp 811–814
119. Storm TL, Sorensen OH, Lund BJ et al (1983) Vitamin D metabolism in insulin-dependent diabetes mellitus. Metab Bone Dis Relat Res 5:107–110

120. Nyomba BL, Bouillon R, Bidingija M, Kandjingu K, De Moor P (1986) Vitamin D metabolites and their binding protein in adult diabetic patients. Diabetes 35:911–915
121. Ishida H, Cunningham NS, Henry HL, Norman AW (1988) The number of 1,25-dihydroxyvitamin D_3 receptors is decreased in both intestine and kidney of genetically diabetic db/db mice. Endocrinology 122:2436–2443
122. Wu K, Schubek KE, Frost HM, Villanueva A (1970) Haversian bone formation rates determined by a new method in a mastodon, and in human diabetes mellitus and osteoporosis. Calcif Tissue Res 6:204–219
123. Andress DL, Herez G, Kopp JB et al (1987) Bone histomorphometry of renal osteo-dystrophy in diabetic patients. J Bone Miner Res 2:525–531
124. Aukee S, Alhava EM, Karjalainen P (1975) Bone mineral after partial gastrectomy II. Scand J Gastroenterol 10:165–169
125. Blichert-Toft M, Beck A, Christiansen C, Transbol I (1979) Effects of gastric resection and vagotomy on blood and bone mineral content. World J Surg 3:99–102
126. Inoue K, Shiomi K, Higashide S et al (1992) Metabolic bone disease following gastrectomy: assessment by dual energy X-ray absorpiometry. Br J Surg 79:321–324
127. Mellstrom D, Johansson C, Johnell O et al (1993) Osteoporosis, metabolic aberrations, and increased risk for vertebral fractures after partial gastrectomy. Calcif Tissue Int 53:370–377
128. Nilsson BE, Westlin NE (1971) The fracture incidence after gastrectomy. Acta Chir Scand 137:533–534
129. Baille SP, Davison CE, Johnson FJ, Francis RM (1992) Pathogenesis of vertebral crush fractures in men. Age Aging 21:139–141
130. Caniggia A, Gennari C, Cesari L (1964) Intestinal absorption of 45Ca and dynamics of 45Ca in gastrectomy osteoporosis. Acta Med Scand 176:599–605
131. Arman E, Nilsson LH, Reizenstein P (1970) Studies in the dumping syndrome. VI. Calcium deficiency after partial gastrectomy. Dig Dis 15:455–462
132. Recker R (1985) Calcium absorption and achlorhydria. N Engl J Med 11:70–73
133. Bo-Linn GW, Davis GR, Buddrus DJ, Morawski SG, Santa Ana C, Fordtran JS (1984) An evaluation of the importance of gastric acid secretion in the absorption of dietary calcium. J Clin Invest 73:640–647
134. Fries W, Rumenapf G, Schwille PO (1992) Disturbances of mineral and bone metabolism following gastric antrectomy in the rat. Bone Miner 19:245–25
135. Nilas L, Christiansen C, Christiansen J (1985) Regulation of vitamin D and calcium metabolism after gastrectomy. Gut 26:252–257
136. Bisballe S, Eriksen EF, Melsen F, Moseklide L, Sorensen OH, Hessov I (1991) Osteopenia and osteomalacia after gastrectomy: interrelations between biochemical markers of bone remodeling, vitamin D metabolites, and bone histomorphometry. Gut 32:1303–1307
137. Clements D, Motley RJ, Evans WD et al (1992) Longitudinal study of cortical bone loss in patients with inflammatory bowel disease. Scand J Gastroenterol 27:1332–1336

138. Motley RJ, Clements D, Evans WD et al (1993) A four-year longitudinal study of bone loss in patients with inflammatory bowel disease. Bone Miner 23:95–104

139. Compston JE, Judd D, Crawley EO et al (1987) Osteoporosis in patients with inflammatory bowel disease. Gut 28:410–415

140. Pigot F, Roux C, Chaussade S et al (1992) Low bone mineral density in patients with inflammatory bowel disease. Dig Dis Sci 37:1396–1403

141. Roux C, Abitol V, Chaussade S et al (1995) Bone loss in patients with inflammatory bowel disease: a prospective study. Osteoporosis Int 5:156–160

142. Mahida YR, Scott E, Kurlak L, Gallagher A, Hawkey CJ (1992) Interleukin 1 beta, tumor necrosis factor alpha and interleukin 6 synthesis by circulating mononuclear cells isolated from patients with active ulcerative colitis and Crohn's disease. Eur J Gastroenterol Hepatol 6:501–507

143. Silvennoinen J (1996) Relationship between vitamin D, parathyroid hormone and bone mineral density in inflammatory bowel disease. J Int Med 239:131–137

144. Johnell O, Nilsson BE, Wiklund PE (1982) Bone morphometry in alcoholics. Clin Orthop 165:253–258

145. Bikle DD, Genant Hk, Cann C et al (1985) Bone disease in alcohol abuse. Ann Intern Med 103:42–48

146. Crilly RG, Anderson C, Hogan D et al (1988) Bone histomorphometry, bone mass, and related parameters in alcoholic males. Calcif Tissue Int 43:269–276

147. Nuti R, Martini G, Frediani B et al (1992) Effects of alcohol abuse on bone metabolism. Eur J Exp Musculoskel Res 1:81–85

148. Seeman E, Melton LJ, O'Fallon WM, Riggs BL (1983) Risk factors for spinal osteoporosis in men. Am J Med 75:977–983

149. Lalor BC, France MW, Powell D, Adams PH, Counihan TB (1986) Bone and mineral metabolism in chronic alcohol abuse. Q J Med 59:497–511

150. Spencer H, Rubio N, Rubio E, Indreika M, Seitam A (1986) Chronic alcoholism: frequently overlooked cause of osteoporosis in men. Am J Med 80:393–397

151. Feitelberg S, Epstein S, Ismail F et al (1987) Deranged bone mineral metabolism in chronic alcoholism. Metabolism 36:322–326

152. Stevenson JC, Lees B, Devemport M et al (1989) Determinants of bone density in normal women: risk factors for future osteoporosis? Br J Med 298:924–928

153. Laitnen K, Karkkainen M, Lalla M et al (1993) Is alcohol an osteoporosis-inducing agent for young and middle-aged women? Metabolism 42:875–881

154. de Vernejoul MC, Bielakoff J, Herve M et al (1983) Evidence for defective osteoblastic function. A role for alcohol and tobacco consumption in osteoporosis in middle-aged men. Clin Orthop 179:107–115

155. Diamond T, Stiel D, Lunzer M, Wilkinson M, Posen S (1989) Ethanol reduces bone formation and may cause osteoporosis. Am J Med 86:282–288

156. Pepersack T, Fuss M, Otero J, Bergmann P, Valsamis J, Corvilain J (1992) Lon-

gitudinal study of bone metabolism after ethanol withdrawal in alcoholic patients. J Bone Miner Res 7:383–387

157. Bannister P, Handley T, Chapman C, Losowsky MS (1986) Hypogonadism in chronic liver disease. BMJ 293:1191–1193

158. Editorial (1987) Calcium and chronic liver disease. Lancet 2:1065–1066

159. Whedon GD, Schorr E (1957) Metabolic studies in paralytic acute anterior poliomyelitis. II. Alterations in calcium and phosphorus metabolism. J Clin Invest 36:966–981

160. Alffram PA (1964) An epidemiologic study of cervical and trochanteric fractures of the femur in an urban population: analysis of 1,664 cases with special reference to etiologic factors. Acta Orthop Scand 65 [Suppl]:1–109

161. Mulley G, Espley AJ (1979) Hip fracture after hemiplegia. Postgrad Med J 55:264–265

162. Prince RL, Price RI, Ho S (1988) Forearm bone loss in hemiplegia: a model for the study of immobilization osteoporosis. J Bone Miner Res 3:305–310

163. Kronler B, Toft B (1983) Vertebral bone loss: an unheeded side effect of terapeutic bed rest. Clin Sci 64:537–540

164. Leblanc AD, Schneider VS, Evans HJ, Engelbreston DA, Krebs JM (1990) Bone mineral loss and recovery after 17 weeks of bed rest. J Bone Miner Res 5:843–850

165. Minaire M, Meunier P, Edouard C, Bernard J, Courpron P, Bourret J (1974) Quantitative histological data on disuse osteoporosis. Calcif Tissue Res 17:53–73

166. Stewart AF, Adler M, Byers CM, Segre GV, Brodaus AE (1982) Calcium homeostasis in immobilization: an example of resorptive hypercalciuria. N Engl J Med 306:1136–1140

167. Poplingher AR, Pillar T (1985) Hip fracture in stroke patients: epidemiology and rehabilitation. Acta Orthop Scand 56:226–227

168. White HC (1988) Post stroke hip fractures. Arch Orthop Trauma Surg 107:345–347

169. Rambaut PC, Johnston RS (1979) Prolonged weightlessness and calcium loss in man. Acta Astronaut 6:1313–1322

170. Anderson SA, Cohn SH (1985) Bone demineralization during space flight. Physiologist 28:212–217

171. Buchner DM Larson EB (1987) Falls and fractures in patients with Alzheimer-type dementia. JAMA 257:1492–1495

172. Melton LJ III, Beard CM, Kokmen E, Atkinson EJ, O'Fallon WM. (1994) Fracture risk in patients with Alzheimer's disease. J Am Geriatr Soc 42:614–619

173. Ishizaki F, Harada T, Katayama S, Abe H, Nakamura S (1993) Relationship between osteopenia and clinical characteristics of Parkinson's disease. Mov Disord 80:507–511

174. Revilla M, de la Sierra G, Aguado F, Varela L, Jiménez-Jiménez FJ, Rico H (1995) Bone mass in Parkinson's disease: a study with three methods. Calcif Tissue Int 58:311–315

175. American Psychiatric Association (1987) Diagnostic and statistical manual of mental disorders (DSM-III-R), 3rd rev edn. American Psychiatric Association, Washington DC
176. Biller BMK, Saxe V, Herzog DB, Rosenthal DI, Holzman S, Klibanski A (1989) Mechanisms of osteoporosis in adult and adolescent women with anorexia nervosa. J Clin Endocrinol Metab 68:548–554
177. Bacharch LK, Guido D, Katzman D, Litt IF, Marcus R (1990) Decreased bone density in adolescent girls with anorexia nervosa. Pediatrics 86:440–447
178. Seeman E, Szmukler GI, Formica C, Tsalamandris C, Mestrovic R (1992) Osteoporosis in anorexia nervosa: the influence of peak bone density, bone loss, oral contraceptive use, and exercise. J Bone Miner Res 7:1467–1474
179. Herzog W, Minne H, Deter C et al (1993) Outcome of bone mineral density in anorexia nervosa patients 11.7 years after first admission. J Bone Miner Res 8:597–605
180. Sowers MF (1996) Pregnancy and lactation as risk factors for subsequent bone loss and osteoporosis. J Bone Miner Res 11:1052–1060
181. Christiansen C, Rodbro R, Heinlind B (1976) Unchanged total body calcium in normal human pregnancy. Acta Obstet Gynecol Scand 55:141–143
182. Sowers MF, Crutchfield M, Jannausch M (1991) A prospective evaluation of bone mineral change in pregnancy. Obstet Gynecol 77:841–845
183. Kent GN, Rice RI, Gutteridge DH et al (1993) Effect of pregnancy and lactation on maternal bone mass and calcium metabolism. Osteop Int 3 (S1):44–47
184. Cross NA, Hillman LS, Allen SH, Krause GF, Viera NE (1995) Calcium homeostasis and bone metabolism during pregnancy, lactation, and postweaning: a longitudinal study. Am J Clin Nutr 61:514–523
185. Lamke B, Brundin J, Moberg P (1977) Changes of bone mineral content during pregnancy and lactation. Acta Obstet Gynecol Scand 56:217–219
186. Drinkwater BL, Chesnut CH III (1991) Bone density changes during pregnancy and lactation in active women: a longitudinal study. Bone Miner 14:153–160
187. Chan GM, McMurry M, Westover K et al (1987) Effects of increased dietary calcium intake upon the calcium and bone mineral status of lactating adolescent and adult women. Am J Clin Nutr 46:319–323
188. Kent GN, Price RI, Gutteridge DH et al (1990) Human lactation: forearm trabecular bone loss, increased bone turnover, and renal conservation of calcium and inorganic phosphate with recovery of bone mass following weaning. J Bone Miner Res 5:361–369
189. Sowers MF, Corton G, Shapiro B et al (1993) Changes in bone density with lactation. JAMA 269:3130–3135
190. Prentice A, Landing MAJ, Cole TJ, Stirling DM, Dibba B, Fairweather-Tait S (1995) Calcium requirements of lactating Gambian mothers: effects of a calcium supplement on breastmilk calcium concentration, maternal bone mineral content, and urinary calcium excretion. Am J Clin Nutr 62:58–67
191. Kritz-Silverstein D, Barrett-Connor E, Hollenbach KA (1992) Pregnancy and lactation as determinants of bone mineral density in postmenopausal women. Am J Epidemiol 136:1052–1059

192. Fox KM, Magaziner J, Shervin R et al (1993) Reproductive correlates of bone mass in elderly women. J Bone Miner Res 8:901–908
193. Johnell O, Nilsson BE (1984) Lifestyle and bone mineral mass in perimenopausal women. Calcif Tissue Int 36:354–356
194. Koetting CA, Wardlaw GM (1988) Wrist, spine and hip bone density in women with variable histories of lactation. Am J Clin Nutr 48:1479–1481
195. Feldblum PJ, Zhang J, Rich LE, Fortney JA, Talmage RV (1992) Lactation history and bone mineral density among perimenopausal women. Epidemiology 3:327–331
196. Ribot C, Tremollieres F, Pouilles JM et al (1993) Risk factors for hip fracture. Bone 14:S77–S80
197. Specker BL, Tsang R, Ho ML (1991) Changes in calcium homeostasis over the first year postpartum: effect of lactation and weaning. Obstet Gynecol 78:56–62

27 Assessing the Response to Treatment for Osteoporosis

R. Nuti, G. Martini, and C. Gennari

The objective of long-term drug treatment of osteoporosis is the prevention and reduction of the effects of bone loss on the quality of life and life expectancy. This means that the agent should reduce the lifetime risk of fracture. Clinical trials have demonstrated that an agent can be considered effective in the treatment of osteoporosis when it reduces the risk of new fractures [1]. Once it has been established that a drug is able to prevent or reduce osteoporotic fractures, the problem is how to monitor the efficacy of individuals' treatment. Of course evaluating atraumatic fracture of the axial and appendicular skeleton is not feasible for this purpose, even if determining the presence of a fracture is important on clinical grounds. This is also true for vertebral fractures. The difficulty in deciding whether a specific treatment is indeed capable of avoiding the appearance of vertebral deformities results from technical limitations. It is widely known that variations may be caused by differences, firstly, in the manner in which radiographs are taken at individual centers and, secondly, in the way in which the radiographs are assessed. Standard radiographic protocols have been utilized to reduce differences in technique between centers.

Nevertheless, we must bear in mind that for an individual patient there are often different views between physicians and radiologists regarding the presence of borderline deformities. It is also possible that a vertebra has more than one type of deformity, for example, both wedge and compression. In certain circumstances such as severe scoliosis or osteoarthritis it is impossible to assess accurately the presence or progression of vertebral deformity secondary to osteoporosis. Various classification systems have been proposed with the aim of defining the type, degree, and number of deformities [2–5]. Qualitative or semiquantitative and quantitative assessement (morphometry) of vertebral fractures have been used to determine the prevalence of vertebral deformity in epidemiological studies [6] and to validate the efficacy of specific treatments in clinical trials [7–9]. No data are currently available concerning their value in monitoring the efficacy of a drug in an individual subject.

Fracture is considered a stochastic event related to several parameters that indicate risk: bone mineral density (BMD), postural inability, and presumably falls [10]. Although all of these variables could be targeted, BMD is the most obvious. Many prospective studies indicate that the risk of fragility fractures increases progressively and continuously as BMD declines [11–13].

Dual energy X-ray absorptiometry (DXA) has become the reference in clinical practice for evaluating osteoporosis [14]. Because of the very accurate absorptiometric techniques for measuring bone mineral mass, these can be used both as a prognostic tool to predict fractures and as a test for the presence of osteoporosis. A reduction in bone mass may be considered osteoporosis when a value for BMD or bone mineral content (BMC) is 2.5 SD or more below the young adult mean value (T score ≤ 2.5). It is calculated that the risk of fracture increases 1.5- to 3-fold or more for each decrease of 1 SD in BMD [15]. The average lifetime risk of the common osteoporotic fractures in white men and women is about 13% and 40%, respectively, at the age of 50 years with average BMD for that age [16]. On the other hand, for an osteoporotic population with a BMD 2 SD below average the risk increases more than fourfold.

Other than as a diagnostic and prognostic tool, BMD measurements may be used to gauge the response to antiosteoporotic treatment. Previously bone density measurements with a photon-emitting source were associated with large precision errors relative to estimate rates of bone change and could not reliably monitor changes in bone density in individual patients. With the arrival of X-ray absorptiometry and the refinements in measurement precision, monitoring of certain medical regimens in individual patients may be considered. However, closely following the efficiency of a treatment for osteoporosis is not as straightforward as monitoring the efficacy of an antihypertensive drug. The ability of a technique to monitor changes in skeletal status (longitudinal sensitivity) is based on assessment of the precision or reproducibility, that is, the ability to obtain the same result from repeated measurements [17]. Therefore monitoring BMD changes correctly requires high precision because of the relatively small variations in BMD with aging or therapy. Indeed, normal changes in the mineral content of skeletal tissue proceed at a relatively slow rate, ranging from 0.5%–1% per annum for most of the adult lifespan of healthy individuals to 2%–5% in early postmenopausal women [18].

Other methods for monitoring the progression of the disease or its therapy today available in addition to DXA are: single X-ray absorptiometry (SXA), quantitative computed tomography (QCT), and ultrasound. DXA enables us to measure axial (spine, femur), appendicular (forearm), and the entire skeleton with good precision and low-dose exposure. Single and dual QCT are the sole methods of measuring only the trabecular bone of the vertebral spongiosum, while DXA measures both compact and trabecular bone. The precision error of spine QCT is 2%–4%. QCT can also be used to measure forearm bone density (peripheral QCT), but its advantage over SXA or DXA is yet to be demonstrated. Ultrasound-based techniques are promising methods of evaluating bone mass and, probably, bone quality.

In clinical practice same-day precision has been used to assess whether changes between period measurements carried out in patients months apart truly represent actual changes or are merely random variability. The precision errors are usually calculated by expressing the standard deviation as a percentage of the average number of repeated measurements on the same day, known as the coefficient of variation or CV%. Typically any change between two measurements exceeding 2√2 CV% has been considered a true or "significant change": with a 2% precision error a change in bone density in individual patients must be greater than 5.5% to be detected within 95% confidence limits [19]. Monitoring bone mass changes in the individual patient can also be adequate using a one-tailed test of significance and a 90% confidence level; a technique with 2% precision error can demonstrate changes in bone mass greater than 3.6% with 90% confidence [20]. However, expressing precision errors on a percentage basis is not always appropriate because, for example, in elderly and osteoporotic individuals the precision error is greater than expected because the SD is divided by a smaller mean [21]. For a clearer understanding of the rate of change of BMD between two measurements it has been proposed that the SD of the annualized ratio of BMD change be considered. A rate that is twice the SD is considered significant [22]. To judge a technique's ability in monitoring changes in BMD, an agreement on how to measure and calculate reproducibility is required. The short-term precision errors must be calculated in the correct fashion, i.e., using the correct degrees of freedom and averaging based on root mean squared averages. Employing arithmetic means, precision errors would be underestimated by as much as 25%. For long-term precision it is better to calculate the standard errors of the estimate of changes in bone density with time [18].

There is a great body of literature on the effects of various treatments upon bone mass. A critical question here is whether changes in BMD, a powerful index of fracture risk in epidemiological studies, can be used as an alternative for fracture risk alterations. In some situations, for example, in early postmenopausal women, prevention of bone loss measured by BMD seems a reasonable surrogate since we are trying to conserve existing bone structure. On the other hand, with treatment of osteoporosis following substantial loss of bone density and structural integrity this assumption is more difficult.

With fluoride salts a substantial increase in BMD has been observed without comparable increase in bone strength or reduction in fracture incidence [23–25]. However, a re-analysis of data suggested that the lower doses of the drug increase BMD and reduce fracture incidence. By contrast, controlled trials have demonstrated both a beneficial effect upon bone density and a decrease in spinal fracture for etidronate [7, 8], alendronate [26], transdermal estrogen treatment [27], salmon calcitonin [28, 29], and vitamin D metabolites [30]. Accordingly, changes in bone mass or density have become the standard means of assessing and reporting the effects of all bone-active agents from exercise to sodium fluoride [31].

However, what is the best site for assessing the efficacy of treatment? Total-body determinations of BMC and BMD have a low precision error, and the results are almost independent of operator analysis, making this a strong clinic test. Until 20 years ago total-body measurements using neutron activation in vivo were thought to be the best obtainable, and only therapies which increased total-body bone mass were considered effective [32, 33]. This has been forgotten over the past 20 years as researchers have devoted more attention to the effects of various agents on the spine – quite responsive; the proximal femur – intermediate in response; and the peripheral skeleton and total-body BMD – the least responsive.

Cortical and trabecular bone have a heterogeneous biochemical composition [34] and can react differently to specific treatments [35]. For example, fluoride may affect only trabecular bone [24] and another drug, such as parathormone, may induce positive effects on trabecular bone and negative effects on cortical bone [36]. For this reason it is important to evaluate osseous response to treatment at both cortical and trabecular level because these differences may determine whether the treatment of osteoporosis is beneficial.

Total-body BMC, because of its constant calcium proportion, reveals changes in skeletal calcium content. The total-body BMD differences found with respect to basal values were small using calcitonin [37], calcitriol [38, 39], and bisphosphonates [26] but always significant compared to control groups. Total-body DXA also enables us to evaluate major anatomical areas such as the spine and pelvis (axial bone) and the arms and legs (compact bone). The reproducibility of bone density of a single region is higher than that of the total body, ranging between 1% and 2% [40]. In addition, more bone is measured than in the regional analysis of the distal radius, representative of cortical bone (1g vs 1500 g), or the lumbar spine, as trabecular bone (40 g vs 1000 g). The pelvic region of whole-body density, composed mainly of trabecular bone, has been revealed to be more sensitive to hormonal changes, either spontaneous or induced by therapeutic intervention [37–41].

Precision of lumbar spine BMD measurements is sufficiently good (about 1%) to ascertain the changes in BMD in the follow-up of treated patients. Problems arise when the lumbar spine cannot be measured because of degenerative changes of the spine, frequent after 60 years, with extraskeletal calcification and changes in the distribution of fat and width of bones [42–44]. All of this makes the interpretation of changes in bone density at lumbar level difficult.

The QCT of the lumbar vertebrae could be the method of choice to monitor longitudinal changes in BMD due to the high responsiveness of this technique to detect change in trabecular bone, although it has a relatively high precision error. The high sensitivity of QCT in measuring age-related bone loss has been demonstrated in cross-sectional study. Generally bone loss rate in women is about 1.2%/year, about twice that found with posteroanterior lumbar DXA [45, 46]. The limiting factor is attendant radiation exposure, about 60 Sv including the dose for the localization radiograph, which is acceptable as a diagnostic test but is not compatible with serial measurements.

An alternative measurement site is the femoral neck, but although the changes in the BMD tend to be similar to those at lumbar spine, the precision error is higher [47].

Forearm BMD, especially the midradius, represents a measure of cortical bone, and it can be used to monitor BMD changes as another site because of small changes which can be detected after therapy. Morever, forearm BMD does not change with the same treatment that increases lumbar BMD, such as fluoride [24]. The radius may be measured at a more distal site which contains amounts of cancellous bone. It is uncertain whether cancellous bone at this site responds to therapeutic interventions in a manner similar to cancellous bone of the spine [48].

New approaches such as lateral DXA, peripheral QCT and quantitative ultrasound have recently been introduced, but their value in monitoring response to treatment has yet to be defined. The precision error (2%–4%) of lateral spine DXA is greater than that of anteroposterior spine BMD, and this offsets the advantages that it theoretically would have for monitoring loss or gain of bone [47], i.e., measuring bone with more metabolic activity in the body where fractures occur. Lateral spine DXA may be advantageous in the diagnostic approach to osteoporosis in older men and women characterized by a higher anteroposterior lumbar BMD due to osteophytes [49]. QCT of the peripheral skeleton is relatively insensitive to aging bone loss, and no data are available on therapy [50]. Ultrasound parameters, speed of sound (SOS) and broadband ultrasound attenuation (BUA), obtained with measurements at the os calcis have been demonstrated to be useful for diagnosis of osteoporosis and to evaluate fracture risk [51, 52]. The reproducibility is about 1% for SOS, 1.2%–2.5% for BUA, and 2% for stiffness, which represents a combination of SOS and BUA [53]. Stiffness has been demonstrated to increase with intranasal salmon calcitonin [54]. Since the magnitude of the increase results in about twice the precision error, stiffness could potentially be used for monitoring efficacy. Nevertheless other results indicated that long-term users of estrogen may be nonresponders with regards to the effect of estrogen on bone quality expressed in heel ultrasound values [55].

The method of choice for monitoring the effect of a treatment also depends on the treatment. Hormone replacement therapy prevents bone loss in all areas of the skeleton [56] and may thus be monitored by any BMD measurements; the technique used would therefore be the most precise method available. Considering that nonresponders to hormone replacement therapy are relatively rare [57], the question is whether bone density needs monitoring at all during such treatment. Repeating densitometric evaluation is justified in the presence of complicating factors, such as malabsorption or corticosteroid therapy, or to aid compliance [58]. With other antiosteoporotic drugs such as fluoride and calcitonin it may be necessary to measure BMD at several sites more often to identify non responders. The response to treatment at the lumbar spine tends to be the greatest of any skeletal site [59]. Newer bisphosphonates such as alendronate caused significant increases in BMD of 2.2%–8.8% to all skeletal sites, the effect being the most marked at the spine, with a mean percentage gain at 12 months of about 6% [60]. Hormone therapy increases spine BMD by 3.5%–5%, particularly during the first year of therapy, while the increase at femoral sites is only 1.5% [61]. The injection of salmon calcitonin at the dose of 50 U every other day for 1 year has shown to increase spine BMD by about 7%, while femur BMD is decreased by 3% [62]. The dose-related response to nasal calcitonin was manifested by an increase at lumbar spine level of 1% bone mineralization/100 UI calcitonin over 2 years [63]. Fluoride treatment promoted an increase in L2–L4 bone mass of 4%–5% per year and a mean increase in femural neck BMD of 2.4% per year [64]. After treatment with vitamin D analogs the spine BMD was increased by only a few percentage points (0.2%–0.6%) [65, 66].

In general bone mass, which should always be measured at baseline, should be monitored after 12 months of therapy has been completed. A decrease in bone mass of 2% or more indicates the need for a change in therapy, either a change in dosage or a change in medication. After a patient has experienced 1 full year of successful therapy, with either an increase in bone mass or a decrease of less than 2%, monitoring could be repeated yearly. Attention should be paid to the fact that the occurrence of an osteoporotic fracture within the first 6–12 months of therapy should not be taken as an indication of failed therapy [67].

The interpretation of BMD changes during therapy with antireabsorptive drugs must consider the "bone remodeling transient" [31]. The increase in BMD that is usually found after 1 year of therapy can be due to the filling of bone spaces that are undergoing remodeling: in the subsequent years we must expect less increase with respect to the first year.

For many physicians, and indeed many patients, a wait of up to 1 year to evaluate the efficacy of treatment is not welcome. A suitable alternative for measuring the response to therapy may be the use of biochemical markers of bone turnover [68]. These markers can reflect the enzymatic activity of the osteoblast and the osteoclast, for example, alkaline or acid phosphatase activity. They can be proteins synthesized by the bone forming cells, for example, osteocalcin and procollagen 1 extension peptides, or bone matrix components released into the circulation during resorption phase, such as hydroxyproline and the pyridinoline cross-links (urinary free pyridinoline and pyridinoline-containing type I collagen crosslinks peptides as serum C-telopeptide or urinary C-telopeptide and N-telopeptide). The most common markers currently used to assess formation are alkaline phosphatase, osteocalcin, and procollagen 1 extension peptides, all of which are serum measurements. Serum tartrate resistant phosphatase, urinary hydroxyproline, and pyridinoline cross-links are currently employed markers of bone resorption. The rate of bone turnover can be studied by measuring levels of one or more of the biochemical markers. Testing for biochemical markers is noninvasive and relatively inexpensive. Prospective studies over a 12-year period suggest that 80% of women can be correctly defined as fast or slow bone losers from the initial bone marker measurements [69]. The biochemical tests have 50% efficiency or more compared with direct methods of assessment by repeated measurements of bone loss [15]. Therefore the clinical utility of these techniques is twofold: they identify adults at high risk for the development of osteoporosis, and older adults with established osteoporosis and high rate of bone loss, so that aggressive therapy can be instituted to prevent or limit the disorder [70–72]. Bone formation and resorption markers are increased about 30% and 60%, respectively, in postmenopausal women, with higher values in subjects with the lowest BMD levels [73]. They also provide a noninvasive, sensitive, and dynamic tool for monitoring the clinical course and effect of therapy.

Serum alkaline phosphatase and osteocalcin levels are increased in osteoporotic patients treated with fluoride, and these measurements have been proposed for monitoring the efficacy of this drug to stimulate bone formation [74]. Also the administration of calcitriol promotes bone formation as shown by the increase in osteocalcin [75,76]. Estrogens induce a significant decrease in both the formation and the resorption markers that fall in the premenopausal range [77–81]. Nevertheless a transient decrease of 30% was found during estrogen therapy on bone resorption markers, with return to baseline after treatment was stopped. Also in older women, those aged over 70 years, conjugated estrogens reduce markers of bone turnover. This change is considered useful in assessing the response to treatment in this age group [82]. Salmon calcitonin is able to decrease bone markers [83]. It is known that high bone turnover patients, assessed by a number of biochemical bone markers, respond better to intramuscularly administered salmon calcitonin than those characterized as normal or low bone turnover patients [62, 84]. On the other hand, a recent study comparing various doses of alendronate found a clear dose-dependent decrease in serum osteocalcin and urinary pyridinoline at the end of the 6-week treatment [85]. Moreover, in late postmenopausal osteoporotic women with alendronate treatment the levels of bone markers were reduced to the normal premenopausal range, and this steady state was maintained from 6–15 months [86]. The behavior of free and peptide-bound cross-link excretion varies with the treatment: bisphosphonate therapy decreases markedly cross-linked peptides without change in free cross-link excretion while with estrogen therapy a decrease in both free and peptide-bound cross-links was found [87].

These results suggest that bone turnover markers can be used to predict the bone mass response to antireabsorptive therapy. On the other hand, other studies have shown that the measure of individual serum and urine markers of bone turnover cannot predict variance in bone density change at spine and femur sites in estrogenized women [88].

The typical reduction in bone resorption markers with antireabsorptive therapy has been found to be in the order of 30%–60%. Given the good precision of the majority of the bone markers, about 10% for serum markers, the effect of the treatment can be detected after a short period of time (3–6 months).

However, most of the biochemical markers are currently limited to the research area. Among bone formation markers, osteocalcin is preferred to alkaline phosphatase and carboxyterminal propeptide of type I procollagen because of ease of assay and sensitivity [80]. All of these serum markers show high variability among subjects (20%–45%) but low temporal variation (5%–10%) [89]. As regards resorption markers, clinical use in individual assessment is made difficult by large day-to-day variability [90–92], especially all for urinary markers (from 20% to 35%). For example, N-telopeptide of type I collagen has proven valuable for monitoring changes in bone turnover in individual patients when a 50% reduction in bone turnover is possible as a result of therapy [93]. Bone markers are also influenced by circadian rhythms with a wider variation in markers of bone resorption than of bone formation. The nocturnal increase in urinary deoxypyridinoline and cross-linked N-telopeptide of type I collagen is about 30%, while the increase in osteocalcin and procollagen type I carboxyl-terminal propeptides is 10%–20% [94–97]. The problem of circadian rhythm in turnover markers is confounded by a rhythm in creatinine, which is often used to normalize resorption markers [98]; thus the daily variation in urinary N-telopeptide is reduced from 30% to 20%. In order to use the result normalized for creatinine it is necessary to sample at the same time each day, preferably in the morning [99]. On average a urine sample collected early in the afternoon gives a 22% higher N-telopeptide/creatinine value than in the early evening and 22% lower than in the morning [98]. Another way to reduce day-to-day variability is to obtain at least two measurements after starting therapy; for this purpose it has been suggested to pool urine samples for a week and then perform one assay [100].

Reliable and convenient tests for quantifying bone turnover would be of help in measuring the response to therapy in osteoporosis. Immunoassays for novel bone metabolites have been reported in research literature, with data indicating improved specificity and responsiveness. The transfer of research methods to clinical care is often difficult. Indeed, performance data for longitudinal studies on individual subjects are few. However, bone markers are likely to improve the efficacy of assessing the effect of an antiosteoporotic agent. We believe that to optimize the approach to monitoring treatment it is necessary to integrate the use of bone markers with the evaluation of bone density which still remains an irreplaceable measure.

References

1. Reginster JY, Compston JE, Jones EA et al (1995) Recommendations for the registration of new chemical entities used in the prevention and treatment of osteoporosis. Calcif Tissue Int 57:247–250
2. Eastell R, Cedel SL, Wahner HW, Riggs BL, Melton LJ III (1991) Classification of vertebral fractures. J Bone Miner Res 6:207–215
3. McCloskey EV, Spector TD, Eyres KS et al (1993) The assessement of vertebral deformity. A method for use in population studies and clinical trials. Osteoporosis Int 3:138–147
4. National Osteoporosis Foundation Working Group on Vertebral Fractures (1995) Assessing vertebral fractures. J Bone Miner Res 10:518–523
5. Genant HK, Jergas M, Palermo L et al (1996) Comparison of semiquantitative visual and quantitative morphometric assessement of prevalent and incident vertebral fractures in osteoporosis. J Bone Miner Res 11:984–996
6. O'Neill TW, Felsenberg D, Varlow J, Cooper C, Kanis JA, Silman AJ (1996) The prevalence of vertebral deformity in European men and women: the European Vertebral Osteoporosis Study. J Bone Miner Res 11:1010–1018
7. Storm T, Thamsborg G, Steiniche T, Genant HK, Sorenson OH (1990) Effect of intermittent cyclical etidronate therapy on bone mass and fracture rate in women with postmenopausal osteoporosis. N Engl J Med 322:1265–1271

8.　Watts NB, Harris ST, Genant HK et al (1990) Intermittent cyclical etidronate treatment of postmenopausal osteoporosis. N Engl J Med 323:73–79

9.　Leidig-Bruckneer G, Genant HK, Minne HW et al (1994) Comparison of a semi-quantitative and quantitative method for assessing vertebral fractures in osteoporosis. Osteoporosis Int 3:154–161

10.　Nguyen T, Sambrook P, Kelly P et al (1993) Prediction of osteoporotic fractures by postural instability and bone density. Br Med J 307:1111–1115

11.　Hui SL, Slemenda CW, Johnston CC (1988) Age and bone mass as predictors of fracture in a prospective study. J Clin Invest 81:1804–1809

12.　Wasnich RD, Ross PD, Heirbrum LK, Vogel JM (1987) Selection of the optimal site for fracture risk prediction. Clin Orthop 216:262–268

13.　Gardsell P, Johnell O, Nilsson BE (1991) The predictive value of bone loss for fragility fractures in women: a longitudinal study over 15 years. Calcif Tissue Int 49:90–94

14.　Kanis JA, Melton LJ III, Christiansen C, Johnston CC, Khaltaev N (1994) The diagnosis of osteoporosis. J Bone Miner Res 9:1137–1141

15.　Kanis JA, WHO Study Group (1994) Assessement of fracture risk and its application to screening for postmenopausal osteoporosis: synopsis of a WHO report. Osteoporosis Int 4:368–381

16.　Melton LJ, Atkinson EJ, O'Fallon WM, Wahner HW, Riggs BL (1993) Long-term fracture prediction by bone mineral assessed at different skeletal sites. J Bone Miner Res 8:1227–1233

17.　Genant HK, Engelke K, Fuerst T et al (1996) Noninvasive assessment of bone mineral and structure: state of the art. J Bone Miner Res 11:707–730

18.　Gluer CC, Blake G, Lu Y, Blunt BA, Jergas M, Genant HK (1995) Accurate assessment of precision errors: how to measure the reproducibility of bone densitometry techniques. Osteoporosis Int 5:262–270

19.　Hassager C, Jensen SB, Gotfredsen A, Christiansen C (1991) The impact of measurement errors on the diagnostic value of bone mass measurements: theoretical considerations. Osteoporosis Int 1:250–256

20.　Genant HK, Block JE, Steiger P, Gluer CC, Ettinger B, Harris ST (1988) Appropriate use of bone densitometry. Radiology 170:817–822

21.　Ryan PJ, Blake GM, Herd R, Parker J, Fogelman I (1993) Spine and femur BMD by DXA in patients with varying severity spinal osteoporosis. Calcif Tissue Int 52:263–268

22.　Fuleihan GE-H, Testa MA, Angell JE, Porrino N, Leboff MS (1995) Reproducibility of DXA absorptiometry: a model for bone loss estimates. J Bone Miner Res 10:1004–1014

23.　Eisman JA (1995) Efficacy of treatment of osteoporotic fractures. Am J Med 98(S2A):17S–23S

24.　Riggs BL, Hodgson SF, O'Fallon WM et al (1990) Effect of fluoride treatment on fracture rate in postmenopausal women with osteoporosis. N Engl J Med 332:802–809

25.　Kleerekoper M, Peterson EL, Nelson DA et al (1991) A randomized trial of sodium fluoride as a treatment for postmenopausal osteoporosis. Osteoporosis Int 1:155–161

26. Lieberman UA, Weiss SR, Broll J et al (1995) Effect of oral alendronate on bone mineral density and the incidence of fractures in postmenopausal osteoporosis. N Engl J Med 333:1437–1443

27. Lufkin EG, Wahner HW, O'Fallon WM (1992) Treatment of postmenopausal osteoporosis with transdermal estrogen. Ann Intern Med 117:1–9

28. Gennari C, Chierichetti SM, Bigazzi S et al (1985) Comparative effects on bone mineral content of calcium plus salmon calcitonin given in two different regimens in postmenopausal osteoporosis. Curr Ther Res 38:455–464

29. Rico H, Hernandez ER, Revilla M, Gomez-Castresana F (1992) Salmon calcitonin reduces vertebral fracture rate in postmenopausal crush fracture syndrome. Bone Miner 16:131–138

30. Gallagher JC, Riggs BL, Recker RR, Golgar D (1989) The effect of calcitriol on patients with postmenopausal osteoporosis with special reference to fracture frequency. Proc Soc Exp Biol Sci 191:287–292

31. Heaney RP (1995) Interpreting trials of bone-active agents. Am J Med 98:329–330

32. Cohn SH (1982) Techniques for determining the efficacy of treatment of osteoporosis. Int J Calcif Tissue 34:433–438

33. Gruber HE, Ivey JL, Baylink DJ et al (1984) Long-term calcitonin therapy in postmenopausal osteoporosis. Metabolism 33:295–303

34. Ninomiya JT, Tracy RP, Calore JD, Gendreau MA, Kelm RJ, Mann KG (1990) Heterogenity of human bone. J Bone Miner Res 5:933–938

35. Laan RFJM, Buijs WCAM, van Erning LJTO et al (1993) Differential effects of glucocorticoids on cortical appendicular and cortical vertebral bone mineral content. Calcif Tissue Int 52:5–9

36. Reeve J, Davies UM, Hesp R, McNally E, Katz D (1990) Treatment of osteoporosis with human parathyroid peptide and observation on effect of sodium fluoride. Br J Med 301:314–318

37. Rico H, Revilla M, Hernandez ER, Villa LF, Alvarez de Buergo M (1995) Total and regional bone mineral content and fracture rate in postmenopausal osteoporosis treated with salmon calcitonin: a prospective study. Calcif Tissue Int 56:181–185

38. Gallagher JC, Goldgar D (1990) Treatment of postmenopausal osteoporosis with high doses of synthetic calcitriol. Ann Intern Med 113:649–655

39. Nuti R, Martini G, Valenti R, Giovani (1996) Open-label, controlled study on the metabolic and absorptiometric effects of calcitriol in involutional osteoporosis. Clin Drug Invest 11:270–277

40. Nuti R, Martini G, Righi G, Frediani B, Turchetti V (1991) Comparison of total body measurements by dual-energy X-ray absorptiometry and dual-photon absorptiometry. J Bone Miner Res 6:681–687

41. Rico H. Revilla M, Hernandez ER, Villa LF, Alvarez de Buergo M (1992) Is pelvic bone mineral content assessed through dual energy X-ray absorp-

tiometry a good measure of bone mass loss in women? Clin Rheumatol 11:508–511

42. Orwoll ES, Oviatt SK, Mann T (1990) The impact of osteophytic and vascular calcifications on vertebral mineral density measurements in men. J Clin Endocrinol Metab 70:1202–1207

43. Reid IR, Evans MC, Ames R, Wattie DJ (1991) The influence of osteophytes and aortic calcification on spinal mineral density in postmenopausal women. J Clin Endocrinol Metab 72:1372–1374

44. Yu W, Gluer CC, Fuerst T et al (1995) Influence of degenerative joint disease on spinal bone mineral measurements in postmenopausal women. Calcif Tissue Int 57:169–174

45. Genant HK, Steiger P, Block JE et al (1987) Quantitative computed tomography: update 1987. Calcif Tissue Int 41:179–186

46. Guglielmi G, Grimston SK, Fischer KC, Pacifici R (1994) Osteoporosis: diagnosis with lateral and posteroanterior dual X-ray absorptiometry compared with quantitative CT. Radiology 192:845–850

47. Mazess RB, Barden HS, Eberle RW, Drue Denton M (1995) Age changes of spine density in posterior-anterior and lateral projections in normal women. Calcif Tissue Int 56:201–205

48. Riis BJ, Christiansen C (1988) Measurements of spinal or peripheral bone mass to estimate early postmenopausal bone loss ? Am J Med 84:646–653

49. Slosman DO, Rizzoli R, Donath A, Bonjour J-P (1990) Vertebral bone mineral density measured laterally by dual-energy X-ray absorptiometry. Osteoporosis Int 1:23–29

50. Grampp S, Jergas M, Lang P et al (1996) Quantitative CT assessement of the lumbar spine and radius in patients with osteoporosis. AJR 167:133–140

51. Heaney RP, Avioli LV, Chesnut CH III, Lappe J, Recker RR, Brandenburger GH (1995) Ultrasound velocity through bone predicts incident vertebral deformity. J Bone Miner Res 10:341–345

52. Hans D, Dargent-Molina P, Schott AM et al (1996) Ultrasonographic heel measurements to predict hip fracture in the elderly women: the EPIDOS prospective study. Lancet 348:511–514

53. Cepollaro C, Zacchei F, Borracelli D et al (1992) Precision of new ultrasound bone densitometers: correlation with absorptiometry methods. In: Proceedings of ultrasonic assessement of bone II, Bath, 23 June, p 19

54. Gonnelli S, Cepollaro C, Pondrelli C, Martini S, Rossi S, Gennari C (1996) Ultrasound parameters in osteoporotic patients treated with salmon calcitonin: a longitudinal study. Osteoporosis Int 6:303–307

55. Naessen T, Mallmin H, Ljunghall S (1995) Heel ultrasound in women after long-term ERT compared with bone densities in the forearm, spine and hip. Osteoporosis Int 5:205–210

56. Gotfredsen A, Riis BJ, Christiansen C (1986) Total and local bone mineral during estrogen treatment: a placebo controlled trial. Bone Miner 1:167–173

57. Hassager C, Jensen SB, Christiansen C (1994) Non-responders to hormone

replacement therapy for the prevention of postmenopausal bone loss. Do they exist ? Osteoporosis Int 4:36–41

58. Kanis JA, Devogelaer JP, Gennari C (1996) Practical guide for the use of bone mineral measurements in the assessement of treatment of osteoporosis: a position paper of the European Foundation for Osteoporosis and Bone Disease. Osteoporosis Int 6:256–261

59. Eastell R (1996) Assessement of bone density and bone loss. Osteoporosis Int [Suppl] 2:S3–S5

60. Tucci JR, Tonino RP, Emkey RD et al (1996) Effect of three years of oral alendronate treatment in postmenopausal women with osteoporosis. Am J Med 101:488–501

61. PEPI Trial Writing Group (1996) Effects of hormone therapy on bone mineral density. JAMA 276:1389–1396

62. Civitelli R, Gonnelli S, Zacchei S et al (1988) Bone turnover in postmenopausal osteoporosis: effect of calcitonin treatment. J Clin Invest 82:1268–1274

63. Overgaard K, Hansen MA, Jensen SB, Christiansen C (1992) Effect of salcatonin given intranasally on bone mass and fracture rates in established osteoporosis: a dose-response study. Br Med J 305:556–561

64. Pak CYC, Sakhaee K, Adams-Huet B, Piziack V, Peterson RD, Poindexter JR (1995) Treatment of postmenopausal osteoporosis with slow-release sodium fluoride. Ann Intern Med 123:401–408

65. Aloia JF, Vaswani A, Yeh JK, Ellis K, Yasumura S, Cohn SH (1988) Calcitriol treatment of postmenopausal osteoporosis. Am J Med 84:401–408

66. Orimo H, Shiraki M, Hayashi Y et al (1994) Effects of 1α-hydroxyvitamin D3 on lumbar bone mineral density and vertebral fractures in patients with postmenopausal osteoporosis. Calcif Tissue Int 54:370–376

67. Kleerekoper M, Avioli LV (1996) Evaluation and treatment of postmenopausal osteoporosis. In: Favus MJ (ed) Primer on the metabolic bone diseases and disorders of mineral metabolism. Lippincott-Raven, Philadelphia, pp 264–271

68. Eastell R (1994) Biochemical markers. Spine State Art Rev 8:155–170

69. Hansen M, Overgard K, Riis B, Christiansen C (1991) Role of peak bone mass and bone loss in postmenopausal osteoporosis. BMJ 303:961–964

70. Christiansen C, Riis BJ, Rodbro P (1987) Prediction of rapid bone loss in postmenopausal women. Lancet 1:1105–1108

71. Uebelhart D, Schlemmer A, Johansen JS, Gineyts E, Christiansen C, Delmas PD (1991) Effect of menopause and hormone replacement therapy on the urinary excretion of pyridinoline cross-links. J Clin Endocrinol Metab 72:367–373

72. Dresner-Pollak R, Parker RA, Poku M, Thompson J, Seibel MJ, Greenspan SL (1996) Biochemical markers of bone turnover reflect femoral bone loss in elderly women. Calcif Tissue Int 59:328–333

73. Garnero P, Sornay-Rendu E, Chapuy MC, Delmas PD (1996) Increased bone turnover in late postmenopausal women is a major determinant of osteoporosis. J Bone Miner Res 11:337–349

74. Boivin G, Dupuis J, Meunier PJ (1993) Fluoride and osteoporosis. In: Simopoulos AP, Galli C (eds) Osteoporosis: nutritional aspects. World Rev Nutr Diet 73:80–103

75. Geusens P, Vanderschueren D, Verstraeten A, Dequeker J, Devos P, Bouillon R (1991) Short term course of 1,25(OH)2D3 stimulates osteoblasts but not osteoclasts in osteoporosis and osteoarthritis. Calcif Tissue Int 49:168–173

76. Caniggia A, Nuti R, Galli M, Lorè F, Turchetti V, Righi G (1986) Effect of a long-term treatment with 1,25 dihydroxyvitamin D3 on osteocalcin in postmenopausal osteoporosis. Calcif Tissue Int 38:328–332

77. Hasling C, Eriksen EF, Melkko J et al (1991) Effects of a combined estrogen-gestagen regimen on serum levels of the carboxy-terminal propeptide of human type I procollagen in osteoporosis. J Bone Miner Res 6:1295–1300

78. Seibel MJ, Cosman F, Shen V et al (1993) Urinary hydroxypyridinium crosslinks of collagen as markers of bone resorption and estrogen efficacy in postmenopausal osteoporosis. J Bone Miner Res 8:881–889

79. Hassager C, Jensen LT, Podenphant J, Thomsen K, Christiansen C (1994) The carboxy-terminal pyridinoline cross-linked telopeptide of type I collagen in serum as a marker of bone resorption: the effect of nandrolone decanoate and hormone replacement therapy. Calcif Tissue Int 54:30–33

80. Alexandersen P, Hassager C, Riis BJ (1995) The effect of menopause and hormone replacement therapy on bone alkaline phosphatase. Scand J Clin Lab Invest 55:571–576

81. Riis BJ, Overgaard K, Christiansen C (1995) Biochemical markers of bone turnover to monitor the bone response to postmenopausal hormone replacement therapy. Osteoporosis Int 5:276–280

82. Prestwood KM, Pilbeam CC, Burleson JA et al (1994) The short term effects of conjugated estrogen on bone turnover in older women. J Clin Endocrinol Metab 79:366–371

83. Nielsen NM, von der Recke P, Hansen MA, Overgaard K, Christiansen C (1994) Estimation of the effect of salmon calcitonin in established osteoporosis by biochemical bone markers. Calcif Tissue Int 55:8–11

84. Lyritis GP, Magiasis B, Tsakalakos N (1995) Prevention of bone loss in early nonsurgical and nonosteoporotic high turnover patients with salmon calcitonin: the role of biochemical bone markers in monitoring high turnover patients under calcitonin treatment. Calcif Tissue Int 56:38–41

85. Harris ET, Gertz BJ, Genant HK et al (1993) The effect of short term treatment with alendronate on vertebral density and biochemical markers of bone remodeling in early postmenopausal women. J Clin Endocrinol Metab 76:1399–1403

86. Garnero P, Shih WJ, Gineyts E, Karpf DB, Delmas PD (1994) Comparison of new biochemical markers of bone turnover in late postmenopausal osteoporotic women in response to alendronate treatment. J Clin Endocrinol Metab 79:1693–1700

87. Garnero P, Gineyts E, Arbault P, Christiansen C, Delmas PD (1995) Different

effects of bisphosphonate and estrogen therapy on free and peptide-bound bone cross-links excretion. J Bone Miner Res 10:641–649

88. Cosman F, Nieves J, Wilkinson C, Schnering D, Shen V, Lindsay R (1996) Bone density change and biochemical indices of skeletal turnover. Calcif Tissue Int 58:236–243

89. Panteghini M, Pagani F (1995) Biological variation in bone-derived biochemical markers in serum. Scand J Lab Invest 55:609–616

90. Beck Jensen JE, Kollerup G, Sorensen HA, Thamsborg G, Sorensen HA (1994) Biological variation of biochemical bone markers. Scand J Clin Lab Invest 54 [Suppl 219]:36–39

91. Morris HA, Cleghom DB, Need AG, Horowitz M, Nordin BEC (1995) The 5-year reproducibility of calcium-related biochemical variables in post-menopausal women. Scand J Clin Lab Invest 55:383–389

92. Blumshon A, Hannon RA, Al-Dehaimi AW, Eastell R (1994) Short-term intraindividual variability of markers of bone turnover in healthy adults. J Bone Miner Res 9 [Suppl 1]:S153

93. Gertz BJ, Shao P, Hanson DA et al (1994) Monitoring bone resorption in early postmenopausal women by an immunoassay for cross-linked collagen peptides in urine. J Bone Miner Res 9:135–142

94. Hassager C, Risteli J, Risteli L, Jensen SB, Christiansen C (1992) Diurnal variation in serum markers of type I collagen synthesis and degradation in healthy premenopausal women. J Bone Miner Res 7:1307–1311

95. Eastell R, Simmons PS, Colwell A et al (1992) Nyctohemeral changes in bone turnover assessed by serum bone Gla-protein concentrations and urinary deoxypyridinoline excretion: effects of growth and ageing. Clin Sci 83:375–382

96. Blumshon A, Herrington K, Hannon RA, Shao P, Eyre DR, Eastell R (1994) The effect of calcium supplementation on the circadian rhythm of bone resorption. J Clin Endocrinol Metab 79:730–735

97. Pedersen BJ, Schlemmer A, Rosenquist C, Hassager C, Christiansen C (1995) Circadian rhythm in type collagen formation in postmenopausal women with and without osteopenia. Osteoporosis Int 5:472–477

98. Bollen AM, Martin MD, Leroux BG, Eyre DR (1995) Circadian variation in urinary excretion of bone collagen cross-links. J Bone Miner Res 10:1885–1890

99. Panteghini M, Pagani F (1996) Biological variation in urinary excretion of pyridinium crosslinks: reccomendations for the optimum specimen. Ann Clin Biochem 33:36–42

100. Popp-Snijders C, Lips P, Netenlenbos JC (1996) Intra-individual variation in bone resorption markers in urine. Ann Clin Biochem 33:347–348

28 Periprosthetic Bone Mineral Density and Other Orthopedic Applications

C. Trevisan and S. Ortolani

Introduction

Bone quality is a crucial concept in orthopedic practice. When implanting a total hip prosthesis or placing a transpeduncular screw, one needs to know the mechanical consistency and biological reactivity of the host bone. These two components, the mass-related mechanical properties and the biological ability to remodel and adapt, are what have been called bone quality [155]. They have been studied extensively histologically, roentgenographically, and scintigraphically since fracture fixation devices, prosthetic implants, and limb lengthening instrumentaries were introduced into the orthopedic surgery [32, 83, 106, 155]. In this regard a noninvasive and quantitative measurement of bone mass should have been considered a major advance for further insight into bone quality. However, after its development bone densitometry found early but few applications in the orthopedic field.

Single-photon absorptiometry (SPA) was used in some investigations despite the intrinsic limits of the method such as the low spatial resolution, its necessity of a standardized overall thickness of soft tissues, and its low accuracy [114]. The greatest disadvantage of SPA, the impossibility of measuring bone mass when soft tissues of different composition and thickness are present, was solved by dual-photon absorptiometry (DPA), but DPA had drawbacks in terms of space resolution, precision and scan time so that bone densitometry diffusion in orthopedics remained confined to few studies.

A critical step in the field was represented by the introduction of dual X-ray absorptiometry (DXA) for fast and quantitative measurement of bone mass at several skeletal sites. The use of roentgenographic tubes as photon generators provides higher beam intensity and improved spatial resolution, precision, and accuracy [114, 129]. Eventually DXA instruments were provided with metal-removal software which allows the evaluation of bone mineral content (BMC) and density (BMD) in the proximity of metal implants by their automatic insulation through recognition of extreme density outside the normal range of bone. In recent years these advancements have led to a widespread use of DXA in fields other than metabolic bone disease.

Several studies on accuracy and precision have recognized the validity of DXA in the field of metabolic bone diseases. Its feasibility in the orthopedic field has been proven in methodological studies on specific applications, and this is discussed in the following sections.

Bone densitometry was also compared with other semiquantitative and quantitative methods for a noninvasive assessment of bone mass described in the orthopedic literature: visual and computer-processing of roentgenograms, quantitative computed tomography (QCT), magnetic resonance imaging (MRI) and three-dimensional finite element models generated from CT data.

Roentgenographic visual inspection, computer processing of roentgenograms, and DXA were compared ex vivo in their ability to disclose bone loss in the presence of a knee prosthesis by Robertson et al. [140]. In this study visual processing of roentgenograms and computer processing of roentgenograms detected losses of, respectively, 25% or more and 8% or more whereas DXA was able to disclose bone losses below 8%. The determination of BMC by DXA was highly correlated with ash content (r=1.00, p<0.001), and the difference between the measurements made by DXA with the prosthesis in place and those made without it in place was below 4% (Fig. 28-1). The determination of bone mass with DXA and computer processing of roentgenograms was, respectively, seven times and three times more accurate than the visual readings. The authors concluded that DXA was superior to the other methods considered, and that it may be used to quantify accurately bone mineral changes in metaphyseal regions after a joint replacement.

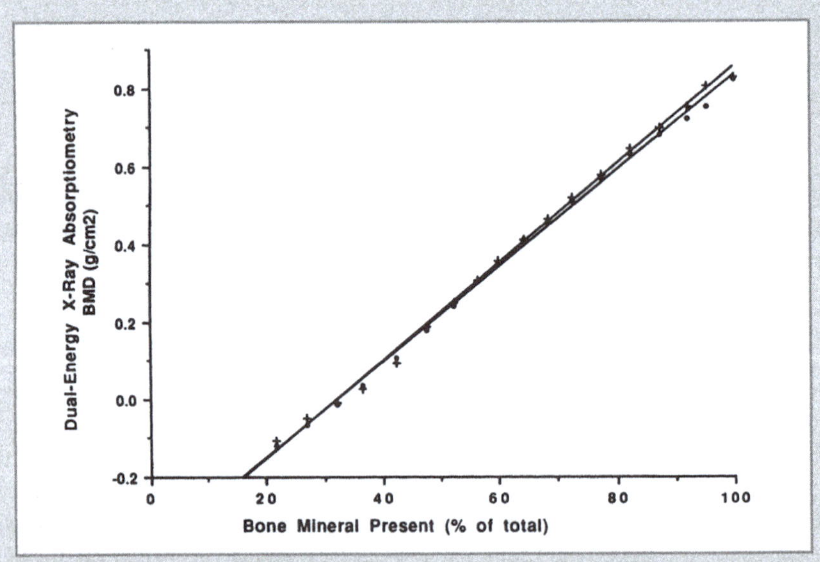

Fig. 28-1 Current bone densitometers are equipped with specific software which allows the removal of metal objects from the analysis of bone mineral content, retaining excellent characteristics of accuracy. In this study there was a substantial equivalence of the bone density measured in autoptic specimens of distal femora with (+) or without (−) the femoral prosthetic component in place. Furthermore, there was a high linear correlation between the bone density measured by DXA and the percentage of bone mineral at each measurement as determined by ash weight (r=0.998, p<0.001). (From [140])

In another study, Markel et al. [109] compared bone densitometry techniques (SPA and DXA) with other noninvasive imaging modalities (QCT, MR) in their ability to quantitatively evaluate tibial osteotomy healing in dogs. Correlations were evaluated of the four techniques with the torsional properties and with the local stiffness properties and calcium content of the healing bone (as determined by invasive techniques). Eighteen very small regions of interest (ROIs) in the coronal plane were considered for invasive and noninvasive determinations: six areas of periostal callus, six of endostal callus, four of cortex, and two of gap tissue. Despite the modest correlations with calcium content, which ranged from 0.16 to 0.69 and were probably due to the very small ROIs used, SPA and DXA showed significant correlations with torsional and local stiffness properties not different from those observed with QCT (r=0.18–0.73). MR showed the poorest associations with the local parameters studied. Markel et al. concluded that the possibility to predict the ultimate torque of the healing bone by noninvasive bone mass measurement techniques could lead to very interesting clinical applications.

Skinner et al. combined the results of finite element stress analysis of uncemented femoral stems implanted ex vivo with quantitative BMD measured in vivo by DXA at periods after implantation and found a significant correlation between finite element models and DXA data (Fig. 28-2) [149]; in one case the superimposition of calculated stress values and bone density data from DXA was impres-

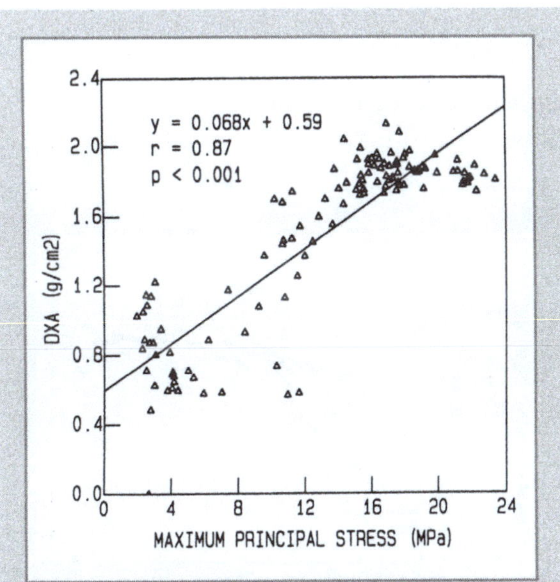

Fig. 28-2 Bone redistribution after THA as determined by DXA is mainly affected by stress parameters, as shown by linear regression between bone density values measured by DXA and absolute value of maximum principal stress generated by finite element stress analysis at different levels of an uncemented femoral stem. (From [149])

sive (Fig. 28-3). Their results confirm that the bone mass redistribution after stem insertion is driven mainly by stress redistribution, and that DXA is effective in the monitoring of stress and bone rearrangement after total hip arthroplasty.

The main limitation of DXA is that measured bone density is a function of the projected area of the scanned bone, therefore a two-dimensional density and not a true volumetric density. In a study of six femoral specimens retrieved from three patients treated with unilateral uncemented prosthesis, McGovern et al. compared true volumetric bone density measured by calibrated videodensitometry with two-dimensional bone density measured by DXA in different transverse sections perpendicular to the long axis of the diaphysis of the femur [118]. A strong correlation was found between DXA analysis of intact specimens and the quadrant analysis of the sectioned femora by calibrated videodensitometry ($R^2 = 0.80$, $p < 0.001$) showing that periprosthetic bone density measured by DXA is closely related to the volumetric cortical density and confirming the clinical role of DXA for quantification of remodeling after total hip arthroplasty (Fig. 28-4).

The number of dedicated methodological investigations and their results fully support the interest arisen in bone densitometry in the orthopedic field. The different DXA applications recently emerged can be arranged in two main areas: the assessment of bone reaction to metal implants and the assessment of bone healing and bone regeneration. Specific applications are recognized for each area:
- Assessment of bone reaction to metal implants
    - Total hip arthroplasty
    - Total knee arthroplasty
    - Other implants
- Assessment of bone healing and bone regeneration
    - Bone healing after fracture

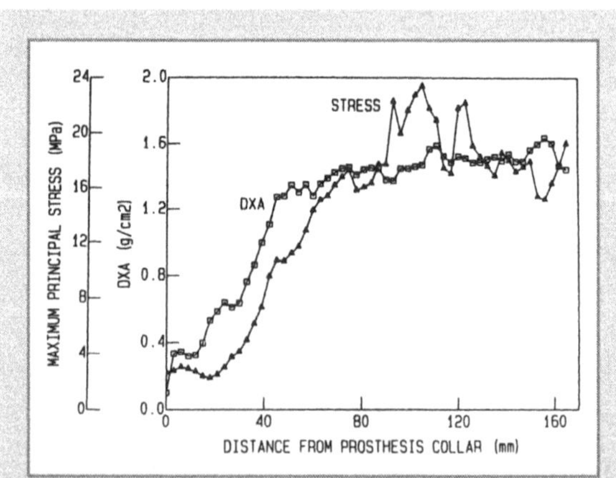

Fig. 28-3 The relationship between bone redistribution and absolute values of maximum principal stress after femoral stem insertion is striking when data are scaled and superimposed. (From [149])

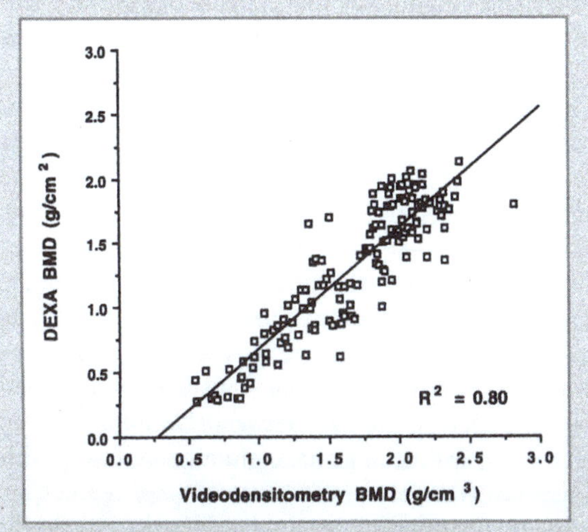

Fig. 28-4 A limitation of DXA is that measured bone density is a two dimensional density and not a true volumetric density. Nevertheless, there is a significant correlation between DXA analysis of intact specimens and the quadrant analysis of the sectioned femora by calibrated videodensitometry of slab radiographs, confirming the efficiency of DXA for the quantification of remodeling after THA. (From [118])

- New bone formation during limb lengthening
- Post-traumatic osteopenia

Assessment of Bone Reaction to Metal Implants

Joint replacement has become a common procedure for the treatment of degenerative joint diseases. Every year over 300 000 total hip arthroplasties (THA) and total knee arthroplasties (TKA) are implanted in the United States [66]. The considerable improvements in surgical and anesthesiological techniques and in prosthetic biomaterials and design make joint replacement a safe procedure. Nevertheless, a lifelong implant does not exist, and early failures are registered in a small but significant number of cases. Moreover, a consistent number of the remaining implants can last for more than 15 years [2, 177], allowing the manifestation of bone aging processes such as bone loss and medullary enlargement which could threaten a longer survival [136]. Considering the large number of patients involved, the impact of the procedure on the quality of life, and the severe consequences of implant failure, the monitoring of prostheses has become mandatory in order to improve their longevity.

The longevity of implants depends on the mechanical stability achieved and on the integration with the hosting bone, that is, the interaction between the quality of the hosting bone and the implant and the adopted surgical procedures

(Fig. 28-5) [56, 107]. At present several diagnostic tools provide direct and indirect information on mechanical stability and biological competence of bone (Fig. 28-6) [107].

Unfortunately there is no a single diagnostic procedure that provides conclusive information on the various potential problems arising from a prosthetic implant or a predictive basis about its durability and final outcome. Traditional roentgenograms give direct information on prosthetic position and bone morphology [38, 81] but semiquantitative information on bone status [21, 36, 174] and indirect and often indefinite information on osseointegration or pathological events [32]. Various scoring scales have been developed based on morphological response, such as osteolysis, medial neck rounding, corticocancellization, bone spur or changes in cortical dimensions, and alterations in visible bone density [31, 57, 60, 67, 141]. Unfortunately, the correspondence between radiographic and histological [97, 155] or clinical [71, 84, 86] findings have often been disappointing even when a recent investigation was able to establish a better correlation between roentgenographic signs and histological findings [34]. Furthermore, the absence of interobserver agreement in the assessment of radiographic outcomes calls into question their reliability [117].

Three phase radionuclide bone scans reflect physiological abnormalities with increased blood flow because of an inflammatory response or increased osteogenic

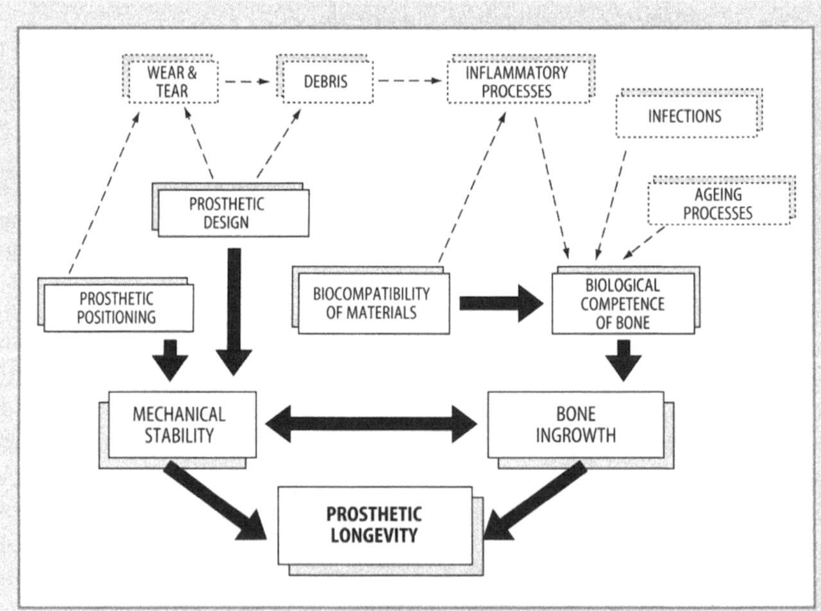

Fig. 28-5 Factors affecting longevity of articular prostheses. Mechanical stability and biological integration are the essential conditions for a positive outcome on which different factors interact. Solid lines, reciprocal interactions; dashed lines, potential pathological events. (From [107])

activity due to abnormal stress or bone repair. Even when a radionuclide bone scan can be useful together with clinical and radiographic examination, its results remain unspecific, and its exact role in prosthesis monitoring has yet to be defined [83]. Histology and mechanical tests are essential but invasive and not feasible for everyday clinical practice. Finally, two- and three-dimensional computed finite element models, now available as experimental source of data, have no diagnostic purposes or clinical applications at present [73, 75].

In this regard, the role of DXA is complementary to the existing techniques which may add valuable direct information on bone mass hence on bone mechanical properties and indirect information on bone biological competence through the monitoring of bone remodeling. In the different phases of joint replacement – before surgery, during prosthetic surveillance, and in the case of revision – this additional information is aimed at different items. Before surgery the bone status evaluation of the patient can lead to the choice of the prosthetic device and to the type of fixation since the mechanical properties of the host bone are related to bone density [25, 63, 110]. In the case of uncemented THA some studies suggest that the osseointegration of the prosthesis is achieved only if micromotions are avoided by means of a strong primary stability [52, 65, 70, 135]. The primary stability is obtained with press-fit design which requires a mechanically sound bone; therefore most surgeons believe that uncemented prostheses are indicated in the

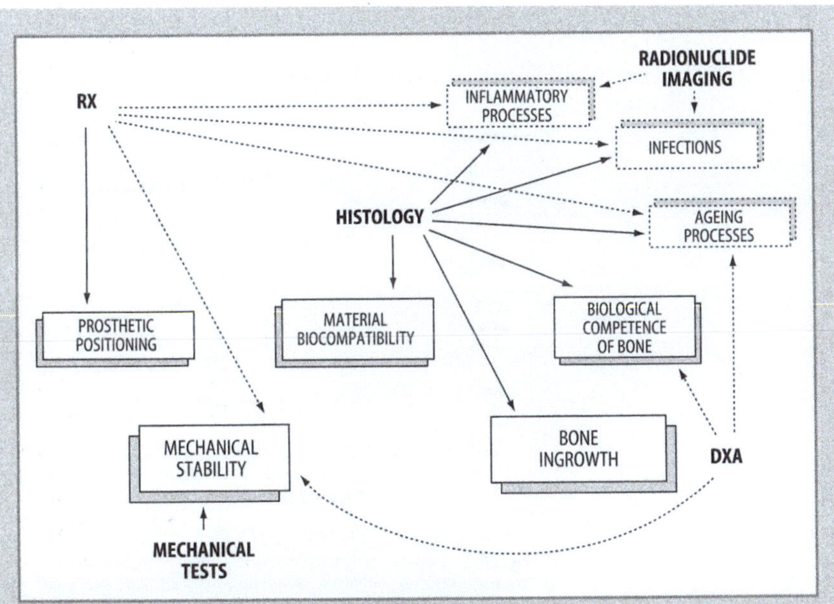

Fig. 28-6 The present diagnostic methods give us direct (solid lines) and indirect (dashed lines) information on some of the factors influencing prosthetic longevity. The less invasive and more available techniques provide mainly indirect information, therefore, an integration of available data is desirable to reduce uncertainty. (From [107])

presence of a valid bone stock [23, 142, 147] while cemented prostheses provide an almost instantaneous stability by means of the cement-bone microinterlock even when osteopenic bone is present.

Other criteria to discriminate between cemented and uncemented prostheses are based on the need to maintain bone status.

Joint replacement should be considered a multistage procedure particularly for younger persons whose life expectancy outreaches the anticipated implant life. In this regard conservation of the bone stock is vital for implant durability and to keep open reconstructive options. The main hazard for bone stock derives from stress-shielding phenomena. When an implant is rigidly fixed or inserted in a bone, part of the stress usually borne by the bone travels through the implant and bypasses the natural way through tissue. As a result of the reduced stimulus, the unloaded part of the bone develops disuse osteopenia. Stress-shielding phenomena following femoral stem insertion are widely described over a wide range of severity and have been considered potentially hazardous for implant stability by several authors [55, 82, 104, 119, 160]. Huiskes et al. demonstrated that the implant stiffness determines the amount of stress-shielding in the proximal femur after THA (Fig. 28-7). They observed that given a certain implant stiffness, the lower the bone density of the host bone, the higher the level of stress shielding [76]. They also calculated that the bone loss around a titanium stem could increase from 4% to 23% depending on the degree of osteopenia at the time of its insertion. It is therefore preferential to use cemented prosthesis when low bone densities are present

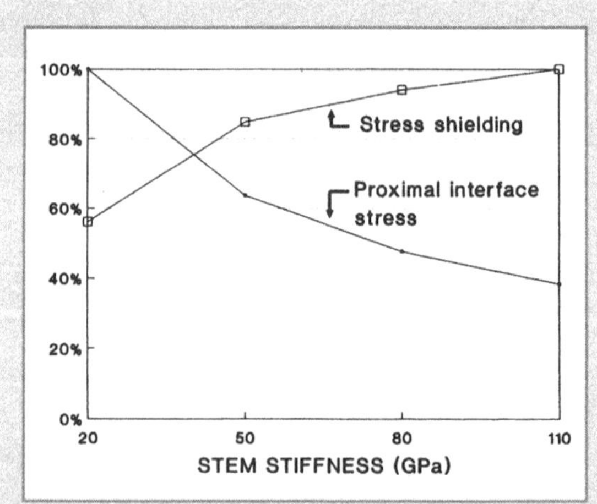

Fig. 28-7 Stress-shielding phenomena following femoral stem insertion are considered potentially hazardous for implant stability and are related to the implant stiffness: the higher the implant stiffness and the lower the bone density of the hosting bone, the higher are the levels of stress-shielding and bone resorption. The measurement of bone density in candidates for prosthetic surgery may be useful to choose the type of implant in relation to the patient bone density. (From [76])

locally due to the fact that flexural rigidity of a cemented stem is 3.6 times lower than that of an uncemented one [74].

Some studies suggeste that bone quality is an important element in the choice of the design and of the type of fixation also in the field of TKA. Lee et al. tested the micromotions of tibial component with various designs and methods of fixation against foam tibial models of variable densities [100]. The efficiency of prosthetic design and type of fixation that resulted were related to bone density. The most rigid implant fixation was achieved using four peripherally placed screws, and the addition of a central stem added stability only in the case of "poor" quality foam. Finally, they found that the use of cement increased stability in "poor" quality foam simulating osteopenic bone. The assessment of bone density is therefore an important consideration in the choice of the design and type of fixation of a tibial component.

Bone status and mechanical properties of the proximal tibia were investigated in other studies [18,78,79] for the important role of bone strength in tibial component stability. Furthermore, when valgus or varus deformities of the knee are present, significant discrepancies in bone distribution between medial and lateral compartments may be expected, as suggested by Wolff's law and the modeling theories [51,78,95] and easily detected preoperatively by densitometry. Krackow suggested that the surgeon should be aware of these situations for a correct preoperatory planning to assure the best implant stability [95].

In the surveillance of prostheses the main role of bone densitometry is in the assessment of bone density redistribution consequent to strain redistribution [106,127]. Stress-related changes in bone density and architecture are a topic of wide investigation in hip surgery. In 1978, as a consequence of the clinical observation of calcar resorption following hip prosthesis, Oh et al. studied the strain redistribution in the proximal part of loaded cadaver femora before and after insertion of cemented stems [127]. They demonstrated a significant strain reduction in the calcar area and different behaviors for different prosthetic designs (Fig. 28-8). Engh et al. compared the theoretical degree of stress-shielding and the relative frequency of different degrees of bone resorption semiquantitatively determined on X-rays to evaluate the influence of stem size and extent of porous coating on femoral bone loss. They concluded that the information gained from this study benefits the design and application of porous-coated femoral implants [33].

Stress patterns of different femoral stems and the consequent bone mass redistribution were inferred by Huiskes using two-dimensional finite element models. His data confirmed the higher reduction in stress in the proximal region of calcar and the differences between cemented, fully coated or partially coated stems (Fig. 28-9) [74]. Using strain-adaptive bone-remodeling theory in combination with finite element models, he also investigated the relationship between implant flexibility and the extent of bone loss around femoral stems [76]. The application of noninvasive, quantitative methods for the assessment of bone mass is an obvious advantage to clinically confirm data obtained from

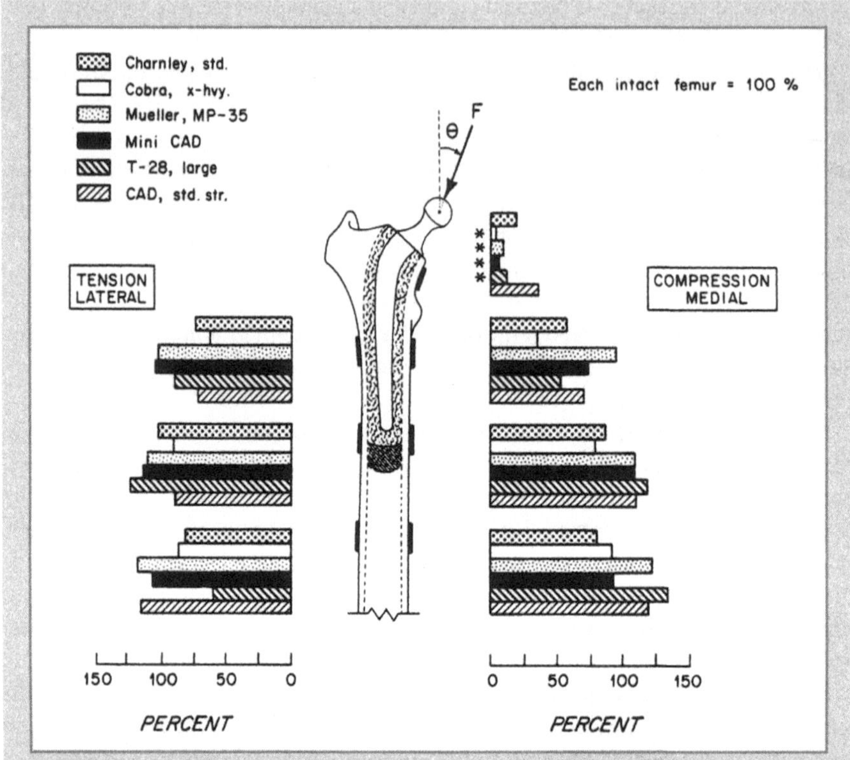

Fig. 28-8 Stress-related changes in bone density and architecture have been a topic of concern as a consequence of the clinical observation of calcar resorption following hip prosthesis. A mechanical test machine was used to study the strain redistribution in the proximal part of loaded cadaver femora before and after insertion of cemented stems and demonstrated different patterns of strain distribution for different prosthetic designs. Similar data may be inferred in clinical settings measuring bone density redistribution by DXA. (From [127])

autopsy specimens or from theoretical models. In fact, recent investigations have coupled invasive histological evaluations and mechanical tests with data obtained by DXA [19, 20, 37].

Stress-shielding phenomena and related concerns are also present in the literature on TKA. Some series of patients operated on for TKA showed roentgenographic evidence of a remarkable osteopenia in the anterior aspect of the distal femur [22,120], an occurrence predicted by finite element models [8,161,172] and determined by stress-shielding. Until now the risk of an early component mobilization does not seem to increase in the presence of an anterior femoral osteopenia, but the relevant bone redistribution may lead to structural collapse for fatigue when abnormal cyclic loads are maintained [120].

The long survival of modern implants poses new threats to their longevity. The perseverance of stress-shielding is not known [106], and bone aging phenomena such as endosteal enlargement [69,126,143,152] and increased cortical porosity could lead to biological failure of the host bone [136].

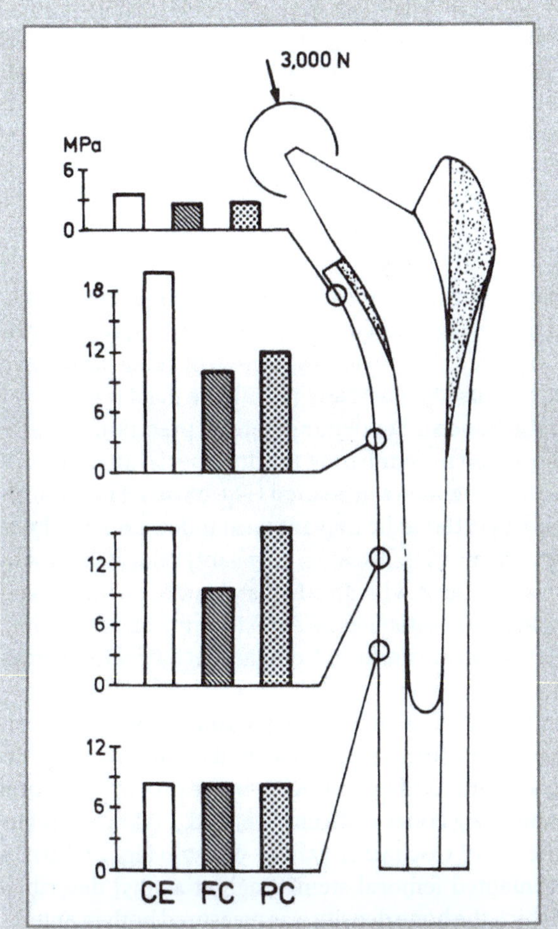

Fig. 28-9 Not only implant flexibility but also the type of bonding is responsible for the degree and the distribution of stress along the femoral cortex after the prosthetic insertion as shown using strain-adaptive bone-remodeling theory in combination with finite element models. CE, Cemented stem; FC, fully coated uncemented stem; PC, partly coated uncemented stem. Measurement of bone density redistribution after THA by DXA may support data obtained by calculations on finite element models. (From [74])

In conclusion, application of DXA in the follow-up of prostheses provides information on the status of the host bone and on bone aging processes and may be useful in evaluating the effect of stem design, type of fixation, and bone-implant stiffness ratio on the strain-related bone density redistribution. At present the value of DXA in predicting the final outcome of implants is under investigation.

Before a revision surgery DXA may tell the surgeon the exact amount of remaining bone stock for a careful preoperative planning.

Adaptive remodeling with local bone loss has also been observed with metal plates and spinal instrumentation methods [3, 115, 131, 159, 167], and most of the considerations expressed for prosthetic monitoring may be applied to other metallic implants currently used in orthopedic surgery. Bone densitometry for assessment of bone changes after fixation can provide data on the impact of the implant on bone structure and on the accidental bone healing processes.

Total Hip Arthroplasty

The first densitometric studies of bone density around the cemented and uncemented femoral stem started at the beginning of the 1990s with anteroposterior scans of the whole femoral component. Some of these were still being performed with DPA [138, 156], and they were used principally to validate densitometry for the assessment of periprosthetic bone and to demonstrate its precision and efficiency. These studies were also aimed at delineating the first special analysis protocols in which bone density and content are measured (Fig. 28-10). Theoretically the choice of the ROIs around an orthopedic implant must follow both methodological and clinical guidelines. Delineated sites must be reliably relocated on subsequent scans. They must be large enough with an adequate number of pixels and relatively uniform in density to assure satisfactory repositioning and precision. They must include bone segments that are uniform from the mechanical and physiological point of view.

Initially these ROIs did not have precise anatomical landmarks but were positioned visually by the operator within bone areas considered distinctive (Fig. 28-11a) [116]. Subsequently some authors codified four ROIs in the proximal femoral metaphysis within the corresponding zones of Gruen 1, 6, and 7, taking as reference point the midpoint of the lesser trochanter [72, 89–91, 137] (Fig. 28-11b). In another recent study on uncemented femoral stems Engh et al. [35] described three proximodistal levels in which the bone density was measured both in anteroposterior (AP) and in laterolateral (LL) projection. For each level they obtained four ROIs: medial and lateral in the AP projection, and anterior and posterior in the LL projection (Fig. 28-11c). Their results showed a strong correlation (R^2 = 0.88) between the losses in BMC as measured in the AP and LL scans, suggesting that just the AP projection may be sufficient for the assessment of the pattern and the extent of remodeling.

Kilgus and colleagues [88] measured periprosthetic bone density in six medial and six lateral ROIs using a distal wider seventh ROI, both medially and laterally, as reference baseline zone because this distal part of the femoral diaphysis showed the least BMD variation within their sample (Fig. 28-11d). In a comparative study of cemented and uncemented prostheses Korovessis et al. [94] used four small ROIs around the femoral stem and three small ROIs around the socket, whose size and position were not clearly established (Fig. 28-11e). In 1993 Trevisan et al. [164] presented an analysis protocol based on the seven zones suggested by Gruen in 1979 for the roentgenographic examination of cemented

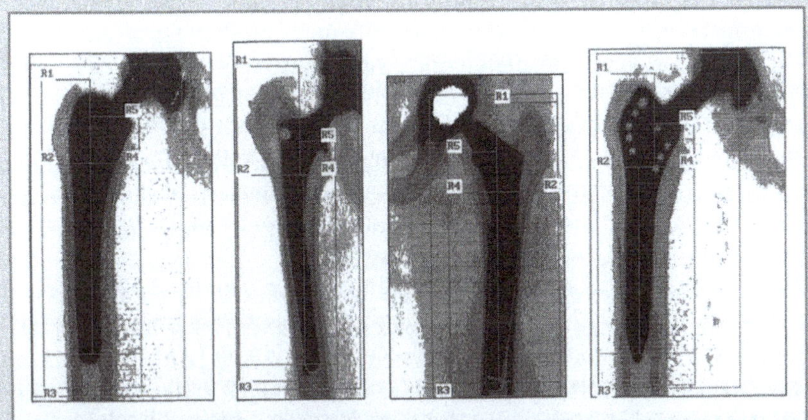

Fig. 28-10 Anteroposterior scans of different uncemented femoral stems. The software automatically removes from the analysis the metal implant and consequently the superimposed parts of bone while BMC (g) and BMD (g/cm²) are precisely measured in the proximity of the implant. Data are expressed as the sum of BMC and average BMD in the whole scanned segment and individually for each ROI outlined by the operator

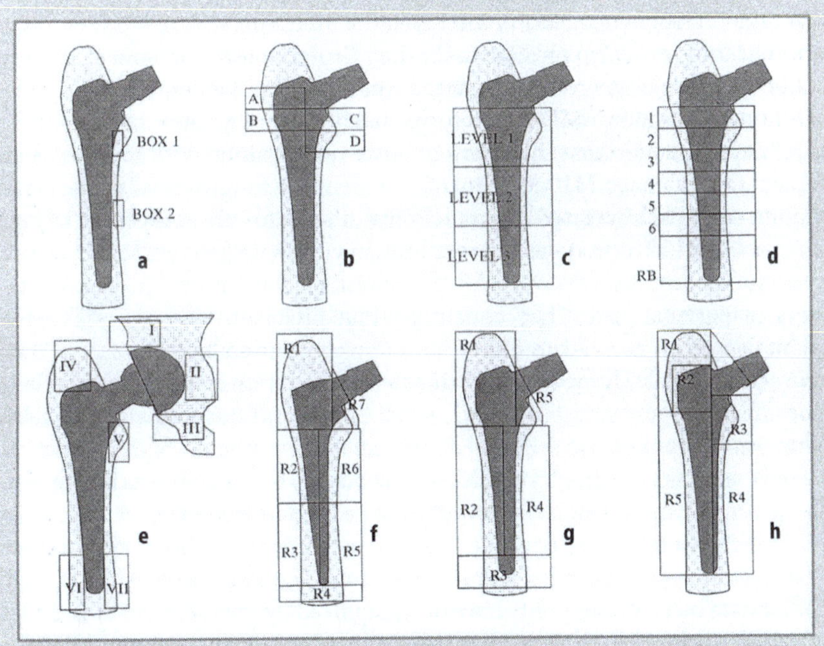

Fig. 28-11 DXA analysis protocols for THA in the literature. **a** McCarthy et al. [116]. **b** Kiratli et al. and others [72, 89–91, 137]. **c** Engh et al. [35]. **d** Kilgus et al. [88]. **e** Korovessis et al. [94]. **f** Cohen and Rushton, Trevisan et al., Petersen et al. [27–29, 132, 164]. **g** Trevisan et al. [163, 165]. **h** Massari et al. [111]

femoral stems [58] (Fig. 28-11f). Taking account of biomechanical studies [20, 74, 127] demonstrating the substantial uniformity in terms of stress-strain relationship of the upper and lower diaphyseal Gruen zones (2 and 3 laterally; 5 and 6 medially), a simplified protocol based on five ROIs, was later introduced by the same group [163, 165] (Fig. 28-11g). Another protocol with 5 ROIs but differently distributed was used by Massari et al. in a longitudinal study of uncemented stems (Fig. 28-11h) [111]. Cohen and Rushton [27, 28] and Petersen et al. [132] adopted the seven-zone Gruen protocol slightly modified in zone 7 whose lower limit was positioned at the distal end of the lesser trochanter.

Most of these protocols were validated by reproducibility data. Despite the use of small ROIs with precarious anatomical landmarks, McCarthy et al. reported a precision error for BMD between 3.7% and 7.5% [116]. Using the same brand of densitometer but a higher scan resolution and a better ROI definition, Kiratli et al found a precision error for BMD lower than 1% on phantom, around 1% ex vivo, and between 2.13% and 5.47% in vivo [91]. They also reported that intraobserver precision errors were small, similar among operators, and similar to the precision error with repeated scans, while in some cases BMD values differed substantially between observers, but interobserver precision errors were not clearly reported in their study. They also evaluated ex vivo the error attributable to femoral rotation (within 5° of medial and 5° of lateral rotation) which caused the greatest effect on precision in the clinical setting. For the BMD of the calcar region (region C) rotation increased the precision error from 1.06 to 5.27. In another study on a hip phantom using the 7 Gruen zones, Mortimer et al. found that between 15° of internal and external rotation from the neutral position the maximum variation in BMD was approximately 5% and greater for regions 2, 5, and 7. They concluded that the extent of observed variation with rotation is not sufficient to influence BMD assessment in patients on longitudinal studies [121].

Cohen and Rushton tested reproducibility of DXA for the assessment of bone density around different types of prosthesis, in vitro with geometric and anthropomorphic phantoms, ex vivo on five femoral specimens, and in vivo on two groups of patients [28]. They concluded that precision was not affected by implant design or material, and they found no correlation between size of BMD and precision error. They confirmed that femoral rotation is the most significant factor affecting reproducibility (Fig. 28-12). Cohen and Rushton also published a comparative study of two different densitometers. Despite the high correlations between the results obtained with the two systems (r=0.94), there was lack of complete agreement, indicating that they may not be used interchangeably (Fig. 28-13) [27]. Similar discrepancies between the two instruments in BMD measurement on lumbar spine and proximal femur were found by other investigators [59, 99].

Other data on reproducibility have been reported by several authors and summarized in Table 28-1. On average the worst precision errors were registered in the region of the lesser trochanter (due to the higher sensitivity to rotation) and on BMC rather than BMD (due to the compensatory effect of projectional area). Accuracy of bone mass evaluation near implants was investigated by Kiratli et al.

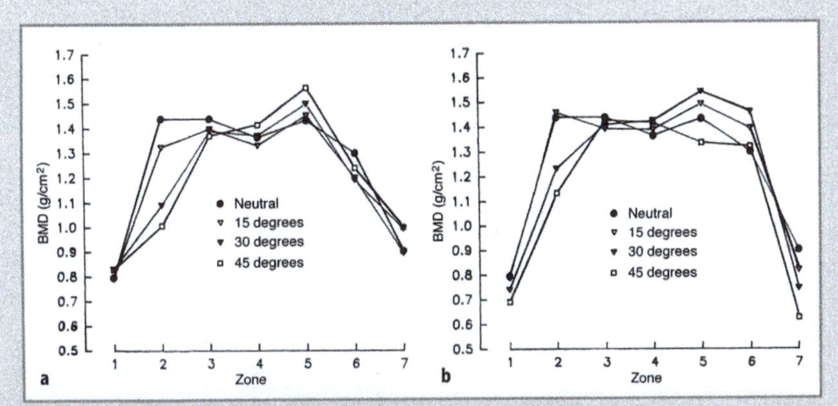

Fig. 28-12 The effect of internal rotation (a) and external rotation (b) on periprosthetic BMD. This study confirms that femoral rotation is the most significant factor affecting reproducibility. (From [28])

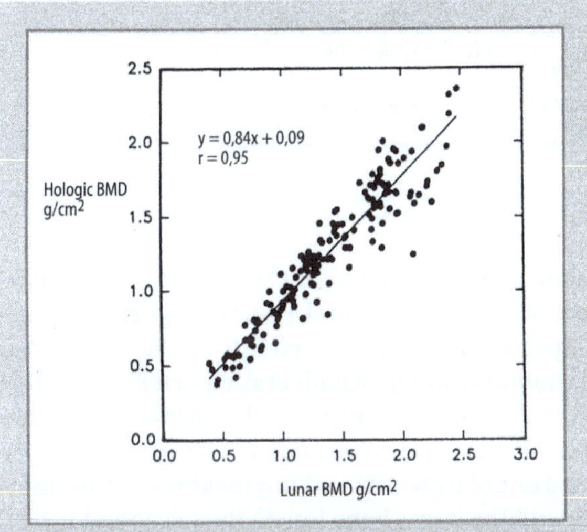

Fig. 28-13 Comparison of two different densitomers found a lack of agreement between the two systems, indicating that they may not be used interchangeably despite the high correlations between their results. (From [27])

[91], Kilgus et al. [88], and Cohen and Rushton [28] with satisfactory results. The presence of the metal device in the scan window and the software procedures for metal removal did not significantly affect the accuracy, which was similar to that reported for standard densitometry examinations of lumbar spine and proximal femur (Table 28-1).

From the clinical point of view, the leading interest of researchers was on the assessment of the amount of bone loss and its main determinants.

Table 28-1 Precision and accuracy errors of DXA in periprosthetic bone mass assessment (if not otherwise specified, precision and accuracy errors are to be intented „in vivo")

Reference	Densitometer	Analysis protocol[a]	Precision error (%)	Accuracy error (% BMD in vitro)
McCarthy et al. [116]	Lunar DPX	11a	Box 1: BMC: 3,8%, BMD: 3,7% Box 2: BMC: 7,5%	–
Kiratli et al. [91]	Lunar DPX	11b	BMD in vitro: 0,3–0,6%; ex vivo: 0,9–1,47% in vivo: 2,68%–4,5%	<1%
Richmond et al. [139]	Lunar DPX	11b	BMD: 2,2%	–
Kilgus et al. [88]	Lunar DPX	11d	BMD: 2,6%–4,7%	5,4%
Hughes et al. [72]	Lunar DPX	11b	BMD: 2%–4%	–
Trevisan et al. [164]	Hologic QDR 1000	11f	BMD: 1,8%–6,8%	–
Trevisan et al. [164]	Hologic QDR 1000	11g	BMD: 1,5%–3%	–
Cohen and Rushton [28]	Hologic QDR 1000	11f	BMD in vitro: 2%–3,3% ex vivo: 0,51–0,87% in vivo: 1,1%–4,5%	–
Massari et al. [111]	Hologic QDR 1000	11h	BMD: 1,34%	–
Petersen et al. [132]	Hologic QDR 2000	11f	BMD: 2,2–4,9%	–

[a] See Fig. 28-11 for reference.

All the published investigations agree that significant bone loss follows implant insertion. The onset of this loss is fast. Richmond et al. [138,139] reported a reduction in periprosthetic BMD, especially in the calcar region, from 5% to 31% 1 year after surgery in uncemented femoral stem, and Kiratli et al. reported a 13% – 24% bone reduction after 2 years [92]. The early onset of bone loss has also been confirmed in longitudinal studies. Massari et al. found a bone reduction of 1%–8% within 45 days after surgery and one of 1.5%–21% within 3 months after the insertion of an uncemented stem, with the larger bone loss in the calcar and medial cortex regions [111]. Our group [165] and Kiratli et al. [93] reported rates of bone loss higher in the first 3 months after surgery. Cohen and Rushton [29] studied bone redistribution for 1 year after the insertion of a cemented Charnley prosthesis and found the greater bone loss within the first 6 months.

This early phase of bone loss is related to the surgical insult and to the subsequent bed rest and weight-bearing delay. The bone reaming procedures may in some way give rise even to a paradoxical increase in bone density at the metaphyseal region of the proximal femur due to trabecular compression, as suggested by Kiratli et al. [93] and Niinimaki and Jalovaara [122], who compared preoperative BMD values with those measured within 5 days from the operation. Later bone redistribution is related to the stress redistribution induced by the prosthesis or by pathological events.

It is controversial as to the time at which a steady state is reached. From the examination of plain radiographs Engh et al. concluded that in their experience most of the implants induce bone changes within 2 years after surgery [33]. Several DXA studies suggest that most of the bone redistribution occurs within the first 6–12 months but that the progression of bone loss persists well over 2 years. In their group of patients 4–7 years after surgery Kiratli et al. found a reduction of up to 50%, larger than that found in the group at 2 years, suggesting a progression beyond this limit [90]. In the medial region of proximal femur McCarthy et al. found a greater decrease in periprosthetic BMC and BMD in patients with a longer follow-up [116]. Similarly, cross-sectional data collected by Kilgus et al. suggest that bone loss persists over 2 years after surgery with greater variations in the proximal regions (Fig. 28-14) [88]. In the longitudinal study of Massari et al. the endpoint was at 2 years. During the second year the BMD of the distal cortical regions did not change significantly whereas a persisting bone loss was present in the proximal regions of the great trochanter and calcar [111].

In the study of Trevisan et al. whose endpoint was at 4 years after surgery a steady state was reached at 24–36 months, after which a slow negative trend, suggesting bone aging rather than stress-induced redistribution, affected the three distal cortical regions. In the calcar region an accelerated bone loss persisted over 36 months under the probable influence of stress-shielding phenomena [165]. A similar pattern was expressed in the study of Kiratli et al. [93] with most of the bone changes occurring within the first 6 months and a persistent bone loss detected up to 8 years after surgery.

In these clinical investigations there is a great variability of the assessed bone loss from study to study (Table 28-2) and also from patient to patient within uniform samples [29, 35]. A first explanation of this variability is the reference system adopted to estimate bone loss. Evaluation of the amount of bone loss was calculated mainly by comparing the THA side with the contralateral side or with non-operated femora in healthy controls in which the same sections of bone shielded by the femoral implant were shielded, transposing the scan image of the implant via software. In both cases an inevitable degree of uncertainty is introduced due to the fact that difference in bone status between sides or between different individuals could be remarkable. In our experience, a difference in BMD values of over 10% in at least two regions of the standard DXA hip examination is present in over 18% of the population [162]. Similarly, McCarthy et al. reported an average percentage difference between sides in their age-matched controls of around 10% (with a large standard deviation induced by the small ROIs used) that were not statistically different in their study but were also not definitively equal [116].

Preoperatively the average BMD difference between healthy and affected sides varied from +3.9% to +6.4% in the study by Kiratli et al. [93] and from −3.0% to +4.9% in the study by Niinimaki and Jalovaara [122]. These findings suggest a disuse osteopenia in the affected side and also uncertainty in the relationship between sides.

                                                                C. Trevisan, S. Ortolani

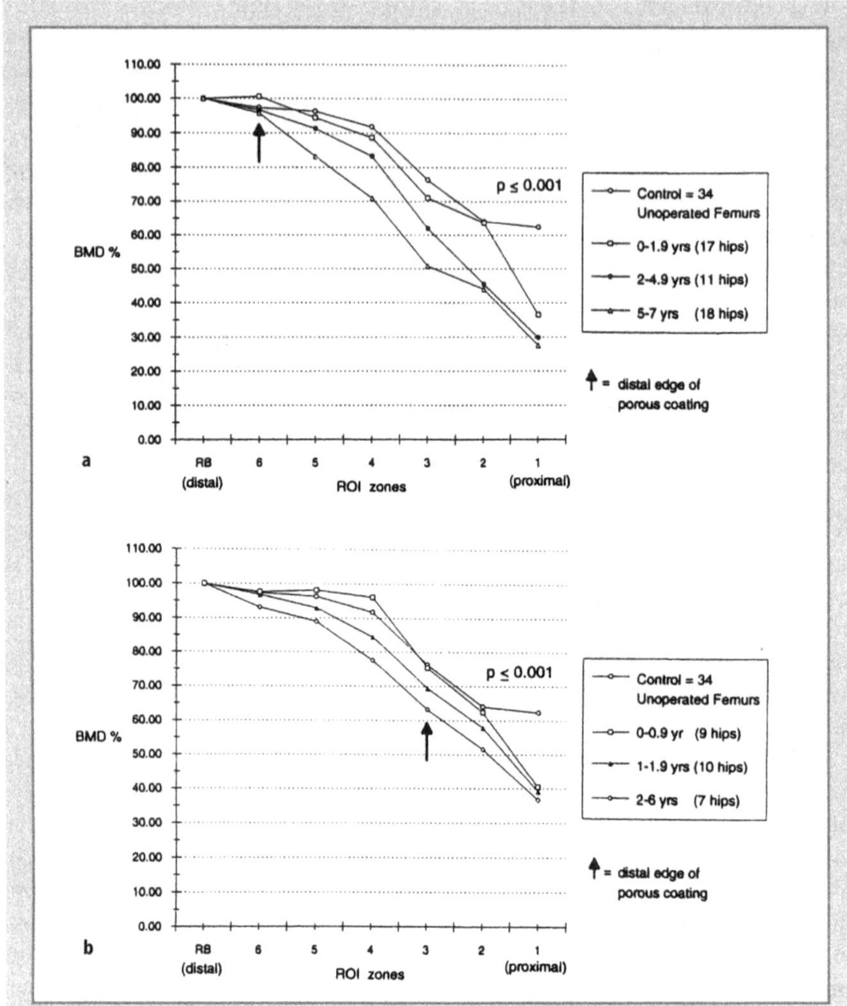

Fig. 28-14 Regional periprosthetic BMD of the medial femoral cortices related to time interval since operation in extensively **a** and proximally coated **b** stems. In both cases data suggest that bone loss persisted over 2 years since surgery with greater variations in the proximal regions and in extensively coated stems. (From [88])

Other sources of variability in the assessment of bone loss are the analysis protocols with their differently sized and positioned ROIs. If some common features must be delineated, it should be said that despite the unhomogeneity of reference systems and analysis protocols the amount of bone loss was greater the longer one moved from distal to proximal, being the greatest in the calcar region in almost all the published studies.

In conclusion, in the distal cortical regions around the femoral stem which have a relative biological inertia and sustain a lower biomechanical derangement

Table 28-2 Bone loss after total hip arthroplasty in the literature

Reference	Analysis protocol[a]	Materials	Reference values	Bone loss
McCarthy et al. [116]	11a	28 pts. with cem. THA TAS: >14 yrs	Contralateral femur	Box 1: BMC 40.3%–40.8% Box 1: BMD 39.6%–43.6% Box 2: BMC 43.1%–49%
Kilgus et al. [88]	11d	46 pts. with FC uncem. THA 26 pts. with PC uncem. THA TAS: 0–7yrs	Values as % BMD of a reference baseline region and compared with contralateral shielded femur	FC stems: 1.6%–34.8%, calcar 34.8% PC stems: 0.9%–21.8%, calcar 21.8% Greater bone loss with larger stems and FC stems
Hughes et al. [72]	11b	15 pts. with Ti uncem. stem TAS: 36–48 months	Index: ratio of BMD operated/healthy side	Comparison of Ti vs. CoCr stems: ROI A: Ti 10%, CoCr 18% ROI B: Ti 18%, CoCr 30% ROI C: Ti 15%, CoCr 34% ROI D: Ti 7%, CoCr 17%
Pritchett [137]	11a,b	50 pts. with 5 different types of femoral stems TAS: > 3 yrs	Contralateral shielded femur	Proximal bone loss from 8%–57% correlated with the estimated degree of stress shielding due to each stem
Korovessis et al. [94]	11e	52 pts. with THA 19 cem. and 33 uncem. sockets; 18 cem. and 34 uncem. stems. TAS: 1 month to 10 yrs	Contralateral femur	Socket: 2.1%–17.6% Stem: 11.5%–24.6% Significant differences in bone redistribution for uncem. and cem. sockets and stems
Trevisan et al. [164]	11f	14 pts. with uncem. THA TAS: < 18 months	Z score from contralateral femur	Recalculated after normalization of BMD for ROI 4 BMD: 1.8%–12.7%, with the greater bone loss proximally
Trevisan et al. [165]	11g	20 pts. with uncem. THA 4 yrs longitudinal study	Percentage change from baseline measurement (within 30 days from surgery)	Bone loss at 3 months R1–R4: 6%–14% then partial recovery; calcar > 20% at 2 yrs (no recovery)
Engh et al. [35]	11c	5 autoptic speciments of femora with uncem. THA implanted in vivo and contralateral sides implanted ex vivo TAS: 17–84 months	Contralateral ex vivo implanted femur	Level 1: AP 24%–72%, LL 28%–83% Level 2: AP 2%–62%, LL 8%–67% Level 3: AP 0%–29%, LL 5%–38% Strong correlation between AP and LL; relationship between initial bone mass and consequent loss

cem., cemented; uncem., uncemented; FC, fully coated; PC, partly coated; TAS, time after surgery; Ti, titanium; CoCr, cobalt chromium.

[a] See Fig. 28-11 for reference.

Table 28-2 Continued: Bone loss after total hip arthroplasty in the literature

Reference	Analysis protocol[a]	Materials	Reference values	Bone loss
Massari et al. [111]	11h	40 pts. with uncem. THA 2 yrs longitudinal study	Percentage change from baseline measurement (within 15 days from surgery)	Greater assessed bone loss: R1: 8.6% at 24 months R2: 23% at 24 months R3: 42% at 24 months R4: 13.8% at 24 months R5: 12.3% at 9–12 months
Kiratli et al. [93]	11b	32 pts with uncem. THA 2 yrs longitudinal study	Percentage change from baseline measurement (within 5 days from surgery)	Higher rates of bone loss in the first 6 months Bone loss at 24 months: A: 9%, B: 29%, C: 25%, D: 24%
Cohen and Rushton [29]	11f	20 pts with cem. THA 1 year longitudinal study	Percentage change from baseline measurement (within 10 days from surgery)	Higher rates of bone loss in the first 6 months. Bone loss at 12 months: cortical regions (R2, R3, R5, R6): 0.76%–8.37%; calcar (R7): 6.74%; BMD increase at the tip (R4): +5%

cem., cemented; uncem., uncemented; FC, fully coated; PC, partly coated; TAS, time after surgery; Ti, titanium; CoCr, cobalt chromium.

[a] See Fig. 28-11 for reference.

it seems that a steady state is reached approximately 2 years after surgery and with limited bone loss, while proximally the higher degree of stress-shielding phenomena leads to a prolonged bone density redistribution with greater bone loss expecially in the calcar region. This suggested pattern fully agrees with several analyses of stress-strain redistribution after stem insertion generated by finite element models [74, 76, 80, 150].

Other factors, such as stem stiffness, design and type of fixation, initial bone mass, and factors related to surgery or postoperative recovery may play an important role in the determination of bone redistribution. Stem stiffness and design and type of fixation were investigated by Kilgus et al. [88], Hughes et al. [72], Pritchett [137], Korovessiss et al. [94] and Niinimaki and Jalovaara [122].

Kilgus showed a significantly greater decrease in regional periprosthetic BMD with larger or extensively coated implants, suggesting different degrees of stress shielding, in accordance with the data elaborated by Huiskes using finite element analysis models [88].

Hughes et al. investigated the effect on periprosthetic BMD of two proximally coated femoral stems, similar in shape and size but differing in material – a cobalt-chromium alloy with higher flexural rigidity versus a titanium stem [72]. The authors concluded that the difference in the modulus of elasticity between the two types of stem had little effect on bone loss since they found significant difference only in the calcar region. In any case, average differences in bone loss between cobalt-chromium and titanium stems ranged from 8% to 19% depending on the selected region. These differences support the assertion of some effect of elasticity, particularly when the reduced statistical power of the study for the high variability in the observed periprosthetic BMD and the small size of the two samples is also considered. Furthermore, in the study of Niinimaki and Jalovaara [122] the percentage of bone loss 9 years after the insertion of an isoelastic stem resulted remarkably lower when compared with that reported in studies concerning stiffer stems [88, 137].

Korovessis et al. [94] and Pritchett [137] compared the bone changes induced by implants with different shape, material, and fixation modalities. In the first study Zweymuller uncemented sockets and stems and Mueller cemented sockets and stems induced statistically different bone mass redistributions. The cemented socket induced an increase in bone density at the cranial acetabular region while bone resorption in the medial and caudal acetabular regions was seen with the uncemented one. With both the cemented and uncemented stems there was found an increase in bone density in the great trochanter region and a decrease in the calcar and distal lateral cortex regions, while the uncemented stem also induced bone resorption at the distal medial cortex region.

Pritchett compared 50 femoral stems of five different types of bone retention in the proximal femur at least 3 years after implantation. The average measured loss of bone density compared with the opposite side ranged from 8% to 43% depending on the type of stem. Stems with a strong extensive bone bonding which loads the femur primarily endosteally and distally (the cemented stems and the uncemented fully coated stems) showed greater bone loss than stems which retain compression stresses and minimize shear stresses on the proximal femur by loading it with an horizontal platform collar. Pritchett concluded that the degree of proximal bone loss was correlated with the degree of stress shielding for the respective types of stem.

The effect of initial bone status on the bone resorption induced by stress shielding was investigated by Engh et al. [35] and Sychterz and Engh [158]. They found a significant inverse correlation between BMC of the control femora and the decrease in bone content of the operated femora (Fig. 28-15). The higher the initial bone mass, the lower was the consequent bone loss due to the fact that the difference in stiffness between implant and bone is lower. Their results agree with the data calculated on three-dimensional finite element models by Huiskes et al. [76]. They also explained the lower bone loss after THA in men that had been observed by McCarthy et al. [116] as due to the fact that average bone density is always higher in men than in women.

Finally, the response of each patient to the insertion of the implant may be affected by the surgical procedures, postoperative course, period of bed rest and load-bearing delay, and present status of bone metabolism. These factors presently remain uninvestigated and may contribute to the variability seen in several samples.

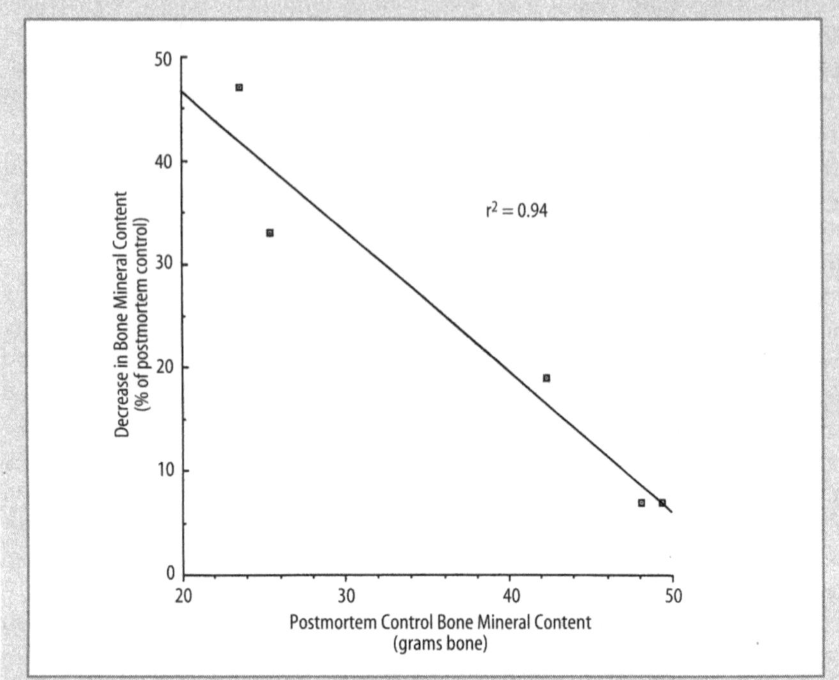

Fig. 28-15 A significant inverse correlation between BMC of the control femora and the decrease in bone content of the operated femora. These results suggest that initial bone status is a determinant of the bone resorption induced by stress shielding: the higher the initial bone mass is, the lower the consequent bone loss due to th fact that the difference in stiffness is lower between implant and bone. (From [35])

Despite the crucial acceleration of the DXA employment in the THA field and the growing number of published studies there is still a substantial lack of standardization on analysis protocols and reference values. Some of these problems could be solved by improvements in software and agreements among manufacturers. A precise assessment of bone mass variation is difficult when a preoperative scan is lacking, and the use of shielded femurs from the opposite side or from a control population involves an uncertainty that degrades the otherwise excellent measurement features. Therefore performing preoperative scans is highly desirable for future investigations.

Total Knee Arthroplasty

Bone mineral assessment around knee arthroplasty is at its very beginning. The effect of bone status on the stability of tibial components [18, 78, 79, 100] and the roentgenographic occurrence of significant osteopenia in the anterior part of the proximal femur after TKA [8, 22, 120] are the main incentives for the assessment of bone mass.

The first report of local bone density changes after TKA was by Seitz et al. [148] in 1987 using QCT. They observed a significant reduction in the mean BMD and in the cortical thickness at the proximal tibia with higher rates soon after the implantation. Other studies of bone density after TKA using DPA or DXA have been published only since 1995. Some evidence of the feasibility of DXA in this field is suggested by the studies of Robertson et al. [140], in which DXA was superior to other methods in assessing bone mineral changes in proximity of TKA. Also, Banks et al. [11] developed the application of orthopedic software for the hip in patients with TKA.

As for densitometry after THA, the assessment of bone density changes around TKA may provide information on the bone response to surgical procedures, bed rest, weight-bearing delay, and stress redistribution. In the case of TKA, however-er, the sometimes considerable rearrangement of the mechanical axis of lower limb to correct for varus or valgus deformities may play a primary role in deter-mining stress redistribution.

Bone changes in the distal femur after TKA were investigated by Liu et al. [103] using DXA and Petersen et al. [134] using a custom-made knee DPA. In their 1-year follow-up studies they found a greater BMD decrease within the first 6 months after surgery, similarly to that which was observed by Seitz et al. and in the lon-gitudinal studies on THA. In the study by Petersen et al. the amount of bone loss reached 44% in the region anterior to the fixation peg and 19% distally to the fix-ation peg [134]. Petersen et al. also investigated the tibial site and reported an aver-age BMD decrease of 8% 1 year after surgery [133].

Levitz et al. measured the bone changes in the proximal tibia by DPA and DXA in 31 patients 1 year after surgery and extended their observation to 8 years in 7 patients [101]. They found no statistical difference between the BMD measured 1 week after surgery and those measured after 1 year, but after 8 years the aver-age decrease in BMD below the tibial component was over 36% with a rate of loss of 5% per year.

A precise analysis protocol was not clearly delineated in any of these studies. Moreover, almost all studies were performed using only AP scans, but patients with TKA may be placed in lateral decubitus on the examining side at fixed knee flexion for an additional LL scan. In both projections the rotation is more diffi-cult to control than in the case of hip scans, and positioning devices are advis-able. In this regard the recent introduction of DXA machines with a rotating arm which allow scans to be performed with different projections without reposi-tioning the patient may be a significant improvement.

An analysis protocol for AP and LL scans of the knee joint after TKA was recently suggested (Fig. 28-16) [107, 166]. For the AP scan of the proximal femur one medial and one lateral ROI were identified in the metaphyseal region taking as landmark the edge of the prosthetic femoral shield. In the LL scan an anteri-or and a posterior ROI were recognized using as boundary the long axis of the femoral diaphysis. For the tibia three ROIs were characterized for both AP and LL scans: in the AP scan one medial, one lateral, and one distal region; in the LL

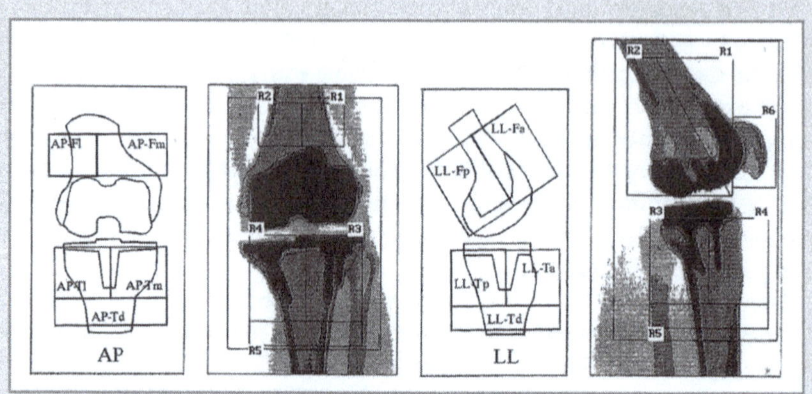

Fig. 28-16 Analysis protocol for the densitometric evaluation of periprosthetic bone status after TKA. For the AP scan of the proximal femur one medial and one lateral ROI were identified in the metaphyseal region taking as landmark the edge of the prosthetic femoral shield. In the LL scan an anterior and a posterior ROI were recognized using as boundary the long axis of the femoral diaphysis. For the tibia three ROIs were characterized for both AP and LL scans: in the AP scan one medial, one lateral, and one distal region; for the LL scan one anterior, one posterior, and one distal region. The midpoint to divide medial and lateral or anterior and posterior regions was calculated in the proximal limit of these ROIs for the femur and in its distal limit for the tibia. (From [107])

scan one anterior, one posterior, and one distal region. The short-term in vivo reproducibility of BMC and BMD in the femoral and tibial ROIs ranged, respectively, from 2.1% to 4.1% and from 0.9% to 2.6% for the AP scan and from 2.7% to 5.6% and from 2.3% to 4.7% for the LL scan [166].

Another main feature of knee scans is the scarce amount of soft tissues around the joint, which can affect measurement reproducibility. A soft tissue equivalent material in the form of rice bags may be used to provide an adequate soft tissue baseline. In the near future this method will provide useful data for clinical investigation.

Other Implants

The number of fractures surgically treated increases year by year, and the variety of available fixation devices increases accordingly. The presumed advantage of one system over another lies in the ease and flexibility of the involved surgical procedures and the promise of strong and secure fixation. Mechanical tests have been used extensively on autopsy specimens to compare various devices in several experimental studies, but despite the importance of bone quality for a successful surgical fracture fixation clinical studies on the relationship between bone density and efficacy of fixation devices are few [4]. Moreover, fragility fractures deserve special care, and a high degree of osteoporosis can lead to unexpected, disastrous situations in which the most advanced and tested implants fail to work: screws do not hold, and bone cracks during reduction and fixation attempts. A number of solutions have been suggested: screw fixed with nuts, cerclage wiring instead of screws, and polymethylmethacrylate to strengthen bone structure [12, 64, 146]. However, there have been no systematic investigations on special strategies to treat fragile fractures.

Despite the number of mechanical comparisons between instrumentations, studies examining performance in relation to different bone densities are scarce. With femoral fixation devices Laros and Moore [98] found that under their laboratory conditions internal fixation of intertrochanteric fracture failed in more than 80% cases when a bone with a Singh grade 3 or less was used while 80% of successful fixation was achieved with bone grade 4 or more. More recently Husby et al. [77] found a correlation between bone density and the load resistance of implant-bone constructs using autoptic specimens of the proximal femur. Conversely, the effect of bone density on the fixation strength of implants was extensively investigated for different spinal instrumentation systems.

In 1988 Smith et al. were the first to use DPA to assess the occurrence of stress-shielding phenomena in response to rigid Steffee pedicular instrumentation in dogs [151]. One year later McAfee et al. investigated the bone remodeling after spinal instrumentation in an animal model with traditional radiography, biomechanical tests, quantitative histomorphometry, and microradiography and confirmed the relationship between rigidity of spinal instrumentation and the device-related osteoporosis in the spine [115].

Coe et al. tested the ultimate failure from a posteriorly directed load of four different types of spinal implants in seven fresh-frozen cadaveric spines. They considered bone density measured by DPA as an independent variable and found that, in contrast to spinous process wires and pedicular screws, loads to failure for laminar hooks were not affected by low BMD. They concluded that laminar hooks are superior in patients with decreased BMD due to osteoporosis, osteomalacia, or other forms of metabolic bone diseases [26].

In human lumbosacral spines instrumented with three different systems, Wittenberg et al. confirmed that the fixation strength of the intrapedicular screws is correlated with the equivalent mineral density as measured by QCT. The screw design was less important, and screw loosening occurred in spines with equivalent mineral density below 74 ± 17 mg/cm^3 regardless of the screw type. Their results led to a recommendation against intrapedicular screw fixation in vertebral bodies with low BMD [176].

Performing pull-out tests on cadaveric lumbar vertebrae, Soshi et al. investigated the relationship between degree of osteoporosis – evaluated by a semiquantitative roentgenographic scale, a microdensitometry method, and by DPA or DXA – and the fixation strength of pedicle screws [154]. They reported a strong positive correlation between pull-out force and BMD, with the correlation coefficient ranging for 0.65 to 0.85 (Fig. 28-17) and confirmed that the transpedicular screw fixation method is not indicated when low BMD is present.

The effects of depth of penetration, screw orientation, and bone density on sacral screw fixation were evaluated by Smith et al. in 25 human cadaveric sacra whose regional BMD was measured by QCT [153]. They found that intraspeci-

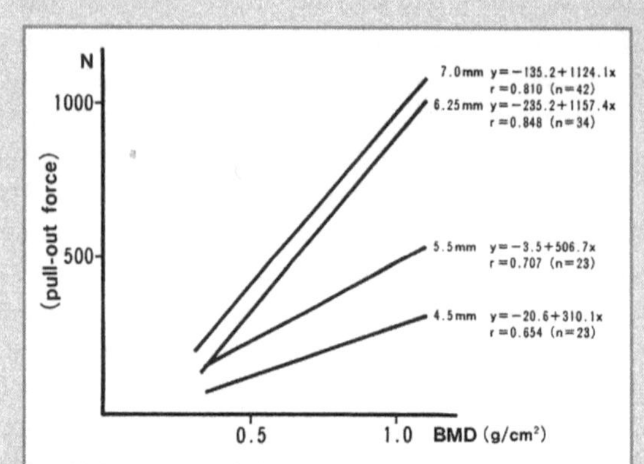

Fig. 28-17 Positive correlation between BMD measured by DPA or DXA and the fixation strength of a pedicle screw on cadaveric lumbar vertebrae. Data from various studies such as this one concluded that bone density is a relevant factor for the success of instrumented spinal fixation. (From [154])

men bone densities may account for differences in screw fixation strength. The medially directed screws placed in the centrum region of the sacrum where the BMD was approximately 60% more dense than the bone in the lateral sacral alar region sustained the maximum load. Increased bone density was correlated with greater fixation strength of the bone-screw interface, as previously suggested by Zindrick et al. [179] and Carlson et al. [24]. The authors suggested that this finding would support the clinical use of bone density determination in patients who may be candidates for sacral screw fixation.

Dalenberg et al. studied by DXA the bone changes after the implantation of stiff spinal instrumentation in dogs. They found that bone loss was uniform at 3 months postoperatively and persisted to 6 and 9 months only when the implants were loosening, while in secure implants the BMD did not worsen [30]. Interestingly, in their sham-operated group there was an average vertebral bone loss of 4.7% at 3 months, 4.6% at 6 months, and 5.4% at 9 months, suggesting a small effect of the stress of operation.

Kumano et al. studied the relationship between BMD of the lumbar spine measured by QCT and the rate of successful fusion and screw problems in 35 patients operated on for spinal canal stenosis due to degenerative lumbar disorders [96]. They failed to find any difference in rate of fusion or screw loosening or breakage between one group of patients with low BMD and another group with high BMD. They concluded that decompression and pedicle screw fixation can be performed safely with one-level fusion in patients with decreased BMD if patients with advanced osteoporosis and spinal compression fractures are excluded. They also suggested performing a preoperative evaluation of BMD in patients with osteoporosis. Their results partially disagree with the experimental findings from

Coe et al., Wittenberg et al., and Soshi et al., and they suggested that the construction of the Cotrel-Debousset system may explain its good performance in osteoporotic bone. However, the size of the sample and the limited follow-up (28 months) argue for further clinical observation.

Assessment of Bone Healing and Bone Regeneration

Bone Healing After Fracture and New Bone Formation During Limb Lengthening

The assessment of bone healing after fracture is a major topic in orthopedic practice and is currently performed mostly on subjective criteria, such as the manual evaluation of fracture stability, elapsed time, local pain and tenderness, and radiographic evidence of callus [108]. Noninvasive methods to quantify new bone formation have been extensively used, but a resolvent technique is still lacking [108]. Plain radiographs detect only a large amount of bone formation, and not in a quantitative way [130,178]. Vibration and wave-propagation techniques have been used experimentally to provide quantitative information on the mechanical properties of bone [102,144], but their clinical use is restricted to bone with accessible landmarks, the presence of surgical implants produces poor evaluations [144], and the results are affected by surrounding soft tissues because the device is not in immediate contact with the bone [128]. Measuring the speed of sound and comparing the ratio of the bone wave amplitude through a fractured bone to that through the contralateral bone [53, 54] have been used, as has been ultrasound imaging, to quantify bone healing [17,105,130,178]. Measurements with these techniques show significant fluctuations due to the diffraction of low-frequency ultrasound and to the variability in repositioning and amount of overlying soft tissues. Radiographic photodensitometry suffers from the unstable broad-spectrum output of X-ray tube and from the film sensitivity to exposure and development conditions [112,174].

A strong need for noninvasive methods to evaluate bone healing remains. Markel and Chao have argued their value on the following grounds: (a) the timing of fixation device removal; (b) recommendation for progression from non-weight bearing to full weight bearing; and (c) the prediction of abnormal fracture healing such as delayed union or nonunion [108].

Newer methods for BMD measurements, QCT and bone densitometry, may play a complementary role to other diagnostic procedures, considering the actual resolution characteristics and the limited iconographic properties.

QCT was used to study bone regeneration in animal limb lengthening by Aronson et al. [10], Markel et al. [109], and van Roermund et al. [170, 171]. SPA was used to monitor fracture mineralization by Beljan et al. who studied the effect of calcium deficiency on healing in experimental fractures of the avian tarsus [14]. It has also been used by Hellewell in the metatarsus of chickens [68], by Aro et al. [9] in the rat tibiofibular bone, and by Svesnikov and Oficerova [157]. DPA has been used to monitor mineralization after mid-diaphyseal tibial osteotomy in sheep by Kenwright and Goodship [87] and after limb lengthening in man by Peretti et al. [130].

As noted above, Markel et al. compared QCT, SPA, and DXA for the quantitative description of the mechanical properties of the callus in healing canine tibial osteotomies [109]. SPA and QCT showed the highest correlations with torsional and stiffness properties and with the calcium content of the healing bones, but the authors suggested that the lower correlations of DXA are due to the resolution used (2 mm) to study a very small fracture gap. The current fourfold increase in resolution of DXA instruments suggests a similar improvement in predictive power.

DXA was also used in an experimental animal model to study the effect of bone marrow cell transplantation or electrical stimulation on the mineralization processes of the callus after lengthening of the tibia [61, 62].

An excellent description of DXA application for the monitoring of new bone formation during leg lengthening was presented by Eyres et al. [39]. Preoperative and postoperative sequential measurements of bone density in the longitudinal and transverse axes of the femur and tibia were performed in six patients. On DXA images new bone could be seen within 1–2 weeks from the start of distraction while on plain radiographs no new bone appeared before 3–6 weeks. The bone generation during lengthening, the bone loss in distal segments, and the return to a normal pattern of BMD across the diameter of the lengthened bone were clearly delineated quantitatively and in their time sequence (Fig. 28-18). The rate of mineralization of the regenerating bone was assessed in the femur (0.8 ± 0.08 g/cm^2

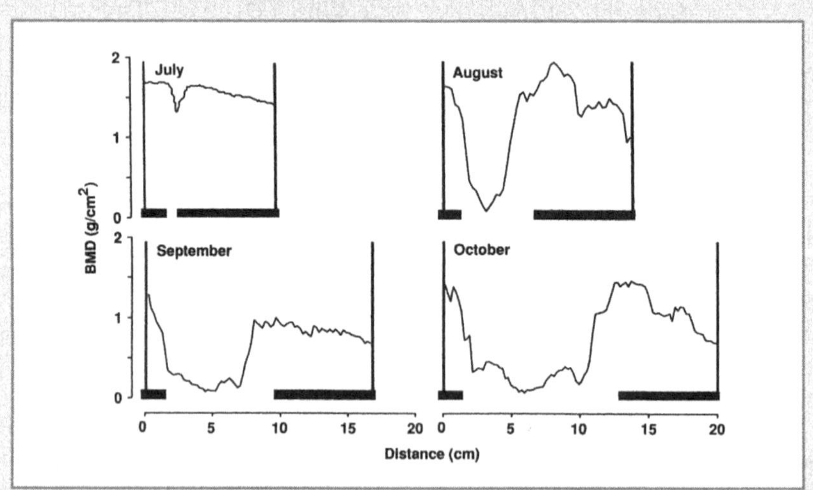

Fig. 28-18 Sequential BMD measurements in the long axis of the femur during distraction at the time of osteotomy (July) and after 1, 2, and 4 months. Bone density fell at the site of osteotomy; then as the limb was distracted, bone was generated from each end of the corticotomy. Vertical bars, site of fixator pin; horizontal bars, bone proximal and distal to the distraction gap. Bone generation during lengthening and bone loss in distal segments of the lengthened bone are clearly delineated quantitatively and in their time sequence by DXA. (From [39])

per month) and in the tibia (0.6±0.07 g/cm² per month) and final consolidation was estimated at 3–4 months after maximal distraction.

In a subsequent study the same authors compared ultrasound, radiography, and DXA for assessing bone formation in ten patients during leg lengthening [40]. Ultrasound proved useful in detecting cysting filling defects in the regenerate which was not recognized by radiography or DXA, and radiography was useful in evaluating small cortical defects unruled by the other two techniques. The obvious advantage of DXA over ultrasound and radiography lay in the possibility to determine the quantity and the rate of bone formation. Furthermore, they demonstrated that distraction achieved could be reliably measured by DXA since the correlation between interpin distance as measured by DXA and by a ruler on the skin surface was very high ($R^2 = 0.99$). They concluded that ultrasound complements DXA during limb lengthening, and that the use of both can reduce the need of traditional radiography [40].

Post-traumatic Osteopenia

The loss of bone after a fracture is a well-known phenomenon. An increase in the rate of bone turnover after fracture was first described in 1954 by Bauer [13] and later confirmed by others [50, 173], and the consequent bone loss was thoroughly investigated. The occurrence of osteopenia was also reported in the distal end of the femur after meniscectomy [124], in the proximal tibia after repair of injured knee ligaments [5], and in amputation stumps [16] and may be regarded as the result of regional acceleratory phenomena increasing bone remodeling activities with the contemporary contribution of vascular or soft tissue damages and disuse [50, 131].

The degree of demineralization was measured by several authors with various techniques (Table 28-3). Nilsson performed the first study using bone densitometry, an SPA with americium-241 source, finding a 25% BMC decrease in the distal femur years after ipsilateral tibial fracture [123]. Other investigations with the same technique [1, 5–7, 42, 43, 46, 47, 124, 125, 175], with DPA [49, 168] and with DXA [41, 85, 145, 169] followed. The amount of measured bone loss after fracture in the various studies was 15%–25% in the upper limb and 4%–50% in the lower limb depending on the site measured, technique used, time elapsed from fracture, and other variables (Table 28-3). After the trauma a bone loss was detected at the site of the fracture [41, 43, 47, 125], proximally [6, 7, 124, 175] or distally to it [41, 43, 125], and also in adjacent bones [46, 47, 85].

The bone loss is greater particularly when measured closer to the site of fracture and in bone regions with prevalent trabecular composition as the metaphysis or the epiphysis. Finsen and Haave [47] evaluated the bone changes after 16–68 months from tibial shaft fractures at different levels. They found an average 7%–8% bone loss at the metaphysis of distal femur and of proximal and distal tibia while the femoral and tibial diaphysis showed a 3% bone loss. In a similar study on ankle fractures Finsen and Benum [46] found a bone loss at the meta-

Table 28-3 Posttraumatic bone loss reported in literature

Reference	Technique	Site of injury	Site of measurement	Time (years)	Bone loss (%)
Nilsson 1966 [123]	SPA	Tibia	Distal femur	15	25
Bjork and Lemperg 1967 [16]	CW	Below knee amputation	Tibial stump	-	50
Nilsson and Westlin 1969 [124]	SPA	Postmeniscectomy	Distal femur	5	7
Westlin 1974 [175]	SPA	Colles' fracture	Midshaft radio Distal radio	1 1	18 18
Nilsson and Westlin 1977 [125]	SPA	Midshaft radius and ulna	Distal radius	5	15
Andersson and Nilsson 1977 [6]	SPA	Tibia	Proximal tibia	1	25
Andersson and Nilsson 1979 [5]	SPA	Ligamentous knee injury	Proximal tibia	1	18
Andersson and Nillson 1979 [7]	SPA	Tibia	Proximal tibia	1	25
Finsen and Benum 1986 [43]	SPA	Colles' fracture	Distal radio	2.5	+36a
Finsen and Haave 1987 [47]	SPA	Tibia	Distal tibia Distal femur	2.5 2.5	7 9
Ahl et al. 1988 [1]	SPA	Ankle	Calcaneus	3	7
Finsen 1988 [42]	SPA	Tibial osteotomy	Distal tibia	2	10
Finsen et al. 1988 [49]	DPA	Femur	Femur	2	12
Finsen and Benum 1989 [46]	SPA	Ankle	Distal tibia	2	3–9
Ulivieri et al. 1990 [168]	DPA	Tibia	Distal tibia	0.3	50
Karlsson et al. 1993 [85]	DXA	Lower extremity trauma	Trochanter Femoral condyle	15–38 15–38	1.2 4.4
Bickerstaff et al. 1993 [15]	SPA	Colles' fracture	Metacarpals	1	25
Sarangi et al. 1993 [145]	DXA	Tibia	Distal tibia Calcaneus	0.3 0.3	34.5–49.5 24.4–45.1
Van der Wiel et al. 1994 [169]	DXA	Tibia	Lumbar spine Femur Trochanter, femur neck	1 1 1	1 9 5
Eyres and Kanis 1995 [41]	DXA	Tibia	Site of fracture Distal tibia	5–11 5–11	+72a 46.5

CW, Cortical width on radiographs.

[a] Bone density measured at fracture level after complete recovery.

physis of the distal femur and proximal tibia of 5% and 9%, respectively, after 2 years while the corresponding values at the femoral and tibial diaphysis were 3.5% and 6%. One year after unstable fractures of the leg van der Wiel et al. [169] found a greater bone loss in the mainly trabecular trochanteric region than in the mainly cortical neck region of the proximal femur (9% vs. 5%).

When the repairing processes are completed, the BMD at the site of the fracture is greater than on the contralateral healthy site. This increase was found after diaphyseal radial fractures by Nilsson and Westlin [125], after Colles' fractures by Finsen and Benum (+39%) [43], after tibial fractures by Finsen and Haave (+28%) [47], and by Eyers and Kanis (+72% in adults, +30% in children) [41]. The longitudinal studies also presented a substantial agreement on the chronological succession of the repairing events. The lowest values of bone mass are reached 4–12 months after injury [6, 41, 46, 168, 175] and a complete recovery is possible in children [41] but not in adults [41, 47, 85]. More severe injuries were correlated with greater bone loss [1, 123], and there was only scarce evidence of a negative effect of older age [46] and duration of unloading [169]. Early weight bearing and movement did not seem to reduce bone loss [1, 7, 46, 49], and the type of treatment was barely significant in one study [41] and was not significant in others [49, 168].

The body of information obtained with these studies is in a strict agreement with some epidemiological data. The increase in bone density at the fracture site seems to exert a protective effect, as suggested by the marked reduction in the incidence of ipsilateral refracture after both previous Colles' and hip fractures [44, 45, 48], and the enduring lower limb reduction of BMD after certain types of fractures, such as the tibial fractures, is linked to a higher probability of subsequent ipsilateral fractures at a different level [48].

DXA has been used in this field since 1992. Sarangi et al. published a prospective study of the natural history of algodystrophy after tibial shaft fractures, measuring BMD in the distal tibial metaphysis and calcaneus of both legs in 60 consecutive patients [145]. The average percentage difference between fractured and healthy sides was around 45%–50% in the patients with algodystrophy and around 24%–34% in those without. Karlsson et al. measured residual bone loss 15–38 years after lower extremity trauma; the measured regions included the neck, trochanteric, and Ward regions of the hip and three other areas on femoral and tibial condyles and tibial diaphyses [85]. The bone loss was estimated comparing the values of the injured and uninjured sides, and they concluded that post-traumatic osteopenia was still evident decades after the injury [85]. Van der Wiel et al. used DXA to evaluate bone loss at the lumbar spine and both femora in 25 adult patients who sustained a tibial fracture [169]. In the ipsilateral but not in the contralateral bone proximal to the fractured bone they confirmed a significant bone loss that was more evident in the great trochanter region, and that showed no signs of recovery at 1 year. Finally, DXA was also used by Eyres and Kanis to evaluate bone loss after tibial fractures at the site of fracture and distal to it [41]. In addition to the data obtained following BMD changes over time and comparing BMD measured in selected regions of the fractured and healthy sides, Eyres and Kanis used the linear BMD measurements across the bone to enlighten remodeling activities at the site of the fracture.

All the investigations discussed above have strengthened the use of densitometry in this field, where it is still only marginally applied in spite of the necessity to verify bone fracture healing management procedures in an ever more aged population.

References

1. Ahl T, Sjoberg H, Dalen N (1988) Bone mineral content in the calcaneus after ankle fracture. Acta Orthop Scand 59:173–175
2. Ahnfelt L, Herberts P, Malchau H, Andersson GBJ (1990) Prognosis of total hip replacement: a Swedish multicenter study of 4.664 revisions. Acta Orthop Scand 238 [Suppl 61]:1–25
3. Akeson WH, Woo SL, Rutherford L et al (1976) The effects of rigidity of internal fixation plates on long bone remodeling. A biomechanical and quantitative histologic study. Acta Orthop Scand 47:241–249
4. Alho A (1993) Mineral and mechanics of bone fragility fractures. A review of fixation methods. Acta Orthop Scand 64:227–232
5. Andersson SM, Nilsson BE (1979) Changes in bone mineral content following ligamentous knee injuries. Med Sci Sports 11:351–354
6. Andersson SM, Nilsson BE (1979) Changes in bone mineral content following tibial shaft fractures. Clin Orthop 144:226–229
7. Andersson SM, Nilsson BE (1979) Posttraumatic bone mineral loss in tibial shaft fractures treated with a weightbearing brace. Acta Orthop Scand 50:689–691
8. Angelides M, Chan M, Ahmed AM, Joly L (1988) Effect of total knee arthroplasty on distal femur stress. Trans Orthop Res Soc 13:475–483
9. Aro HT, Wippermann BW, Hodgson SF, Wahner HW, Lewallen DG, Chao EYS (1989) Prediction of properties of fracture callus by measurement of mineral density using micro-bone densitometry. J Bone Joint Surg Am 71:1020–1030
10. Aronson J, Harrison BH, Steward CL, Harp JH (1989) The histology of distraction osteogenesis using different external fixators. Clin Orthop 241:106–116
11. Banks LM, Fowler CP, Robertson I, Thomas R, Whittle M, Strachan R (1994) DXA and total knee replacement – an initial experience. Bone Miner 25 [Suppl 2]:s3 (abstract)
12. Bartucci EJ, Gonzales MH, Cooperman DR, Freedberg HI, Barmada R, Laros GS (1985) The effect of adjunctive methylmethacrylate on failures of fixation and function in patients with intertrochanteric fractures and osteoporosis. J Bone Joint Surg Am 67:1094–1107

13. Bauer GCH (1954) Rate of bone salt formation in healing fractures determined in rats by means of radiocalcium. Acta Orthop Scand 23:169–191

14. Beljan JR, Hellewell AB, Goldman M (1971) The effect of calcium deficiency on healing of experimental fractures in the avian tarsus as determined by the fracture repair ratio. Clin Orthop 78:277–285

15. Bickerstaff DR, O'Doherty DP, Kanis JA (1993) Changes in cortical and trabecular bone in algodystrophy. Br J Rheumatol 32:46–51

16. Bjork L, Lemperg R (1967) Radiographic determination of the bone mineral content in amputation stumps. Acta Radiol Diagn (Stockh) 6:575–578

17. Blane CE, Herzenberg JE, DiPietro MA (1991) Radiographic imaging for Ilizarov limb lengthening in children. Pediatr Radiol 21:117–120

18. Bloebaum RD, Bachus KN, Mitchell W, Hoffman G, Hofmann AA (1995) Analysis of the bone surface area in resected tibia. Clin Orthop 309:2–10

19. Bobyn JD, Glassman AH, Goto H, Krygier JJ, Miller JE, Brooks CE (1990) The effects of stem stiffness after canine porous-coated total hip arthroplasty. Clin Orthop 261:196–213

20. Bobyn JD, Mortimer ES, Glassman AH, Engh CA, Miller JE, Brooks CE (1992) Producing and avoiding stress shielding: laboratory and clinical observations of noncemented total hip arthroplasty. Clin Orthop 274:79–96

21. Brand RA, Yoder SA, Pedersen DR (1985) Intraobserver variability in interpreting radiographic lucencies aboult total hip reconstructions. Clin Orthop 192:237–239

22. Cameron HV, Cameron GI (1987) Stress relief osteoporosis of the anterior femoral condyles in total knee replacement. A study of 185 patients. Orthop Rev 16:449–456

23. Capello WN (1990) Technical aspects of cementless total hip arthroplasty. Clin Orthop 261:102–106

24. Carlson GD, Abitbol JJ, Anderson DR et al. (1992) Screw fixation in the human sacrum: an in vitro study of the biomechanics of fixation. Spine 17:S1–S8

25. Carter DR, Hayes WC (1976) Bone compressive strength: the influence of density and strain rate. Science 194:1174–1176

26. Coe JD, Warden KE, Herzig MA, McAfee PC (1990) Influence of bone mineral density on the fixation of thoracolumbar implants: a comparative study of transpedicular screws, laminar hooks, and spinous process wires. Spine 15:902–907

27. Cohen B, Rushton N (1994) A comparative study of peri-prosthetic bone mineral density measurement using two different dual-energy X-ray absorptiometry systems. Br J Radiol 67:852–855

28. Cohen B, Rushton N (1995) Accuracy of DEXA measurement of bone mineral density after total hip arthroplasty. J Bone Joint Surg Br 77:479–483

29. Cohen B, Rushton N (1995) Bone remodelling in the proximal femur after Charnley total hip arthroplasty. J Bone Joint Surg Br 77:815–819

30. Dalenberg DD, Asher MA, Robinson RG, Jayaraman G (1993) The effect of a stiff spinal implant and its loosening on the bone mineral content in canines. Spine 18:1862–1866

31. Engh CA (1983) Hip arthroplasty with a Moore prosthesis with porous coating: a five year study. Clin Orthop 176:53–66

32. Engh CA, Bobyn JD, Glassman AH (1987) Porous-coated hip replacement: the factors governing bone ingrowth, stress shielding, and clinical results. J Bone Joint Surg Br 69:45–55

33. Engh CA, Bobyn JD (1988) The influence of stem size and extent of porous coating on femoral bone resorption after primary cementless hip arthroplasty. Clin Orthop 231:7–28

34. Engh CA, Massin P, Suthers KE (1990) Roentgenographic assessment of the biologic fixation of porous-surfaced femoral component. Clin Orthop 257:107–128

35. Engh CA, McGovern TF, Bobyn JD, Harris WH (1992) A quantitative evaluation of periprosthetic bone-remodeling after cementless total hip arthroplasty. J Bone Joint Surg Am 74:1009–1020

36. Engh CA, McGovern TF, Schmidt LM (1993) Roentgenographic densitometry of bone adjacent to a femoral prosthesis. Clin Orthop 292:177–190

37. Engh CA, Hooten Jr JP, Zettl-Schaffer KF, Ghaffarpour M, McGovern TF, Macalino GE, Zicat BA (1994) Porous coated total hip replacements. Clin Orthop 298:89–96

38. Ewald FC (1989) The Knee Society total knee arthroplasty roentgenographic evaluation and scoring system. Clin Orthop 248:9–12

39. Eyres KS, Bell MJ, Kanis JA (1993) New bone formation during leg lengthening. J Bone Joint Surg Br 75:96–106

40. Eyres KS, Bell MJ, Kanis JA (1993) Methods of assessing new bone formation during limb lengthening: ultrasonography, dual energy X-ray absorptiometry and radiography compared. J Bone Joint Surg Br 75:358–364

41. Eyres KS, Kanis JA (1995) Bone loss after tibial fracture: evaluated by dual-energy X-ray absorptiometry. J Bone Joint Surg Br 77:473–478

42. Finsen V (1988) Osteopenia after osteotomy of the tibia. Calcif Tissue Int 42:1–4

43. Finsen V, Benum P (1986) Refracture rare after removal of fixation device from healed hip fractures. Acta Orthop Scand 57:434–435

44. Finsen V, Benum P (1986) The second hip fracture: an epidemiologic study. Acta Orthop Scand 57:431–433

45. Finsen V, Benum P (1987) The interrelationship of past and present fractures of the forearm and hand. Acta Orthop Scand 58:370–372

46. Finsen V, Benum P (1989) Osteopenia after ankle fractures: the influence of early weight bearing and muscle activity. Clin Orthop 245:261–268

47. Finsen V, Haave O (1987) Changes in bone-mass after tibial shaft fracture. Acta Orthop Scand 58:369–371

48. Finsen V, Haave O, Benum P (1989) Fracture interaction in the extremities: the possible relevance of post-traumatic osteopenia. Clin Orthop 240:244–249

49. Finsen V, Svenningsen S, Harnes OB, Nesse O, Benum P (1988) Osteopaenia after plated and nailed femoral shaft fractures. J Orthop Trauma 2:13–17

50. Frost HM (1989) The biology of fracture healing: an overview for clinicians, part. 1. Clin Orthop 248:283–293
51. Frost HM (1990) Structural adaptations to mechanical usage (SATMU): 1. Redefining Wolff's Law: the bone modeling problem. Anat Rec 226:403–413
52. Galante JO, Rostoker W, Lueck R, Ray RD (1971) Sintered fiber composites as a basis for attachment of implants to bone. J Bone Joint Surg Am 53:101–108
53. Gerlanc M, Haddad D, Hyatt GW, Langloh JT, St Hilaire P (1975) Ultrasonic study of normal and fractured bone. Clin Orthop 111:175–184
54. Gill PJ, Kernohan G, Mawhinney IN, Mollan RA, McIlhagger R (1989) Investigation of the mechanical properties of bone using ultrasound. Proc Inst Mech Eng 203:61–63
55. Glassman AH, Engh CA, Griffin WL (1990) Removal of porous coated femoral hip stem. In: Proceedings of AADS 57th Annual Meeting, New Orleans, Louisiana, p 199
56. Gristina AG (1994). Implant failure and the immuno-incompetent fibro-inflammatory zone. Clin Orthop 298:106–118
57. Gruen T (1987) Radiographic criteria for the clinical performance of uncemented total hip replacements. In: Lemons JE (ed) Quantitative characterization and performance of porous implants for hard tissue applications. American Society for Testing and Materials, Philadelphia, pp 207–218
58. Gruen TA, McNeice GM, Amstutz HC (1979) "Modes of failure" of cemented stem-type femoral components: a radiographic analysis of loosening. Clin Orthop 141:17–27
59. Gundry CR, Miller CW, Ramos E (1990) Dual-energy radiographic absorptiometry of the lumbar spine: clinical experience with two different systems. Radiology 174:539–541
60. Haddad RJ, Cook SD, Brinker MR (1990) A comparison of three varieties of uncemented porous-coated hip replacement. J Bone Joint Surg Br 72:2–8
61. Hamanishi C, Kawabata T, Yoshii T, Tanaka S (1995) Bone mineral density changes in distracted callus stimulated by pulsed direct electrical current. Clin Orthop 312:247–252
62. Hamanishi C, Yoshii T, Totani Y, Tanaka S (1994) Bone mineral density of lengthened rabbit tibia is enhanced by transplantation of fresh autologous bone marrow cells: an experimental study using dual X-ray absorptiometry. Clin Orthop 303:250–255
63. Hansson T, Roos B, Nachemson A (1980) The bone mineral content and ultimate compressive strength of lumbar vertebrae. Spine 5:46–54
64. Harrington KD (1975) The use of methylmethacrylate as an adjunct in the internal fixation of unstable comminuted intertrochanteric fractures in osteoporotic patients. J Bone Joint Surg Am 57:744–750
65. Harris WH, Jasty M (1985) Bone ingrowth into porous coated canine acetabular replacements: the effect of pore size, apposition and dislocation. In: Fitzgerald RH (ed) The hip. Proceedings of the 13th open scientific meeting of the hip society. Mosby, St Louis, pp 214–234

66. Healy WL (1995) Economic considerations in total hip arthroplasty and implant standardization. Clin Orthop 311:102–108

67. Hedley AK, Gruen TA, Borden LS (1986) Two year follow-up of the PCA non-cemented total hip replacement. In: Brand RA (ed) The hip. Proceedings of the 14th open scientific meeting of the hip society. Mosby, St Louis, pp 225–250

68. Hellewell AG (1980) Absorptiometric quantitation of experimental fracture mineralization. In: 4th International Conference on Bone Mineral Measurement. NIH publication 80-1938:121–125

69. Hofmann AA, Wyatt RW, France EP, Bigler GT, Daniels AU, Hess WE (1987) Endosteal bone loss after total hip arthroplasty. Clin Orthop 245:138–144

70. Hollis JM, Hofmann OE, Steward CL, Flahiff CM, Nelson CL (1992) Effect of micromotion on ingrowth into porous coated implants using a transcortical model. In: Transactions of the 4th World Biomaterials Congress, p 258

71. Hozack WJ, Booth RE Jr (1990) Clinical and radiographic results with the trilock femoral component: a wedge-fit porous ingrowth stem design. Semin Arthroplasty 1:64–69

72. Hughes SS, Furia JP, Smith P, Pellegrini VD Jr (1995) Atrophy of the proximal part of the femur after total hip arthroplasty without cement. J Bone Joint Surg Am 77:231–239

73. Huiskes R (1980) Some fundamental aspects of human-joint replacement. Acta Orthop Scand 51 [Suppl 1]:1

74. Huiskes R (1990) The various stress patterns of press-fit, ingrown, and cemented femoral stems. Clin Orthop 261:27–38

75. Huiskes R, Chao EYS (1989) A survey of finite element methods in orthopaedic biomechanics. J Biomech 16:385–394

76. Huiskes R, Weinans H, van Rietbergen B (1992) The relationship between stress shielding and bone resorption around total hip stems and the effects of flexible materials. Clin Orthop 274:124–134

77. Husby T, Hoiset A, Alho A (1987) Osteoporosis and stability of osteosynthesis of the femoral neck. Trans Orthop Res Soc 12:236

78. Hvid I (1988) Trabecular bone strength of the knee. Clin Orthop 227:210–222

79. Hvid I, Hansen SL (1985) Trabecular bone strength patterns at the proximal tibial epiphysis. J Orthop Res 3:462–470

80. Jasty M, O'Connor DO, Henshaw RM, Harrigan TP, Harris WH (1994) Fit of uncemented femoral component and the use of cement influence the strain transfer to the femoral cortex. J Orthop Res 12:648–656

81. Jiang CC, Insall JN (1989) Effect of rotation on the axial alignment of the femur. Clin Orthop 248:50–56

82. Johnston RC, Crowninshield RD (1983) Roentgenologic results of total hip arthroplasty: a ten-year follow-up study. Clin Orthop 181:92–102

83. Kantor SG, Schneider R, Insall JN, Becker MW (1990) Radionuclide imaging of asymptomatic versus syptomatic total knee arthroplasties. Clin Orthop 260:118–123

84. Kaplan PA, Montesi SA, Jardon OM (1988) Bone-ingrowth hip prostheses in asymptomatic patients: radiographic features. Radiology 169:221–227

85. Karlsson MK, Nilsson BE, Obrant KJ (1993) Bone mineral loss after lower extremity trauma. Acta Orthop Scand 64:362–364

86. Kattapuram SV, Lodwick GS, Chandler H (1990) Porous coated total hip prostheses: radiographic analysis and clinical correlation. Radiology 174:861–864

87. Kenwright J, Goodship AE (1989) Controlled mechanical stimulation in the treatment of tibial fractures. Clin Orthop 241:36–47

88. Kilgus DJ, Shimaoka EE, Tipton JS, Eberle RB (1993) Dual-energy X-ray absorptiometry measurement of bone mineral density around porous-coated cementless femoral implants. J Bone Joint Surg Br 75:279–287

89. Kiratli BJ, Heiner JP, McBeath AA (1991) Bone mineral density response after total hip arthroplasty: one year follow up. J Bone Miner Res 6 [Suppl 1]:S110 (abstract)

90. Kiratli BJ, Heiner JP, McKinley N, Wilson MA, McBeath AA (1991) Bone mineral density of the proximal femur after uncemented total hip arthroplasty. Trans Orthop Res Soc 16:545

91. Kiratli BJ, Heiner JP, McBeath AA, Wilson MA (1992) Determination of bone mineral density by dual X-ray absorptiometry in patients with uncemented total hip arthroplasty. J Orthop Res 10:836–844

92. Kiratli BJ, Heiner JP, McKinley N, Wilson MA, McBeath AA (1992) Bone mineral density of the proximal femur after uncemented total hip arthroplasty. Trans Orthop Res Soc 17:238

93. Kiratli JB, Checovic MM, McBeath AA, Wilson MA, Heiner JP (1996) Measurement of bone mineral density by dual-energy X-ray absorptiometry in patients with the Wisconsin hip, an uncemented femoral stem. J Arthroplasty 11:184–192

94. Korovessis P, Piperos G, Michael A (1994) Prosthetic bone mineral density after Mueller and Zweymueller total hip arthroplasties. Clin Orthop 309:214–221

95. Krackow KA, Jones MM, Teeny SM, Hungerford DS (1991) Primary total knee arthroplasty in patients with fixed valgus deformity. Clin Orthop 273:9–18

96. Kumano K, Hirabayashi S, Ogawa Y, Aota Y (1994) Pedicle screws and bone mineral density. Spine 19:1157–1161

97. Kwong LM, Jasty M, Mulroy RD, Maloney WJ, Bragdon C, Harris WH (1992) The histology of the radiolucent line. J Bone Joint Surg Br 74:67–73

98. Laros GS, Moore JF (1974) Complications of fixation in intertrochanteric fractures. Clin Orthop 101:110–116

99. Laskey MA, Flaxman ME, Barber RW (1991) Comparative performance in vitro and in vivo of Lunar DPX and Hologic QDR 1000 dual energy X-ray absorptiometers. Br J Radiol 64:1023–1029

100. Lee RW, Volz RG, Sheridan DC (1991) The role of fixation and bone quality on the mechanical stability of tibial knee components. Clin Orthop 273:177–189

101. Levitz CL, Lotke PA, Karp JS (1995) Long-term changes in bone mineral density following total knee replacement. Clin Orthop 321:68–72

102. Lewis JL (1975) A dynamic model of a healing fractured long bone. J Biomech 8:17–24

103. Liu TK, Yang RS, Chieng PU, Shee BW (1995) Periprosthetic bone mineral density of the distal femur after total knee arthroplasty. Int Orthop 19:346–351

104. Lord J, Marotte JH, Guillamon JL, Blanchard JP (1988) Cementless revisions of failed aseptic cemented and cementless total hip arthroplasties: 284 cases. Clin Orthop 235:67–74

105. Maffulli N, Hughes T, Fixsen JA (1992) Ultrasonographic monitoring of limb lengthening. J Bone Joint Surg Br 74:130–132

106. Maloney WJ, Jasty M, Burke DW, O'Connor DO, Zalenski EB, Bragdon C, Harris WH (1989) Biomechanical and histologic investigation of cemented total hip arthroplasty: a study of autopsy-retrieved femurs after in vivo cycling. Clin Orthop 249:129–140

107. Marinoni EC, Trevisan C, Bigoni M, Castellano S, Ortolani S, Peretti G (1994) Metodiche di valutazione strumentale nel follow-up delle protesi totali di ginocchio. In: Monteleone A (ed) International meeting knee prosthesis, microprint SBR, Napoli 1994, pp 195–204

108. Markel MD, Chao EY (1993) Noninvasive monitoring techniques for quantitative description of callus mineral content and mechanical properties. Clin Orthop 293:37–45

109. Markel MD, Wikenheiser MA, Morin RL, Lewallen DG, Chao EYS (1990) Quantification of bone healing. Comparison of QCT, SPA, MRI and DEXA in dog osteotomies. Acta Orhtop Scand 61:487–498

110. Martin B (1993) Ageing and strengh of bone as a structural material. Calcif Tissue Int 53 [Suppl 1]:s34–s40

111. Massari L, Mura P, Giancolo R, Biscione R, Bagni B, Villani C, Gallazzi MB (1994) Valutazione con DEXA dell'osteointegrazione nelle componenti protesiche rivestite con idrossiapatite. Ital J Orthop Traumatol 20 [Suppl 1]: 93–100

112. Mazess RB (1983) Noninvasive bone measurement. In: Kunin A (ed) Skeletal research II. Academic, New York, p 277

113. Mazess RB, Barden HS (1988) Measurement of bone by dual-photon absorptiometry (DPA) and dual-energy X-ray absorptiometry (DEXA). Ann Chirur Gynaecol 77:197–203

114. Mazess RB, Wahner HM (1988) Nuclear medicine and densitometry. In: Riggs BL, Melton LJ III (eds) Osteoporosis, aetiology, diagnosis and management. Raven, New York, pp 251–295

115. McAfee PC, Farey ID, Sutterlin CE, Gurr KR, Warden KE, Cunningham BW (1989) Device-related osteoporosis with spinal instrumentation. Spine 14:919–926

116. McCarthy CK, Steinberg GG, Agren M, Leahey D, Wyman E, Baran DT (1991) Quantifying bone loss from the proximal femur after total hip arthroplasty. J Bone Joint Surg Br 73:774–778

117. McCaskie AW, Brown AR, Thompson JR, Gregg PJ (1996) Radiological evaluation of the interfaces after cemented total hip replacement: interobserver and intraobserver agreement. J Bone Joint Surg Br 78:191–194

118. McGovern TF, Engh CA, Zettl-Schaffer K, Hooten JP (1995) Cortical bone density of the proximal femur following total hip arthroplasty. Clin Orthop 306:145–154

119. Miller JE, Kelebay LC (1981) Bone ingrowth-disuse osteoporosis. Trans Orthop Res Soc 5:380–386

120. Minzer CM, Robertson DD, Rackemann S, Ewald FC, Scott RD, Spector M (1990) Bone loss in the distal anterior femur after total knee arthroplasty. Clin Orthop 260:135–143

121. Mortimer ES, Rosenthall L, Paterson I, Bobyn JD (1996) Effect of rotation on periprosthetic bone mineral measurements in a hip phantom. Clin Orthop 324:269–274

122. Niinimaki T, Jalovaara P (1995) Bone loss from the proximal femur after arthroplasty with an isoelastic femoral stem: BMD measurements in 25 patients after 9 years. Acta Orthop Scand 66:347–351

123. Nilsson BE (1966) Post-traumatic osteopenia: a quantitative study of the bone mineral mass in the femur following fracture of the tibia in man using americium-241 as a photon source. Acta Orthop Scand 37 [Suppl]:91

124. Nilsson BE, Westlin NE (1969) Osteoporosis following injury to the semilunar cartilage. Calcif Tissue Res 4:185–187

125. Nilsson BE, Westlin NE (1977) Bone mineral content in the forearm after fracture of the upper limb. Calcif Tissue Res 22:329–331

126. Noble PC, Box GG, Kamaric E, Fink MJ, Alexander JW, Tullos HS (1995) The effect of aging on the shape of the proximal femur. Clin Orthop 316:31–44

127. Oh I, Harris WH (1978) Proximal strain distribution in the loaded femur: an in vitro comparison of the distributions in the intact femur and after insertion of different hip replacement femoral components. J Bone Joint Surg Am 60:75–83

128. Orne D (1974) The in vivo driving point impedance of the human ulna: a viscoelastic beam model. J Biomech 7:249–254

129. Ortolani S, Trevisan C, Montesano A, Gandolini G, Bianchi ML, Caraceni MP, Ulivieri FM (1990) Comparison between 153-Gd and X-ray dual photon absorptiometry. Ital J Miner Electrolyte Metab 4:37–42

130. Peretti G, Memeo A, Paronzini A, Marinoni EC (1988) Methods for the study of bone regeneration in lengthening of the limbs. Ital J Orthop Traumatol 15:217–221

131. Perren SM, Cordey J, Rahn BA, Gautier E, Schneider E (1987) Early temporary porosis of bone induced by internal fixation implants. A reaction to necrosis, not to stress protection? Clin Orthop 232:139–151

132. Petersen MB, Kolthoff N, Eiken P (1995) Bone mineral density around femoral stems: DXA measurements in 22 porous-coated implants after 5 years. Acta Orhtop Scand 66:432–434

133. Petersen MM, Nilsen PT, Lauritzen JB, Lund B (1995) Changes in bone density of the proximal tibia following uncemented knee arthroplasty: a 3 years follow-up of 25 knees. Acta Orthop Scand 66:513–516

134. Petersen MM, Lauritzen JB, Pedersen JG, Lund B (1996) Decreased bone density of the distal femur after uncemented knee arthroplasty. Acta Orthop Scand 67:339–344

135. Pilliar RM, Cameron HU, Welsh RP, Binnington AG (1981) Radiographic and morphologic studies of load-bearing porous-surfaced structured implants. Clin Orthop 156:249–254

136. Poss R (1992) Natural factors that affect shape and strength of the ageing human femur. Clin Orthop 274:194–201

137. Pritchett JW (1995) Femoral bone loss following hip replacement. A comparative study. Clin Orthop 314:156–161

138. Richmond BJ, Bauer TW, Stulberg BN, Fox JS (1990) Bone mineral in patients undergoing uncemented total hip arthroplasty. Calcif Tissue Int 46:145 (abstract)

139. Richmond BJ, Eberle RW, Stulberg BN, Deal CL (1991) DEXA measurement of peri-prosthetic bone mineral density in total hip arthroplasty. J Bone Miner Res 6 [Suppl 1]:S241 (abstract)

140. Robertson DD, Minzer CM, Weissman BN, Ewald FC, LeBoff M, Spector M (1994) Distal loss of femoral bone following total knee arthroplasty. J Bone Joint Surg Am 76:66–76

141. Rosenberg A (1989) Cementless total hip arthroplasty: femoral remodelling and clinical experience. Orthopaedics 12:1223–1233

142. Rosenberg AG, Andriacchi TP, Barden R, Galante JO (1988) Patellar component failure in cementless total knee arthroplasty. Clin Orthop 236:106–114

143. Ruff CB, Hayes WC (1982) Subperiosteal expansion and cortical remodelling of the human femur and tibia with ageing. Science 217:945–946

144. Saha S, Lakes RS (1977) The effect of soft tissue on the wave-propagation and vibration tests for determining the in vivo properties of bone. J Biomech 10:393–398

145. Sarangi PP, Ward AJ, Smith EJ, Staddon GE, Atkins RM (1993) Algodystrophy and osteoporosis after tibial fractures. J Bone Joint Surg Br 75:450–452

146. Sarmiento A (1973) Unstable intertrochanteric fractures of the femur. Clin Orthop 92:77–85

147. Scott RD, Volatile TB (1986) Twelve years' experience with posterior cruciate-retaining total knee arthroplasty. Clin Orthop 205:100–114

148. Seitz P, Ruegsegger P, Gschwend N, Dubs L (1987) Changes in local bone density after knee arthroplasty. J Bone Joint Surg Br 69:407–411

149. Skinner HB, Kilgus DJ, Keyak J, Shimaoka EE, Kim AS, Tipton JS (1994) Correlation of computed finite element stresses to bone density after remodelling around cementless femoral implant. Clin Orthop 305:178–189

150. Skinner HB, Kim AS, Keyak JH, Mote CD (1994) Femoral prosthesis implantation induces changes in bone stress that depend on the extent of porous coating. J Orthop Res 12:553–563

151. Smith KR, Hunt TR, Asher MA, Anderson HC, Robinson R, Carson WL (1988) Study of bone stress shielding in the canine lumbar spine. Presented

at the annual meeting of the Scoliosis Research Society, Baltimore, Maryland, 29 Sept–2 Oct

152. Smith RW, Walker RR (1964) Femoral expansion in ageing women: implication for osteoporosis and fractures. Science 145:156–158

153. Smith SA, Abitbol JJ, Carlson GD, Anderson DR, Taggart KW, Garfin SR (1993) The effects of depth of penetration, screw orientation and bone density on sacral screw fixation. Spine 18:1006–1010

154. Soshi S, Shiba R, Kondo H, Murota H (1991) An experimental study on transpedicular screw fixation in relation to osteoporosis af the lumbar spine. Spine 16:1335–1341

155. Stulberg BN, Bauer TW, Watson JT, Richmond B (1989) Bone quality: roentgenographic versus histologic assessment of hip bone structure. Clin Orthop 240:200–205

156. Stulberg BN, Eberle RW, Fox JS, Richmond BJ (1989) The technical aspects of peri-prosthetic bone mineral density in uncemented total hip arthroplasty. In: 2nd International Symposium for Custom Prostheses, Chicago, IL, p 23 (abstract 70)

157. Svesnikov AA, Oficerova NV (1985) Mineralstoffwechsel bei Knochenbrüchen nach den Ergebnissen Photonen-Absorptionsmessung. Radiol Diagn (Berl) 26:407–412

158. Sychterz CJ, Engh CE (1996) The influence of clinical factors on periprosthetic bone remodeling. Clin Orthop 322:285–292

159. Terjesen T, Benum P (1983) The stress protecting effect of metal plates on the intact rabbit tibia. Acta Orthop Scand 54:810–818

160. Thomas BJ, Salvati EA, Small RD (1986) The CAD hip arthroplasty: five to ten year follow-up. J Bone Joint Surg Am 68:640–651

161. Tissakht M, Ahmed AM, Chan KC (1993) Stress-shielding in the distal femur following TKR: effect of bone/implant interface condition. Trans Orthop Res Soc 18:426

162. Trevisan C, Caraceni MP, Gandolini G, Montesano A, Ortolani S (1990) Bone density of dominant and nondominant hip measured by dual-energy X-ray absorptiometry. In: Christiansen C, Overgaard K (eds) Osteoporosis 90. Handelstrykkeriet Aalborg, Aalborg, pp 863–865

163. Trevisan C, Bigoni M, Cherubini R, Randelli G, Ortolani S (1992) Longitudinal assessment of periprosthetic bone mineral density by DXA in total hip arthroplasty. Bone Miner 17 [Suppl 1]:225 (abstract)

164. Trevisan C, Bigoni M, Cherubini R, Steiger P, Randelli G, Ortolani S (1993). Dual X-ray absorptiometry for the evaluation of bone density from the proximal femur after total hip arthroplasty: analysis protocols and reproducibility. Calcif Tissue Int 53:158–161

165. Trevisan C, Bigoni M, Randelli G, Marinoni EC, Peretti G, Ortolani S (1997) Periprosthetic bone density around fully hydrohyapatite coated femoral stem. Clin Orthop 340:109–117

166. Trevisan C, Bigoni M, Benti M, Marinoni EC, Ortolani S (1997) Bone assess-

ment after total knee arthroplasty by dual-energy X-ray absorptiometry: analysis protocol and reproducibility. Calcif Tissue Int (in press)

167. Uhthoff HK, Boisvert D, Finnegan M (1994) Cortical porosis under plates. J Bone Joint Surg Am 76:1507–1512

168. Ulivieri FM, Bossi E, Azzoni R, Ronzani C, Trevisan C, Montesano A, Ortolani S (1990) Quantification by dual photonabsorptiometry of local bone loss after fracture. Clin Orthop 250:291–296

169. Van der Wiel HE, Lips P, Nauta J, Patka P, Haarman HJThM, Teule GJJ (1994) Loss of bone in the proximal part of the femur following unstable fractures of the leg. J Bone Joint Surg Am 76:230–236

170. Van Roermund PM, Ter Haar Romeny BM, Hoekstra A, Schoonderwoert GJ, Brandt CJ, van der Steen SP, Roelofs JMM, Scholten F, Visser WJ, Renoij W (1991) Bone growth and remodeling after distraction epiphysiolysis of the proximal tibia of the rabbit. Clin Orthop 266:304–312

171. Van Roermund PM, Ter Haar Romeny BM, Schoonderwoert GJ, Brandt CJ, Sijbrandij S, Renooij W (1987) The use of computed tomography to quantitate bone formation after distraction epiphysiolysis in the rabbit. Skeletal Radiol 16:52–56

172. Walker PS, Granholm J, Lowrey R (1982) The fixation of femoral components of condylar knee prostheses. Eng Med 11:135–140

173. Wendeberg B (1961) Mineral metabolism of fractures of the tibia in man studied with external counting of Sr^{85}. Acta Orthop Scand [Suppl] 52:130

174. West JD, Mayor MB, Collier JP (1987) Potential erors inherent in quantitative densitometric analysis of orthopaedic radiographs: a study after total hip arthroplasty. J Bone Joint Surg Am 69:58–64

175. Westlin NE (1974) Loss of bone mineral after Colles' fracture. Clin Orthop 102:194–199

176. Wittenberg RH, Shea M, Swartz DE, Lee KS, White AA, Hayes WC (1991) Importance of bone mineral density in instrumented spine fusions. Spine 16:647–652

177. Wrobleski BM (1986) 15–21 year results of the Charnley low-friction arthroplasty. Clin Orthop 211:30–42

178. Young JWR, Kostrubiak IS, Resnick CS, Paley D (1990) Sonographic evaluation of bone production at the distraction site in Ilizarov limb-lengthening procedures. AJR 154:125–128

179. Zindrick MR, Wiltse LL, Widell EH, Thomas JC, Holland WR, Field BT, Spencer CW (1986) A biomechanical study of intrapeduncular screw fixation in the lumbosacral spine. Clin Orthop 203:99–112

29 Osteoporosis and Oral Bone Loss: Mandibular Bone Density and Its Relationship to Systemic Osteoporosis in Edentulous Women

M. T. DiMuzio, K. Houki, C. B. Westlund, C. Berkovich, and L. K. Fattore

Introduction

The contribution of oral bone loss to the overall morbidity in the aging population cannot be underestimated, and the amount of alveolar bone loss after tooth extraction may also limit the overall retention and stability of dentures. This fact alone increases the difficulty in the construction of the prosthesis. For many years the gradual resorption of the alveolar bone was thought to be due only to local factors such as the loss of the functional influence of the teeth on the surrounding tissues, direct loading of the alveolus by complete dentures, continuous wearing of ill-fitting dentures, and periodontal disease. Currently the literature suggests a relationship between systemic bone loss from osteoporosis and the resorption of the edentulous alveolar ridge.

Evidence of such a relationship was provided in 1978 by Rosenquist et al. who compared the bone calcium mass of the radius in two groups of edentulous men (those needing vestibuloplasty of the mandible, and an age-matched control group). They found that the patients with mandibular atrophy had a lower bone calcium mass than their age-matched controls. Kribbs et al. (1983) reported a significant correlation between skeletal osteopenia and mandibular density in the edentulous mandible of women subjects. Habets et al. (1988) examined iliac crest biopsies of 74 patients with severe mandibular atrophy and found evidence of systemic osteoporosis. In a 1990 study Kribbs et al. observed that osteoporosis adversely affects mandibular bone by decreasing its bone mass and density. These studies suggest that alveolar ridge reduction is an oral manifestation of osteoporosis, and the preponderance of postmenopausal women with this condition gives some credence to this theory.

Radiological methods [dual-photon absorptiometry, dual energy X-ray absorptiometry (DXA)], originally used to assess the bone mineral content (BMC) and the bone mineral density (BMD) of the lumbar spine, hip, and forearm, have been used by several investigators to measure the BMD of the mandible. Their studies have examined the relationship of BMD and BMC of the jaws with other skeletal sites. Kribbs et al. (1989) reported a positive correlation between mandibular bone mass, as measured by microdensitometry, and total body calcium in a population of osteoporotic women. Kribbs' study suggested that mandibular bone mass may better reflect the status of the entire skeleton rather than merely the bone mass or mineral content of the wrist and vertebrae. Von Wowern and Hjorting-Hansen (1991), using dual-photon absorptiometry to measure the BMC of edentulous mandibles, reported that mandibular BMC measurements can be used to predict the rate of residual ridge resorption. In a 1992 study Von Wowern and Kollerup found that the BMC, as measured by a dual-photon scanner, was significantly lower in the mandibles and forearm bones of a small group of osteoporotic women than in a control group. Klemetti et al. in a series of 1993 studies used single-energy quantitative computed tomography to determine the BMD of the cortical bone of the mandible (Klemetti et al. 1993a,b). Corten et al. (1993) developed a new method to measure the mandibular BMD using DXA (Hologic QDR-1000). The conflict over interpreting these studies is due to the fact that comparisons are difficult because of a lack of standardization of radiological technique and patient positioning.

The present study was conducted to test the following hypotheses of a positive correlation between mandibular bone density and the bone density of other skeletal sites, and of osteoporosis as a risk factor for severe alveolar ridge atrophy. The specific aims were: (a) to demonstrate the stability, reproducibility, and reliability of DXA measurements of mandibular bone; (b) to compare BMD, BMC, and the residual alveolar ridge height of the mandible in women with and without osteoporosis; (c) to determine the relationship of mandibular bone density to that of the hip, spine, and wrist; and (d) to determine the relationship, if any, of mandibular bone density with residual alveolar ridge height in osteoporotic women.

Materials and Methods

Subjects

Subjects for the study were selected from the patient population of the geriatric dental clinic of Northwestern University Dental School and from the community and resident populations of the United Methodist Home, an affiliated teaching nursing home. All case and control patients had to be 55 years of age or older, edentulous for a minimum of 5 years, and of white or Asian race. Only edentulous patients were selected in order to eliminate periodontal disease as a confounding factor. A diagnosis of osteoporosis was made by measuring the BMD of the femoral neck and lumbar spine, which reflect the osteoporosis status of the whole body. All subjects with secondary osteoporosis were excluded from this study as well as those who had a known history of any physical condition that was associated with bone mass loss or gain.

Of the 13 participating patients 10 were diagnosed with osteoporosis; their ages were 57, 71 (n=4), 75, 76, 81 (n=2), and 84 years. The remaining 3 were diagnosed as being normal; their ages were 61, 81, and 91 years.

Bone Densitometry

DXA measurements were made with a Hologic QDR-2000 bone densitometer (Hologic, Waltham, Mass.). The QDR-2000 uses a multiple detector fan beam, and while providing equivalent information, differs in a number of ways from earlier single-beam DXA systems such as the Hologic QDR-1000 (which was used by Corten, 1993). Compared to the latter, the QDR-2000 provides faster scan times, higher image resolution, and improved reproducibility for lateral lumbar spine scans.

DXA analyses in all subjects were performed in the Nuclear Medicine Clinic of Children's Memorial Hospital, an affiliated hospital of Northwestern University Medical Center. In addition to the mandible, the hip, spine, and forearm were scanned in each patient for BMC (in grams) and BMD (in grams per square centimeters). DXA analyses were used to confirm the clinical diagnosis of primary osteoporosis according to the World Health Organization guidelines. These criteria define osteoporosis with BMD values less than or equal to 2.5 SD from the young peak bone mass of a valid reference population of healthy sex- and race-matched individuals. The BMD values of the femoral neck and lumbar spine of each patient were thus compared to age-matched values (Z) and young peak bone mass values (T). The Z score is used to compare the amount of bone loss to the expected amount of loss for peers of the same age. The T score is used to compare the BMD value to peak bone mass and serves as an indicator of bone health and fracture risk. The T score is determined by the distance between the patient's actual BMD and the peak bone mass for a young normal patient, expressed as a standard deviation and as a percentage value. A diagnosis of osteoporosis was made if the bone density of the femoral neck and lumbar spine was less than that of an age-matched reference population by more than 2.5 SD (T value <2.50).

The location of the mandibular sites to be measured using DXA are shown in Fig. 29-1. Mandibular DXA measurements were analyzed with the forearm analy-

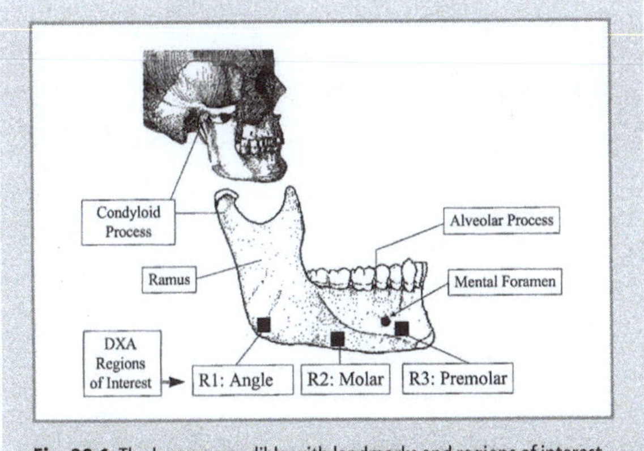

Fig. 29-1 The human mandible with landmarks and regions of interest chosen for DXA analysis

sis software, which is well-suited for mandibular densitometry because of the similar relationship of thin skin and bone. Three areas of the mandible were scanned for BMD measurements: R1 was defined as the site located at the angle of the mandible, R2 as the site located at the molar region of the mandible, and R3 as the site located at the premolar region which contains the mental foramina landmark.

Patient Positioning

Proper and reproducible patient positioning was an important variable. Precise positioning of the patient was possible because of special positioning marks printed on the mattress surface, positioning aids such as cushions, and the alignment laser. The latter projects a laser dot onto the patient during the positioning procedure; the dot denotes the position of the photon beam. The mandible had to be oriented with respect to the photon beam in order to achieve a projection which images one side of the mandible while avoiding superimposition of the contralateral side. The patient was positioned as follows. The patient removed the dentures, and then lay on the table in a lateral oblique position. The head was centered in the active region scan and was allowed to rest on the table. The mandible was tilted such that the portion which was closest to the table was parallel to the limit

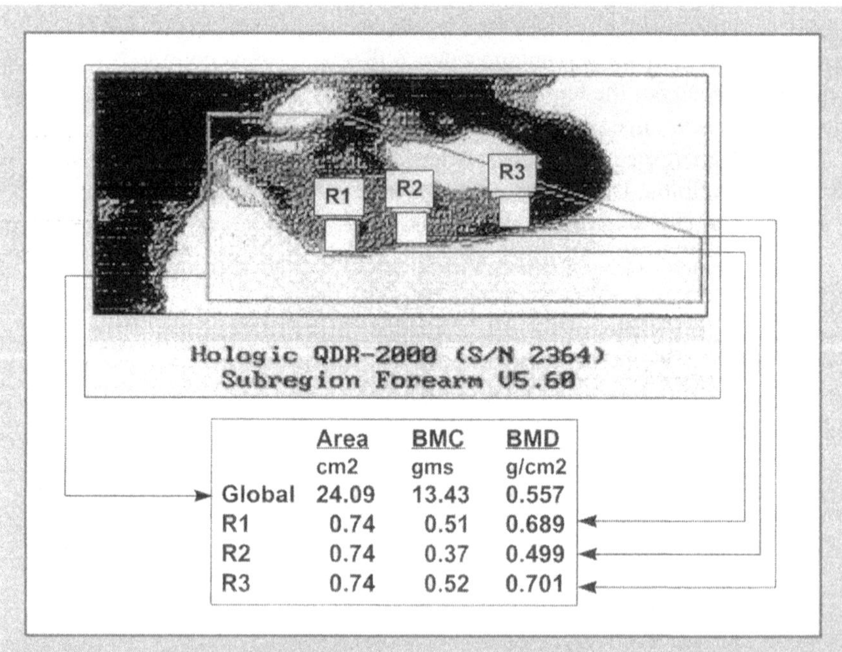

	Area cm2	BMC gms	BMD g/cm2
Global	24.09	13.43	0.557
R1	0.74	0.51	0.689
R2	0.74	0.37	0.499
R3	0.74	0.52	0.701

Fig. 29-2 Reproducibility of patient positioning and DXA evaluation of mandibular regions of interest R1, R2, and R3

lines drawn on the mattress or perpendicular to the long axis of the scan table. The segment of the mandible which was closest to the table was the one imaged. Figure 29-2 represents a typical DXA image of a single mandible determination.

One measurement of the mandible took about 5 or 6 min. According to the information supplied by the manufacturer, the entrance dose for the patient under all operating conditions was 0.02–0.05 mSv per scan, which is equal to about the exposure of one or two bitewing radiographs.

Results

All patient data were analyzed using Pearson's correlation test. Significant correlations were found between the BMD of the premolar region of the mandible (R3) and the BMD at each site of the hip. The results of these correlations in 12 subjects (the data for one subject was deleted because of the inability to get a R3 measurement) are as follows [correlations between the BMD (g/cm^2) of the premolar region of the mandible (R3) and the BMD (g/cm^2) at each site of the hip]:

- Neck: $r=0.551, p=0.063$
- Trochanter: $r=0.345, p=0.271$
- Intertrochanter: $r=0.629, p=0.028$
- Ward's triangle: $r=0.663, p=0.018$
- Total hip: $r=0.582, p=0.047$

The strongest correlation was that between the BMDs of R3 and Ward's triangle ($r=0.663; p=0.187$); the linear regression with 95% confidence limits is shown in Fig. 29-3.

No significant correlation was found between the mandibular BMD and the lumbar and forearm BMDs. When comparisons were made between the BMD at

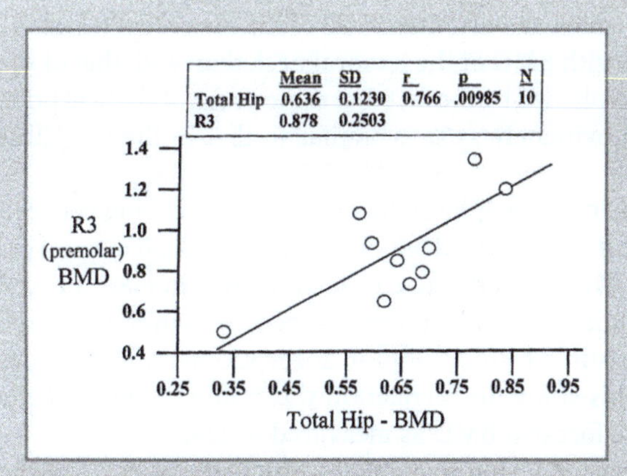

Fig. 29-3 Comparative analysis of mandibular site R3 BMD vs. total hip BMD

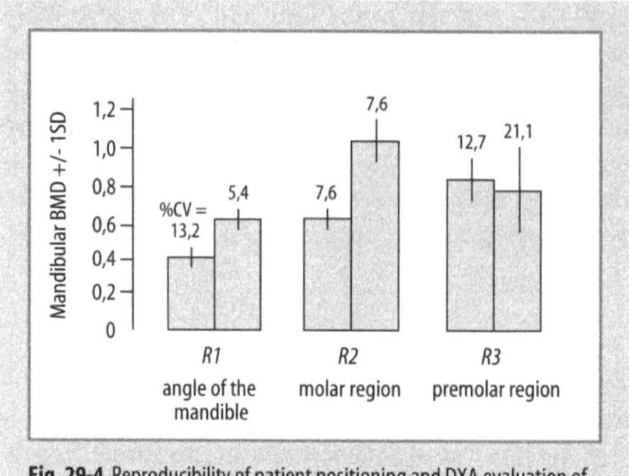

Fig. 29-4 Reproducibility of patient positioning and DXA evaluation of mandibular regions of interest R1, R2, and R3

the individual sites of the mandible (R1, R2, R3), no significant correlation was found. The BMD values of the other skeletal sites were also not correlated with each other.

Reproducibility and precision of the DXA measurements was expressed by standard deviations and coefficient of variation based on a set of repeated BMD measurements. The reproducibility of three independent BMD measurements at mandibular sites R1, R2, and R3 is shown in Fig. 29-4.

Discussion

In this study a strong correlation was found between the BMD of the hip and that of the premolar region of the mandible (R3). These findings support those in the 1993 study by Klemetti et al. which showed that BMD of the buccal cortex of the mandible is better correlated with BMD of the femoral neck than with that of the lumbar spine. This might be explained by the fact that the amount of cortical bone in the femoral collumn, approximately 75 %, is similar to that in the mandible (Wahner et al. 1983).

Previous studies on normal individuals have shown a weak correlation between BMC of the mandible and that of other cortical bones, such as the second metacarpal and the forearm bones (Von Wowern and Stolze 1979; Von Wowern 1985). In 1988 Von Wowern et al. found no significant correlation between the mandibular BMC and the forearm BMC, as measured by dual-photon absorptiometry and single-photon absorptiometry. In this study no correlation was found either between the mandibular BMD and the forearm BMD as measured by DXA.

In 1986 and 1988 Von Wowern et al. found no relationship between BMC of the mandible and that of the lumbar spine; they also found that changes in mandibular bone mass were not related to changes in trabecular bone mass (Von Wowern 1986; Von Wowern et al. 1988). The results of this study confirm the findings of both Von Wowern studies.

The lack of correlation between the percentage of resorption and the mandibular BMD is consistent with results of previous studies on the relationship between alveolar ridge height and mandibular bone mass. Elders et al. (1992) did not find a significant correlation between the height of the alveolar crest and bone mass measurements. Klemetti and Vainio (1993) found no significant relationship between the clinical height of the residual alveolar ridge and mandibular BMD. However, their study showed a correlation with the BMD of the femoral collum, as did this study. Klemetti and Vainio (1993) commented that, "Bone density may remain constant even though there is a decrease in the volume of the mandible, and the bone may lose minerals without changes in the ridge shape."

Originally the Hologic QDR was designed for studies on the bone density of the lumbar spine, and the in vivo precision was found to be approximately 1% for lumbar BMD (Pouilles et al. 1991). According to Haddaway et al. (1992) the reproducibility is usually highest for femur BMD. Indeed, they found a coefficient of variation in Ward's triangle of 4.29%. Larcos and Wahner (1991) compared the precision of DXA and single-photon absorptiometry for bone mineral analysis of the forearm. The mean short-term precision of DXA was 0.9% in vitro and about 1.5% in vivo. However, the reproducibility was shown not to be as good for osteoporotic patients (Pouilles et al. 1991). Corten et al. (1993) used DXA to measure the mandibular bone mass and found a SD of 3% in vivo. In this study the reproducibility of the DXA measurement of the bone density of the mandible was inconclusive. The BMD measurements at R3 were less precise than those at R1 and R2. These findings may reflect the difficulty in positioning the patient.

Due to the difficulty in patient positioning to avoid overlapping images of the mandible, future studies may require that a devise be used to position the head. Use of a light cast (strips of fabric that are embedded in a light-curing acrylic that is polymerized once the head position has been established) may be a viable technique to adapt to the DXA technique for measuring mandibles. In addition, allowing the patient to wear her dentures aids in keeping the patient in rest position.

One problem that arose in this study was that patients tended to move the jaw while the machine was scanning it. This necessitated multiple retrials to obtain the proper records. By keeping the dentures in the mouth patients may be able to keep the mandible in the proper position for the required 6 min of scan time.

A noteworthy feature of this study is that it was the first using DXA to measure BMC and BMD of the mandible in multiple subjects and without superimposition of the mandible. Corten et al. in their 1993 study looked at only two subjects and had the problem of superimposition of the mandible with which to contend.

Limitations of the Study
- The sample size of subjects was small: ten osteoporotic and three normals.
- The group of subjects was nonhomogeneous, including subjects with very severe osteoporosis and those with borderline osteoporosis. Within the osteo-

porotic population, some had very severe alveolar atrophy while others had retained a fair amount of bone.
- Because some of the subjects had severe alveolar ridge atrophy, the mental foramen could not be located on panoramic radiographs.
- Positioning of the mandible during DXA scans was extremely difficult because some patients had conditions that limited their mobility (e.g., severe osteoporosis, fractures, osteoarthritis of the neck, and severe kyphosis). The data for one subject was deleted because of the inability to obtain an R3 measurement.

Acknowledgements. This work was presented in part at the 1994 16th Meeting of the American Society for Bone and Mineral Research in Kansas City, Missouri, and the 1995 11th International Meeting on Bone Densitometry in Gleneden Beach, Oregon.

References

Corten FG, Van't Hof MA, Buijs WC, Hoppenbrouwers P, Kalk W, Corsten FH (1993) Measurement of mandibular bone density ex vivo and in vivo by dual energy X-ray absorptiometry. Archs Oral Biol 38:215–219

Elders PJ, Habets LL, Netelenbos JC, Van der Linden LW, Van der Stelt PF (1992) The relation between periodontitis and systemic bone mass in women between 46 and 55 years of age. J Clin Periodont 19:492–496

Habets LL, Bras J, Merkesteyn JP (1988) Mandibular atrophy and metabolic bone loss. Histomorphometry of iliac crest biopsies in 74 patients. Int J Oral Maxillofac Surg 17:325–329

Haddaway MJ, Davie MW, McCall IW (1992) Bone mineral density in healthy normal women and reproducibility of measurements in spine and hip using dual-energy X-ray absorptiometry. Br J Radiol 65:213–217

Larcos G, Wahner HW (1991) An evaluation of forearm bone mineral measurement with dual-energy X-ray absorptiometry. J Nucl Med 32:2101–2106

Klemetti E, Vainio P (1993) Effect of bone mineral density in skeleton and mandible on extraction of teeth and clinical alveolar height. J Prosthet Dent 70:21–25

Klemetti E, Vainio P, Lassila V, Alhava E (1993a) Trabecular bone mineral density of mandible and alveolar height in postmenopausal women. Scand Dent 101:166–170

Klemetti E, Vainio P, Lassila V, Alhava E (1993) Cortical bone mineral density in the mandible and osteoporosis status in postmenopausal women. Scand J Dent Res 101:219–223

Kribbs PJ, Smith DE, Chestnut CH (1983) Oral findings in osteoporosis. II. relationship between residual ridge and alveolar bone resorption and generalized skeletal osteopenia. J Prosthet Dent 50:719–724

Kribbs PJ, Chestnut CH, Ott SM (1989) Relationships between mandibular and skeletal bone in an osteoporotic population. J Prosthet Dent 62:703–707

Kribbs PJ, Chesnut CH, Ott SM, Kilcoyne RF (1990) Relationships between mandibular and skeletal bone in a population of normal women. J Prothet Dent 63:86–89

Pouilles JM, Tremollieres F, Todorovsky N, Ribot C (1991) Precision and sensitivity of dual-energy X-ray absorptiometry in spinal osteoporosis. J Bone Miner Res 6:997–1002

Rosenquist JB, Baylink DJ, Berger JS (1978) Alveolar atrophy and decreased skeletal mass of the radius. Int J Oral Surg 7:479–481

Von Wowern N (1985) In vivo measurement of bone mineral content of mandibles by dual-photon absorptiometry. Scand Dent Res 93:162–168

Von Wowern N (1986) Bone mass of mandibles. In vitro and in vivo analyses. Dan Med Bull 33:23–44

Von Wowern N, Hjorting-Hansen E (1991) The mandibular bone mineral content in relation to vestibulolingual sulculoplasty. A 2-year follow-up. J Prosthet Dent 65:804–808

Von Wowern N, Kollerup G (1992) Symptomatic osteoporosis: a risk factor for residual ridge reduction of the jaws. J Prosthet Dent 67:656–660

Von Wowern N, Stoltze K (1979) Comparative bone morphometric analysis of mandibles and 2nd metacarpals. Scand J Dent Res 87:134–136

Von Wowern N, Storm TL, Olgaard K (1988) Bone mineral content by photon absorptiometry of the mandible compared with that of the forearm and the lumbar spine. Calcif Tissue Int 42:157–161

Wahner HW, Dunn WL, Riggs BL (1983) Non invasive bone mineral measurements. Semin Nucl Med 13:282–289

Wical KE, Swoope CC (1974) Studies of residual ridge resorption. I Use of panoramic radiographs for evaluation and classification of mandibular resorption. J Prosthet Dent 32:7–12

Subject Index

Springer
and the
environment

At Springer we firmly believe that an international science publisher has a special obligation to the environment, and our corporate policies consistently reflect this conviction.

We also expect our business partners – paper mills, printers, packaging manufacturers, etc. – to commit themselves to using materials and production processes that do not harm the environment. The paper in this book is made from low- or no-chlorine pulp and is acid free, in conformance with international standards for paper permanency.

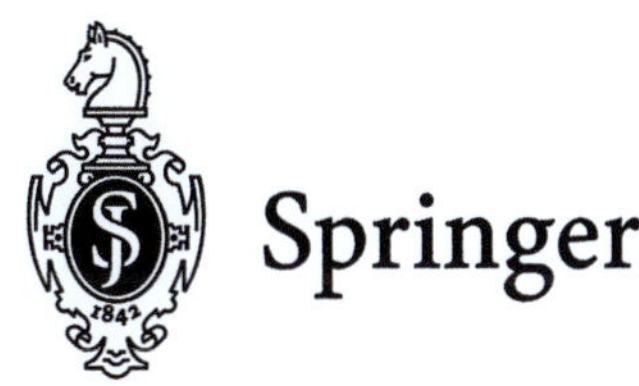